约翰·霍普金斯 糖尿病指南
糖尿病的治疗与管理

主编：【美】克里斯托弗（Christopher D. Saudek）
　　　卡利亚尼（Rita Rastogi Kalyani）
　　　弗雷德里克（Frederick L. Brancati）

主译：郭晓蕙

译者：丁荣晶　陈丽竹　葛　庆　顾　楠
　　　高元丰　陆迪菲　梁瑞娟　李　昂
　　　刘　雯　马鲁峰　田新利　王慧丽
　　　薛　超　袁晓勇　向晓莉　于　楠
　　　于利平　杨　渊

科学技术文献出版社
·北京·

Original English Language Jones&Bartlett Learning, LLC. 5 Wall Street Burlington, MA01803.
© Copyright year Jones&Bartlett Learning LLC. All Rights Reserved
Simplified Chinese Language edition published by pharma-service,
owned by Buclas·布克（北京）文化传播有限公司 .Chinese translation rights © 2014 pharma-service,
owned by pharma-service Buclas·布克（北京）文化传播有限公司
出版的各类医学教育图书和各种产品均可在大多数网站及Buclas·布克网站购买。

若制药公司、医疗器械公司、医学院校、专业协会和其他的认证机构大量购买pharma-service的出版物，将会有更多的价格优惠。欲了解具体和详细的信息，可以通过以下的联系信息或者发送邮件marketing@buclas.com或联系在pharma-service的销售部门。

版权所有，违者必究。在没有获得版权所有者的书面同意下，在版权保护下的任何资料均不可以任何形式，包括影印、录音或者任何信息存储和恢复系统等电子的或者机械的形式，复制或者利用。

作者、编者和出版人员已尽力提供准确的信息。然而，对于错误、遗漏或者任何使用书中内容造成的后果概不负责，并且对于书中描述的产品和方法的使用也不负责。在本书中描述的治疗方法和不良反应可能并非适用于所有人，同理，部分人群的适宜剂量或者发生的不良反应可能与此书所描述的不完全一致。书中所提及的药物和医疗装置的使用范围可能受到食品药品监督管理局（FDA）的控制，只能用于学术研究或者临床试验。研究结果、临床实践和国家的规章制度经常改变本领域内已被公认的标准。临床上考虑使用某个药物时，医务工作者和读者需参考FDA对该药物的审批情况，同时也要阅读药品说明书，浏览和掌握关于用药剂量、预防措施和禁忌证等方面的最新资料和推荐意见，然后做出恰当的临床决策。对于新药和罕用药物，以上做法尤为重要。

我们的目标是以医务人员为重点，提供便捷、系统和准确的核心处方信息。本指南的目的在于支持，而非取代存在于患者或网页浏览者与临床医生之间的纽带。书中的内容有助于读者温习已掌握的知识，而不能够取代培训、实践、继续教育或学习最新文献所起的作用。

图书在版编目（CIP）数据

约翰·霍普金斯糖尿病指南：糖尿病的治疗与管理／（美）克里斯托弗（Saudek, C.D.），（美）卡利亚尼（Kalyani, R.R.），（美）弗雷德里克（Brancati, F.L.）主编；郭晓蕙，丁荣晶译．—北京：科学技术文献出版社，2015.4

书名原文：Johns Hopkins Diabetes Guide 2012：Treatment and Management of Diabetes
ISBN 978-7-5023-9727-2

Ⅰ.①约…Ⅱ.①克…②卡…③弗…④郭…⑤丁…Ⅲ.①糖尿病—诊疗—指南 Ⅳ.① R587.1-62

中国版本图书馆CIP数据核字（2015）第001231号
著作权合同登记号 图字：01-2014-8137

书　　　名：	约翰·霍普金斯糖尿病指南——糖尿病的治疗与管理
编　　　著：	Christopher D. Saudek　Rita Rastogi Kalyani　Frederick L. Brancati
主　　　译：	郭晓蕙
总　策　划：	刘伟鹏
策划编辑：	孔荣华
责任编辑：	车宜平
文字编辑：	王继珍　胡馨予
美编·策划：	魏青青　韩颖颖　张海雪　乔博才
出　版　者：	科学技术文献出版社
地　　　址：	北京市复兴路15号
发　行　者：	布克（北京）文化传播有限公司
版　　　次：	2015年4月第1版 2018年12月第2次印刷
印　刷　厂：	北京蓝图印刷有限公司
开　　　本：	787×1092 1/32
印　　　张：	22.25
字　　　数：	430千
定　　　价：	168.00元

策划执行：Pharma-service Buclas·布克 医学教育事业部
团购电话：+86-10-51284280.87952148
个人订购：布克的礼物（淘宝网）官方网址 buclas.taobao.com（成为布克会员，享受更多优惠）
网址：www.Buclas.com/www.pharma-service.com.cn
如有质量问题，请直接与我公司联系调换。

All rights reserved.No part of this publication may be reproduced or transmitted in any form or by any means, electronic or mechanical,without written permission of the publisher.

参与贡献人员

主编

Christopher D. Saudek, MD
(in memoriam)Professor of Medicine Division of Endocrinology and Metabolism The Johns Hopkins University School of Medicine Baltimore, MD

Rita Rastogi Kalyani, MD, MHS
Assistant Professor of Medicine Division of Endocrinology and Metabolism The Johns Hopkins University School of Medicine Baltimore, MD

Frederick L. Brancati, MD, MHS
Professor of Medicine and Epidemiology Director, Division of General Internal Medicine Director, Diabetes Prevention & Control Core, Baltimore DRTC The Johns Hopkins University School of Medicine Baltimore, MD

著者

Bassam G. Abu Jawdeh, MD
Postdoctoral Fellow Division of Nephrology The Johns Hopkins University School of Medicine Baltimore, MD

Nada Alachkar, MD
Assistant Professor Division of Nephrology The Johns Hopkins University School of Medicine Baltimore, MD

Reza Alavi, MD, MHS, MBA
Postdoctoral Fellow Division of General Internal Medicine The Johns Hopkins University School of Medicine Baltimore, MD

Martinson K. Arnan, MD, MPA
Resident Division of Neurology The Johns Hopkins University School of Medicine Baltimore, MD

Douglas W. Ball, MD
Associate Professor of Medicine and Oncology Division of Endocrinology and Metabolism The Johns Hopkins University School of Medicine Baltimore, MD

Nancyellen Brennan, CRNP, CDE
Senior Diabetes Nurse Practitioner The Johns Hopkins Comprehensive Diabetes Center Division of Endocrinology and Metabolism The Johns Hopkins University School of Medicine Baltimore, MD

Todd T. Brown, MD, PhD
Assistant Professor of Medicine Division of Endocrinology and Metabolism The Johns Hopkins University School of Medicine Baltimore, MD

Kathleen Burks, MSN, CRNP
Nurse Practitioner Division of Neurology The Johns Hopkins University School of Medicine Baltimore, MD

Shivam Champaneri, MD
Postdoctoral Fellow Division of Endocrinology and Metabolism The Johns Hopkins University School of Medicine Baltimore, MD

Gregory O. Clark, MD
Assistant Professor Division of Endocrinology and Metabolism University of Texas Southwestern Medical Center Dallas, TX

Jeanne M. Clark, MD, MPH
Associate Professor of Medicine and Epidemiology Division of General Internal Medicine The Johns Hopkins University School of Medicine Baltimore, MD

David W. Cooke, MD
Associate Professor of Pediatrics Division of Pediatric Endocrinology The Johns Hopkins University School of Medicine Baltimore, MD

Rachel Derr, MD, PhD
Adult Endocrinologist Center for Medicine, Endocrinology and Diabetes Atlanta, GA

Joanne Dintzis, CRNP, CDE
Senior Diabetes Nurse Practitioner The Johns Hopkins Inpatient Diabetes Management Service Division of Endocrinology and Metabolism The Johns Hopkins University School of Medicine Baltimore, MD

Ari Eckman, MD
Adult Endocrinologist Chief, Division of Diabetes, Endocrinology & Metabolism Trinitas Regional Medical Cente Elizabeth, NJ

Ana Emiliano, MD
Adult Endocrinologist Sinai Hospital of Baltimore Baltimore, MD

Rebecca Gottesman, MD, PhD
Assistant Professor of Neurology Cerebrovascular Division The Johns Hopkins University School of Medicine Baltimore, MD

Sheldon H. Gottlieb, MD
Associate Professor of Medicine Division of Cardiology The Johns Hopkins University School of Medicine Baltimore, MD

Sherita Hill Golden, MD, MHS
Associate Professor of Medicine and Epidemiology Director, Inpatient Diabetes Management Service Division of Endocrinology and Metabolism The Johns Hopkins University School of Medicine Baltimore, MD

Nadeen Hosein, MD, MS
Adult Endocrinologist San Diego, CA

Mary Huizinga, MD, MPH
Assistant Professor (Parttime) Division of General Internal Medicine The Johns Hopkins University School of Medicine Associate, McKinsey & Company Washington, DC

Sachin D. Kalyani, MD
Ophthalmologist Rutzen Eye Specialists & Laser Center Severna Park, MD

Mariana Lazo, MD, ScM, PhD
Postdoctoral Fellow Clinical Epidemiology The Johns Hopkins University Bloomberg School of Public Health Baltimore, MD

Emily Loghmani, MS, RD, LDN, CDE
Senior Nutritionist The Johns Hopkins Comprehensive Diabetes Center Division of Endocrinology and Metabolism The Johns Hopkins University School of Medicine Baltimore, MD

Simeon Margolis, MD, PhD
Professor Emeritus of Medicine Division of Endocrinology and Metabolism The Johns Hopkins University School of Medicine Baltimore, MD

Nisa M. Maruthur, MD, MHS
Assistant Professor Division of General Internal Medicine The Johns Hopkins University School of Medicine Baltimore, MD

Nestoras Mathioudakis, MD
Postdoctoral Fellow Division of Endocrinology and Metabolism The Johns Hopkins University School of Medicine Baltimore, MD

Ali Mohamadi, MD
Pediatric Endocrinologist Chevy Chase, MD Kendall F. Moseley, MD Postdoctoral Fellow Division of Endocrinology and Metabolism The Johns Hopkins University School of Medicine Baltimore, MD

Donna I. Myers, MD
Assistant Professor of Medicine Division of Nephrology The Johns Hopkins University School of Medicine Baltimore, MD

Wanda K. Nicholson, MD, MPH, MBA
Associate Professor of Obstetrics and Gynecology University of North Carolina School of Medicine at Chapel Hill Chapel Hill, NC

Octavia Pickett-Blakely, MD, MHS
Instructor of Medicine Division of Gastroenterology University of Pennsylvania Philadelphia, PA

Brian Pinto, PharmD, MBA
Clinical Pharmacist Division of Clinical Pharmacology Assistant Director, Medication Policy and Clinical Informatics The Johns Hopkins Hospital Baltimore, MD

Michael Polydefkis, MD, MHS
Associate Professor of Neurology Director, Johns Hopkins Cutaneous Nerve Laboratory Director, Bayview EMG Laboratory The Johns Hopkins University School of Medicine Baltimore, MD

Naresh Punjabi, MD, PhD
Professor of Medicine and Epidemiology Division of Pulmonary and Critical Care Medicine The Johns Hopkins University School of Medicine Baltimore, MD

Amin Sabet, MD
Instructor in Medicine Division of Endocrinology, Diabetes & Metabolism Beth Israel Deaconess Medical Center, Harvard Medical School Boston, MA

Lipika Samal, MD, MPH
Instructor of Medicine Division of General Internal Medicine and Primary Care Brigham and Women's Hospital, Harvard Medical School Boston, MA

Lee J. Sanders, DM
Clinical Professor (Adjunct) Department of Podiatric Medicine Temple University School of Podiatric Medicine Consultant, Veterans Affairs Medical Center Podiatry Service Lebanon, PA

Vanessa Walker Harris, MD
Postdoctoral Fellow Division of Endocrinology and Metabolism The Johns Hopkins University School of Medicine Baltimore, MD

Donna Westervelt, CRNP, MS, CDE
Diabetes Nurse Practitioner Johns Hopkins Bayview Diabetic Neuropathy Center The Johns Hopkins University School of Medicine Baltimore, MD

Melissa Yates, MD
Assistant Professor of Gynecology and Obstetrics Division of Reproductive Endocrinology The Johns Hopkins University School of Medicine
Baltimore, MD

Hsin–Chieh Yeh, PhD
Assistant Professor of Medicine and Epidemiology Division of General Internal Medicine The Johns Hopkins University School of Medicine
Baltimore, MD

中文版序言

糖尿病这一犹如洪水猛兽般蔓延的慢性疾病正在不断影响着医疗环境、医疗决策的判断，进而影响到医疗质量以及医疗结局。

糖尿病是一个终身存在的疾病，又是一个影响全身的疾病，临床医生会碰到各种复杂的疾病状况。上个世纪胰岛素的出现使糖尿病患者的寿命延长，但并没有减慢糖尿病患病率迅速增长的趋势。

由于糖尿病患者群增长迅速，近30余年涌现出非常多的糖尿病治疗药物，糖尿病治疗方案以及慢性并发症的防治方案。临床医生特别是初出茅庐的年轻医生往往很困惑应该如何选择合适的治疗方案。而内科学教科书糖尿病的章节受篇幅所限，其内容往往医学生一毕业就不够用了；糖尿病学专著虽既有基础又有临床但却过丁冗长，与临床实践连接不够密切。

本书将可以解决临床医生以上的困惑。本书是美国著名的约翰·霍普金斯医院的临床专家们为了解决临床医生每日碰到的实际问题而撰写的。书中没有长篇大论的说教，对每个问题仅寥寥数语，但字字珠玑，几乎每句话都可解决临床工作中的一个问题。且每一句话的背后都有着非常扎实的理论基础。在每个短小精悍的章节后面是非常丰富的参考文献，提示读者如果想知道得更多就去看原文。处于工作中的临床医生在这本书中可以迅速找到问题的答案而不必花费大量的时间去从大部头著作中找到所需的内容。

这本书还有一个特点是包罗万象，一个患者从血糖发生异常到其生命走到尽头时会发生的各种并发症状况及解决办法都有涉及。书中还涉及如何对糖尿病患者进行教育和管理。最重要的是文中所有的观点来源都有循证医学证据的支持，很多观点来源于权威糖尿病治疗指南，临床医生以此内容为鉴，可以免受商业推广的影响，做出正确的临床决策。

可以说本书是约翰·霍普金斯医院专家们数十年临床心血的结晶。作为一本手边书，会使临床医生的每一个决策都得到专家团队的支持，犹如站在巨人的肩膀上一样。

感谢本书的版权所有者同意将此书译成中文，让更多的临床医生学到临床医学殿堂之巅——约翰·霍普金斯医院的糖尿病诊疗指南。也感谢译者团队的辛勤工作。

愿本书能够为临床医生所用，帮助更多的糖尿病患者。

北京大学第一医院
2015年4月于北京

目录

参与贡献人员 iii
中文版序言 vii
序言 xiii
致谢 xv

第一部分 概述 1

糖尿病简介 3
糖尿病概述 3
糖尿病的并发症与合并症 3
糖尿病及其并发症的管理 4
糖尿病的临床试验 5

糖尿病的诊断与分型 6
分型 6
诊断 6

1 型糖尿病的流行病学 9
美国 1 型糖尿病发病率与患病率 9
美国青少年 T1DM 的管理与预后 9
全球 T1DM 的发病率与患病率 . 9

2 型糖尿病的流行病学 12
美国 2 型糖尿病的患病率 ... 12
美国糖尿病经济负担 12
全球 2 型糖尿病的患病率 ... 12
全球糖尿病经济负担 13
全球糖尿病的发病率和死亡率 13

糖尿病治疗相关的重要研究：预防与血糖控制 15
糖尿病的预防 12
长期血糖控制的益处 16
住院患者血糖控制的益处 .. 16

糖尿病治疗的关键研究：控制并发症 22
视网膜病变 22
肾脏病变 24
神经病变 25

高血压病 26
血脂 26
心血管疾病 27

糖尿病治疗的关键研究：治疗效果 33
1 型糖尿病和 2 型糖尿病的药物治疗 33
妊娠期糖尿病的药物治疗 .. 36
糖尿病及其并发症的外科治疗 36

第二部分 管理 43

突发事件 45
糖尿病酮症酸中毒 45
高血糖高渗状态（HHS） ... 51

主要原则 56
黎明现象 56
低血糖症：预防和治疗 ... 60
夜间低血糖 64
餐后低血糖 67
糖尿病和急性疾病的院外管理 70
日常预防保健 72
糖尿病疫苗指导 76

医院管理和外科手术 78
医院糖尿病管理 78
糖尿病患者围手术期护理 .. 91
胰腺切除术后糖尿病 95
减肥手术 98

生活方式和健康教育 102
营养：关于糖尿病的综述 .. 102
1 型糖尿病的营养 105
营养：碳水化合物计数 .. 108
2 型糖尿病的营养 112
营养：流行的糖尿病食疗法 116
体力活动和锻炼 119
患者教育：糖尿病概述 .. 124

患者教育：糖尿病的课程主题 127
患者教育：克服糖尿病障碍 . 130

糖尿病前期 134
糖尿病前期或增加患糖尿
病的风险类别 134

怀孕 138
妊娠糖尿病 138
妊娠与糖尿病 142

社会/法律 146
糖尿病对驾驶的影响 146
就业和歧视 151

特殊人群或亚型 153
儿童及2型糖尿病 153
青年人中的成年发病型
糖尿病（MODY）..... 156
线粒体糖尿病 159
成人隐匿性自身免疫
糖尿病（LADA）..... 162
老年糖尿病 166
激素诱发糖尿病 171

1型糖尿病 174
1型糖尿病：危险因素 ... 174
1型糖尿病：胰岛素治疗 ... 177
胰岛素泵的管理 181
胰腺移植 185

2型糖尿病 188
2型糖尿病：
环境危险因素与筛查 ... 188
2型糖尿病：遗传危险因素 .. 192
2型糖尿病：序贯疗法 ... 194
2型糖尿病：胰岛素治疗 ... 197

第三部分 并发症和伴随疾病 .201

心血管疾病、肥胖和危险因素 203
心血管疾病的筛查和治疗 ... 203
脂代谢紊乱 212
心力衰竭 217
高血压 224

代谢综合征 227
肥胖 231
周围血管疾病 236

内分泌疾病 243
肢端肥大症 243
库欣综合征 247
胰高血糖素瘤 250
胰岛素瘤 254
施密特综合征 260
生长抑制素瘤 263

女性疾病 266
绝经期对高血糖的影响 ... 266
绝经期前妇女的
月经周期和高血糖 ... 269
多囊卵巢综合征 272

消化道疾病 275
乳糜泻与1型糖尿病 275
胃轻瘫 278
非酒精性脂肪肝 281
胰腺炎 286

血液系统疾病/恶性肿瘤 289
癌症和糖尿病 289
胰腺癌 294

感染性疾病 297
截肢 297
足部溃疡 301
艾滋病毒相关糖尿病 306
感染性疾病和糖尿病 309
骨髓炎 313
伤口愈合 318

男性疾病 330
勃起功能障碍 330
男性性腺功能减退症 332

肌肉、皮肤及骨骼疾病 336
骨骼疾病 336
Charcot关节病 341
糖尿病患者的皮肤表现 .. 346

坏疽和严重肢体缺血 350
肌肉骨骼疾病 354

神经系统疾病 359
周围神经病变 359
肌萎缩 362
自主神经病变 365
卒中 369

眼科疾病 376
视网膜病变 376
黄斑水肿 381
白内障 384

耳科疾病 386
听力障碍 386

精神疾病 389
糖尿病相关抑郁 389
糖尿病的饮食紊乱 393

肺疾病 398
囊性纤维化相关糖尿病 398
睡眠呼吸暂停 401

肾和泌尿系统疾病 404
肾病 404
糖尿病中的肾脏疾病 410
透析开始和管理 416
肾移植 423
糖尿病的膀胱疾病 429

第四部分 药物 431

心血管疾病 433
抗凝药物使用 433

补充和替代医学 440
草药 440
非草药方面 443

脂代谢紊乱 445
胆汁酸螯合剂 445
依泽替米贝 448

纤维酸衍生物 451
烟酸类 456
OMEGA-3脂肪酸（鱼油） 460
他汀类药物和联合药物 463

勃起功能障碍 469
昔多芬 469

胃轻瘫 473
多潘立酮 473
红霉素 476
甲氧氯普胺 479

降糖治疗 482
α糖苷酶抑制剂 482
DPP-IV抑制剂 485
肠促胰素类似物和胰淀粉样
多肽类似物 489
二甲双胍 494
磺脲类降糖药和其他促泌剂 498
噻唑烷二酮类药物 503
胰岛素（基础）：
中效和长效胰岛素 508
胰岛素（餐时）：速效和短效 512
预混胰岛素 516
胰岛素：其他形式和
可植入式的胰岛素泵 521

升高血糖 523
糖尿病患者需谨慎使用抗生素 523
抗精神病药 529

高血压 545
血管紧张素转换酶
（ACE）抑制剂 545
血管紧张素
受体阻断剂（ARBs） 557
β受体阻滞剂 565
钙通道阻滞剂 576
利尿剂 581

肾病 ... 587
乙酰半胱氨酸 ... 587

神经病变 ... 590
神经性疼痛的治疗 ... 590

肥胖 ... 595
奥利司他 ... 595
苯丁胺 ... 598

泌尿系统 ... 601
氨甲酰甲胆碱 ... 601
奥昔布宁 ... 604

第五部分 临床试验 ... 607

骨骼系统 ... 609
骨骼矿物质密度 ... 609
维生素 D ... 613

内分泌系统 ... 617
醛固酮减少症 ... 617
性激素 ... 619

消化系统 ... 623
肝功能 ... 623

血糖监测 ... 626
动态血糖监测 ... 626
果糖胺，血清 1,5 - A G ... 629
糖化血红蛋白 ... 633
自我血糖监测 ... 637

血液系统 ... 640
贫血 ... 640

免疫学 ... 655
1 型糖尿病的自身免疫性抗体 643
胰岛素抗体 ... 648

血脂 ... 652
血脂 ... 652

肾脏 ... 656
肾功能 ... 656
蛋白尿 ... 661

附录

附录 1：
2 型糖尿病高血糖治疗路径 ... 667

附录 2：GFR 和白蛋白尿网格 . 668

附录 3：
2015 ADA EASD 立场声明对
2 型糖尿病降糖治疗的推荐 ... 670

附录 4：
2015 AACE/ACE 血糖控制流程图 672

序言

你手中这本书是独一无二的。它不是一本糖尿病的教科书,但它囊括了多数你希望在教科书中找到的详尽的知识。它也不仅仅是指南的汇总,而是包括了所有相关的指南的内容。它不是一套评论证据等级的综述,尽管其内容列出了来自专家们的有循证医学证据的信息。故而你最终得到的是不受设备仪器或药品赞助商所影响的信息。

这本糖尿病学指南是一本十分全面、独立而简明扼要的对于临床相关知识的总结,尤其为繁忙的专业医护人员提供了简单便捷地获取知识的途径。

即使与近几年前相比,糖尿病的诊治已变得更加复杂。诊断标准已被修订,新的血糖监测方法不断涌现,口服降糖药种类不断增多,新型胰岛素制剂和新的饮食推荐建议、甚至胰岛素泵已被广泛使用。这本糖尿病学指导视角综合、全面,以覆盖上述这些新进展。本书包括140余个不同章节,每章书写时深入浅出,让你在掌握基本知识的同时了解糖尿病治疗进展的细节。

当你有一些相对简要、直接的问题时也可查阅本书,比如说:新的肠促胰素类似物艾塞那肽的剂量是什么?其潜在的不良反应是什么?你可能需要回顾复习糖尿病诊治的最新指南,进一步学习糖尿病的某种并发症,或明确某一实验室检查结果的意义。无论是什么问题,这本糖尿病学指导都可以像我们预期的那样帮助你在几分钟内找到答案,而无须费力地遍阅那些连篇累牍。

每章由以下分类内容组成:概况,治疗,并发症与合并症,药物和临床检查。你会立刻发现本书全部用短句和短语而非长句写成。但这些短句绝不会减少其全面、准确和严谨,它们仅仅会减少你的阅读时间、加速你学习的进度。如果你想进一步寻找原始数据,我们也提供了相关文献。此外,有一章节概述了有关糖尿病的重要临床研究,详尽总结了50个以上里程碑式的临床研究的结论,而这些研究也作为目前临床建议的根据而被广泛引用。本书的另一个特点是专家建议部分,其中作者们深刻阐述了在临床实践中糖尿病治疗的实际情况。同样,每一章节都被大规模、认真地编辑和审阅。

作者们都是规律出诊的临床医师。他们都是目前在职或曾经在约翰·霍普金斯的全职员工,同时是他们所著章节相关领域的专家。他们代表了多种学科,包括内科医师、药剂师、足部疾病医师、护士、营养师和教育工作者。

这本糖尿病学指导建立在 John Bartlett 医师所著的约翰·霍普金斯《ABX 指南——感染性疾病的诊断与治疗》一书的概念上。特尼达岛和多巴哥岛的专业医疗工作者首先开始发展、资助这本糖尿病学指导的雏形,并提供在线版本,包括特尼达岛和多巴哥岛的专门章节及作者。我们在此感谢特尼达岛和多巴哥岛政府对本书作出的支持。

致谢

我们在此感谢约翰·霍普金斯内分泌与代谢学系专业及其主任 Paul Ladenson 对本书的鼓励和指导。同时感谢内科学系主任 Myron Weisfeldt 对本书的支持。尤其感谢 POC-IT 中心团队全体人员——Nicole Sokol, Danielle Meinsler, Steve Libowitz 和 Paul Auwaerter,他们在幕后投入了大量的时间和精力。同样感谢 Jones & Bartlett 出版社,尤其是 Laura Almozara, Daniel Stone 和 Nancy Duffy,他们在本书的出版过程中付出了努力和高效的组织工作。

在此特别感谢我们的作者们,他们对糖尿病领域的热情和广泛的专业知识最终成就了这部独一无二的指导书。同时对 Ron Daniel 主席诚恳的前言表示无尽谢意。

从个人的角度上,我们要感谢 Susan Saudek 和孩子们,Mark、Debbie、Tina 和 Tony,以及其他为 C.D.S 的生活带来欢乐的家庭成员们。

R.R.K 在此感谢她的家人,包括父母,Ashok 和 Kanchan,以及哥哥 Kapil 和他们无条件的支持;尤其要感谢她的丈夫 Sachin 和孩子们,Shaan 和 Sonia,他们每天为她的生活带来灵感与鼓舞。

F.L.B 在此感谢他的两个家庭——一个是他的小家,一个是霍普金斯的大家庭。

最后,我们要感谢我们的患者们,他们是我们最好的老师,也是我们写这本书的原动力。

编者

第一部分

概述

糖尿病简介	3
糖尿病的诊断与分型	6
1 型糖尿病的流行病学	9
2 型糖尿病的流行病学	12
糖尿病治疗相关的重要研究：预防与血糖控制	15
糖尿病治疗的关键研究：控制并发症	22
糖尿病治疗的关键研究：治疗效果	33

糖尿病简介

Christopher D. Saudek, MD, and Rita Rastogi Kalyani, MD, MHS

糖尿病概述

- 糖尿病是一种常见的慢性疾病,其定义为高血糖(血中葡萄糖升高)并常伴多种其他代谢紊乱(如酸中毒)。
- 糖尿病的病理生理学特征为胰岛素敏感性降低和/或胰岛素分泌不足引起的胰岛素相对或绝对缺之。
- 胰岛素是调节大多数细胞从血液中摄取葡萄糖的关键激素(主要是骨骼肌细胞和脂肪细胞,不包括中枢神经系统细胞)。当血糖升高时,例如进食之后,胰腺中的胰岛 β 细胞释放胰岛素入血。胰岛素同时还调控葡萄糖转化为糖原储存于肝脏和骨骼肌细胞中。高胰岛素水平增加合成代谢,如细胞生长、蛋白质合成、脂肪储存等。低胰岛素水平则导致分解代谢,尤其是触发酮症或脂肪分解。
- 糖尿病与尿崩症无关联,唯一的共同点是二者均可引起多尿。
- 据疾病预防控制中心(Centers for Disease Control, CDC)统计,2007 年美国约有 2 360 万人被诊断为糖尿病,占美国总人口的 7.8%。其中超过 40% 的患者在 20 岁时就诊断为糖尿病或糖尿病前期(Cowie)。总人群中大约 1/4 的糖尿病患者未能确诊。
- 25 年后美国糖尿病人数将增加一倍,达到 4 410 万(Huang)。
- 糖尿病是美国第七大死亡原因,耗费约 1/3 的医疗保险开支,是工作年龄段成年人口致盲(由于糖尿病视网膜病变和黄斑水肿)、非创伤性截肢、终末期肾病和透析以及外周神经病变的首要原因。
- 诊断与分型:2 型糖尿病(胰岛素抵抗及相对胰岛素分泌不足)占总例数的 90%~95%,1 型糖尿病(绝对胰岛素分泌不足)占 5%~10%,其他类型(如不常见的遗传缺陷)占 1%~5%。妊娠糖尿病是指在妊娠期间首次诊断的糖尿病。
- 2 型糖尿病与脂肪增加,尤其是向心性肥胖(腹型肥胖)以及阳性家族史高度相关。
- 1 型糖尿病与特异性遗传标志物相关,并且在北欧人种中更为多发。

糖尿病的并发症与合并症

- 急性并发症:高血糖和其他代谢紊乱所引起的直接、快速的临床后果,需要及时纠正。例如:过度口渴(烦渴)、尿频(多尿症)、视力模糊、疲乏、酮症酸中毒等。
- 多尿症和烦渴往往发生在血糖超出肾糖阈(180mg/dl)时。视力模糊是由于血糖升高引起晶状体内渗透压的改变。
- 慢性并发症:糖尿病存在数年或数十年后发生,且往往难以或不可逆转,其中包括微血管并发症(即小血管病变)如视网膜病变、神经病变、肾脏病变,大血管并发症(即大血管病变)如冠心病、外周血管疾病、卒中。
- 发生大血管和微血管并发症的病理生理学基础相似;长期控制不佳的高血糖状态使大、小血管发生氧化损伤,进而导致斑块形成、血管狭窄引起远端组织器官的缺血性损伤。
- 心血管疾病可致死,糖尿病人群患心血管疾病的概率较普通人群增加2~4倍。
- 其他常见并发症包括伤口不易愈合、易于感染、勃起功能障碍以及糖尿病性胃轻瘫等。
- 有些合并症可能会影响糖尿病的治疗,如艾滋病(human immunodeficiency virus, HIV)、囊胞性纤维症、多囊卵巢综合征(polycystic ovarian syndrome, PCOS)、胰切除术后糖尿病以及库欣综合征等。睡眠呼吸暂停和抑郁症往往对其治疗也有影响。
- 妊娠期间糖尿病若控制不佳,可能会使新生儿和孕产妇出现并发症。

糖尿病及其并发症的管理
- 依靠健康的生活方式和控制肥胖来预防糖尿病或防止糖尿病前期进展为糖尿病是最为理想的。
- 一旦确诊为糖尿病,治疗内容包括医学营养治疗、运动锻炼和药物治疗。其中药物治疗包括口服降糖药(磺脲类、促泌剂、α-糖苷酶抑制剂、噻唑烷二酮类、二甲双胍、二肽基肽酶-4抑制剂)和非胰岛素注射剂(肠促胰岛素类似物)或胰岛素(基础胰岛素和餐时胰岛素),并由专业医疗人员定期监测。最重要的是糖尿病患者的教育。
- 2004-2006年,57%的糖尿病患者仅采用口服降糖药治疗,16%仅采用胰岛素治疗,13%采用口服降糖药和胰岛素联合治疗,14%没有采取药物干预(CDC)。
- 对于严重肥胖的糖尿病患者,可以通过外科减肥手术来改善病情。
- 一些用于治疗糖尿病并发症和合并症的药物可能会使血糖升高加剧,包括抗精神病药、噻嗪类利尿剂、β受体阻滞剂、烟酸以及部分抗生素。
- 胰岛素泵对治疗1型糖尿病更为有效和适用。
- 糖尿病引起的慢性微血管并发症可以通过良好的血糖控制(即糖化血红蛋白<7%)来延迟或预防,这一观点在针对1型糖尿病的糖尿病控制与并发症试验(Diabetes Control and Complications Trial, DCCT)和针对2型糖尿病的英国前瞻性糖尿病研究(The United Kingdom Prospective Diabetes Study, UKPDS)中均已证实。
- 良好的血糖控制对减少视网膜病变、神经病变以及肾病发生至关重要。
- 控制滥用烟草、肥胖、高血压(目标血压<130/80mmHg)和血脂异常(目标LDL<100mg/dl)有助于减少心血管疾病。DCCT/糖尿病干预与并发症流行病学研究(The Epidemiology of Diabetes Interventions and Complications Study, EDIC),以及UKPDS研究长期随访结果表明,控制血糖对减少心血管疾病也很重要。
- 应同时治疗高血糖和其他心血管危险因素以减少心血管疾病的发生。
- 对儿童和老年人而言,糖化血红蛋白目标值可以略高一些。
- 对于糖尿病的急性并发症,如酮症酸中毒、严重高血糖、糖尿病足、心肌梗死等,应定期随访以建立良好的门诊治疗服务。
- 最好能建立一个包括护理教育家、营养学家、主治医生、足病学家、眼科学家及其他专科学家的小组,以便满足患者的需求。
- 值得一提的是,患者参与是每个糖尿病治疗计划成功的核心。

糖尿病的临床试验

- 纵向监测包括患者自我血糖监测和专业医疗人员行预防性筛查，包括血压、糖化血红蛋白、血脂、尿微量白蛋白、视网膜以及足部检查。
- 应进行流感和肺炎的例行性疫苗接种。
- 可采用其他实验室检查对糖尿病合并症进行评估，如通过性激素评估性腺机能减退，通过维生素 D 和骨密度评估骨质疾病，通过肝功检查评估非酒精性脂肪肝及贫血等。
- 自身抗体有助于区别 1 型和 2 型糖尿病。
- 对于难治性糖尿病而言，采用动态血糖监测系统有助于改善血糖控制。

专家意见

- 糖尿病是可控的，在血糖及心血管危险因素控制良好的情况下并发症是可以避免的，并且这些并发症是可以治疗的。
- 若不采取治疗措施，糖尿病仍然是一种严重的疾病，它可以导致严重的并发症以及过早死亡。
- 糖尿病长期的并发症、长期的护理以及老年人口的增加，这些都给社会带来了沉重的负担，且日益严重。
- 与糖尿病有关的社会问题包括就业歧视和人群排斥等仍有待解决。

参考文献

Cowie CC, Rust KF, Ford ES, et al. Full accounting of diabetes and pre-diabetes in the U.S. population in 1988-1994 and 2005-2006. Diabetes Care, 2009; Vol. 32: pp. 287-94.
  Comments: A recent publication from NIDDK reporting an alarming 40% of people age > 20 years in the U.S. with either diabetes or pre-diabetes.

Huang ES, Basu A, O'Grady M, et al. Projecting the future diabetes population size and related costs for the U.S. Diabetes Care, 2009; Vol. 32: pp. 2225-9.
  Comments: Modeled projection of rates of diabetes in the U.S. over the next 25 years.

American Diabetes Association. http://www.diabetes.org/.
  Comments: The American Diabetes Association is a reliable source of diabetes information, and has multifaceted programs for people with diabetes.

Centers for Disease Control and Prevention. Diabetes Data and Trends.http://apps.nccd.cdc.gov/DDTSTRS/ default.aspx.
  Comments: Centers for disease Control and Prevention (CdC) is an excellent source of reliable data on diabetes in the US.

International Diabetes Federation. Diabetes Facts and Figures. http://www.idf.org/Facts_ and_Figures.
  Comments: International Diabetes Federation (IDF) is an excellent source of reliable data on diabetes worldwide, as well as educational programs.

Juvenile Diabetes Research Foundation International. http://www.jdrf.org/.
  Comments: The Juvenile Diabetes Research Foundation is an important funder of diabetes research, as well as source of reliable diabetes information.

National Diabetes Education Program. http://www.ndep.nih.gov/.
  Comments: The National Diabetes Education Program has useful, multicultural education information and resources.

National Diabetes Information Clearinghouse (NDIC). http://diabetes.niddk.nih.gov/.
  Comments: The National Institute of Diabetes, Digestive and Kidney Diseases has reliable diabetes information.

糖尿病的诊断与分型

Christopher D. Saudek, MD

分型

- 糖尿病分为1型糖尿病（既往称为青少年型或胰岛素依赖型糖尿病）、2型糖尿病（既往称为成人型或非胰岛素依赖型糖尿病）、妊娠糖尿病以及其他特殊类型糖尿病。
- 1型糖尿病：胰岛素完全或几乎完全缺乏，常由自身免疫性疾病引起。临床表现（常见但不限于30岁以下）：体重正常，既往无糖尿病家族史，需即刻或在一年之内进行胰岛素治疗，谷氨酸脱羧酶（Glutamic acid decarboxylase, GAD）抗体、胰岛细胞抗原2（islet antigen-2, IA2）抗体和/或胰岛细胞抗体阳性（参见1型糖尿病的自身抗体，643页），容易出现酮症酸中毒（见45页）和血糖不稳。
- 1b型或特发性糖尿病：1型糖尿病中罕见的亚型，胰岛素几乎完全缺乏，与遗传高度相关，无自身免疫征象。主要见于非洲和亚洲人群。
- 成人隐匿性自身免疫性糖尿病（latent autoimmune diabetes of adulthood, LADA）：1型糖尿病中由成人起病的一种亚型，疾病进展缓慢，起始药物治疗可能有效，但最终需要采用胰岛素治疗，一般不出现酮症酸中毒，GAD、IA2和/或胰岛细胞抗体阳性（见LADA，162页）。
- 2型糖尿病：内源性分泌的胰岛素不能完全对抗机体对胰岛素的抵抗，该类型大约占糖尿病总数的90%，在亚洲和非洲人中更为常见。临床表现：起病较晚（多在>35岁发病，近来趋向年轻化），超重或肥胖，与糖尿病家族史相关，数年内对口服降糖药敏感，血糖水平相对稳定。
- 存在其他急性疾病，或当2型糖尿病患者的胰岛素缺乏加剧时，可能会出现酮症酸中毒（"酮症倾向的2型糖尿病"）(Umpierrez)。
- 妊娠糖尿病（gestational diabetes mellitus, GDM）：妊娠期初次确诊的糖尿病。通常是2型糖尿病的发病前兆，也有可能是1型糖尿病首次发病。
- 其他特殊类型糖尿病：其他病因明确的糖尿病，如胰切除术后糖尿病，库欣综合征，HIV相关糖尿病，囊性纤维化相关糖尿病，某些药物如糖皮质激素引发的糖尿病，遗传综合征如青少年发病的成人型糖尿病（maturity onset diabetes in young, MODY），柯萨奇病毒B等感染型糖尿病（见美国糖尿病协会特殊类型糖尿病的诊断与分类指南明细表）。

诊断

- 非妊娠成年人稳定状态（非急病）的糖尿病诊断标准：（1）空腹血糖（fasting plasma glucose, FPG）≥126mg/dl（7mmol/L）；（2）伴有高血糖症状者随机血糖≥200mg/dl（11.1mmol/L）；（3）口服葡萄糖耐量试验（oral glucose tolerance test, OGTT）2小时血糖>200mg/dl（11.1mmol/L）；或（4）近来推荐的诊断标准：糖化血红蛋白≥6.5%（美国糖尿病协会糖尿病诊疗标准）。
- FPG和OGTT检测前，患者需至少8小时无热量摄入，并且在检测前数天应保持足够的碳水化合物摄入。

糖尿病的诊断与分型

- 理想的糖尿病诊断应在不同日期再次确诊。
- "糖尿病前期"或"糖尿病风险增加"的诊断标准包括空腹血糖受损（impaired fasting glucose, IFG）即 FPG 100~125mg/dl，糖耐量受损（impaired glucose tolerance, IGT）即 OGTT 后 2 小时血糖 140~199mg/dl。二者满足其一即可。近来推荐的诊断标准为糖化血红蛋白 5.7%~6.4%。
- ≥ 45 岁或 BMI ≥ 25kg/m^2 的成人，以及具有其他糖尿病危险因素的人应接受糖尿病筛查。
- GDM 的诊断标准另有详述（见 138 页）。

专家意见

- 可通过具体的葡萄糖水平来确诊糖尿病或糖尿病前期。
- 糖尿病分型通常十分明显，但也不绝对。
- 1 型和 2 型糖尿病的临床表现也会出现例外。例如，部分 2 型糖尿病患者的体重正常并且伴有酮症酸中毒，而部分 1 型糖尿病患者则超重。
- 当存在疑问时，可以检测 GAD、IA2 和 / 或胰岛细胞抗体。如若为阳性，往往诊断为 1 型糖尿病；即使为阴性，也不能排除 1 型糖尿病的可能。
- 大部分 2 型糖尿病患者最终需要采用胰岛素治疗，但并非全部如此。因此，非胰岛素依赖不能作为 2 型糖尿病的定义。
- 不同类型的糖尿病应鉴别诊断以便进行适当的针对性治疗，例如，1 型糖尿病必须使用胰岛素治疗，而且绝大多数为多次给药。
- 我们尚未发现胰岛素水平或 C- 肽（C-peptide）有助于诊断糖尿病，因为在 2 型糖尿病或 1 型糖尿病"蜜月期"，胰岛素分泌量可以是正常的。
- 最好不要使用"1.5 型"或"3 型"糖尿病这样的词。虽然有些病例无法明确诊断，但这些规定之外的术语不具有明确含义。
- 在临床实践中，检测 FPG（或近来推荐的糖化血红蛋白）比完整的 OGTT 更为便利。

参考文献

American Diabetes Association. Standards of medical care in diabetes—2011. Diabetes Care, 2011; Vol. 34 Suppl 1:pp. S11–61.
Comments: The annually updated standards of medical care, which include diagnosis and classification.

American Diabetes Association. Diagnosis and classification of diabetes mellitus. Diabetes Care, 2010; Vol. 33 Suppl 1: pp. S62–9.
Comments: The annually updated diagnosis and classification of diabetes including a complete etiological classification of diabetes with subtypes.

International Expert Committee International Expert Committee report on the role of the A1C assay in the diagnosis of diabetes. Diabetes Care, 2009; Vol. 32: pp. 1327–34.
Comments: An ADA committee that recently recommended use of A1c for diagnosis; not officially endorsed by ADA.

Saudek CD, Herman WH, Sacks DB, et al. A new look at screening and diagnosing diabetes mellitus. J Clin Endocrinol Metab, 2008; Vol. 93: pp. 2447–53.

Comments: Publication by a panel that reviews the literature and presents arguments in favor of use of A1c for diagnosis.

Genuth S, Alberti KG, Bennett P, et al. Follow-up report on the diagnosis of diabetes mellitus. Diabetes Care, 2003; Vol. 26: pp. 3160–7.
Comments: A follow-up expert committee report that lowered the criterion for IFG to 100 mg/dl.

Report of the Expert Committee on the Diagnosis and Classification of Diabetes Mellitus. Diabetes Care, 1997; Vol. 20: pp. 1183–97.
Comments: This committee report established diagnostic criteria for the modern era, changing the FPG criterion to 126 mg/dl, and establishing the names type 1 and type 2, and impaired fasting glucose (IFG).

Umpierrez GE, Casals MM, Gebhart SP, et al. Diabetic ketoacidosis in obese .African-Americans. Diabetes, 1995; Vol. 44: pp. 790–5.
Comments: A description of type 2 diabetes presenting with diabetic ketoacidosis ("ketosis-prone type 2 diabetes").

1型糖尿病的流行病学

Rita Rastogi Kalyani,MD,MHS

美国1型糖尿病（T1DM）发病率与患病率
- SEARCH青少年糖尿病研究结果显示，在2002-2003年，10~14岁青少年的1型糖尿病发病率最高（25.9例/10万人年）。
- 男女发病率相近（发病率比值接近于1）。
- 总体来说，在各个年龄层中，非西班牙裔白种青少年的T1DM发病率最高（15.1/10万人年~32.9/10万人年）。
- 2001年美国T1DM患病率约为0.15%。
- 0~9岁年龄段T1DM患病率（0.78例/1 000名青少年）低于10~19岁年龄段（2.28例/1 000名青少年）。
- 从各个年龄层来看，非西班牙裔白种人的T1DM患病率最高（低年龄组和高年龄组分别为1.03例/1 000名青少年和2.88例/1 000名青少年）。
- 所有种族中，< 10岁的青少年糖尿病类型均以T1DM最为常见（> 85%）。> 10岁的青少年中，非西班牙裔白种人青少年患T1DM更为常见（85.1%），高于其他多个种族的青少年患者，包括西班牙裔（53.9%）、非裔美国人（42.2%）、亚裔/太平洋岛（30.3%）以及美洲印第安人（13.8%）；在这些种族中2型糖尿病更为常见。

美国青少年T1DM的管理与预后
- 威斯康星州糖尿病注册队列研究中，1987-1992年期间纳入诊断的T1DM患者进行20年随访，患者年龄均≤30岁（Palta）。
- 血糖监测和控制在青春期均出现明显恶化。
- 在患糖尿病14~20年之后（平均年龄30岁），仅有22%的患者糖化血红蛋白< 7%。
- 96%的患者需要使用胰岛素泵或进行每日3次以上胰岛素注射。
- 22%的患者出现肥胖（BMI ≥ 30kg/m^2），36%出现超重（BMI为25~29kg/m^2）。
- 76%的患者每日监测血糖至少3次。
- 低血糖发生较为常见，26%~32%的患者每周出现≥ 2~4次低血糖。
- 视网膜病变在这二十年中出现的时间较晚且严重程度较低。
- 在威斯康星州，十年内T1DM年发病率增加了2倍，主要发生于年幼和体重超重的少年（Evertsen）。

全球T1DM的发病率与患病率
- 经过年龄校正后T1DM的发病率从中国和委内瑞拉的每年0.1例/10万人到芬兰的每年40.9例/10万人不等（DIAMOND项目组）。
- 1990-1999年，全世界的T1DM发病率每年增加2.8%（95%CI:2.4%~3.2%）。
- 在此期间，各大洲绝大多数发病率均显著增加且具有统计学差异（亚洲为4.0%，欧洲为3.2%，北美洲为5.3%），除外中美洲和西印度群岛发病率降低了 3.6%。
- 在大多数人群中,男女发病率相当。
- 1990–1999 年间年龄最低组人群的发病率增长最多。
- 有研究表明,早期的环境危险因素可能会增加发病率,包括孕妇肠病毒感染、高龄产妇(39~42 岁)、先兆子痫、剖宫产分娩、出生体重增加、早期摄入牛乳蛋白以及出生后生长过快(包括体重和身高)等。补充维生素 D 可能会起到保护作用。病毒感染可能触发对 β 细胞的自身免疫,同时其他暴露因素则可能加重 β 细胞的负担,从而加速糖尿病进展(Soltesz)。
- 一般来说,发病率随着年龄的增加而增加,在青春期达到顶峰。青春期后,年轻女性的发病率显著下降,而男性的发病率则保持在较高水平直至 29–35 岁。在芬兰,男孩与女孩的整体发病率比为 1.1,而在 13 岁时这一比例为 1.7(1.4~2.0)(Harjutsalo)。
- 按照欧洲目前的发展趋势,基于 20 项以人群为基础的 EURODIAB 注册机构,科学家们预测,2005–2020 年欧洲 <5 岁儿童的 T1DM 患病率将新增一倍,其中年龄低于 15 岁患者的患病率将增加 70%(Patterson)。

参考文献

American Diabetes Association. Standards of medical care in diabetes—2011. Diabetes Care, 2011; Vol. 34 Suppl 1: pp. S11–61.
Comments: Outlines standards of medical care for diabetes including A1c goals by age group for T1DM.

Evertsen J, Alemzadeh R, Wang X. Increasing incidence of pediatric type 1 diabetes mellitus in Southeastern Wisconsin: relationship with body weight at diagnosis. PLoS ONE, 2009; Vol. 4: p. e6873.
Comments: Describes increasing incidence of type 1 diabetes between 1995 and 2004 in Wisconsin youth.

Palta M, LeCaire T. Managing type 1 diabetes: trends and outcomes over 20 years in the Wisconsin Diabetes Registry cohort. WMJ, 2009; Vol. 108: pp. 231–5.
Comments: Describes diabetes management and acute and chronic complications from diabetes among youth with type 1 diabetes followed for up to 20 years in Wisconsin Diabetes Registry cohort.

Patterson CC, Dahlquist GG, Gyürüs E, et al. Incidence trends for childhood type 1 diabetes in Europe during 1989–2003 and predicted new cases 2005–20: a multicentre prospective registration study. Lancet, 2009; Vol. 373: pp. 2027–33.
Comments: Population-based study of 20 EURODIAB registers in 17 countries that registered children diagnosed with diabetes before their 15th birthday between 1989–2003. Describes trends in incidence during this time and predicted new cases in 2005–2020.

Harjutsalo V, Sjöberg L, Tuomilehto J. Time trends in the incidence of type 1 diabetes in Finnish children: a cohort study. Lancet, 2008; Vol. 371: pp. 1777–82.
Comments: Children with newly diagnosed type 1 diabetes in Finland who were listed on public registers in 1980–2005 were included in a cohort study and followed for trends in diabetes incidence.

Soltesz G, Patterson CC, Dahlquist G, et al. Worldwide childhood type 1 diabetes incidence—what can we learn from epidemiology? Pediatr Diabetes, 2007; Vol. 8 Suppl 6: pp. 6–14.
Comments: Describes global epidemiology of type 1 diabetes, and trends in incidence and risk factors in early life.

Writing Group for the SEARCH for Diabetes in Youth Study Group, Dabelea D, Bell RA, et al. Incidence of diabetes in youth in the United States. JAMA, 2007; Vol. 297: pp. 2716–24.
Comments: Estimates incidence rates for youth <20 years of age in the US for years 2002–2003 by age, gender, race/ethnicity, and type of diabetes.

SEARCH for Diabetes in Youth Study Group, Liese AD, D'Agostino RB, et al. The burden of diabetes mellitus among US youth: prevalence estimates from the SEARCH for Diabetes in Youth Study. Pediatrics, 2006; Vol. 118: pp. 1510–8.
Comments: Estimates national prevalence of diabetes in youth <20 years of age in 2001 in the United States according to age, gender, race/ethnicity, diabetes type.

DIAMOND Project Group. Incidence and trends of childhood type 1 diabetes worldwide 1990–1999. Diabet Med, 2006; Vol. 23: pp. 857–66.
Comments: The incidence of type 1 diabetes was analyzed in children aged ≤ 14 years from 114 populations in 112 centers in 57 countries. A total of 43,013 cases were diagnosed in the 84 million children. Average annual increase in incidence 2.8%.

2 型糖尿病的流行病学

Rita Rastogi Kalyani, MD, MHS

美国 2 型糖尿病的患病率
- ≥ 20 岁成人已确诊的 2 型糖尿病粗患病率从 1988–1994 年的 5.1% 上升至 2005–2006 年的 7.7%（Cowie）。
- 2005–2006 年，≥ 20 岁成人全部 2 型糖尿病的粗患病率为 12.9%，其中 40% 为未诊断患者（空腹血糖 ≥ 7mmol/L 和／或 2 小时血糖 ≥ 11.1mmol/L）。
- ≥ 20 岁成人，空腹血糖受损的粗患病率为 25.7%，糖耐量受损为 13.8%，二者任有其一的粗患病率为 30%。
- 三分之一的老年人患有糖尿病，四分之三的老年人患有糖尿病或糖尿病前期。
- 非西班牙裔黑人和墨西哥裔美国人年龄和性别标化后已确诊的 2 型糖尿病患病率是非西班牙裔白人的两倍。

美国糖尿病经济负担
- 糖尿病人群的医疗费用大约是非糖尿病人群的 2.3 倍。
- 在美国，大约 1/5 的医疗支出用于对糖尿病患者的护理，1/10 用于对糖尿病的直接治疗。
- 新近研究表明，2007 年糖尿病的总花费为 2 180 亿美元，其中 1 530 亿美元为额外的医疗费用，650 亿美元为降低的国民生产力。
- 糖尿病的医疗费用中，270 亿美元用于糖尿病的直接治疗，580 亿美元用于糖尿病相关慢性并发症的治疗，310 亿美元为常规医疗费用。
- 糖尿病的主要医疗支出包括：住院治疗（占总花费的 50%）、糖尿病药品和物料（12%）、治疗并发症的零售处方（11%）、医生门诊（9%）。
- 平均每例患者的医疗成本：未诊断糖尿病患者 2 864 美元，已确诊糖尿病患者 9 975 美元（2 型糖尿病 9 677 美元，1 型糖尿病 14 856 美元），糖尿病前期患者 443 美元（以上仅为医疗成本）。
- 不考虑糖尿病疾病状态的情况下，每个美国人每年的花费大约为 700 美元。
- 间接花费包括旷工、工作能力下降、伴随疾病导致的失业、由于过早死亡导致生产力下降。
- 具有医疗保险的人群中，糖尿病人群将从 2009 年的 8 200 万增加至 2034 年的 14 600 万，据估算，相关费用将从 450 亿美元增加至 1 710 亿美元。
- 以上信息来自美国糖尿病协会；DallTM, Zhang Y, Chen YJ 等，以及 Basu A, O'Grady M 等。

全球 2 型糖尿病的患病率
- 2010 年全球成年人（20~79 岁）的糖尿病患病率为 6.4%，即 2.85 亿人（Shaw）。
- 到 2030 年，糖尿病患病率将增至 7.7%，即 4.39 亿人。
- 预计 2010 年至 2030 年，发展中国家糖尿病人群将增加 69%，发达国家增加 20%。

2 型糖尿病的流行病学

- 2010 年糖尿病患病率位居前十的国家是：瑙鲁（31%），阿拉伯联合酋长国（19%），沙特阿拉伯（17%），毛里求斯（16%），巴林（15%），留尼汪岛（15%），科威特（15%），阿曼（13%），汤加（13%），马来西亚（12%）。
- 2010 年 20~79 岁人群糖尿病患病人数位居前十的国家是（单位为百万人）：印度（50.8），中国（43.2），美国（26.8），俄罗斯（9.6），巴西（7.6），德国（7.5），巴基斯坦（7.1），日本（7.1），印度尼西亚（7.0），墨西哥（6.8）。
- 到 2030 年，预计患病人数排名仍将靠前的国家是（单位为百万人）：印度（87），中国（62.6），美国（36）。

全球糖尿病经济负担

- 2010 年，全球约有 12% 的医疗开支（1 330 美元/人）用于糖尿病（Zhang）。
- 2010 年全球用于糖尿病的医疗开支总和达 3 760 亿美元，到 2030 年预计达到 4 900 亿美元。
- 据估算，2010 年国家总医疗开支数额最高的前十个国家是（单位为美元）：美国（1 970 亿），德国（280 亿），日本（220 亿），法国（170 亿），加拿大（110 亿），意大利（110 亿），英国（80 亿），西班牙（70 亿），中国（50 亿），墨西哥（50 亿）。
- 2010 年用于糖尿病的人均国民医疗开支前十名是：美国（7 383 美元），卢森堡（7 268 美元），冰岛（7 001 美元），挪威（6 933 美元），瑞士（5 995 美元），摩纳哥（5 866 美元），爱尔兰（5 035 美元），奥地利（4 007 美元），加拿大（3 914 美元），斯洛文尼亚（1 626 美元）。
- 糖尿病开支占国民医疗开支比例最高的前十名是：瑙鲁（41%），沙特阿拉伯（21%），毛里求斯（20%），图瓦卢（19%），巴林（19%），汤加（18%），阿曼（18%），卡塔尔（18%），塞舌尔（18%），马来西亚（16%）。
- 预计到 2030 年，美国仍然位居糖尿病医疗支出总额首位，约为 2 640 亿美元或世界总支出的 54%。

全球糖尿病的发病率和死亡率

- 根据 WHO 疾病的电脑模型计算，2010 年全球由糖尿病引起的 20~79 岁年龄人群的非自然死亡总数为 396 万人（占全球全部年龄死亡率的 6.8%）（Roglic）。
- 2001 年高收入国家疾病负担（残疾相关校正生命年）的前十名为：（1）缺血性心脏病，（2）脑血管疾病，（3）单相抑郁症，（4）痴呆，（5）肺癌，（6）失聪，（7）慢性阻塞性肺病（Chronic obstructive pulmonary disease, COPD），（8）糖尿病，（9）酒精滥用，（10）骨关节炎（Lopez）。
- 2001 年中低收入国家的相对负担更多的是传染病（如 HIV/AIDS、呼吸道感染、腹泻、疟疾、结核）和围产期疾病。
- 糖尿病死亡人数占成年人总死亡人数的比例为：非洲 6%，北美洲 15.7%。
- 在不同地区，49 岁以上人群中女性糖尿病致死率高于男性，在部分地区部分年龄段甚至达到 25%。
- 由于糖尿病患病率增加，糖尿病引起的总病死率和死亡率也将增加，在中低收入国家尤为明显。

参考文献

Roglic G, Unwin N. Mortality attributable to diabetes: estimates for the year 2010. Diabetes Res Clin Pract, 2010; Vol. 87: pp. 15–9.
Comments: Estimates of underlying mortality and relative risk of dying for people with diabetes compared to those without diabetes using a computerized disease model.

Shaw JE, Sicree RA, Zimmet PZ. Global estimates of the prevalence of diabetes for 2010 and 2030. Diabetes Res Clin Pract, 2010; Vol. 87: pp. 4–14.
Comments: Based on studies from 91 countries, estimated prevalence of diabetes for 216 countries for 2010 and 2030.

Zhang P, Zhang X, Brown J, et al. Global healthcare expenditure on diabetes for 2010 and 2030. Diabetes Res Clin Pract, 2010; Vol. 87: pp. 293–301.
Comments: Country-by-country expenditures for 193 countries estimated based on diabetes prevalence, population estimates, and healthcare expenditures for years 2010 and 2030.

Cowie CC, Rust KF, byrd-Holt dd, et al. Prevalence of diabetes and high risk for diabetes using A1c criteria in the U.S. population in 1988–2006. diabetes Care, 2010; Vol. 33: pp. 562–8.
Comments: using data from National Health and Nutrition Examination Survey 1988–2006, provides estimates for prevalence of diabetes and high risk for diabetes using HbA1c. The authors conclude that HbA1c alone detects much lower prevalence of diabetes than glucose criteria.

Dall TM, Zhang Y, Chen YJ, et al. The economic burden of diabetes. Health aff (Millwood), 2010; pp. 297–303.
Comments: Provides more updated estimates of spending on diabetes in 2007 for U.S.

Cowie CC, Rust KF, Ford ES, et al. Full accounting of diabetes and pre-diabetes in the U.S. population in 1988–1994 and 2005–2006. diabetes Care, 2009; Vol. 32: pp. 287–94.
Comments: using data from National Health and Nutrition Examination Survey in 1988–2004 and 2005–2006, provides estimates for prevalence of diabetes and prediabetes in the U.S using glucose criteria.

Huang ES, Basu a, O'Grady M, et al. Projecting the future diabetes population size and related costs for the U.S. Diabetes Care, 2009; Vol. 32: pp. 2225–9.
Comments: using a novel population-level model, projected that the number of people with diagnosed and undiagnosed diabetes will increase from 23.7 million (2009) to 44.1 million (2034), and annual diabetes-related spending is expected to increase from $113 billion to $336 billion in US. For the Medicare-eligible population, associated spending is estimated to rise from $45 billion to $171 billion.

American diabetes association. Economic costs of diabetes in the U.S. in 2007. Diabetes Care, 2008; Vol. 31: pp. 596–615.
Comments: using a prevalence-based approach, estimates health care costs attribute able to diabetes in the US.

Lopez ad, Mathers Cd, Ezzati M, et al. Global and regional burden of disease and risk factors, 2001: systematic analysis of population health data. Lancet, 2006; Vol. 367: pp. 1747–57.
Comments: The global burden of disease and risk factors for 2001 was calculated for 136 diseases, including diabetes, using mortality, incidence, prevalence, and disability-adjusted life years.

糖尿病治疗相关的重要研究：预防与血糖控制

Christopher D. Saudek, MD, and Rita Rastogi Kalyani, MD, MHS

目的

- 将编者认为最重要的糖尿病原始研究进行总结，为读者提供方便。
- 方便大家在研究糖尿病循证医学证据时快速获取原始数据。

糖尿病的预防

- 2型糖尿病（大庆糖耐量受损与糖尿病研究，1997）：该研究将中国大庆557例IGT患者随机分为饮食治疗组、运动组、饮食运动治疗组或对照组。6年后对照组有67.7%进展为糖尿病；饮食治疗组则降低至44%，运动组降低至41%，饮食运动治疗组降低至46%。在校正基线BMI和空腹血糖的差异后，饮食治疗和/或运动组糖尿病发病率一共降低了31%（Pan）。长期随访结果显示，坚持良好的生活方式干预可以使20年内糖尿病相对风险降低40%（Li）。
- 2型糖尿病（糖尿病预防计划，DPP，2002）：该计划纳入3 234例糖耐量受损和空腹血糖>95mg/dl的成年人（平均年龄51岁，BMI 34kg/m²），随机给予强化生活方式辅导（intensive lifestyle counseling，ILS）、二甲双胍850mg每天2次或安慰剂。平均随访2.8年后，研究结果显示，接受ILS的患者糖尿病发病率降低58%，接受二甲双胍治疗者降低31%（Knowler）。
- 2型糖尿病（芬兰糖尿病预防研究，2002）：将552例糖耐量受损者随机分为生活方式干预组和对照组。3.2年后，对照组有23%发展为糖尿病，生活方式干预组为11%。与DPP显示的降低效果一致（Tuomilento）。
- 2型糖尿病[曲格列酮预防糖尿病发生的作用（Troglitazone In the Prevention of Diabetes，TRIPOD），2002]：对既往患有妊娠糖尿病的133名女性随机给予曲格列酮或安慰剂治疗。30个月后，安慰剂组中12.1%发生糖尿病，曲格列酮组则为5.4%。随后曲格列酮由于肝脏毒性作用被撤市，该研究揭盲后使用吡格列酮继续进行，仍表明可降低糖尿病发病率和保护β细胞功能（Buchanan）。
- 2型糖尿病[雷米普利和罗格列酮降低糖尿病风险的试验（Diabetes REduction Assessment with ramipril and rosiglitazone Medication trial，DREAM），2008]：该试验纳入5 269例糖耐量受损或空腹血糖异常，但无心血管疾病或肾功能不全的患者。随机分为雷米普利与安慰剂组、罗格列酮与安慰剂组。罗格列酮可以增加心力衰竭（OR=7.04，95%CI:1.60~31.0），并降低肾脏事件风险20%（P=0.01）。糖尿病预防与改善肾脏预后作用独立相关（P < 0.001）（Dagenais）。
- 1型糖尿病[1型糖尿病预防试验研究组（Diabetes Prevention Trial-Type 1 Study Group，DPT-1），2002]：DPT-1研究了超高危人群口服胰岛素或非肠道给予低剂量长效胰岛素对预防1型糖尿病进展的作用。结果显示，在患糖尿病之前口服胰岛素或进行胰岛素注射不能延迟或预防T1DM起病（DPT-1 Study Group）。
- 1型糖尿病（Herold等，2002）：2005年，这一小型研究证实了一个理论，即免疫调节可以延缓1型糖尿病的胰岛素减少。24名受试者在诊断为T1DM后六周内接受了人灭活CD3-hOKT3gamma1单克隆抗体(Ala-Ala)或安慰剂治疗。接受抗体治疗的12名患者中有9名患者胰岛素反应改善，接受安慰剂的12名患者中有2名患者胰岛素反应改善。研究中患者出现了发热、皮疹和肌肉疼痛。该研究引发了一系列对新近诊断T1DM采用免疫调节来改善胰岛素反应的尝试研究。

- 1型糖尿病（Keymeulen等，2005）：人源无糖基化抗CD3抗体（ChAglyCD3）的2期安慰剂对照试验，80例T1DM患者分别给予连续6天的CD3抗体或安慰剂。18个月后，CD3抗体组残留β细胞功能更好，安慰剂组胰岛素剂量需要增加，而抗体组不增加。试验开始时，β细胞功能残留≥50%的患者中，CD3抗体组平均胰岛素剂量为0.22IU/（kg·d），安慰剂组为0.61IU/（kg·d）（$P < 0.001$）。

长期血糖控制的益处

- 血红蛋白作为评价血糖控制的一项指标（Koenig等，1976）：早期研究中，应用血红蛋白A1c（与A1a和1b相比）作为血糖控制的指标。5名血糖控制不佳的受试者在接受3个月的强化治疗后显示，血红蛋白A1c水平降低。血红蛋白A1c反映了检测之前数周至数月的平均血糖水平，被推荐作为监测血糖控制程度的有效方法。

- 1型糖尿病［糖尿病控制与并发症试验（Diabetes Control and Complications Trial, DCCT），1993］：该试验由美国国家卫生研究院（National Institutes of Health, NIH）赞助，是探讨血糖控制对并发症影响的决定性研究。基线时无视网膜病变（一级预防组）和轻度视网膜病变（二级预防组）的1 441例1型糖尿病患者随机分为"强化治疗组"或"常规治疗组"进行血糖控制。平均随访6.5年后，强化治疗组的平均血红蛋白A1c为7.2%，传统治疗组为9.1%。一级预防组强化治疗后糖尿病视网膜病变的进展降低了76%，二级预防组降低54%。两个队列合并后，强化治疗可减少尿微量白蛋白排泄达39%，减少蛋白尿达54%，以及减少临床神经病变达60%。然而，强化治疗组低血糖增加2~3倍。许多更早的或随后的研究报道源自DCCT(DCCT)。

- 1型糖尿病，长期随访［糖尿病控制与并发症的流行病学研究小组（Epidemiology of Diabetes Interventions and Complications Research Group, EDIC），2000］：EDIC首次报道了DCCT试验结束后的患者长达4年的随访结果。研究结果显示，尽管强化治疗组和常规治疗组的血红蛋白A1c水平已经趋于一致，但两者的视网膜病变和肾脏病变进展的差异性仍然存在，结果更有利于强化治疗组（DCCT/EDIC）。

- 2型糖尿病（Kumamoto试验，1995）：110例2型糖尿病患者随机采用多次胰岛素注射（MIT）或常规胰岛素注射治疗6年。在一级预防队列中，MIT组的视网膜病变（7.7% vs 32%）和肾脏病变（7.7% vs 28.0%）显著低于常规治疗组。在二级预防队列中，MIT组的视网膜病变（19.2% vs 44.0%）和肾脏病变（11.5% vs 32.0%）的进展显著低于常规治疗组。基于这项研究，预防糖尿病微血管病变发生或进展的血糖阈值被界定为HbA1c<6.5%，空腹血糖<110mg/dl，餐后2小时血糖<180mg/dl（Ohkubo）。

- 2型糖尿病［英国前瞻性糖尿病研究33（UK Prospective Diabetes Study

Group 33, UKPDS 33），1998］：该研究纳入了3 867例新诊断2型糖尿病患者，采用磺脲类或胰岛素对其进行血糖控制，评价疗效及并发症进展风险。10年后，强化治疗组平均HbA1c为7.0%，常规治疗组为7.9%。强化治疗组的糖尿病相关终点事件降低12%（P=0.029）；糖尿病相关死亡降低10%（P=0.34）；微血管终点事件降低25%（P=0.009 9）。降低心肌梗死风险的统计学差异处于临界水平（P=0.052）。磺脲类与胰岛素之间疗效无显著性差异，强化组的低血糖更多（P < 0.000 1）。总之，采用磺脲类或胰岛素进行强化血糖控制可以大幅减少2型糖尿病的微血管而非大血管并发症风险（UKPDS 33）。

- 2型糖尿病，长期随访（UKPDS，2008）：在UKPDS中接受强化血糖控制或常规血糖控制之后，3 277例再度接受临床治疗，对这些患者进行长期随访，评估后续6~10年的结果。尽管第一年以后两组之间的A1c水平就不存在差异，但磺脲类-胰岛素组表现为所有糖尿病终点事件风险降低9%（P=0.04），微血管病变风险降低24%（P=0.01）。同时，心肌梗死风险降低15%（P=0.01），全因死亡风险降低13%（P=0.001）。二甲双胍强化治疗组也表现出相似或更有效的风险降低。这一随访表明，即使短暂的早期强化治疗也对2型糖尿病终点事件具有改善作用（Holman）。

- 2型糖尿病，多因素干预（Steno-2，2003）：该试验检测了多因素干预对2型糖尿病心血管病变发展的影响，有别于单独血糖控制对并发症影响的试验。160例持续性微白蛋白尿患者分为常规治疗组或采用行为干预和药物联合强化治疗组。7.8年随之后，强化治疗组的心血管病变和微血管并发症均降低50%（Gaede）。

- 2型糖尿病，多因素干预长期随访（Steno-2，2008）：与DCCT（EDIC）和UKPDS的长期随访结果相似，该试验结果表明，多个危险因素控制对2型糖尿病具有延长效益，包括降低全因死亡率和心血管疾病（Gaede）。

- 强化治疗的局限性［控制糖尿病心血管风险试验（Action to Control Cardiovascular Risk in Diabetes Study Group, ACCORD），2008］：ACCORD研究纳入10 251例具有心血管病高危因素的糖尿病患者随机分为强化治疗组（A1c<6.0%）或常规治疗组（A1c7.0%~7.9%）。该研究由于强化治疗组的死亡率较高（253 vs 207，P=0.04）而提前终止。但是，强化治疗组的非致死性心血管疾病事件更少，药物副作用更多。强化治疗引起死亡率升高的原因仍有争议，一些相似的研究［糖尿病和血管疾病的行动：百普乐和达美康缓释控制评价试验（The Action in Diabetes and Vascular Disease：Preterax and Diamicron Modified Release Controlled Evaluation (ADVANCE) trial, ADVANCE），退伍军人糖尿病研究（Veterans Affairs Diabetes Trial, VADT）］并不支持ACCORD的结论。可能的推断是，通过药物治疗使A1c低于6%并不合适，尤其是对有心脏疾病风险的老年人。

- 强化治疗的局限性（ADVANCE，2008）：该试验将11 140例2型糖尿病患者随机分为标准治疗组（A1c 7.3%）和强化治疗组（A1c 6.5%），使用格列齐特（缓释剂型）和其他所需药物进行血糖控制。5年后，强化治疗组的主要大血管和微血管事件复合终点较标准治疗组降低了10%。这主要是因为肾病发病率降低了21%。对视网膜病变的发病率没有显著影响。两组间的死亡率也没有显著差别。强化治疗组出现严重低血糖事件较标准治疗组多（2.7% vs 1.5%，OR=1.86，

95%CI:1.42~2.40）（ADVANCE）。
- 强化治疗的局限性（VADT,2009）：随机将1 791例患有2型糖尿病的退伍军人分为强化治疗组（A1c 6.9%）或标准治疗组（8.4%）。经过中位随访5.6年之后，首次主要心血管事件风险减少了12%。除蛋白尿外，两组间的死亡率和微血管并发症均没有显著性差异。然而，强化治疗组的低血糖发生率为24.1%，显著高于标准治疗组的17.6%（Duckworth）。

住院患者血糖控制的益处

- 强化治疗（van den Berghe等，2001）：通过这项纳入单中心重症监护室（Intensive Care Unit，ICU）中采用机械通气的1 548例患者的研究，Van den Berghe转变了住院治疗的观点。患者随机接受强化胰岛素治疗（血糖维持在80~110mg/dl）或传统治疗（只有当血糖超过215mg/dl时才给予胰岛素，目标血糖为180~200mg/dl）。仅13%的患者曾诊断为糖尿病，5%的患者曾使用胰岛素。1年后，传统治疗组死亡率降低4.6%，强化胰岛素治疗死亡率降低8.0%（P<0.04）。这些降低的死亡率主要源于入住ICU 5天以上的患者。强化胰岛素治疗组的其他发病率同样降低，包括血液感染（降低46%），急性肾衰竭需要透析或血液滤过（降低41%），红细胞输注数量（降低50%），重症多发性神经病变（降低44%）。在Van den Berghe随后进行的研究中，她将这些研究发现扩展到了其他ICU住院患者。
- 强化治疗［危重患者强化或常规血糖控制研究（Normoglycemia in Intensive Care Evaluation – SurVival Using Glucose Algorithm Regulation, NICE-SUGAR），2009］：这是一项大型多中心试验，纳入6 104例在ICU治疗3天以上的患者，随机采取强化血糖控制（目标血糖81~108mg/dl）或常规血糖控制（目标血糖<180mg/dl）。常规血糖控制的死亡率（24.9%）低于强化血糖控制组（27.5%，P<0.02）。强化血糖控制组的严重低血糖发生率也更多（6.8% vs 0.5%，P<0.001）。这一研究对在ICU进行强化胰岛素控制有益的观点提出了挑战（Finfer）。
- 强化治疗（临床综述，2009）：Van den Berge教授在NICE-SUGAR之前的已经开启了对ICU患者进行强化血糖控制的序幕。回顾之前的文献，她提出一个规避先前研究中所存在矛盾的有效方法。她建议，就目前的证据而言，不能仅单纯控制血糖的一个指标，较为合适的做法是在ICU患者中应使血糖维持在尽可能接近于正常的水平，避免引起太大的波动、低血糖或低血钾（Van den Berghe）。

专家意见

- 上述研究，以及更多尚未提及的研究均支持如下观点：糖尿病前期（早期葡萄糖耐受不良）向2型糖尿病转变的概率是可以减少的。改变生活方式是最有效的干预措施，许多口服降糖药，尤其是二甲双胍，也具有同样的效果。
- 预防1型糖尿病往往更加困难。普遍认同的干预时机介于发现阳性胰岛标志物证实自身免疫进程激活（例如IA2）到确诊为1型糖尿病之间。

多项正在进行的研究从一定程度上认为关键在于调控免疫系统对 β 细胞破坏的进展。
- 早期研究先后在 1、2 型糖尿病中证实，更好的血糖控制可以有效降低视网膜病变和肾脏病变发生风险。不可避免的，紧接着就需要通过降低血糖水平，甚至低到 ACCORD 中的 HbA1c<6% 来研究解决"应该控制到多低的水平？"这一问题。上述所提到的这些研究对这一问题的回答模棱两可，主要是因为当 HbA1c<6% 时，低血糖的发生率和死亡率抵消了血糖控制带来的益处。
- Van den Berge 等进行的原创、单中心研究开启了对住院患者强化血糖控制的新篇章。随后的多中心 NICE-SUGAR 研究发现，严重低血糖风险超出了血糖控制带来的益处，从而使许多医院对住院患者的血糖控制变得不那么严格。

参考文献

Duckworth W, Abraira C, Moritz T, et al. Glucose control and vascular complications in veterans with type 2 diabetes. NEJM, 2009; Vol. 360: pp. 129–39.
Comments: A summary of the results of the VADT study.

Knowler WC, Fowler SE, Hamman RF, et al. 10-year follow-up of diabetes incidence and weight loss in the Diabetes Prevention Program Outcomes Study. Lancet, 2009; Vol. 374: pp. 1677–86.
Comments: A summary of the results of the DPPOS follow-up study.

NICE-SUGAR Study Investigators, Finfer S, Chittock DR, et al. Intensive versus conventional glucose control incritically ill patients. NEJM, 2009; Vol. 360: pp. 1283–97.
Comments: A summary of the results of the NICE-SUGAR study.

Van den Berghe G, Schetz M, Vlasselaers D, et al. Clinical review: Intensive insulin therapy in critically ill patients: NICE-SUGAR or Leuven blood glucose target? J Clin Endocrinol Metab, 2009; Vol. 94: pp. 3163–70.
Comments: Clinical review comparing NICE-SUGAR and the Leuven study.

DREAM Trial Investigators, Dagenais GR, Gerstein HC, et al. Effects of ramipril and rosiglitazone on cardiovascular and renal outcomes in people with impaired glucose tolerance or impaired fasting glucose: results of the Diabetes REduction Assessment with ramipril and rosiglitazone Medication (DREAM) trial. Diabetes Care, 2008; Vol. 31: pp. 1007–14.
Comments: A summary of the results of the DREAM Trial Study.

Li G, Zhang P, Wang J, et al. The long-term effect of lifestyle interventions to prevent diabetes in the China Da Qing Diabetes Prevention Study: a 20-year follow-up study. Lancet, 2008; Vol. 371: pp. 1783–9.
Comments: A summary of the results of the Da Qing follow-up study.

Holman RR, Paul SK, Bethel MA, et al. 10-year follow-up of intensive glucose control in type 2 diabetes. NEJM, 2008; Vol. 359: pp. 1577–89.
Comments: A summary of the results of the UKPDS follow-up study.

Action to Control Cardiovascular Risk in Diabetes Study Group, Gerstein HC, Miller ME, et al. Effects of intensive glucose lowering in type 2 diabetes. NEJM, 2008; Vol. 358: pp. 2545–59.
Comments: A summary of the results of the ACCORD study.

Gaede P, Lund-Andersen H, Parving HH, et al. Effect of a multifactorial intervention on mortality in type 2 diabetes. NEJM, 2008; Vol. 358: pp. 580–91.
Comments: A summary of the results of the Multifactorial Intervention Long-term Follow-up (Steno-2) study.

AD VANCE Collaborative Group, Patel A, MacMahon S, et al. Intensive blood glucose control and vascular outcomes in patients with type 2 diabetes. NEJM, 2008; Vol. 358: pp. 2560–72.
Comments: A summary of the results of the ADVANCE study.

Lindströn J, Ilanne-Parikka P, Peltonen M, et al. Sustained reduction in the incidence of type 2 diabetes by lifestyle intervention: follow-up of the Finnish Diabetes Prevention Study. Lancet, 2006; Vol. 368: pp. 1673–9.
Comments: A summary of the results of the Finnish Diabetes Prevention follow-up study.

Keymeulen B, Vandemeulebroucke E, Ziegler AG, et al. Insulin needs after CD3-antibody therapy in new-onset type 1 diabetes. NEJM, 2005; Vol. 352: pp. 2598–608.
Comments: A hallmark study describing use of CD3-antibody for type 1 diabetes prevention.

Gaede P, Vedel P, Larsen N, et al. Multifactorial intervention and cardiovascular disease in patients with type 2 diabetes. NEJM, 2003; Vol. 348: pp. 383–93.
Comments: A summary of the results of the Multifactorial Intervention (Steno-2) study.

Knowler WC, Barrett-Connor E, Fowler SE, et al. Reduction in the incidence of type 2 diabetes with lifestyle intervention or metformin. NEJM, 2002: Vol. 346; pp. 393–403.
Comments: A summary of the results of the Diabetes Prevention Program (DPP).

Buchanan TA, Xiang AH, Peters RK, et al. Preservation of pancreatic beta-cell function and prevention of type 2 diabetes by pharmacological treatment of insulin resistance in high-risk hispanic women. Diabetes, 2002; Vol. 51: pp. 2796–803.
Comments: A summary of the results of the TRIPOD Study.

Diabetes Prevention Trial—Type 1 Diabetes Study Group. Effects of insulin in relatives of patients with type 1 diabetes mellitus. NEJM, 2002; Vol. 346; pp. 1685–91.
Comments: A summary of the results of the DPT Study.

Herold KC, Hagopian W, Auger JA, et al. Anti-CD3 monoclonal antibody in new-onset type 1 diabetes mellitus. NEJM, 2002; Vol. 346: pp. 1692–8.
Comments: A hallmark study describing use of anti-CD3 antibody for type 1 diabetes prevention.

Tuomilehto J, Lindstr, Eriksson JG, et al. Prevention of type 2 diabetes mellitus by changes in lifestyle among subjects with impaired glucose tolerance. NEJM, 2001; Vol. 344: pp. 1343–50.
Comments: A summary of the results of the Finnish Diabetes Prevention Study.

Van den Berghe G, Wouters P, Weekers F, et al. Intensive insulin therapy in the critically ill patients. NEJM, 2001; Vol. 345: pp. 1359–67.
Comments: A summary of the results of the Leuven study.

The Diabetes Control and Complications Trial/Epidemiology of Diabetes Interventions and Complications Research Group. Retinopathy and nephropathy in patients with type 1 diabetes four years after a trial of intensive therapy. NEJM, 2000; Vol. 342: pp. 381–9.
Comments: A summary of the results of the EDIC Study.

UK Prospective Diabetes Study (UKPDS) Group. Intensive blood-glucose control with sulphonylureas or insulin compared with conventional treatment and risk of complications in patients with type 2 diabetes (UKPDS 33). Lancet, 1998; Vol. 352: pp. 837–53.Comments: A summary of the results of UK Prospective Diabetes Study Group 33.

Pan XR, Li GW, Hu YH, et al. Effects of diet and exercise in preventing NIDDM in people with impaired glucose tolerance. The Da Qing IGT and Diabetes Study. Diabetes Care, 1997; Vol. 20: pp. 537–44.

Comments: A summary of the results of the Da Qing IGT and Diabetes Study.

Ohkubo Y, Kishikawa H, Araki E, et al. Intensive insulin therapy prevents the progression of diabetic microvascular complications in Japanese patients with non-insulin-dependent diabetes mellitus: a randomized prospective 6-year study. Diabetes Res Clin Pract, 1995; Vol. 28: pp. 103–17.

Comments: A summary of the results of the Kumamoto Trial study.

The Diabetes Control and Complications Trial Research Group. The effect of Intensive treatment of diabetes on the development and progression of long-term complications in insulin-dependent diabetes mellitus. NEJM, 1993; Vol. 329: pp. 977–86.

Comments: A summary of the results of the Diabetes Control and Complications Trial Research Group (DCCT) Study.

Koenig RJ, Peterson CM, Jones RL, et al. Correlation of glucose regulation and hemoglobin A1c in diabetes mellitus. NEJM, 1976; Vol. 295: pp. 417–20.

Comments: One of the earliest studies describing use of hemoglobin A1c as an index of glycemic control.

糖尿病治疗的关键研究：控制并发症

Christopher D. Saudek, MD, and Rita Rastogi Kalyani, MD, MHS

视网膜病变

- 糖化血红蛋白A1c对视网膜病变的预测作用（Wisconsin研究，1988）：本研究对891例年轻糖尿病患者和987例老年糖尿病患者进行了超过4年随访，并应用立体眼底成像法对视网膜病变进行了判定。研究者在年轻患者中比较了糖化血红蛋白最高与最低四分位数，各种视网膜病变的相对风险（relative risk，RR）如下：任意一种视网膜病变为1.9%，增殖性视网膜病变为21.8%，病情进展的风险为4.0%。在应用胰岛素治疗的老年糖尿病患者中，相应的相对风险分别为1.9%、4.0%和2.1%。以上数据表明视网膜病变的发生率和进展情况与糖化血红蛋白A1c呈相关性，即使在控制混杂变量后依然如此。这些结果可强化DCCT研究的效力，并具有重要意义（Klein）。

- 血糖控制对1型糖尿病的作用（糖尿病控制与并发症工作组，1995）：DCCT研究中包含1 441名1型糖尿病患者，该研究更加详细地关注了强化降糖治疗对糖尿病视网膜病变的改善作用。强化治疗可将任意视网膜病变的风险降低27%。虽然该疗法尚不能完全预防视网膜病变，但它可在治疗3年后为患者带来获益（DCCT）。

- 血糖控制对1型糖尿病的作用（糖尿病干预和并发症流行病研究组，2000）：在DCCT试验结束4年后，EDIC研究首次报导了DCCT试验的长期随访结果；EDIC研究发现，尽管强化治疗组和传统控制组的血红蛋白A1c水平趋于一致，但患者视网膜病变（N=1 208）和肾脏病变（N=1 302）的进展情况却存在差别，其中接受强化治疗者可获益（DCCT/EDIC）。

- 血糖控制对2型糖尿病的作用（Kumamoto试验，1995）：该随机试验包含110例2型糖尿病患者，这些患者分别接受了多次胰岛素注射（MIT）治疗和常规胰岛素注射治疗，治疗时间为6年。在一级预防队列中，MIT组患者的视网膜病变率显著低于常规治疗组（前者为7.7%，后者为32%）。在二级预防队列中，MIT组患者视网膜病变进展率显著低于常规治疗组（前者为19.2%，后者为44.0%）。以上研究结果表明，能够预防视网膜病变进展和糖尿病微血管病变的血糖阈值分别为：HbA1c<6.5%，空腹血糖<110mg/dl，餐后2小时血糖<180mg/dl（Ohkubo）。

- 血糖控制对2型糖尿病的作用（英国前瞻性糖尿病研究50，2001）：UKPDS研究对1 919例患者进行了随访，这些患者在确诊为糖尿病时和确诊6年后均接受了视网膜成像检查。63%患者在确诊时无视网膜病变、但在确诊6年后发生了视网膜病变，其中22%患者视网膜病变有所加重。37%患者在确诊时即患有视网膜病变，其中29%患者的视网膜病变进展了2级或2级以上。糖尿病视网膜病变的发生率与基础血糖水平、高血糖6年以上、高血压以及不吸烟相关。高血糖也是导致视网膜病变加重的危险因素（UKPDS 50）。

- 血糖控制对1型糖尿病的作用（肾素-血管紧张素系统研究，2009）：该研究纳入了285例血压和尿蛋白正常的1型糖尿病患者，比较氯沙坦、依那普利和安慰剂的作用。研究者仔细评估了糖尿病肾病的进展情况，并发现两种药物对此并无作用。然而，氯沙坦和依那普利能够显著降低视网膜病变的发病率（前者降低70%、后者降低65%；Mauer）。

- 血压控制对2型糖尿病的作用（英国前瞻性糖尿病研究38，1998）：该随机试验包含1 148例高血压伴2型糖尿病的患者，这些患者分别接受了严格血压控制（<150/85mmHg；N=758）与非严格血压控制（<180/105mmHg；N=390），中位随访时间为8.4年；本研究具有多个终点，视网膜病变（通过视网膜成像检查来判定）也属于其中之一。严格控制组患者的视网膜病变发生率降低了34%，病变程度降低了2级；根据糖尿病视网膜病变早期治疗研究（Early Treatment Diabetic Retinopathy Study, ETDRS）中的视力表显示，患者视敏度提高了三行，恶化风险降低了47%（UKPDS 38）。
- 血脂控制对2型糖尿病的作用[非诺贝特干预与减少糖尿病事件研究（Fenofibrate Intervention and Event Lowering in Diabetes, FIELD），2005]：FIELD研究纳入了9 795例2型糖尿病患者，患者经随机分配进入非诺贝特组与安慰剂组。经过5年随访发现，非诺贝特可降低总体心血管事件发生率（$P=0.035$）；但在两组之间，冠状动脉事件这一主要终点却并无显著差别。在非诺贝特组，需要通过激光治疗视网膜病变的患者也少于安慰剂组（$P=0.0003$）（Keech）。
- 药物治疗对2型糖尿病的作用（控制糖尿病心血管风险试验，2010）：该随机试验纳入了10 251例2型糖尿病患者，这些患者发生心血管疾病的危险较高，并接受了强化降糖治疗（A1c<6%）和标准降糖治疗（A1c7.0%~7.9%），其目的为降低血糖、降低血脂[非诺贝特（160mg/d）联合辛伐他汀与安慰剂联合辛伐他汀]以及控制收缩压（分别为<120mmHg和<140mmHg）。通过ETDRS严重程度量表评估了2 856例患者糖尿病视网膜病变的进展情况（由立体眼底成像法判定）。在第4年，强化降糖治疗组患者的视网膜病变进展率降低33%，非诺贝特和他汀类药物强化降脂组降低40%；强化降压治疗未见明显疗效（Chew）。
- 全视网膜激光光凝治疗[糖尿病视网膜病变研究（Diabetic Retinopathy Study, DRS），1981]：DRS研究首次表明全视网膜激光光凝治疗可使严重视力损害的风险降低50%或更多，并为糖尿病增殖性视网膜病变的治疗提供了依据，也阐明了对糖尿病患者进行视力筛查的合理性，后者有助于增殖性视网膜病变的及时诊断。然而，氙弧光凝法常可导致视敏度降低和周围视野受损等。以上结果表明，若糖尿病患者视网膜病变有所加重，则应立即进行治疗（DRS研究组）。
- 焦点激光凝固治疗（糖尿病视网膜病变早期治疗研究，1985）：ETDRS研究检测了激光凝固治疗能否使增殖性视网膜病变前期患者获得受益。经随机分配，754例患有轻至中度糖尿病视网膜病变、伴黄斑水肿的患者接受了焦点氩激光凝固治疗；1 490例患者接受了延迟激光治疗。本研究的主要结果包括黄斑水肿因焦点激光凝固治疗（而非全视网膜激光凝固治疗）而获益，以及激光治疗未能有效改善增殖性视网膜病变（ETDRS）。
- 玻璃体切除治疗[糖尿病视网膜病变玻璃体切除研究报告（Diabetic Retinopathy Vitrectomy Study Report），1988]：该随机试验纳入了375例视力较差的增殖性视网膜病变（proliferative diabetic retinopathy,

PDR）患者，并比较了玻璃体切除术与观察等待之间的差别。经4年随访发现，玻璃体切除组患者视力可恢复至10/20、甚至更佳；而传统治疗组中只有28%患者的视力有所恢复。PDR的严重程度越高，玻璃体切除治疗的价值也越高。

肾脏病变

- 2型糖尿病患者肾病进展情况（英国前瞻性糖尿病研究64，2003）：UKPDS研究纳入了5 097例2型糖尿病患者，并经过10年研究观察了糖尿病肾脏的自然病程。由确诊为糖尿病至微量白蛋白尿的进展率为2.0%/年，由微量白蛋白尿至大量白蛋白尿的进展率为2.8%/年，由大量白蛋白尿至血浆肌酐水平增高或肾脏替代治疗的进展率为2.3%/年。10年之后，微量白蛋白尿的发生率为24.9%，大量白蛋白尿的发生率为5.3%，血浆肌酐水平增高或肾脏替代治疗率为0.8%。需要接受肾脏替代治疗的患者死亡率较高（19.2%）（UKPDS 64）。

- 血糖控制对1型糖尿病的作用（糖尿病并发症与控制试验，1995）：该研究随访了1 441例1型糖尿病患者，这些患者均来自DCCT试验；该研究详细关注了强化胰岛素治疗对糖尿病肾病进展的有益作用。在一级预防队列中，经第1年强化胰岛素治疗后，微量白蛋白尿的累积发生率显著降低了34%，白蛋白排泄率显著降低了15%。在二级预防队列中，强化胰岛素治疗使微量白蛋白尿的累积发生率显著降低了43%，使微量白蛋白尿的进展率显著降低了56%，并使临床白蛋白尿显著降低了56%（DCCT）。

- 血糖控制对1型糖尿病的作用（糖尿病干预和并发症流行病研究组，2000）：在DCCT试验结束4年后，EDIC研究首次报导了DCCT试验的长期随访结果；EDIC研究发现，尽管强化治疗组和传统控制组的血红蛋白A1c水平趋于一致，但患者视网膜病变（N=1 208）和肾脏病变（N=1 302）的进展情况却存在差别，其中接受强化治疗者可获益（DCCT/EDIC）。

- 血糖控制对2型糖尿病的作用（Kumamoto试验，1995）：该随机试验包含110例2型糖尿病患者，这些患者分别接受了多次胰岛素注射（MIT）治疗和常规胰岛素注射治疗，治疗时间为6年。在一级预防队列中，MIT组患者的视网膜病变率显著低于常规治疗组（前者为7.7%，后者为32%）。在二级预防队列中，MIT组患者肾病进展率显著低于常规治疗组（前者为11.5%，后者为32.0%）。以上研究结果表明，能够预防糖尿病微量白蛋白尿进展的血糖阈值分别为：HbA1c<6.5%，空腹血糖<110mg/dl，餐后2小时血糖<180mg/dl（Ohkubo）。

- 血糖控制对2型糖尿病的作用（英国前瞻性糖尿病研究33，1998）：在UKPDS 33研究中，更加严格的血糖控制使微量白蛋白尿的发生率降低了24%，使大量白蛋白尿的发生率降低了33%，并使9年血浆肌酐倍增率降低了24%（以上结果均具有统计学差异）。更加严格的血糖控制也使微量白蛋白尿有所降低，但对6年血浆肌酐水平并无作用（UKPDS 33）。

- 血管紧张素转换酶抑制剂（Angiotensin-converting enzyme inhibitors，ACEI）对1型糖尿病的作用（协作研究组，1993）：该随机对照试验纳入了尿蛋白排出量大于500mg/d的1型糖尿病患者，并比较了卡托普利和安慰剂（允许应用其他降压药物）的作用。卡托普利与联合终点事件（死亡、透析及肾脏移植）发生率降低50%相关，且与血压变化无关。

对肾脏功能进行精细检测（尿蛋白、血浆肌酐倍增时间）后发现，卡托普利对肾脏功能具有益处。以上结果首次表明ACEI可为高血压合并糖尿病患者带来获益。

- 血压控制对1型糖尿病的作用（肾素-血管紧张素系统研究，2009）：该研究纳入了285例血压和尿蛋白正常的1型糖尿病患者，并比较了氯沙坦、依那普利和安慰剂的作用。在该研究当中，两种药物对肾病进展均无明显作用（Mauer）。
- 血脂控制对2型糖尿病的作用（非诺贝特干预与减少糖尿病事件研究，2005）：FIELD研究纳入了9 795例2型糖尿病患者，患者经随机分配进入非诺贝特组与安慰剂组。经过5年随访发现，非诺贝特可降低总体心血管事件发生率（P=0.035）；但在两组之间，冠状动脉事件这一主要终点却并无显著差别。在非诺贝特组，蛋白尿的进展率亦有所降低（P=0.002）（Keech）。

神经病变

- 2型糖尿病神经病变的危险因素（San Luis Valley糖尿病研究，1997）：对231例患者进行了平均4.7年随访，结果发现糖尿病感觉神经病变的发生率为6.1%。高血糖、近期吸烟史和心肌梗死均为神经病变进展的独立危险因素（Sands）。
- 2型糖尿病神经病变的危险因素（Seattle前瞻性糖尿病足研究，1997）：该前瞻性研究纳入了288例患有糖尿病、但无神经病变的美国退伍军人，经10年随访发现，20%患者发生了糖尿病神经病变。糖尿病神经病变的危险因素包括年龄、基线糖化血红蛋白A1c水平、身高、足部溃疡病史、饮酒、近期吸烟史和尿中白蛋白水平（ALDER）。
- 1型糖尿病神经病变的危险因素（EURODIAB IDDM并发症研究，1996）：在3 250例胰岛素依赖性糖尿病患者中，神经病变的发生率为28%，并与年龄、身高、糖尿病病程、糖化血红蛋白A1c、伴发视网膜病变、吸烟、高密度脂蛋白、心血管疾病、舒张压增高、严重酮症酸中毒、空腹甘油三酯水平增高、以及微量白蛋白尿相关（Tesfaye）。
- 血糖控制对1型糖尿病的作用（糖尿病控制与并发症试验，1993）：DCCT研究纳入了伴或不伴轻度视网膜病变（diabetic retinopathy，DR）的1型糖尿病患者，本研究由NIH资助；患者被随机分入"强化降糖治疗组"和"常规降糖治疗组"。在一级和二级预防队列中，强化治疗使神经病变发生率降低了60%，但低血糖的发生率也增加了2~3倍（DCCT）。
- 血糖控制对1型糖尿病的作用（糖尿病干预和并发症流行病研究组，2010）：在DCCT研究结束前对603例强化治疗者和583例常规治疗者进行了长达13~14年的随访。结束时强化治疗组和常规治疗组患者的糖化血红蛋白A1c水平十分相似；在强化治疗组患者中，神经病变的发病率由9%增加至25%；在常规治疗组，神经病变的发病率由17%增加至35%，两组之间差异仍具有显著性。与曾接受传统治疗的患者相比，强化治疗者的神经病变发生率较低（前者为28%，后者为22%；P=0.01）（ALBERS）。
- 血糖控制对1型糖尿病的作用（糖尿病干预和并发症流行病研究组，2009）：对DCCT试验患者进行了长达13~14年的随访。与常规治疗相比，强化治疗降低了心脏自主神经病变的发生率（前者为35.2%，后者为 28.9%；P =0.02）。与常规治疗组患者相比，强化治疗组患者发生心脏自主神经病变的几率也较低（OR=0.69，95%CI:0.51~0.93）（Pop-busui）。

高血压病

- ACEI 对 1 型糖尿病神经病变的作用（协作研究组，1993）：该随机对照试验纳入了尿蛋白排出量大于 500mg/d 的 1 型糖尿病患者，并比较了卡托普利和安慰剂（允许应用其他降压药物）的作用。卡托普利与联合终点事件（死亡、透析及肾脏移植）发生率降低 50% 相关，且与血压变化无关。对肾脏功能进行精细检测（尿蛋白、血浆肌酐倍增时间）后发现，卡托普利对肾脏功能具有益处。以上结果首次表明 ACE 抑制剂可为高血压合并糖尿病的患者带来获益（Lewis）。

- 对 1 型糖尿病肾病和视网膜病变的作用（肾素 – 血管紧张素系统研究，2009）：该研究纳入了 285 例血压和尿蛋白正常的 1 型糖尿病患者，并比较了氯沙坦、依那普利和安慰剂的作用。研究者仔细评估了糖尿病肾病的进展情况，并发现两种药物对此并无作用。然而，氯沙坦和依那普利能够显著降低视网膜病变的发病率（前者降低 70%、后者降低 65%；Mauer）。

- 对 2 型糖尿病微血管和大血管并发症的作用（英国前瞻性糖尿病研究 38，1998）：UKPDS 38 是一项比较强化降压治疗和常规降压治疗的随机对照研究，使用 ACE 抑制剂或 β – 受体阻滞剂。该随机试验包含 1 148 例高血压伴 2 型糖尿病的患者，这些患者分别接受了严格血压控制（<150/85mmHg；N=758）与非严格血压控制（<180/105mmHg；N=390），中位随访时间为 8.4 年；本研究具有多个终点，视网膜病变（通过视网膜成像检查来判定）也属于其中之一。严格控制组患者的视网膜病变发生率降低了 34%，病变程度降低了 2 级；根据 ETDRS 中的图表显示，患者视敏度提高了三行，视敏度恶化的风险降低了 47%。严格和非严格血压控制与糖尿病相关终点事件发生率降低 24% 相关。收缩压由 170mmHg 降至 120mmHg 与风险降低呈线性相关。有趣的是，后续文章表明 ACEI 和 β – 受体阻滞剂可同等程度地降低心血管事件风险，这打破了"β – 受体阻滞剂对高血压病合并糖尿病患者无效"的观点（UKPDS 38）。

- 对 2 型糖尿病心血管疾病预防的作用（控制糖尿病心血管风险试验，2010）：在 ACCORD 血压控制试验中，4 733 例亚组人群被随机分入"血压 <120mmHg 组"和"血压 <140mmHg 组"，分组以非盲方式进行。在两组患者之间，多数心血管事件发生率并无显著差异；但非致命性卒中发病率不同，强化治疗组患者的卒中发病率低于标准血压控制组患者（P=0.03）。然而，在强化治疗组患者中严重不良事件（如低血压、晕厥等）的发生率也增高了 3 倍（P <0.001）。以上结果表明不必将糖尿病患者血压降至 120mmHg 以下，这可能为患者带来身体损害（Cushman）。

血脂

- 普伐他汀对心血管疾病的预防作用［胆固醇和复发事件研究（The Cholesterol And Recurrent Events Study，CARE），1996］：CARE 研究包含 4 159 例患者，这些患者被随机分入普伐他汀组和安慰剂组，研究时间为5年。总体而言，在普伐他汀组，致命性冠状动脉事件或非致命性心肌梗死的发生率显著降低了24%。在586例糖尿病患者中，该风险降低了25%，其统计学差异处于临界水平（$P=0.05$）（Sacks）。

- 辛伐他汀对2型糖尿病心血管疾病的预防作用[Scandinavian生存研究（4S），1997]：在4S试验中，对202例糖尿病亚组人群进行了分析；经中位随访5.4年发现，辛伐他汀使重大心血管事件的发病风险显著降低了55%。相比之下，在无糖尿病的患者中，重大心血管事件的发病风险显著降低了32%（Pyorala）。
- 阿托伐他汀对2型糖尿病心血管疾病的预防作用[阿托伐他汀糖尿病合作研究（Collaborative Atorvastatin Diabetes Study，CARDS），2009]：CARDS研究纳入了2838例不伴有心血管疾病的2型糖尿病患者，患者被分为阿托伐他汀组和安慰剂组，研究时间为3.9年。在伴或不伴肾小球滤过率降低的患者中，阿托伐他汀组患者的重大心血管事件发生率降低了42%（Colhoun）。
- 非诺贝特对2型糖尿病心血管事件的预防作用（非诺贝特干预与减少糖尿病事件研究，2005）：FIELD研究纳入了9795例2型糖尿病患者，这些患者被随机分入非诺贝特组和安慰剂组。经5年随访发现，非诺贝特虽可降低总体心血管事件发生率（$P=0.035$），但它并未显著降低主要终点（冠状动脉事件）发生率。
- 非诺贝特对2型糖尿病心血管疾病的预防作用（控制糖尿病心血管风险试验，2010）：ACCORD试验第三支包含5518名糖尿病患者（其余为高血糖组和高血压组患者），这些患者入组前已接受了他汀类药物治疗，他们被随机分入联合应用非诺贝特组或安慰剂组。结果显示非诺贝特并未降低心血管事件的发生率。以上结果表明，虽然某些亚组人群（如高甘油三酯水平人群、低高密度脂蛋白水平人群）会因联合应用他汀类药物和非诺贝特而获益，但在总体上对糖尿病患者并无额外获益（ACCORD）。

心血管疾病

- 糖尿病是心血管疾病的等危症（芬兰以人群为基础的研究，1998）：该研究在1373例无糖尿病者和1059例糖尿病患者中比较了心肌梗死（myocardial infarction，MI）的发生率，研究时间超过7年。在无糖尿病的受试者中，既往MI者的MI发病率为18.8%，既往无MI者的MI发病率为3.5%。在糖尿病患者中，既往有MI者的MI发病率为45.0%，既往无MI者的MI发病率为20.2%。校正混杂变量后发现，在既往无MI的糖尿病患者中，其MI发病风险与既往患有MI而无糖尿病者相同（危险比接近于1）（Haffner）。
- 空腹血糖、餐后2小时血糖与心血管疾病风险[糖尿病流行病学：欧洲糖尿病诊断标准合作分析（Diabetes Epidemiology Collaborative Analysis of Diagnostic Criteria in Europe，DECODE），2003]：在一项规模更大、前瞻性更强的研究中，DECODE合作组对29714例受试者进行了长达11年的研究；结果表明空腹血糖和餐后2小时血糖高低与否均与心血管疾病风险增高呈直接相关，即使患者血糖水平正常或轻度异常、并对其他已知的心血管危险因素进行调整之后，该结果仍不改变。许多后期分析结果均证实了这一相关性（DECODE研究组）。

糖尿病治疗的关键研究：控制并发症

- 血糖控制对 1 型糖尿病的作用（糖尿病控制与并发症工作组，2005）：在 DCCT 研究中，1983–1993 年 1 441 例 1 型糖尿病患者被随机分入强化治疗组和常规治疗组；患者的平均治疗时间为 6.5 年。EDIC 研究对以上的 93% 患者进行了随访，随访截止至 2005 年 2 月，此时两组患者糖化血红蛋白 A1c 水平相似。在平均 17 年的随访期间，强化治疗使任一心血管事件风险降低了 42%（$P=0.02$），并使非致命性心肌梗死、卒中或心血管疾病死亡率降低了 57%（$P=0.02$）。在 DCCT 研究过程中，与常规治疗组相比，糖化血红蛋白 A1c 水平降低与强化治疗的各种有益作用显著相关（Nathan）。

- 血糖控制对 2 型糖尿病的作用（英国前瞻性糖尿病研究组随访，2008）：在 UKPDS 研究中，3 227 例患者在接受了强化或常规降糖治疗后重新接受了常规治疗，随后对这些患者进行了 6~10 年的长期随访。在第 1 年，两组患者的糖化血红蛋白 A1c 水平相同；但在磺脲类药物联合胰岛素治疗组，患者发生任一糖尿病终点事件的风险降低 9%（$P=0.04$），微血管病变的发生率降低了 24%（$P=0.01$），心肌梗死风险降低了 15%（$P=0.01$），全因死亡率降低了 13%（$P=0.001$）。在二甲双胍强化治疗组，上述风险降低程度与之相似或更高。随访结果表明，即使短暂的早期强化治疗也对 2 型糖尿病终点事件具有改善作用（Holman）。

- 血糖控制对 1 型和 2 型糖尿病的作用（Selvin 等，2004）：该荟萃分析纳入了 3 项 1 型糖尿病研究（N=1 688）和 10 项 2 型糖尿病研究（N=7 435），并分析了糖化血红蛋白 A1c 和心血管疾病之间的相关性。汇总分析显示，2 型糖尿病患者的糖化血红蛋白 A1c 水平每增加 1%，则其心血管事件的风险显著增高 18%。在 1 型糖尿病患者中，糖化血红蛋白 A1c 水平每增高 1%，其心血管事件的风险增高 15%，但该结果并无统计学显著性。相比之下，对于 1 型和 2 型糖尿病患者而言，糖化血红蛋白 A1c 水平每增高 1%，外周动脉疾病的风险可分别显著增高 32% 和 28%。

- 强化血糖控制在 2 型糖尿病治疗中的局限性（控制糖尿病心血管风险试验小组，2008）：ACCORD 研究纳入了 10 251 例 2 型糖尿病患者，这些患者存在较高的心血管疾病风险，患者随机分为强化治疗组（A1c<6.0%）或常规治疗组（A1c7.0%~7.9%）。该研究由于强化治疗组的死亡率较高（253 vs 207，$P=0.04$）而提前终止。但是，强化治疗组的非致死性心血管病事件更少，药物不良反应更多。强化治疗引起死亡率升高的原因仍有争议，一些相似的研究（ADVANCEA 研究、VADT 研究）并不支持 ACCORD 的结论。因此，旨在将糖化血红蛋白 A1c 降至 6% 以下的药物治疗并不适用于患者，在易发生心脏疾病的老年患者中更是如此，或许这才是合理的结论（ACCORD）。

- 强化血糖控制在 2 型糖尿病治疗中的局限性（糖尿病与血管疾病治疗行动：百普乐与达美康缓释片对照评估研究，2008）：ADVANCE 研究纳入了 11 140 例 2 型糖尿病患者，这些患者被随机分入标准降糖治疗组（糖化血红蛋白 A1c 7.3%）和强化降糖治疗组（糖化血红蛋白 A1c 6.5%）；强化降糖治疗由格列齐特（缓释剂）及其他药物组成。5 年以后，与标准治疗组相比，强化降糖治疗组主要大血管和微血管事件共降低 10%；这主要是因为肾脏病变的发生率有所降低（降幅为 21%），但该疗法对视网膜病变无明显改善作用。根据报导，患者死亡率无显著异异。然而与标准治疗组相比，严重低血糖更多见于强化治疗组（前者发生率为1.5%,后者为2.7；OR=1.86,95%CI:1.42~2.40)(ADVANCE)。
- 强化血糖控制在2型糖尿病治疗中的局限性(退伍军人糖尿病试验,2009)：VADT试验纳入了1 791例患有2型糖尿病的退伍军人,这些患者被随机分入强化治疗组(糖化血红蛋白A1c 6.9%)和标准治疗组(糖化血红蛋白A1c 8.4%)。中位随访5.6年后发现,首次严重心血管事件风险降低了12%。在两组患者之间,死亡率或微血管并发症发生率并无差异。然而,强化治疗组的低血糖发病率为24.1%,而在标准治疗组仅为17.6%(Duckworth)。

专家意见

- 上述及其他研究均明确表示,有效控制血糖可降低视网膜病变的发病风险,并延缓本病的进展。专家还认为,适时应用激光凝固术治疗视网膜病变可获得很好的疗效。
- 糖尿病肾脏疾病是另一种严重的微血管并发症,现已证实有效控制血糖可降低本病的发病率(主要还是视网膜病变的发病率)。为防止微量白蛋白尿进展为"临床"蛋白尿以及终末期肾病,血压和血糖控制是主要的治疗目标。
- DCCT和EDIC研究充分表明了血糖控制对神经病变的有益作用,但某些观察性研究也表明在1型和2型糖尿病中,高血糖与神经病变的进展显著相关。
- 高血糖对心血管疾病的独立作用向来是一个难以回答的问题,其可能的原因如下：其他危险因素(如血脂、血压、吸烟、凝血因子等)均与发病风险高度相关,甚至比高血糖更加重要；促进"代谢综合征"(中心性肥胖、高甘油三酯血症、HDL-胆固醇降低、高血压、高血糖等)的各种危险因素也与心血管疾病相关；高血糖的确切发病时间难以判定,且心血管疾病多见于非糖尿病老年人群当中。但对早期研究(DCCT、UKPDS)的长期随访已显示出其相关性。然而,近期研究表明严格的强化降糖治疗对CVD并无有益作用(如ACCORD研究,ADVANCE研究和VADT研究等)。

参考文献

ACCORD Study Group, ACCORD Eye Study Group, Chew EY, et al. Effects of medical therapies on retinopathy progression in type 2 diabetes. NEJM, 2010; Vol. 363: pp. 233–44.
Comments: A summary of the results of the ACCORD study group.

ACCORD Study Group, Cushman WC, Evans GW, et al. Effects of intensive blood-pressure control in type 2 diabetes mellitus. NEJM, 2010; Vol. 362: pp. 1575–85.
Comments: A summary of the results of the ACCORD study on blood pressure.

ACCORD Study Group, Ginsberg HN, Elam MB, et al. Effects of combination lipid therapy in type 2 diabetes mellitus. NEJM, 2010; Vol. 362: pp. 1563–74.
Comments: A summary of the results of the ACCORD study on lipid therapy.

Albers JW, Herman WH, Pop-Busui R, et al. Effect of prior intensive insulin treatment during the Diabetes Control and Complications Trial (DCCT) on peripheral neuropathy in type 1 diabetes during the Epidemiology of Diabetes Interventions and Complications (EDIC) Study. Diabetes Care, 2010; Vol. 33: pp. 1090–6.
Comments: A summary of the results of the DCCT/EDIC research group.

Colhoun HM, Betteridge DJ, Durrington PN, et al. Effects of atorvastatin on kidney outcomes and cardiovascular disease in patients with diabetes: an analysis from the Collaborative Atorvastatin Diabetes Study (CARDS). Am J Kidney Dis, 2009; Vol. 54: pp. 810–9.
Comments: A summary of the results of the CARDS Study.

Duckworth W, Abraira C, Moritz T, et al. Glucose control and vascular complications in veterans with type 2 diabetes. NEJM, 2009; Vol. 360: pp. 129–39.
Comments: A summary of the results of the VADT study.

Mauer M, Zinman B, Gardiner R, et al. Renal and retinal effects of enalapril and losartan in type 1 diabetes. NEJM, 2009; Vol. 361: pp. 40–51.
Comments: A summary of the results of the Renin-Angiotensin System Study.

Pop-Busui R, Low PA, Waberski BH, et al. Effects of prior intensive insulin therapy on cardiac autonomic nervous system function in type 1 diabetes mellitus: the Diabetes Control and Complications Trial/Epidemiology of Diabetes Interventions and Complications study (DCCT/EDIC). Circulation, 2009; Vol. 119: pp. 2886–93.
Comments: A summary of the results of the DCCT/EDIC research group.

Action to Control Cardiovascular Risk in Diabetes Study Group, Gerstein HC, Miller ME, et al. Effects of intensive glucose lowering in type 2 diabetes. NEJM, 2008; Vol. 358: pp. 2545–59.
Comments: A summary of the results of the ACCORD study on glucose lowering.

AD VANCE Collaborative Group, Patel A, MacMahon S, et al. Intensive blood glucose control and vascular outcomes in patients with type 2 diabetes. NEJM, 2008; Vol. 358: pp. 2560–72.
Comments: A summary of the results of the ADVANCE collaborative group.

Holman RR, Paul SK, Bethel MA, et al. 10-year follow-up of intensive glucose control in type 2 diabetes. NEJM, 2008; Vol. 359: pp. 1577–89.
Comments: Results of the UKPDS follow-up of intensive glucose control in T2DM.

Keech A, Simes RJ, Barter P, et al. Effects of long-term fenofibrate therapy on cardiovascular events in 9795 people with type 2 diabetes mellitus (the FIELD study): randomised controlled trial. Lancet, 2005; Vol. 366: pp. 1849–61.
Comments: A summary of the results of the FIELD study.

Nathan DM, Cleary PA, Backlund JY, et al. Intensive diabetes treatment and cardiovascular disease in patients with type 1 diabetes. NEJM, 2005; Vol. 353: pp. 2643–53.
Comments: A summary of the results of the DCCT/EDIC research group.

Selvin E, Marinopoulos S, Berkenblit G, et al. Meta-analysis: glycosylated hemoglobin and cardiovascular disease in diabetes mellitus. Ann Intern Med, 2004; Vol. 141: pp. 421–31.
Comments: Glycosylated hemoglobin and cardiovascular disease meta-analysis.

Adler AI, Stevens RJ, Manley SE, et al. Development and progression of nephropathy in type 2 diabetes: the United Kingdom Prospective Diabetes Study (UKPDS 64). Kidney Int, 2003; Vol. 63: pp. 225–32.
Comments: A summary of the results of the UKPDS 64.

DECODE Study Group, European Diabetes Epidemiology Group. Is the current definition for diabetes relevant to mortality risk from all causes and cardiovascular and noncardiovascular diseases? Diabetes Care, 2003; Vol. 26: pp. 688–96.
Comments: A summary of the results of the DECODE study group.

Stratton IM, Kohner EM, Aldington SJ, et al. UKPDS 50: risk factors for incidence and

progression of retinopathy in Type II diabetes over 6 years from diagnosis. Diabetologia, 2001; Vol. 44: pp. 156–63.
Comments: A summary of the results of the UKPDS 50.

The Diabetes Control and Complications Trial/Epidemiology of Diabetes Interventions and Complications Research Group. Retinopathy and nephropathy in patients with type 1 diabetes four years after a trial of intensive therapy. NEJM, 2000; Vol. 342: pp. 381–9.
Comments: A summary of the results of the DCCT/EDIC research group.

Haffner SM, Lehto S, Rmaa T, et al. Mortality from coronary heart disease in subjects with type 2 diabetes and in nondiabetic subjects with and without prior myocardial infarction. NEJM, 1998; Vol. 339: pp. 229–34.
Comments: A summary of the results of the Finnish Population-Based Study.

UK Prospective Diabetes Study (UKPDS) Group. Intensive blood-glucose control with sulphonylureas or insulin compared with conventional treatment and risk of complications in patients with type 2 diabetes (UKPDS 33). Lancet, 1998; Vol. 352: pp. 837–53.
Comments: A summary of the results of the UKPDS 33.

UK Prospective Diabetes Study Group. Tight blood pressure control and risk of macrovascular and microvascular complications in type 2 diabetes: UKPDS 38. BMJ, 1998; Vol. 317: pp. 703–13.
Comments: A summary of the results of the UKPDS 38.

UK Prospective Diabetes Study Group. Tight blood pressure control and risk of macrovascular and microvascular complications in type 2 diabetes: UKPDS 38. BMJ, 1998; Vol. 317: pp. 703–13.
Comments: A summary of the results of the UK Prospective Diabetes Study 38.

Adler AI, Boyko EJ, Ahroni JH, et al. Risk factors for diabetic peripheral sensory neuropathy. Results of the Seattle Prospective Diabetic Foot Study. Diabetes Care, 1997; Vol. 20: pp. 1162–7.
Comments: A summary of the results of the Seattle Prospective Diabetic Foot Study.

Pyorala K, Pedersen TR, Kjekshus J, et al. Cholesterol lowering with simvastatin improves prognosis of diabetic patients with coronary heart disease. A subgroup analysis of the Scandinavian Simvastatin Survival Study (4S). Diabetes Care, 1997; Vol. 20: pp. 614–20.
Comments: A summary of the results of the Scandinavian Survival Study (4S).

Sands ML, Shetterly SM, Franklin GM, et al. Incidence of distal symmetric (sensory) neuropathy in NIDDM. The San Luis Valley Diabetes Study. Diabetes Care, 1997; Vol. 20: pp. 322–9.
Comments: A summary of the results of the San Luis Valley Diabetes Study.

Sacks FM, Pfeffer MA, Moye LA, et al. The effect of pravastatin on coronary events after myocardial infarction in patients with average cholesterol levels. Cholesterol and Recurrent Events Trial investigators. NEJM, 1996; Vol. 335: pp. 1001–9.
Comments: A summary of the results of the CARE study.

Tesfaye S, Stevens LK, Stephenson JM, et al. Prevalence of diabetic peripheral neuropathy and its relation to glycaemic control and potential risk factors: the EURODIAB IDD M Complications Study. Diabetologia, 1996; Vol. 39; pp. 1377–84.
Comments: A summary of the results of the EURODIAB IDDM Complications Study.

The Diabetes Control and Complications (DCCT) Research Group. Effect of intensive

therapy on the development and progression of diabetic nephropathy in the Diabetes Control and Complications Trial. Kidney Int, 1995; Vol. 47: pp. 1703–20.
Comments: A summary of the results of the DCCT research group.

Diabetes Control and Complications Trial Research Group (DCCT). Progression of retinopathy with intensive versus conventional treatment in the Diabetes Control and Complications Trial. Ophthalmology, 1995; Vol. 102: pp. 647–61.
Comments: A summary of the results of the DCCT research group.

Ohkubo Y, Kishikawa H, Araki E, et al. Intensive insulin therapy prevents the progression of diabetic microvascular complications in Japanese patients with non-insulin-dependent diabetes mellitus: a randomized prospective 6-year study. Diabetes Res Clin Pract, 1995; Vol. 28: pp. 103–17.
Comments: A summary of the results of the Kumamoto Trial.

The Diabetes Control and Complications Trial Research Group. The effect of intensive treatment of diabetes on the development and progression of long-term complications in insulin-dependent diabetes mellitus. NEJM, 1993; Vol. 329: pp. 977–86.
Comments: A summary of the results of the DCCT research group.

Lewis EJ, Hunsicker LG, Bain RP, et al. The effect of angiotensin-converting-enzyme inhibition on diabetic nephropathy. The Collaborative Study Group. NEJM, 1993; Vol. 329: pp. 1456–62. Comments: A summary of the results of the the Collaborative Study Group.

The Diabetic Retinopathy Vitrectomy Study Research Group. Early vitrectomy for severe proliferative diabetic retinopathy in eyes with useful vision. Results of a randomized trial—Diabetic Retinopathy Vitrectomy Study Report 3. Ophthalmology, 1988; Vol. 95: pp. 1307–20.
Comments: A summary of the results of the Diabetic Retinopathy Vitrectomy Study Report 3.

Klein R, Klein BE, Moss SE, et al. Glycosylated hemoglobin predicts the incidence and progression of diabetic retinopathy. JAMA, 1988; Vol. 260: pp. 2864–71.
Comments: A summary of the results of the Wisconsin Study.

Early Treatment Diabetic Retinopathy Study Research Group. Photocoagulation for diabetic macular edema. Early Treatment Diabetic Retinopathy Study report number 1. Arch Ophthalmol, 1985; Vol. 103: pp. 1796–806.
Comments: A summary of the results of the ETDRS research group.

The Diabetic Retinopathy Study Research Group. Photocoagulation treatment of proliferative diabetic retinopathy. Clinical application of Diabetic Retinopathy Study (DRS) findings, DRS Report Number 8. Ophthalmology, 1981; Vol. 88: pp. 583–600.
Comments: A summary of the results of the DRS research group.

糖尿病治疗的关键研究：治疗效果

Christopher D. Saudek, MD, and Rita Rastogi Kalyani, MD, MHS

1型糖尿病和2型糖尿病的药物治疗

- 二甲双胍（多中心二甲双胍研究组，1995）：该随机试验纳入了289例中度肥胖的2型糖尿病患者，并比较了二甲双胍与安慰剂对患者的作用。经过29周治疗，二甲双胍组患者的空腹血糖和糖化血红蛋白水平均低于安慰剂组（空腹血糖值分别为189mg/dl和244mg/dl，糖化血红蛋白值分别为7.1%和8.6%）。与单独应用格列本脲治疗相比，联合治疗可降低空腹血糖和糖化血红蛋白水平（空腹血糖值分别为187mg/dl和261mg/dl，糖化血红蛋白值分别为7.1%和8.7%）。然而，在联合治疗组中低血糖的发生率为18%，在二甲双胍组仅为2%，在格列本脲单药组为3%（DeFronzo）。

- 二甲双胍（英国前瞻性糖尿病研究34，1998）：UKPDS 34试验纳入了新诊断为2型糖尿病的超重患者，研究了二甲双胍强化降糖治疗的作用。1 704例高血糖患者首先进行了3个月饮食控制，随后经随机分配进行常规治疗，所有患者继续接受饮食控制，分别给予二甲双胍或磺脲类药物或胰岛素治疗。二甲双胍降低了任一糖尿病相关终点事件发生率（$P=0.0034$）、全因死亡率（$P=0.021$）和卒中发生率（$P=0.032$）。尽管二甲双胍联合磺脲类药物与死亡风险增加并无相关性，但在磺脲类治疗组中，早期加用二甲双胍却增加了糖尿病相关死亡率（$P=0.039$），这一结果令人感到意外，也难以解释。以上结果表明二甲双胍可能是糖尿病治疗中的一线治疗药物（UKPDS 34）。

- 磺脲类药物［大学组糖尿病研究方案（The University Group Diabetes Program，UGDP），1970］：早期开展的UGDP研究针对新诊断为2型糖尿病的患者，该研究颇具争议；患者经随机分配后进入一代磺脲类药物（SU）治疗组（甲苯磺丁脲）、苯乙双胍治疗组或胰岛素治疗组。在苯乙双胍组发生了乳酸酸中毒死亡事件，且SU组心血管疾病死亡率亦有轻微而显著的增高。各种批评意见纷至沓来，问题的焦点主要为研究方法和研究结论（如A. R. Feinstein曾发表过意见）。在UGDP研究中，SU的不良反应未能得到证实或广泛接受，但该药品的说明书附加了黑框警告。此后，SU已被安全用于各种研究当中（Meinert）。

- 格列本脲（Nathan等，1988）：研究纳入了31例饮食干预后血糖未得到有效控制的2型糖尿病患者；经随机分配后，患者进入鱼精蛋白锌胰岛素（每日1次）组和格列本脲组。两组患者的糖化血红蛋白基线水平为10%。经9个月治疗后，患者糖化血红蛋白水平下降了3%左右。

- 阿卡波糖（Essen研究，1994）：研究纳入了饮食控制失效的96例2型糖尿病患者，这些患者被随机分入阿卡波糖组、格列本脲组和安慰剂组。经过24周治疗，与安慰剂组相比，阿卡波糖组患者糖化血红蛋白降低了1.1%，格列本脲组患者糖化血红蛋白降低了0.9%。阿卡波糖还具有减少餐后胰岛素增加的作用（Hoffman）。

- 曲格列酮（Nolan等，1994）：早期研究纳入了18例葡萄糖耐量正常或受损的肥胖患者，并阐明了噻唑烷二酮类药物（TZDs）（本研究所用药物为曲格列酮）如何减轻胰岛素抵抗效应。曲格列酮现因肝脏不良反应而被停止生产，但其作用代表了 TZDs 类药物的作用机制。

- 吡格列酮（吡格列酮 001 研究组，2000）：研究纳入了 408 例患者，这些患者被随机分入安慰剂组和 4 个不同剂量的吡格列酮单药治疗组。经过 26 周治疗，与安慰剂组相比，三组高剂量吡格列酮组（15mg/d~45mg/d）患者的糖化血红蛋白平均降低了 1%~1.6%。经 2 周治疗即可观察到患者空腹血糖水平有所改善，在第 10 周~第 14 周空腹血糖水平最低，但仅维持至研究结束（与安慰剂组相比降低了 39mg/dl~65mg/dl）。在初次治疗的患者中，血糖改善程度最为明显（与安慰剂组相比，糖化血红蛋白降低了 2.55%）（Aronoff）。

- 吡格列酮［前瞻性吡格列酮大血管事件临床试验（PROspective pioglitAzone Clinical Trial in macroVascular Events, PROactive），2005］：该前瞻性研究纳入了 5 238 例 2 型糖尿病患者，这些患者存在大血管病变风险。患者经随机分配进入吡格列酮组和安慰剂组。主要复合终点包括全因死亡率、非致命性心肌梗死、急性冠脉综合征、冠状动脉或下肢动脉接受血管内或手术干预治疗以及踝关节以上截肢；经过平均 34.5 个月的随访发现，在两组之间初级终点事件的发生率并无差异。然而与安慰剂组相比，吡格列酮组次要终点事件发生率降低了 16%，主要包括全因死亡率、非致命性心肌梗死和卒中（$P=0.027$）（Dormandy）。

- 吡格列酮［吡格列酮对 2 型糖尿病冠状动脉粥样硬化作用的评价研究（Pioglitazone Effect on Regression of Intravascular Sonographic Coronary Obstruction Prospective Evaluation Trial, PERISCOPE），2008］：PERISCOPE 研究纳入了 543 例伴有冠心病的 2 型糖尿病患者，并对这些患者进行了冠脉血管内超声检查（IVUS）。18 个月后复查了血管内超声，并将 360 例患者随机分入格列美脲（一种磺脲类药物）组和吡格列酮（一种噻唑烷二酮类药物）组。在格列美脲组，动脉粥样硬化斑块体积增加了 0.73%（95%CI:0.33%~1.12%），而在吡格列酮组则降低了 0.16%（95%95%CI:-0.57%~0.25%）（$P=0.002$）。上述结果清楚地表明了在延缓冠状动脉粥样硬化的治疗中，吡格列酮的作用优于 SU 类药物（Nissen）。

- 吡格列酮和罗格列酮对血脂代谢的作用比较（Goldberg 等，2005）：研究纳入了血脂异常的 2 型糖尿病患者，这些患者未曾接受过胰岛素治疗或降脂药物治疗；经随机分配后，患者分别进入吡格列酮组（N= 400）和罗格列酮组（N= 402），治疗时间为 12 周。在吡格列酮组，患者甘油三酯水平下降了（51±7.8）mg/dl，而在罗格列酮组则增高了（13.1±7.8）mg/dl，（$P<0.001$）。与罗格列酮相比，吡格列酮增加了 HDL 胆固醇水平［增幅分别为（2.4±0.5）mg/dl 和（5.2±0.5）mg/dl；$P<0.001$］，并降低了 LDL 胆固醇水平［降幅分别为（21±1.6）mg/dl 和（12±1.6）mg/dl，$P<0.001$］。经吡格列酮治疗后，患者 LDL 颗粒密度有所降低、且 LDL 体积有所增加（$P=0.005$），这些变化都对患者有益。以上结果表明，吡格列酮和罗格列酮对脂质代谢的作用不同（吡格列酮获益更多）。

- 罗格列酮（Nissen 等，2007）：该荟萃分析纳入了 42 项已发表和未发表、小规模和大规模研究，结果发现罗格列酮与心肌梗死死亡率显著增高相关（OR = 1.43，95%CI:1.03~1.98；$P=0.03$），并与心血管疾病死亡率增高相关，后者统计学结果显著性处于临界水平（OR=1,

64，95%CI：0.98~2.74；P=0.06）。研究结果立刻陷入争论。
- 罗格列酮［罗格列酮联合口服药物治疗对 2 型糖尿病患者心血管转归的影响（Rosiglitazone Evaluated for Cardiovascular Outcomes in oRal agent Combination therapy for type 2 Diabetes，RECORD），2009］：RECORD 研究为大型随机临床试验（N=4 447），患者在服用二甲双胍或磺脲类药物治疗的基础上加用了罗格列酮，本试验针对心血管事件进行了研究。经过 5.5 年治疗发现，罗格列酮与患者体重显著增加相关（增幅约 4 kg），与心力衰竭风险增加相关（OR = 2.10，95%CI：1.35~3.27），并与总体骨折发生率增加相关（OR=1.57，95%CI：1.26~1.97）骨折主要见于女性、且多为上下肢骨折。然而在本研究中，心血管疾病总体发病率或死亡率并无增加（Home）。该研究属于开放性试验，因此美国食品药品监督管理局（U.S. Food and Drug Administration，FDA）重新判定了研究结果，并表明罗格列酮组患者心肌梗死死亡风险有所增加（Psaty）。
- 罗格列酮（Nissen 等，2010）：这一新的荟萃分析纳入了 56 项与罗格列酮相关的试验，且用药时间至少为 24 周。分析发现罗格列酮显著增加了心肌梗死风险（OR = 1.39，不包括 RECORD 试验，95%CI：1.02~1.89；P=0.04），但并未增加心血管疾病死亡风险 （OR = 1.03，95%CI：0.78~1.36；P=0.86）。
- 口服药物的有效性比较［糖尿病预后进展研究（A Diabetes Outcome Progression Trial，ADOPT），2006］：ADOPT 研究纳入了 4 360 例 2 型糖尿病患者，并比较了几种口服降糖药物的血糖控制时限，研究时间超过 5 年。单药治疗失败的定义为空腹血糖水平超过 180mg/dl。格列本脲的降糖作用最快，但其 5 年失效率最高（34%）。罗格列酮和二甲双胍的治疗失效率分别为 15% 和 21%。罗格列酮与体重增加和水肿相关，并与新发骨折率增高相关（Kahn）。
- 西格列汀（021 研究组，2006）：该试验研究西格列汀单药用于治疗 2 型糖尿病的疗效及安全性。741 例患者被随机分入西格列汀组（100 mg/d 或 200mg/d）和安慰剂组。24 周后，与安慰剂组相比，西格列汀组患者的总体糖化血红蛋白 A1c 水平显著降低，每日服药 100mg 和 200mg 者的降幅分别为 0.79% 和 0.94%。当糖化血红蛋白基线水平大于 9% 时，该药的降糖效果最强（降低程度约为 1.50%）。西格列汀对患者体重无影响，低血糖发生率与安慰剂组相似，胃肠道不良反应率略高（Aschner）。
- 艾塞那肽与甘精胰岛素比较（Barnett 等，2007）：一项早期开放性研究，比较艾塞那肽（一种肠促胰岛素类似物）与甘精胰岛素用于 138 例口服降糖药物治疗失效 2 型糖尿病患者的疗效。治疗 16 周，研究发现艾塞那肽与甘精胰岛素降糖疗效相当（HbA1c<7% 的患者比例为 38%），并且有效减轻体重（较甘精胰岛素组减轻 2.2kg，P<0.001），同时胃肠道不良事件发生率较高（恶心发生率为 42.6%，甘精胰岛素为 3.1%）。
- 吸入式胰岛素（Skyler 等，2007）：该研究纳入了 580 例 1 型糖尿病成年患者，研究吸入式胰岛素的疗效及安全性，治疗时间为 2 年；结果显示吸入式胰岛素安全有效，在治疗前 3 个月可见第 1 秒用力呼气量有所降低，但该现象并无进展，此外还有患者在治疗过程中发生了咳嗽。由于吸入式胰岛素未被广泛接受且销量低，故上市不久即退出市场。FDA 随后发布了令人担忧的消息：虽然本研究中死亡人数很低，但在应用吸入式胰岛素的患者中出现了因肺癌而死亡的不寻常现象。

妊娠期糖尿病的药物治疗

- 格列本脲（Langer 等，2000）：该研究纳入了 404 例患有妊娠期糖尿病的单胎妊娠女性，患者被随机分入格列本脲组和胰岛素组，并于妊娠后第 11~33 周接受了治疗。在两组患者当中，治疗前的平均血糖浓度约为 115mg/dl，治疗后约为 105md/dl。两组之间不良反应无显著差异，不良反应主要包括巨大胎儿、低血糖、肺部并发症、胎儿异常或需要新生儿重症监护等。以上结果表明在妊娠期糖尿病的治疗中，格列本脲可以作为胰岛素的替代药物。但后期研究发现虽然格列本脲与胰岛素一样有效，但它可能与孕妇子痫前期或新生儿光线治疗相关，这些危险因素还有待于进一步研究（Jacobson）。

- 二甲双胍（Moore 等，2010）：研究纳入了 149 例妊娠糖尿病患者，这些患者未能通过饮食干预而有效控制血糖，患者被随机分入二甲双胍组和格列本脲组。在二甲双胍组，35% 患者血糖控制失败，并需要接受胰岛素治疗；这一比率在格列本脲组为 16%。

糖尿病及其并发症的外科治疗

- 胰岛移植（Shapiro 等，1975）：本研究首次表明胰岛移植是可行的治疗方法。研究包含 7 例 1 型糖尿病患者，这些患者具有严重的代谢紊乱和低血糖病史，并接受了 2~3 个供者的胰腺移植。术后给予了西罗莫司、他克莫司和达利珠单抗进行治疗，未应用激素。1 年以后，所有患者均不再依赖胰岛素治疗，长期随访显示患者病情有所恶化。胰腺分离技术的提高以及无需激素的免疫抑制治疗方案可能促进了患者的初期好转。

- 胰岛移植（Edmonton 计划，2006）：Edmonton 胰岛移植计划为一项大型国际试验，本研究纳入了 36 例 1 型糖尿病患者。1 年以后，16 例患者（44%）不再依赖胰岛素并获得了充分的血糖控制，10 例患者（28%）的胰腺功能部分性恢复，10 例患者（28%）移植治疗完全失败。第 2 年，在 16 例不再依赖胰岛素的患者中有 5 人（31%）仍然无胰岛素治疗。研究者认为患者在接受胰岛移植后可以不再依赖胰岛素治疗，但其成功性尚不够稳定；但胰腺功能持续性恢复可防止严重低血糖的发生，并改善糖化血红蛋白的水平（Shapiro）。

- 植入胰岛素泵（退伍军人事务部植入胰岛素泵研究组，1996）：研究纳入了 171 例男性 2 型糖尿病患者，被随机分入植入胰岛素泵（implantable insulin pump，IIP）组和每日多次注射胰岛素组（MDI）。1 年后发现两组患者血糖降低水平（约 8mmol/L）和糖化血红蛋白降低水平相似。IIP 明显减少血糖波动，虽然患者发生了轻度低血糖和体重增加，但 IIP 可以明显改善患者生存质量。然而，25% 患者因胰岛素泵内形成了微小沉淀而未能得到足量注射（Saudek）。

- 胃束带手术（大学肥胖研究中心，澳大利亚，2008）：腹腔镜下可调式胃束带手术（减重手术）用于治疗 2 型糖尿病的研究为数不多，本研究属于其中之一。在 60 例肥胖患者中，73% 手术组患者的 2 型糖尿病病情缓解，而在生活方式治疗组仅有 13% 患者的病情得到缓解（OR = 5.5，95%CI:2.2~14.0）。患者的获益与体重降低直接相关。手术组患者的体重平均降低了 20.7%，而生活方式治疗组患者体重仅降低了 1.7%（Dixon）。

- 减重手术（Adams 等，2007）：最常用的减重手术方法为胃旁路术，与对

糖尿病治疗的关键研究：治疗效果

照组的回顾性评估结果相比（N=9 628），胃旁路术（N=9 949）后7年的长期死亡率降低了40%（P<0.001）；在因糖尿病、心脏病以及肿瘤死亡的患者中更是如此。然而与对照组相比，手术组患者因事故和自杀的死亡率增加了58%（P=0.04）。

- 减重手术［瑞典肥胖受试者研究（Swedish Obesity Subjects study, SOS），2007］：SOS研究对4 047例肥胖受试者进行了长达11年的随访，其中2 010人接受了减重手术，2 037人接受了传统治疗。经15年随访发现传统治疗组患者体重降低幅度为±2%，在手术治疗1~2年后和10年后的体重降幅分别为：胃旁路术（32%、25%）、垂直束带胃成形术（25%、16%）、束带手术（20%、14%）。经年龄、性别和危险因素调整后，手术组患者的死亡率比传统治疗组低29%（P=0.01）（Sjöström）。

- 减重手术［减重手术手术纵向评估联盟（Longitudinal Assessment of Bariatric Surgery Consortium，LABS），2009］：LABS联盟报告评估了减重手术在4 776例患者中的安全性，其中3/4患者接受了Roux-en-Y胃旁路手术，其余患者接受了经腹腔镜可调节式胃束带手术。总体而言，4.3%患者发生了至少1种严重不良反应，30日死亡率为0.3%。极度肥胖与预后不良风险增高相关（Flum）。

- 冠状动脉旁路移植手术［旁路血管成形术血运重建研究（The Bypass Angioplasty Revascularization Investigation，BARI），1996］：BARI试验纳入了1 892例多支血管病变的患者，并比较了冠状动脉旁路移植手术（coronary-artery bypass grafting，CABG）和经皮冠状动脉腔内成形术（percutaneous transluminal coronary angioplasty，PTCA）的疗效。经过平均5.4年的随访发现，两组患者的死亡率无显著差异。然而，对于患有糖尿病的患者（N=353）而言（事先并未设定这一亚组），CABG治疗后的生存率显著优于PTCA组（生存率分别为80.6%和65.5%，P=0.003）。该研究针对PTCA在糖尿病患者中的应用提出了质疑，并指出PTCA技术也处于不断完善的过程中（BARI研究人员）。

- 冠状动脉旁路移植手术（2型糖尿病旁路血管成形术血运重建研究，2009）：BARI 2D研究纳入了2 368例伴有稳定性缺血性心脏病的2型糖尿病患者。患者被随机分入快速血运重建干预（CABG）组或快速经皮冠状动脉干预组（PCI），以及最优药物治疗组。根据患者病情的严重程度来选择快速干预的方式。经过平均5年随访发现，除接受CABG治疗外（患者病情较重），最优药物治疗组和快速干预组之间死亡率并无差异；在CABG组，严重心血管事件发生率低于药物治疗组（分别为22.4%和30.5%，P=0.01）（Frye）。

专家意见

- 值得注意的是，多种胰岛素治疗方案评估相关疗效的研究未包含在上述研究目录中。

- 药物有效性试验可能会受到出版偏差的影响。但几种主流医学杂志要求临床试验于开始时就应当在公共数据库进行注册，从而降低只有阳性结果才被公开发表的可能性。

- 对于糖化血红蛋白基线水平较高（如>9%）或未经治疗的患者而言，其降糖治疗效果相对更为明显。

- 目前，关于罗格列酮和吡格列酮的应用尚有争议。此两种药物均属于噻唑烷二酮类降糖药，其副作用已经十分明确：二者均可导致体液潴留，增加充血性心力衰竭的发病率，增加体重，并增加骨折的发病率。一项头对头研究（Goldberg等）发现，吡格列酮可显著改善患者的血脂水平。然而与吡格列酮相比，罗格列酮能否增加心血管疾病的发生率，这一点还尚有争议。其证据主要来源于Nissen教授的荟萃分析。2010年10月，由FDA组成的专家团体宣称罗格列酮将继续上市，但其应用将受到严格限制。
- 外科治疗方法主要用于糖尿病并发症的治疗（如肥胖、心血管疾病等），但新型治疗方法（如1型糖尿病胰岛移植治疗）仍处于开发阶段。

参考文献

Psaty BM, Prentice RL. Minimizing bias in randomized trials: the importance of blinding. JAMA, 2010; Vol. 304:pp. 793–4.
Comments: A commentary on bias in clinical trials, specifically addressing the RECORD trial.

Moore LE, Clokey D, Rappaport VJ, et al. Metformin compared with glyburide in gestational diabetes: a randomizedcontrolled trial. Obstet Gynecol, 2010; Vol. 115: pp. 55–9.
Comments: An original study comparing metformin versus glyburide for treatment of gestational diabetes.

Nissen SE, Wolski K. Rosiglitazone revisited: an updated meta-analysis of risk for myocardial infarction and cardiovascular mortality. Arch Intern Med, 2010; Jun 28 [Epub ahead of print].
Comments: Updated meta-analysis of 52 trials.

BARI 2D Study Group, Frye RL, August P, et al. A randomized trial of therapies for type 2 diabetes and coronary artery disease. NEJM, 2009; Vol. 360: pp. 2503–15.
Comments: A summary of results from the BARI 2D Study Group.

Home PD, Pocock SJ, Beck-Nielsen H, et al. Rosiglitazone evaluated for cardiovascular outcomes in oral agent combination therapy for type 2 diabetes (RECORD): a multicentre, randomised, open-label trial. Lancet, 2009; Vol. 373: pp. 2125–35.
Comments: A summary of the results of the RECORD Study.

Longitudinal Assessment of Bariatric Surgery (LABS) Consortium, Flum DR, Belle SH, et al. Perioperative safety in the longitudinal assessment of bariatric surgery. NEJM, 2009; Vol. 361: pp. 445–54.
Comments: Results from a study of bariatric surgery from the LABS Consortium.

Dixon JB, O'Brien PE, Playfair J, et al. Adjustable gastric banding and conventional therapy for type 2 diabetes: a randomized controlled trial. JAMA, 2008; Vol. 299: pp. 316–23.
Comments: Results from the University Obesity Research Center.

Nissen SE, Nicholls SJ, Wolski K, et al. Comparison of pioglitazone vs glimepiride on progression of coronary atherosclerosis in patients with type 2 diabetes: the PERISCOPE randomized controlled trial. JAMA; 2008; Vol. 299: pp. 1561–73.
Comments: A summary of the results of the PERISCOPE Study.

Adams TD, Gress RE, Smith SC, et al. Long-term mortality after gastric bypass surgery. NEJM, 2007; Vol. 357: pp. 753–61.

Comments: Results of a study examining gastric bypass surgery long-term mortality.

Barnett AH, Burger J, Johns D, et al. Tolerability and efficacy of exenatide and titrated insulin glargine in adult patients with type 2 diabetes previously uncontrolled with metformin or a sulfonylurea: a multinational, randomized, open-label, two-period, crossover noninferiority trial. Clin Ther, 2007; Vol. 29: pp. 2333–48.
Comments: Results of a study of exenetide versus insulin glargine.

Nissen SE, Wolski K. Effect of rosiglitazone on the risk of myocardial infarction and death from cardiovascular causes. NEJM, 2007; Vol. 356: pp. 2457–71.
Comments: Meta-analysis of rosiglitazone on cardiovascular outcomes.

Sjöström L, Narbro K, Sjöström CD, et al. Effects of bariatric surgery on mortality in Swedish obese subjects. NEJM, 2007; Vol. 357: pp. 741–52.
Comments: A summary of results from the Swedish Obesity Subjects study.

Skyler JS, Jovanovic L, Klioze S, et al. Two-year safety and efficacy of inhaled human insulin (Exubera) in adult patients with type 1 diabetes. Diabetes Care, 2007; Vol. 30: pp. 579–85.
Comments: Safety study of the effects of inhaled insulin in adult patients with type 1 DM.

Aschner P, Kipnes MS, Lunceford JK, et al. Effect of the dipeptidyl peptidase-4 inhibitor sitagliptin as monotherapy on glycemic control in patients with type 2 diabetes. Diabetes Care, 2006; Vol. 29: pp. 2632–7.
Comments: An early study of sitagliptin as monotherapy for T2DM patients.

Kahn SE, Haffner SM, Heise MA, et al. Glycemic durability of rosiglitazone, metformin, or glyburide monotherapy. NEJM, 2006; Vol. 355: pp. 2427–43.
Comments: A summary of the results from the ADOPT study.

Shapiro AM, Rocordi C, Hering BJ, et al. International trial of the Edmonton protocol for islet transplantation. NEJM, 2006; Vol. 355: pp. 1318–30.

Nissen SE, Wolski K. Rosiglitazone revisited: an updated meta-analysis of risk for myocardial infarction and cardiovascular mortality. Arch Intern Med, 2010; Jun 28 [Epub ahead of print].
Comments: Updated meta-analysis of 52 trials.

BARI 2D Study Group, Frye RL, August P, et al. A randomized trial of therapies for type 2 diabetes and coronary artery disease. NEJM, 2009; Vol. 360: pp. 2503–15.
Comments: A summary of results from the BARI 2D Study Group.

Home PD, Pocock SJ, Beck-Nielsen H, et al. Rosiglitazone evaluated for cardiovascular outcomes in oral agent combination therapy for type 2 diabetes (RECORD): a multicentre, randomised, open-label trial. Lancet, 2009; Vol. 373: pp. 2125–35.
Comments: A summary of the results of the RECORD Study.

Longitudinal Assessment of Bariatric Surgery (LABS) Consortium, Flum DR, Belle SH, et al. Perioperative safety in the longitudinal assessment of bariatric surgery. NEJM, 2009; Vol. 361: pp. 445–54.
Comments: Results from a study of bariatric surgery from the LABS Consortium.

Dixon JB, O'Brien PE, Playfair J, et al. Adjustable gastric banding and conventional therapy for type 2 diabetes: a randomized controlled trial. JAMA, 2008; Vol. 299: pp. 316–23.
Comments: Results from the University Obesity Research Center.

Nissen SE, Nicholls SJ, Wolski K, et al. Comparison of pioglitazone vs glimepiride on progression of coronary atherosclerosis in patients with type 2 diabetes: the

PERISCOPE randomized controlled trial. JAMA; 2008; Vol. 299: pp. 1561–73.
Comments: A summary of the results of the PERISCOPE Study.

Adams TD, Gress RE, Smith SC, et al. Long-term mortality after gastric bypass surgery. NEJM, 2007; Vol. 357: pp. 753–61.
Comments: Results of a study examining gastric bypass surgery long-term mortality.

Barnett AH, Burger J, Johns D, et al. Tolerability and efficacy of exenatide and titrated insulin glargine in adult patients with type 2 diabetes previously uncontrolled with metformin or a sulfonylurea: a multinational, randomized, open-label, two-period, crossover noninferiority trial. Clin Ther, 2007; Vol. 29: pp. 2333–48.
Comments: Results of a study of exenetide versus insulin glargine.

Nissen SE, Wolski K. Effect of rosiglitazone on the risk of myocardial infarction and death from cardiovascular causes. NEJM, 2007; Vol. 356: pp. 2457–71.
Comments: Meta-analysis of rosiglitazone on cardiovascular outcomes.

Sjöström L, Narbro K, Sjöström CD, et al. Effects of bariatric surgery on mortality in Swedish obese subjects. NEJM, 2007; Vol. 357: pp. 741–52.
Comments: A summary of results from the Swedish Obesity Subjects study.

Skyler JS, Jovanovic L, Klioze S, et al. Two-year safety and efficacy of inhaled human insulin (Exubera) in adult patients with type 1 diabetes. Diabetes Care, 2007; Vol. 30: pp. 579–85.
Comments: Safety study of the effects of inhaled insulin in adult patients with type 1 DM.

Aschner P, Kipnes MS, Lunceford JK, et al. Effect of the dipeptidyl peptidase-4 inhibitor sitagliptin as monotherapy on glycemic control in patients with type 2 diabetes. Diabetes Care, 2006; Vol. 29: pp. 2632–7.
Comments: An early study of sitagliptin as monotherapy for T2DM patients.

Kahn SE, Haffner SM, Heise MA, et al. Glycemic durability of rosiglitazone, metformin, or glyburide monotherapy. NEJM, 2006; Vol. 355: pp. 2427–43.
Comments: A summary of the results from the ADOPT study.

Shapiro AM, Rocordi C, Hering BJ, et al. International trial of the Edmonton protocol for islet transplantation. NEJM, 2006; Vol. 355: pp. 1318–30.

Dormandy JA, Charbonnel B, Eckland DJ, et al. Secondary prevention of macrovascular events in patients with type 2 diabetes in the PROactive Study (PROspective pioglitAzone Clinical Trial In macroVascular Events): a randomised controlled trial. Lancet, 2005; Vol. 366: pp. 1279–89.
Comments: A summary of the results of the PROactive Study.

Goldberg RB, Kendall DM, Deeg MA, et al. A comparison of lipid and glycemic effects of pioglitazone and rosiglitazone in patients with type 2 diabetes and dyslipidemia. Diabetes Care, 2005; Vol. 28: pp. 1547–54.
Comments: A study comparing effects of pioglitazone versus rosiglitazone on lipids.

Jacobson GF, Ramos GA, Ching JY, et al. Comparison of glyburide and insulin for the management of gestational diabetes in a large managed care organization. Am J Obstet Gynecol, 2005; Vol. 193: pp. 118–24.
Comments: A study examining glyburide for treatment of gestational diabetes.

Aronoff S, Rosenblatt S, Braithwaite S, et al. Pioglitazone hydrochloride monotherapy improves glycemic control in the treatment of patients with type 2 diabetes: a 6-month randomized placebo-controlled dose-response study. The Pioglitazone 001 Study Group. Diabetes Care,

2000; Vol. 23: pp. 1605–11.
Comments: A summary of results of the Pioglitazone 001 Study Group.

Langer O, Conway DL, Berkus MD, et al. A comparison of glyburide and insulin in women with gestational diabetes mellitus. NEJM, 2000; Vol. 343: pp. 1134–8.
Comments: A study examining glyburide for treatment of gestational diabetes.

Shapiro AM, Lakey JR, Ryan EA, et al. Islet transplantation in seven patients with type 1 diabetes mellitus using a glucocorticoid-free immunosuppressive regimen. NEJM, 2000; Vol. 343: pp. 230–8.
Comments: A summary of the results of a study of islet transplantation.

UK Prospective Diabetes Study (UKPDS) Group. Effect of intensive blood-glucose control with metformin on complications in overweight patients with type 2 diabetes (UKPDS 34). Lancet, 1998; Vol. 352. pp. 854–65.
Comments: A summary of the results of the UKPDS Group 34 Study.

The Bypass Angioplasty Revascularization Investigation (BARI) Investigators. Comparison of coronary bypass surgery with angioplasty in patients with multivessel disease. NEJM, 1996; Vol. 335: pp. 217–25.
Comments: A summary of the results of The Bypass Angioplasty Revascularization Investigation.

Saudek CD, Duckworth WC, Giobbie-Hurder A, et al. Implantable insulin pump vs multiple-dose insulin for noninsulin-dependent diabetes mellitus: a randomized clinical trial. Department of Veterans Affairs Implantable Insulin Pump Study Group. JAMA, 1996; Vol. 276: pp. 1322–7.
Comments: Department of Veteran Affairs Implantable Insulin Pump Study Group.

DeFronzo RA, Goodman AM. Efficacy of metformin in patients with non-insulin-dependent diabetes mellitus. The Multicenter Metformin Study Group. NEJM, 1995; Vol. 333: pp. 541–9.
Comments: A summary of the results of The Multicenter Metformin Study Group.

Hoffmann J, Spengler M. Efficacy of 24-week monotherapy with acarbose, glibenclamide, or placebo in NIDDM patients. The Essen Study. Diabetes Care, 1994; Vol. 17: pp. 561–6.
Comments: A summary of the results of the Essen Study.

Nolan JJ, Ludvik B, Beerdsen P, et al. Improvement in glucose tolerance and insulin resistance in obese subjects treated with troglitazone. NEJM, 1994; Vol. 331: pp. 1188–93.
Comments: A study of troglitazone benefits on insulin resistance.

Nathan DM, Roussell A, Godine JE. Glyburide or insulin for metabolic control in non-insulin-dependent diabetes mellitus. A randomized, double-blind study. Ann Intern Med, 1988; Vol. 108: pp. 334–40.
Comments: A study examining efficacy of glyburide on glycemic control.

Meinert CL, Knatterud GL, Prout TE, et al. A study of the effects of hypoglycemic agents on vascular complications in patients with adult-onset diabetes. II. Mortality results. Diabetes, 1970; Vol. 19: pp. 789–830.
Comments: A summary of the results of a study from the University Group Diabetes Program.

第二部分

管理

突发事件	45
主要原则	56
医院管理和外科手术	78
生活方式和健康教育	102
糖尿病前期	134
怀孕	138
社会 / 法律	146
特殊人群或亚型	153
1 型糖尿病	174
2 型糖尿病	188

突发事件

糖尿病酮症酸中毒

Rita Rastogi Kalyani, MD, MHS

定义
- 是一种代谢性酸中毒,三项主要特征为高血糖(葡萄糖 > 250mg/dl),代谢性酸中毒(动脉血 pH ≤ 7.3,血清碳酸氢盐 ≤ 18mEq/L)以及中等的酮尿和酮血症。
- 大部分患者患有 1 型糖尿病。
- 2 型糖尿病患者(尤其是非洲裔美国人,或是有西班牙血统的人)急性发病也容易得 DKA,这被称为胰岛素依赖性 2 型糖尿病,其原因可能为大量相对胰岛素缺乏(Linfoot)。

流行病学
- 大部分患者年龄在 18~44 岁(占 56%);2/3 的患者患有 1 型糖尿病,还有 1/3 的患有 2 型糖尿病(Kitabchi;Wang)。
- 成年患者的死亡率为 1%,老年患者的死亡率为 5%,不过更多常见的死亡患者发生在小孩和患有 1 型糖尿病的青少年(疾控中心 CDC)。
- 感染为最常见诱因。
- 其他常见诱因:心肌梗死,胰腺炎,胰岛素泵给药失败,药物依从性,心理因素以及药物(比如类固醇药物、利尿药)。
- 经常表现在新发的 1 型糖尿病中。
- 在美国住院超过十年的 DKA 患者人数从 93 000 人(1995 年)上升到 120 000 人(2005 年),增加了 35%(CDC)。
- 超过 1/3 的住院病人反复发生 DKA(CDC)。
- 平均停留时间从 1980 年的 7.9 天下降到 2005 年的 3.6 天(CDC)。
- 急性 DKA 在年龄、性别、种族上并无明显差异,尽管黑人 DKA 发病有增加的趋势,但可能是由于胰岛素依赖型糖尿病(Ginde)。
- DKA 的发作代表着每 4 美元将有 1 美元用在 1 型糖尿病患者的医疗护理上(Javor)。由于包括 DKA 在内的短期不可控制的糖尿病,可避免的住院费用为 28 亿美元(Kim)。

诊断
- 24 小时内迅速发展,特别是任何原因引起的胰岛素泵停止给药。
- 为寻找更深入的证据,应进行详尽的体格检查,如急促的呼吸(Kussmaul 呼吸)、脱水、血容量不足以及潜在的诱因。
- 动脉血气分析评估酸中毒及呼吸代偿,初步得出静脉 pH 后加 0.03 可以作为检查指标。
- 血清酮体和尿酮体的检测可以证实酮症是引起酸中毒的原因。注意:酮体阳性也可能是由于禁食（碳酸氢钠通常高于 18mEq/L）或酒精引起（血糖很少达到 200mg/dl）；酮体阴性可出现在使用卡托普利和硫基药物。进一步的实验室检查包括全血细胞计数（白细胞通常为 10 000mm^3）、电解质血尿素氮、肌酐、转氨酶、淀粉酶、脂肪酶、心肌酶、乳酸、血浆渗透压、毒性筛选和尿常规。

- 当血糖超过 100mg/dl 时，校正的血钠值对应于每 100mg/dl 血糖将实际测得钠加上 1.6mEq/L，提高的校正钠离子值可以反映脱水情况。
- 由于胰岛素相关的细胞外转移，尽管存在全身消耗，高钾和高磷酸仍可能存在。
- 高阴离子间隙反映酸中毒程度和液体容量，计算公式为：$Na^+ - (Cl^- + HCO_3^-)$ (mEq/L)，其值使用未校正钠离子浓度。正常的阴离子间隙（AG）= 血清白蛋白 ×3。高阴离子间隙为 10~12mEq/L。
- 渗透压的估计值和实测值应进行比较，这样可以排除是否有不可测量的渗透压物质（甲醇、乙醇）等有毒物质的摄入。血清渗透压 (mOsm/L)= $2(Na^+ + K^+)$ (mEq/L) + 葡萄糖 (mg/dl)/18 + 尿素氮 (mg/dl)/2.8。
- 心电图、胸部 X 线检查、尿液、痰或血培养也应该考虑。

体征和症状

- 体征：皮肤弹性减退，黏膜干燥，腋下无汗，心跳过速，直立性低血压，Kussmaul 呼吸（代谢性酸中毒时出现的快而深长的呼吸），酮血症导致的呼气有烂水果味，呕吐和腹肌紧张，出血性胃炎导致的隐血实验阳性。
- 症状：多尿，多饮，体重减轻，皮肤干燥，乏力，疲劳，恶心，呕吐，气短，腹部疼痛，疲劳，嗜睡，昏迷，癫痫发作。
- 精神状态改变（通常当血浆渗透压高于 360mOsm/L），低血压以及严重的合并症，这些是作为识别高死亡风险结果的征状。
- 见表 2-1 为糖尿病酮症酸中毒危险分层

表 2-1. 糖尿病酮症酸中毒危险分层（葡萄糖 >250mg/dl）

	轻度	中度	严重
动脉 pH	7.25~7.30	7.00~7.24	<7.00
血清碳酸氢钠	15~18	10~15	<10
尿酮	阳性	阳性	阳性
血清酮体	阳性	阳性	阳性
血浆有效渗透压	易变的	易变的	易变的
阴离子间隙	>10	>12	>12
精神状态	有意识的	有意识的/昏睡	嗜睡/昏迷

来源：Kitabchi AE, Nyenwe EA. Hyperglycemic crises in diabetes mellitus: diabetic ketoacidosis and hyperglycemic hyperosmolar state. Endocrinol Metab Clin North Am, 2006; Vol. 35(4): pp. 725 - 51, viii. Reprinted with permission from Elsevier

临床治疗

液体疗法

- 目的在于扩充血管，补充组织间隙、细胞内的液体和恢复肾灌注。
- 补液应当纠正 24 小时内丢失量。液体平均丢失量为 6L。

糖尿病酮症酸中毒

- 当钾离子浓度低于 5.2mEq/L 时,补钾应该伴随补液疗法同时进行。
- 没有心脏代偿的情况下,以每小时 15~20ml/(kg·h) 静滴生理盐水溶液(0.9% NaCl)或第一小时补充 1~1.5L 生理盐水,然后按照这个速度补液,防止严重脱水。
- 校正血钠正常或者升高:根据轻度脱水的液体容量,第一小时后以 250~500ml/h 的速度静脉滴注 0.45% NaCl。
- 校正血钠低于正常:轻度脱水,根据脱水情况,第一小时后 0.9% NaCl 以 250~500ml/h 静滴。
- 通过监测血压、液体进出量、实验室检查和体格检查采取有关改善措施。
- 对于有心功能或者肾功能代偿的患者,应更仔细监测以防止医源性的血容量超负荷。
- 高血糖症(血糖高于 250mg/dl)纠正较高血酮快(pH > 7.30,碳酸氢钠 >18mEq/L),平均持续时间分别为 6h 和 12h。
- 一旦血浆血糖低于 200mg/dl,即改为 5% 右旋葡萄糖加上 0.45% NaCl 以 125~250ml/h 静脉滴注,以允许持续胰岛素治疗,直到纠正高酮血症。

胰岛素疗法

- 无论何种途径(静脉、皮下),胰岛素对于治疗酮症酸中毒都有效。
- 由于半衰期短和易滴定,优先选择持续静脉滴注普通胰岛素。当使用胰岛素静脉输注时,应每隔一小时用血糖仪检测血糖,并至少每 2~4 小时实验室检测血糖。急性酮症酸中毒的治疗使用速效胰岛素如诺和锐、优泌乐、谷赖胰岛素可能有效,但需要进一步的观察(Kitabchi;Umpierrez)。
- 0.1U/kg 静脉推注后 0.1U/(kg·h) 静脉持续滴注或者 0.14U/(kg·h) 静脉持续滴注。
- 如果在第一个小时内血糖没有达到每小时降低 50~75mg/dl,那么增加胰岛素用量直到血糖稳定下降。另一方面,如果血糖在第一小时内没有降低 10%,那么静脉推注胰岛素 0.14U/kg 并恢复前面的治疗。
- 当血糖降到 200mg/dl 以下时,降低普通胰岛素至 0.02~0.05 U/(kg·h) 静脉滴注,或者皮下注射速效胰岛素 0.1 U/kg 维持血糖在 125~200mg/dl,直到纠正高酮血症。
- 对于轻度酮症酸中毒,给非重症监护病人皮下注射速效胰岛素的安全性和有效性可能跟静脉输注胰岛素相同。
- 酮症酸中毒的治疗有效包括血糖 <200mg/dl,以及以下两点:血清碳酸氢盐 >15mEq/L,pH>7.3,或者阴离子间隙 <12mEq/L。
- 在纠正酮症酸中毒后,转换为皮下注射胰岛素,在停用胰岛素的静脉输注和开始胰岛素皮下注射之间,至少1~2小时同时给药。人胰岛素(NPH 和普通胰岛素)方案通常每天使用两个或三个剂量。基础剂量的基础胰岛素(来得时和地特胰岛素)和速效胰岛素类似物(诺和锐、优泌乐、谷赖胰岛素)对 1 型糖尿病更符合生理情况。
- 之前胰岛素控制良好的患者,继续前面的治疗;在胰岛素不敏感患者中,胰岛素总剂量应达到 0.5~0.8U/(kg·d),根据住院期间胰岛素需求情况,分次分剂量给予(见 1 型糖尿病:胰岛素治疗,177 页)。

糖尿病酮症酸中毒

纠正电解质

- 钾：首先建立足够的肾功能（尿量 >50ml/h）。如果 K^+ <3.3mEq/L，继续给予胰岛素，并补钾 20~30mEq/L 直到 K^+ >3.3mEq/L。如果 K^+ >5.2mEq/L，停止补钾，但应每 2 小时检查血清钾。如果 K^+ 在 3.3~5.2mEq/L 之间，每升液体补充钾 20~30mEq 以使 K^+ 保持在 4~5mEq/L。
- 碳酸氢钠：如果 pH>6.9，可不补充碳酸氢盐。如果 pH<6.9，以 100mmol 碳酸氢盐 +400mmol 水 +20mEq 氯化钾 2 小时滴注；每隔 2 小时重复一次，直到 pH>7。
- 磷酸盐：当患者有心功能不全、贫血、呼吸代偿或者血清磷 <1.0mg/dl，应该考虑在补充的液体中加入 20~30mEq 磷酸钾（最大耐受量为 4.5mmol/h 或 1.5ml/h）。
- 镁：经常是消耗殆尽的，补液应保持2mg/dl的目标，并有助于纠正低血钾。
- 包括尿素氮和肌酐在内的血清电解质应每 2~4 小时检查一次，以监测电解质失衡和阴离子间隙是否恢复。

并发症

- 常见的有：由于过度补充胰岛素和碳酸氢盐导致的低血糖和低血钾。
- 高氯非阴离子间隙性酸中毒可出现在复苏阶段，并且是自限性的。
- 0.3%~1.0% 的儿童 DKA 发生脑水肿，并且死亡率高，但在成年人中罕见。症状包括头痛，癫痫，大小便失禁，瞳孔变化，血压升高，心率减慢，呼吸抑制以及意识改变。预防措施包括逐渐降低血浆渗透压和葡萄糖，避免水肿进一步发展。治疗包括使用甘露醇和机械通气。

随访

- 在 2 型糖尿病酮症倾向的患者中，有 40% 依然存在 10 年的非胰岛素依赖。

专家意见

- DKA 的治疗过程中低钾是最常见的致死原因，应密切关注补钾。
- 虽然液体治疗可以降低血糖，但是胰岛素对高酮血症的治疗依然是十分必要的。水电解质失衡的纠正对保护心脏、神经、呼吸功能尤其重要。
- 在 DKA 纠正之前，病人往往需要普通病房监测或加护病房监测。
- 血糖正常的 DKA(血糖 ≤ 250mg/dl) 可由多种因素造成，包括院内注射胰岛素或之前食物控制。
- DKA 和高渗状态常常同时发生，伴随某种程度的高渗状态和酮症酸中毒。
- 恶心，呕吐，弥漫性腹痛，常伴随白细胞和肝酶升高，相对高渗高血糖病人更常发生于 DKA 患者（50%）。
- 一个半衰期（约 6min）后，静注胰岛素开始逐渐消失，必须在停止静脉给药前给予皮下注射胰岛素，以避免 DKA 的复发。
- 更好的健康护理，教育（尤其是患者的日常管理）以及保健医师的早期指导，大多数 DKA 的案例是可以预防的。
- 家庭葡萄糖酮监测可以指导家庭胰岛素治疗，避免住院治疗。
- 探寻导致胰岛素治疗自我终止的可能的经济原因，尤其是在少数人群中，并且力图提供资源以克服障碍。

参考文献

Kitabchi AE, Umpierrez GE, Miles JM, etal. Hyperglycemic crises in adult patients with diabetes. Diabetes Care, 2009; Vol. 32: pp. 1335–43.
Comments: ADA consensus statement for management of DKA and HHS.

其他引用

Umpierrez GE, Jones S, Smiley D, et al. Insulin analogs versus human insulin in the treatment of patients with diabetic ketoacidosis: a randomized controlled trial. Diabetes Care, 2009; Vol. 32: pp. 1164–9.
Comments: Regular and glulisine insulin are equally effective during the acute treatment of DKA.

Kitabchi AE, Umpierrez GE, Fisher JN, et al. Thirty years of personal experience in hyporglycomic crises: diabetic ketoacidosis and hyperglycemic hyperosmolar state. J Clin Endocrinol Metab,2008; Vol. 93: pp. 1541–52.
Comments: Summarizes prospective studies on the management and pathophysiology of DKA.

Wang ZH, Kihl-Selstam E, Eriksson JW. Ketoacidosis occurs in both Type 1 and Type 2 diabetes—a population-based study from Northern Sweden. Diabet Med, 2008; Vol. 25: pp. 867–70.
Comments:Contrasts clinical presentation of DKA in type 1 and type 2 diabetes; type 2 diabetes accounted for one-third of all cases.

Kitabchi AE, Nyenwe EA. Hyperglycemic crises in diabetes mellitus: diabetic ketoacidosis and hyperglycemic hyperosmolar state. Endocrinol Metab Clin North Am, 2006; Vol. 35: pp. 725–51, viii.
Comments: Comprehensive technical review of DKA and HHS.

GindeAA,PelletierAJ,CamargoCA.NationalstudyofU.S.emergencydepartmentvisitswithdiabeticketoacidosis, 1993–2003. Diabetes Care, 2006; Vol. 29: pp. 2117–9.
Comments: Describes number of emergency room visits for DKA and demographic trends.

Centers for Disease Control and Prevention (CDC). Diabetes Data and Trends. http://www.cdc.gov/diabetes/ statistics/hospitalization_national.htm. Accessed February 23, 2011.
Comments: Describes US trends for diabetes hospitalizations from 1980–2006, including DKA.

Linfoot P, bergstrom C, Ipp E. Pathophysiology of ketoacidosis in Type 2 diabetes mellitus. Diabet Med,2005; Vol. 22: pp. 1414–9.
Comments:ExplorespossibleexplanationsforDKAintype2diabetesincludingfreefattyacids,growthhormoneandsuppressionofinsulin.Individualswithketosis-pronetype2diabeteshadgreaterinsulinopenia compared to those with nonketosis-prone type 2 diabetes.

Mauvais-Jarvis F, Sobngwi E, Porcher R, et al. Ketosis-prone type 2 diabetes in patients of sub-Saharan African origin:clinicalpathophysiologyandnaturalhistoryofbeta-celldysfunctionandinsulinresistance.Diabetes, 2004; Vol. 53: pp. 645–53.
Comments:Describesprobabilityofremissionandneedforlong-terminsulinamongAfricanpatientswith ketosis-prone type 2 diabetes.

Javor KA, Kotsanos JG, McDonald RC, et al. Diabetic ketoacidosis charges relative to medical charges of adult patients with type I diabetes. Diabetes Care, 1997; Vol. 20: pp. 349–54.

Comments: The direct medical care charges associated with DKA episodes represented 28.1% of the direct medical care charges for a cohort of 228 patients with type I diabetes. The average charge per DKA episode was $6444.

Centers for Disease Control and Prevention (CDC). Hospitalizations for diabetic ketoacidosis—Washington State, 1987–1989. MMWR, 1992; Vol. 41: pp. 837–9.

Comments: Summarizes surveillance of DKA hospitalizations among Washington State residents from 1987 through 1989.

高血糖高渗状态（HHS）

Vanessa Walker Harris, MD, and Rita Rastogi Kalyani, MD, MHS

定义
- 以严重高血糖、高血浆渗透压、脱水为特点，无明显酮症酸中毒（血浆血糖 >600mg/d，动脉 pH > 7.30，HCO_3^- > 18mEq/L，有效血浆渗透压 >320mOsm/kg）（Kitabchi）。
- 由高血糖引起的渗透性利尿。胰岛素水平维持的作用足以防止脂肪降解以及随后的酮体生成，但不足以降低血糖水平（Stoner）。
- 与炎症相关，有效的补液及胰岛素治疗能逆转（Kitabchi）。
- 常见于2型糖尿病患者，并可能为首发症状。极少发生于儿童或1型糖尿病患者（Stoner；Nugent）。

流行病学
- 死亡率为5%~20%，70岁以上明显增加。早期死亡（72小时内）更常见，可能的原因有败血症、休克或潜在的疾病。晚期死亡（72小时后）通常是因为血栓形成或治疗的结果（Kitabchi；Trence；Magee；Nugent）。
- 感染（例如：肺炎、尿路感染）是最常见的诱因。其他常见的因素有：滥用药物、未确诊的糖尿病、心肌梗死、胰腺炎、脑血管意外、药物（钙通道阻滞剂、噻嗪类利尿剂、非典型抗精神病药物），以及使用药物（酒精、可卡因）。内分泌因素包括甲亢、Cushing综合征以及肢端肥大症。
- 长期使用类固醇药物及胃肠炎是儿童患者中的常见诱因（Kitabchi；Stoner；Trence）。
- 潜在的内科疾病可导致严重脱水以及易发生HHS，包括水代谢代偿，拮抗激素如儿茶酚胺、胰高血糖素、皮质醇和生长激素释放增加(Kitabchi)。
- 平均发病年龄57~69岁。
- 常见于居住在疗养院的居民（28%）（Delaney；Nugent）。

诊断
- 通常在几天至几周内发病。
- 通过病史及体格检查，查找症状（如下）和潜在诱因（如上述）。
- 血浆血糖（> 600mg/dl），电解质和阴离子间隙（碳酸氢根 > 18mEq/L），有效血浆渗透压(320mOsm/kg)，动脉血气分析用于评估酸中毒（pH<7.30），血清及尿中酮体含量确定酮症（可能在脱水时出现）。
- 血糖超过100mg/dl时，校正的Na^+浓度计算方法为：对应于每100mg/dl血糖，将测得的Na^+浓度值加上1.6mEq/L。校正血清钠离子浓度升高提示脱水，并可以用来计算自由水丢失量：全身含水量（Total Body Water, TBW）×[(补液前血清钠浓度（校正血清钠）/ 补液后血清钠浓度）−1]，TBW=体重（kg）× 人体含水比例（%）（人体含水比例因性别和年龄不同，约为60%）。现举例说明：TBW = 0.6×70kg，则男性 TBW=42，校正血清钠离子浓度 = 160mEq/L；自由水丢失量

= 42 × [160/140 − 1] = 6L。

- 其他实验室检查：血尿素氮（平均65mg/dl），血清肌酐（平均3mg/dl），血细胞分类计数（即使没有感染白细胞也可能升高），心电图，胸部X线，毒理学，转氨酶（超过1/3的不可控糖尿病患者存在异常），脂肪酶和淀粉酶（升高可提示胰腺炎），肌酸激酶（多达2/3的病人存在异常），尿，痰或血常规以排除感染。

- 阴离子间隙的计算：$Na \times (Cl^- + HCO_3^-)$ (mEq/L)。使用校正Na^+浓度值，正常阴离子间隙 = 血清白蛋白 × 3。大约50%的病患有轻度的阴离子间隙性酸中毒(Stoner; Magee)。

- 有效血浆渗透压反映病情程度，其计算为(2×NamEq/L)+Glucose (mg/dl)/18 + BUN (mg/dl)/2.8。注意血清钠是组成血浆渗透压的主要部分。

- 血浆钾、血清镁和磷酸盐通常是正常或升高，即使由于胰岛素缺乏，导致上述电解质由细胞内向细胞外转移，引起全机体消耗。

- 肾前性氮质血症（尿素升高，与肌酐比不成比例，造成肌酐升高）时常发生。

- 脱水常常引起肌酸激酶的增高，但需要排除横纹肌溶解症。

症状与体征

- 体征：皮肤干燥水肿；黏膜干燥；四肢冰冷；心动过速；低血压；低烧或体温过低；呼吸急促；腹胀（可能由高渗透性诱导的胃轻瘫引起）；局灶性神经系统损害体征，例如：抽搐、偏盲、轻偏瘫、失语症、肌震颤、吞咽障碍（Kitabchi; Stoner; Magee）。

- 症状：多尿、烦渴、虚弱、体重减轻、视力障碍、下肢痉挛、恶心、呕吐以及腹痛（HHS少见但提示腹腔内病变可能）、嗜睡、意识模糊、麻木、昏迷（发生于有效血浆渗透压 >350mOsm/L)(Kitabchi; Stoner; Magee)。

- 昏迷或血压过低提示预后不良。年龄的增加及高水平的血浆渗透压伴随着死亡率的增加（Nugent）。

- 诊断标准见表2-2。

表2-2. 诊断标准

动脉pH	> 7.30
血清碳酸氢钠(mEq/L)	> 18.00
尿酮	少
血清酮体	少
血浆有效渗透压	>320mOsm/kg
阴离子间隙	易变的
精神状态	血浆渗透压高于360mOsm/kg将导致昏迷

来源：Kitabchi AE, Umpierrez GE, Miles JM, Fisher JN.Hyperglycemic crises in adult patients with diabetes.Diabetes Care, 2009; Vol. 32(7): pp. 1335 - 43.Reproduced with permission of The American Diabetes Association

高血糖高渗状态（HHS）

临床治疗

液体疗法
- 目的在于扩充血管，补充组织间隙、细胞内的液体容量和恢复肾灌注(Kitabchi)。
- 平均来说，液体丢失量为100~200ml/kg，占体液的20%~25%，占体重的12%，或大约9L。18到24小时内必须补充一半的丢失量，其余的在接下来的24小时内补完(Kitabchi; Trence; Stoner)。
- 没有心脏代偿的情况下，以每小时15~20ml/（kg·h）静滴生理盐水溶液（0.9% NaCl），或第一小时补充1~1.5L生理盐水。
- 校正血钠正常或者升高：第一小时后以250~500ml/h的速度静脉滴注0.45% NaCl（Kitabchi）。
- 校正血钠低于正常：第一小时后0.9% NaCl以250~500ml/h静滴(Kitabchi)。
- 血流动力学监测可评估补液是否有效，包括液体出入量、实验室评估和临床检查(Kitabchi)。
- 对于有心功能或者肾功能代偿的病人，应更仔细监测血清渗透压和更频繁的临床检查以防止医源性血容量超负荷(Kitabchi)。
- 单纯补液可以降低血糖80~200mg/(dl·h)。一旦血糖高于300mg/dl，需改为5%的葡萄糖+0.45%的NaCl溶液，以防止过快修正高渗状态而导致脑水肿(Delaney; Stoner; Trence)。

胰岛素疗法
- 在给胰岛素前必须补充足够的液体，否则由于体液渗入细胞内，将导致低血压、血管塌陷，或者死亡(Stoner; Kitabchi; Delaney; Trence)。
- 由于半衰期短和容易滴定，优先选择普通胰岛素静脉持续滴注。当使用胰岛素静脉输注时，应每隔一小时用血糖仪检测血糖，并至少每2~4小时实验室检测血糖(Stoner; Kitabchi)。
- 给予0.1U/kg的初始推注剂量，接着给予0.1U/（kg·h）胰岛素持续静脉滴注(Stoner; Kitabchi)。
- 如果第一小时内血糖下降速度没有达到50~75mg/（dl·h），那么应加快胰岛素输注速度，直到血糖稳定下降(Stoner; Kitabchi)。
- 当血糖<300mg/dl，降低胰岛素滴注速度至0.02~0.05U/（kg·h），使血糖维持在250~300mg/dl，直到患者意识清醒(Kitabchi, Stoner)。
- 一旦高渗状态得到解决且病人能够进食，就开始皮下注射胰岛素。为转为皮下注射胰岛素，在开始皮下注射和停止静脉滴注胰岛素之间，有1~2小时两者可以同时使用。如果患者还在禁食，则继续静脉滴注胰岛素(Stoner; Kitabchi)。
- 对于胰岛素缺乏的患者，每天总剂量应为0.5~0.8单位/kg，并分多次进行(Kitabchi)。
- 有些患者的病情通过小剂量的皮下注射胰岛素可得到控制，并且在后期可换成口服的降糖药物来控制疾病(Delaney; Stoner; Kitabchi)。

纠正水电解质平衡
- 钾：首先建立足够的肾功能（尿量>50ml/h）。如果K^+>5.2mEq/L，停止补钾，

高血糖高渗状态（HHS）

但应每2小时检查血清钾。如果 K⁺ 在 3.3~5.2mEq/L 之间，每升液体补充钾 20~30mEq 以使 K⁺ 保持在 4~5mEq/L。如果 K⁺<3.3mEq/L，继续给予胰岛素，并补钾 20~30mEq/L 直到 K⁺>3.3mEq/L。(Kitabchi; Stoner; Delaney)。

- 磷和钙：没有可知的数据表明，补充磷酸盐可以提高治疗效果。但如果血磷水平低于 1mEq/L 且存在肌无力，则考虑补充磷酸钾。由于严重、有症状的低血钙，需仔细监测血清钙 (Delaney; Stoner)。
- 镁：在不可控制糖尿病经常出现缺乏。补充以保持浓度为 2mEq/dl，纠正低镁有助于纠正低钾血症 (Stoner)。
- 碳酸氢钠：没有迹象表示需要补充碳酸氢钠，除非是乳酸中毒导致体液 pH<7 (Magee)。
- 包括尿素氮和肌酐的血清电解质应每隔 2~4 小时检查一次，监测电解质是否失衡 (Kitabchi)。

并发症

- 常见的有：低血糖，低钾血症，血容量不足，大量体液转移，过早停止胰岛素治疗 (Delaney)。
- 由于血液粘度增加且处于高凝状态引起的血管栓塞（肠系膜缺血，心肌梗死，弥漫性血管内凝血）。如果证据表明有血栓形成，则应全剂量使用普通肝素或低分子量肝素进行治疗 (Magee; Stoner)。
- 非创伤性横纹肌溶解伴或不伴急性肾小管坏死可能发生在失代偿性糖尿病患者，并且导致死亡率增加 (Magee; Stoner)。
- 体内水分过多导致的脑水肿和呼吸窘迫综合征罕见，但是在儿童和青年中是致命的。脑水肿的治疗包括静脉滴注甘露醇，机械通气和静脉滴注地塞米松 (Stoner)。

随访

- 患者教育注重鼓励其坚持血糖监测，按时服用规定药物且随时复诊，建立一个持久的糖尿病管理方案 (Delaney; Stoner; Kitabchi)。
- 病期管理教育，鼓励早期医治，接受保健专员指导；回顾血糖控制目标，合理使用胰岛素；感到恶心时，开始进食含有碳水化合物和盐的流质食物 (Kitabchi; Stoner; Trence)。
- 护工应特别检查是否有足够的液体输入，且要严密监测糖尿病患者的液体情况 (Trence; Stoner)。
- 避免使用与胰岛素冲突的相关药物 (Delaney)。

专家意见

- 与糖尿病酮症酸中毒相鉴别，死亡率更高，症状需经过较长的时间才能发觉，一般是血酮偏低而血糖较高。
- 假设患者同时患有 DKA 和 HHS，血 pH 低于 7.3，有高酮血症，血浆渗透压高于 320mOsm/L(Delaney; Magee)。
- 阴离子间隙增大的代谢性酸中毒，应考虑乳酸性酸中毒或者其他非 HHS 疾病 (Trence; Stoner)。

- 补液后如还存在腹胀、腹痛、恶心或呕吐，则考虑是否有急腹症(Stoner；Magee)。
- 局灶性神经系统症状如癫痫发作、偏瘫、嗜睡、昏迷等，需通过补液和降低血糖来治疗(Stoner；Magee)。
- 如果病人血流动力学不稳定，气道受损，意识模糊或有急腹症症状，需在加护病房进行观察(Stoner; Magee)。
- 精神状态改变通常只发生在严重的高渗状态下，渗透压高于360 mOsm/L时会导致昏迷。如果在没有较严重的高渗状态下发生精神改变，则怀疑其他原因，例如中风。

参考文献

Kitabchi AE, Umpierrez GE, Miles JM, et al. Hyperglycemic crises in adult patients with diabetes. Diabetes Care, 2009; Vol. 32: pp. 1335–43.

Comments: Consensus statement outlining precipitating factors and recommendations for the diagnosis, treatment, and prevention of DKA and HHS.

其他引用

Nugent BW. Hyperosmolar hyperglycemic state. Emerg Med Clin North Am, 2005; Vol. 23: pp. 629–48, vii.

Comments: Discussion of the emergency department management of HHS.

Stoner GD. Hyperosmolar hyperglycemic state. Am Fam Physician, 2005; Vol. 71: pp. 1723–30.

Comments: Discussion of precipitating factors, diagnosis, and treatment of HHS.

Magee MF, Bhatt BA. Management of decompensated diabetes. Diabetic ketoacidosis and hyperglycemic hyperosmolar syndrome. Crit Care Clin, 2001; Vol. 17: pp. 75–106.

Comments: Discussion of the management of DKA and HHS.

Trence DL, Hirsch IB. Hyperglycemic crises in diabetes mellitus type 2. Endocrinol Metab Clin North Am, 2001; Vol. 30: pp. 817–31.

Comments: Focuses on management of decompensated diabetes, specifically HHS and DKA.

Delaney MF, Zisman A, Kettyle WM. Diabetic ketoacidosis and hyperglycemic hyperosmolar nonketotic syndrome. Endocrinol Metab Clin North Am, 2000; Vol. 29: pp. 683–705, v.

Comments: Details the pathophysiology, clinical management, and prevention of DKA and HHS.

主要原则

黎明现象

Shivam Champaneri,MD,and Rita Rastogi Kalyani,MD,MHS

定义
- 血糖在 4AM 和 8AM 升高。
- 临床相上表现为,上述时间点血糖增加了 10mg/dl 或需要增加 20% 胰岛素用量(Carroll)。

流行病学
- 1 型糖尿病发生率估计是 29%~91%(Perriello; Koivisto; Edge; Havlin; Bending; Bolli),2 型糖尿病是 6%~89%(Carroll; Atiea; Havlin; Bolli)。总之,大约 55% 的病人可能经历黎明现象(Carroll)。
- 机制:夜间生长激素分泌使得肌肉和肝脏对胰岛素敏感性受损。生长激素缺乏的病人没有黎明现象。黎明现象不能通过抑制糖皮质激素或儿茶酚胺而得到抑制,表明这些激素不参与这一现象(Edge; Carroll)。
- 血糖控制不佳与更高幅度和更多的黎明现象相关。1 型糖尿病患者,血糖控制不佳持续时间越长,黎明现象就越少(Perriello);然而,2 型糖尿病患者 β 细胞功能越差,高血糖以及胰岛素治疗需要的持续时间越长,均促进黎明现象的发生。

诊断
- 睡觉时血糖(10~11PM)以及清晨(2,4,8AM)测量血糖。黎明现象表现为 4AM 到 8AM 之间血糖突然升高,而外源胰岛素作用在 2AM 和 8AM 作用缓慢,效果减弱(见表 2-3)。
- 生长激素或 IGF-1 在诊断黎明现象中的作用还没有得到公认。

症状和体征
- 症状和体征取决于凌晨高血糖的程度。
- 下表表明黎明现象和外源性胰岛素作用减弱的区别。

表 2-3. 黎明现象的鉴别(血糖 mg/dl)

	10PM	2AM	4AM	8AM
黎明现象	100	110	135	250
胰岛素不足	100	160	220	270

Shivam Champaneri 免费提供

临床治疗

1 型糖尿病
- 黎明现象导致血糖控制更差:一项研究中(Atiea),有黎明现象的患者糖化血红蛋白是 9.5%，而没有黎明现象的是 8.4%。
- 治疗包括确定胰岛素治疗已到达更好的血糖控制（Perriello）。
- 除非引起夜间低血糖，睡前增加胰岛素用量可以更有效的控制血糖。
- 使用胰岛素泵治疗，在黎明现象前增加胰岛素基础用量至少 20%。
- 避免后夜吃零食，除非给予适当的速效胰岛素。

2 型糖尿病
- 调整饮食内容（减少碳水化合物），计算晚餐时间，使睡前的血糖水平为 70~110mg/dl。
- 如果单纯调整饮食不够，考虑在晚餐时服用中效或长效磺脲类降糖药。
- 如果黎明现象仍然出现，考虑基础胰岛素。
- 对丁使用胰岛素治疗的 2 型糖尿病患者，治疗同 1 型糖尿病。

随访
- 如果治疗改变以评估饮食或药物调整的有效性监测和必要性，需要持续监测晨起血糖水平。

专家意见
- 甘精胰岛素和地特，由于其作用时间缓慢，较 NPH 胰岛素很少引起夜间低血糖。夜间低血糖导致的晨起反应性的高血糖被称为"苏木杰效应"。但是有证据表明夜间低血糖并不是晨起显著高血糖的原因（Tordjman）。

参考文献

Carroll mF, Schade DS. The dawn phenomenon revisited: implications for diabetes therapy. endocr Pract, 2005; Vol. 11: pp. 55–64.

Comments: This article is an excellent review of the literature that summarizes data on prevalence, pathogenesis, and management of the dawn phenomenon.

Sheehan JP. Fasting hyperglycemia: etiology, diagnosis, and treatment. Diabetes Technol Ther, 2004; Vol. 6: pp. 525–33.

Comments: This is a review of causes and treatment of morning hyperglycemia amongst type 1 and type 2 diabetes patients.

Masharani U, Karam JH. Diabetes mellitus and hypoglycemia. In: Tierney LMJ, McPhee SJ, Papadakis MA, eds. 2002 Current Medical Diagnosis and Treatment: Adult Ambulatory and In-Patient Management. New York: McGraw-Hill; 2002: pp. 1203–1250.

Comments: This is a review of dawn phenomenon and Somogyi efect in type 1 diabetes patients and the

Carroll MF, Hardy KJ, Burge MR, et al. Frequency of the dawn phenomenon in type 2 diabetes: implications for diabetes therapy. Diabetes Technol Ther, 2002; Vol. 4: pp. 595–605.

Comments: This study of 16 type 2 diabetes found that most patients failed to secrete growth hormone during insulin-induced hypoglycemia and noted rare occurrence of the dawn phenomenon.

Bolli GB, Perriello G, Fanelli CG, et al. Nocturnal blood glucose control in type I diabetes mellitus. Diabetes Care,1993; Vol.16 Suppl 3: pp.71–89.

Comments: This is a review of dawn phenomenon and Somogyi effect in type 1 diabetes patients and the limitations of certain insulin treatment modalities.

Atiea JA, Luzio S, Owens DR. The dawn phenomenon and diabetes control in treated NIDDM and IDDM patients. Diabetes Res Clin Pract, 1992; Vol. 16: pp. 183–90.
Comments: This study found that poorly controlled diabetic patients had higher morning hour glucose rises compared to well-controlled patients.

Perriello G, De Feo P, Torlone E, et al. The dawn phenomenon in type 1 (insulin-dependent) diabetes mellitus: magnitude, frequency, variability, and dependency on glucose counterregulation and insulin sensitivity. Diabetologia, 1991; Vol. 34: pp. 21–8.
Comments: This study of 114 type 1 diabetes patients found 101 patients had an increase in insulin requirement in the morning hours, and it correlated inversely with the duration of diabetes.

Bolli GB, Perriello G. Impact of activated glucose counterregulation on insulin requirements in insulin-dependent diabetes mellitus. Horm Metab Res Suppl, 1990; Vol. 24: pp. 87–96.
Comments: This is a review of the role of counterregulatory states in insulin-dependent diabetes for dawn phenomenon and Somogyi effect.

Edge JA, Matthews DR, Dunger DB. The dawn phenomenon is related to overnight growth hormone release in adolescent diabetics. Clin Endocrinol (Oxford, UK), 1990; Vol. 33: pp. 729–37.
Comments: 26 diabetic adolescents were studied in insulin clamp settings with the finding of an increase in insulin infusion rate in the early morning hours with correlation with mean overnight growth hormone concentration. With growth hormone blockade, insulin requirements in the early morning diminished.

Atiea JA, Vora JP, Owens DR, et al. Non-insulin-dependent diabetic patients (NIDDMs) do not demonstrate the dawn phenomenon at presentation. Diabetes Res Clin Pract, 1988; Vol. 5: pp. 37–44.
Comments: This study of 17 newly diagnosed type 2 diabetes patients and 11 patients after 1 year of treatment noted that no dawn phenomenon was noted in new patients, but a significant rise in glucose was observed in patients having been treated for one year.

Atiea JA, Ryder RR, Vora J, et al. Dawn phenomenon: its frequency in non-insulin-dependent diabetic patients on conventional therapy. Diabetes Care, 1987; Vol. 10: pp. 461–5.
Comments: 19 type 2 diabetes patients were studied with 17 noted to have a dawn rise of plasma glucose with a noted rise in insulin during those hours in both diet alone treated and diet plus oral agents.

Havlin CE, Cryer PE. Nocturnal hypoglycemia does not commonly result in major morning hyperglycemia in patients with diabetes mellitus. Diabetes Care, 1987; Vol. 10: pp. 141–7.
Comments: This study of 75 diabetes patients noted that the dawn phenomenon was present in only a third of patients, and nocturnal hypoglycemia did not commonly result in major morning hyperglycemia (Somogyi phenomenon).

Tordjman KM, Havlin CE, Levandoski LA, et al. Failure of nocturnal hypoglycemia to cause fasting hyperglycemia in patients with insulin-dependent diabetes mellitus. NEJM, 1987; Vol. 317: pp. 1552–9.
Comments: A clinical trial inducing nocturnal hypoglycemia under controlled circumstances did not find that it was associated with morning hyperglycemia.

Koivisto VA, Yki-Järvinen H, Helve E, et al. Pathogenesis and prevention of the dawn phenomenon in diabetic patients treated with CSII. Diabetes, 1986; Vol. 35: pp. 78–82.
Comments: This study of 12 type 1 diabetes patients treated with continuous subcutaneous insulin infusion and noted increase in insulin requirement in the early morning hours with higher growth hormone levels compared to controls.

Bending JJ, Pickup JC, Collins AC, et al. Rarity of a marked "dawn phenomenon" in diabetic subjects treated by continuous subcutaneous insulin infusion. Diabetes Care, 1985; Vol. 8: pp. 28–33.
Comments: In studying 41 insulin-dependent diabetes patients treated with insulin pumps, marked dawn phenomenon was rare when a single adequate basal infusion rate was used.

Bolli GB, Gerich JE. The "dawn phenomenon"—a common occurrence in both non-insulin-dependent and insulindependent diabetes mellitus. NEJM, 1984; Vol. 310: pp. 746–50.
Comments: Among 20 insulin-dependent diabetes patients and 13 non-insulin-dependent diabetes patients, 76% were noted to have an increase in insulin requirements in the early morning hours amongst both groups.

Schmidt MI, Hadji-Georgopoulos A, Rendell M, et al. The dawn phenomenon, an early morning glucose rise: implications for diabetic intraday blood glucose variation. Diabetes Care, 1982; Vol. 4: pp. 579–85.
Comments: This is the first description of the dawn phenomenon.

低血糖症：预防和治疗

Ari Eckman, MD, and Sherita Hill Golden, MD, MHS

定义
- 血糖水平 ≤ 70mg/dl（3.9mmol/L）。
- 临床上，出现低血糖的典型症状（震颤，出汗，心动过速或精神状态的变化），摄入碳水化合物可以纠正上述症状。
- 引起低血糖最常见的原因是胰岛素或口服降糖药过量，或摄食不足。

流行病学
- 在接受强化治疗的患者，严重的低血糖的风险增加三倍。
- 1型糖尿病患者平均每周经历2次症状性低血糖，每年会经历一次暂时性致残性低血糖。
- 在糖尿病控制和并发症试验（DCCT）中，强化治疗组有更多的患者至少会发生一次严重的低血糖（65% 比 35% 对照组），低血糖整体发生率分别是61%和19%。
- 危险因素：（1）1型糖尿病患者不仅胰岛素不足，而且对高胰岛素缺乏反应；（2）有低血糖病史，对低血糖不了解或者二者均有；（3）具有较低血糖控制目标的积极降糖治疗；（4）最近中度或剧烈运动；（5）饮食不规律；（6）睡眠；（7）肾衰。

诊断
- 有 Whipple 三联征：低血糖症状，血糖葡萄糖浓度低，血浆葡萄糖浓度升高后症状缓解。
  - 严重的低血糖：需要他人协助摄入碳水化合物，胰高血糖素或者需要复苏。可能发展为严重神经性低血糖从而诱发癫痫或昏迷。
  - 症状性低血糖：典型的低血糖症状，测量血糖浓度是 ≤ 70mg/dl（3.9mmol/L）。
  - 无症状低血糖：没有低血糖症状但是测量血糖浓度是 < 70mg/dl（3.9mmol/L）。
  - 可能是症状性低血糖：低血糖症状不伴血浆葡萄糖降低，可能是血浆葡萄糖浓度是 ≤ 70mg/dl（3.9mmol/L）引起的。不需测量血浆葡萄糖浓度，给予口服碳水化合物治疗低血糖症状。
  - 相对低血糖：典型的低血糖症状，可以用低血糖来解释，但是血浆葡萄糖浓度是 < 70mg/dl（3.9mmol/L）。长期血糖控制不佳的患者在血糖为 < 70mg/dl（3.9mmol/L）时或更低是容易发生低血糖症状。可能并没有直接的危害。
  - 低血糖性意识障碍：通过抑制交感肾上腺及症状性应答以降低前列腺素水平，这是周期性低血糖症所导致的一个结果。

症状和体征
- 可能并不特异。

低血糖症：预防和治疗

- 随着血糖水平下降，开始出现自主（肾上腺）症状，随着血糖水平进一步下降，随后出现神经低血糖症状（精神状态的改变）。
- 症状：出汗和面色苍白非常常见；心动过速和收缩压轻度升高，经常观察到神经性低血糖症状。
- 肾上腺素(自主)症状：心悸，焦虑，震颤，饥饿，感觉温暖，恶心，出汗。
- 神经性低血糖症状：乏力，头晕，头痛，视力障碍，嗜睡，说话费力，注意力不集中，行为异常，记忆减退，思考困难和/或混乱，惊厥，昏迷，甚至死亡。
- 偶尔、短暂的神经功能障碍的发生。永久性的神经损伤罕见。
- 如果患者不了解低血糖，可无症状。

临床治疗

预防

- 预防低血糖发生是最好的治疗方法（Cryer）。
- 患者亲密的朋友或亲戚应该了解低血糖预防战略。
- 积极治疗，包括（1）患者教育，（2）经常自我监测血糖（SMBG），（3）灵活的胰岛素和其他药物疗法，（4）个性化血糖控制目标，（5）持续的专业指导和支持。
- 考虑常规的风险因素和葡萄糖反调节受损的指标。
- 回顾自我血糖监测记录评估低血糖发生的频率和反调节是否充分，尤其对于要开始胰岛素强化治疗以前或者既往有低血糖病史的患者。
- 对于有严重低血糖或者低血糖造成损害的患者，特别是那些无症状的低血糖者，不要太积极的控制糖化血红蛋白的目标值。
- 不断重新评估患者血糖控制的益处及低血糖的风险。
- 医疗报警手镯以方便在急诊室快速治疗。
- 低血糖是促进降低糖化血红蛋白的限制因素。

无症状和有症状的低血糖事件的处理

- 患者应该随时可获得速效碳水化合物（葡萄糖片剂，硬糖，葡萄糖酱或加糖的果汁）。
- 自我血糖监测在 ≤ 70mg/dl（3.9mmol/L）——合理的自我治疗（吃葡萄糖片剂或含碳水化合物的果汁，软饮料，牛奶，糖果，小吃或吃饭）。
- 葡萄糖在成人的推荐剂量为20克（6盎司杯橙汁或可乐或4盎司杯葡萄汁）。
- 应该在15~20分钟内达到临床缓解。
- 因为口服葡萄糖的血糖反应持续大约只有2个小时，在初始治疗后应给予持续零食或者饮食。

严重低血糖的处理

- 训练朋友和亲戚识别和治疗低血糖。
- 朋友和家人应该了解到不要将任何东西放到不能坐起的患者嘴里，或者不要摄取食物和饮料，不要对反应迟钝的人进食蛋糕糊、糖等。
- 如果患者不能安全进食和喝水，使用注射胰高血糖素。

- 胰高血糖素：对于不能进食和喝水的患者，皮下或肌内注射 0.5~1.0mg。一般 10~15min 内恢复意识；可能会导致明显的恶心，60~90min 后高血糖。24 个小时后再给予一个剂量胰高血糖素。
- 定期检查胰高血糖素包，超出其到期日期时更换。
- 在医疗环境（急诊室、办公室、医院），立即给予 25ml 50% 葡萄糖静脉滴注。
- 随后给予葡萄糖输入（对于能进食的患者给予食物），取决于引起低血糖的原因。
- 如果患者可以安全进食应该给予食物。
- 可能需要住院长期治疗和观察。

随访

- 对不认识低血糖的患者，接受 2~3 周避免低血糖的建议，确定了解低血糖（Cryer）。
- 在短期内建立更高的血糖目标。
- 更频繁的自我监测血糖，特别是在驾驶或其他危险的活动之前。
- 对于严重低血糖，尤其是夜间和无症状低血糖，考虑持续血糖监测（见 626 页）。

专家意见

- 对低血糖的确定血糖控制的低限，这有潜在风险，有时是（很少）致命性的。
- 减少低血糖的频率和严重程度，特别是避免夜间低血糖。
- 为了避免低血糖矫枉过正以及反跳性高血糖，进一步治疗前等待 15~20 分钟。
- 低糖化血红蛋白（即 5.5%），可能会显示无法识别的低血糖事件，尤其是两餐之间或过夜，可能表明需要密切监测。

参考文献

Cryer PE, Axelrod L, Grossman AB, et al. Evaluation and management of adult hypoglycemic disorders: an endocrine Society Clinical Practice Guideline. J Clin endocrinol metab, 2009; Vol. 94: pp. 709–28.
Comments: Provides guidelines for evaluation and management of adults with hypoglycemic disorders, including those with diabetes mellitus.

Workgroup on hypoglycemia, american Diabetes association. Defning and reporting hypoglycemia in diabetes: a report from the american Diabetes association workgroup on hypoglycemia. Diabetes Care, 2005; Vol. 28: pp. 1245–9.
Comments: Important discussion on defnition and classifcation of hypoglycemic episodes.

Cryer Pe Diverse causes of hypoglycemia-associated autonomic failure in diabetes. neJm, 2004; Vol. 350: pp. 2272–9.
Comments: Discusses clinical problem of hypoglycemia in diabetes.

Cryer Pe, Davis Sn, Shamoon h. hypoglycemia in diabetes. Diabetes Care, 2003; Vol. 26: pp. 1902–12.
Comments: excellent discussion on benefts and approach to managing and

preventing hypoglycemic unawareness.

The Diabetes Control and Complications Trial Research Group. hypoglycemia in the Diabetes Control and Complications Trial. Diabetes, 1997; Vol. 46: pp. 271–86.

Comments: 65% of patients in the intensive group versus 35% of patients in conventional group had at least one episode of severe hypoglycemia; overall rates of severe hypoglycemia were 61.2 per 100 patient-years versus 18.7 per 100 patient-years in the intensive and conventional treatment groups, respectively, with a relative risk (RR) of 3.28. The relative risk for coma and/or seizure was 3.02 for intensive therapy.

The Diabetes Control and Complications Trial Research Group. The efect of intensive treatment of diabetes on the development and progression of long-term complications in insulin-dependent diabetes mellitus. neJm, 1993; Vol. 329: pp. 977–86.

Comments: In the Diabetes Control and Complications Trial, there was a progressive increase in the incidence of severe hypoglycemic episodes (per 100 patient-years) at lower attained hemoglobin a1c values during intensive insulin therapy in patients with type 1 diabetes.

夜间低血糖

Ari Eckman, MD, and Christopher D. Saudek, MD

定义
- 睡觉期间低血糖[≤70mg/dl(3.9mmol/L)]。
- 对血糖不确定但是出现症状情况下应该怀疑低血糖,如果出现症状和明确的低血糖时明确低血糖,如果低血糖症状严重需要另外一个人协助。

流行病学
- 在糖尿病控制和并发症试验(DCCT),43%的人发生了低血糖,其中55%在睡眠期间发生严重低血糖。
- 同样,在DCCT试验中,胰岛素强化治疗组发生严重低血糖的发生率比胰岛素普通治疗组增加3倍。
- 通常,尤其是在1型糖尿病患者中,血糖变异性大(Yale)。
- 低血糖的发生通常没有症状,不容易被识别,1型糖尿病大多数低血糖症状发生在后半夜(3AM~7AM)(Amin)。

诊断
- 危险因素包括:胰岛素或口服降糖药清楚减慢(例如:肝肾疾病),在晚餐时间使用中效(NPH)胰岛素;遗漏吃放;计划之外的运动;饮酒;感染;减少糖异生底物(例如:从恶病质);长效磺脲类药物,胰岛素合用口服降糖药;低血糖病史;无症状低血糖或者二者兼有;年龄。
- 如果进行Whipple试验诊断明确:低血糖症状及血糖降低,记录到血浆葡萄糖降低,纠正低血糖后上述症状缓解。

症状和体征
- 体征:面色苍白和出汗,心率增快和收缩压上升;低体温;严重时可有不能唤醒,短暂局灶性神经功能异常(例如:复视、偏瘫),或癫痫发作。合作伙伴可能会注意到其呼吸改变,烦躁。
- 症状:从无症状到严重症状,偶尔可以是致命的。患者经常从恶梦中惊醒,伴出汗。
- 神经症状:肾上腺素(儿茶酚胺介导的)——发抖,心悸,焦虑/觉醒;胆碱能——出汗、饥饿和感觉异常。
- 由于无症状低血糖或者睡眠期间意识抑制,也可以是没有症状的。

临床治疗
- 治疗的关键是早期发现。
- 如果患者不能做起来吃饭或者喝水,不要给予任何经口食物(例如果汁),这样可能会导致误吸。
- 对于清醒的患者,优先给予15~20g速效碳水化合物(例如含糖饮料、饼干、糖果和葡萄糖片)。
- 如果症状仍没有改善或者血葡萄糖仍低,自行再监测血糖15~20 min。
- 由于口服葡萄糖的血糖反应是短暂的(2小时),血糖升高后短期内给

夜间低血糖

- 予小吃或进食。
- 避免高脂肪，会延缓葡萄糖吸收。
- 如果患者不能坐起来喝液体，肌注胰高血糖素（1毫克，可以由非专业人士操作）或静脉注射葡萄糖（50%葡萄糖25毫升，由医疗保健专业人士操作）。
- 恶心呕吐是胰高血糖素常见的症状。
- 对于住院的患者，出院前要确保没有夜间低血糖的发生。

随访

- 改变治疗方案，以防止夜间低血糖的发生，减少夜间胰岛素或口服降糖药的剂量，或者睡觉时给予小吃。
- 向患者及其家人提供关于风险和减少风险策略的相关教育。
- 仔细规划膳食和运动。
- 避免晚饭前给予NPH胰岛素，或者在睡觉前给予速效/长效胰岛素，因为胰岛素将在睡眠时间达到峰值。
- 晚饭时使用速效胰岛素类似物（代替普通胰岛素）。
- 如果在睡前给予胰岛素，优选长效胰岛素。
- 如果持续出现夜间低血糖，尝试将睡前长效胰岛素类似物挪用到早晨使用。
- 避免过量饮酒。
- 认真贯彻执行血糖自我监测（SMBG），包括夜间血糖监测，以避免夜间低血糖。
- 强调在例行变化（例如加强在例行的变化，如更改时区、假日、休假）可能增加夜间低血糖的风险。
- 对无症状低血糖和频繁夜间低血糖的病人持续血糖监测是非常有用的。

专家意见

- 夜间低血糖仍然是需要强化血糖控制来避免糖尿病并发症的患者的一个非常大的障碍。
- 尽管夜间低血糖极少导致死亡，但是联合国的研究表明夜间低血糖占1型糖尿病患者意外死亡的50%（Tattersall）。因此需要严肃对待夜间低血糖。
- 夜间低血糖频繁发作可加重无症状低血糖的发生。
- 选择更为认真的胰岛素治疗方案或者使用胰岛素泵可以在不损害血糖控制目标的情况下降低夜间低血糖发生风险。
- 尽管被称为"黎明现象"，夜间低血糖不是晨起或者继发性高血糖的原因（除非过度治疗）（Tordjman；Hirsch）。
- 然而，一种常见的恶性循环是夜间低血糖，过度治疗低血糖，导致白天高血糖。

参考文献

Brunton Sa. nocturnal hypoglycemia: answering the challenge with long-acting insulin analogs. medGenmed, 2007; Vol. 9: p. 38.

Comments: Discusses prevalence, causes, and consequences of nocturnal hypoglycemia; detection and prevention strategies including use of long-acting insulin analogs, ofering more physiologic and predictable timeaction profles than traditional human basal insulin, associated with a lower risk for nocturnal hypoglycemia than NPH without sacrifcing glycemic control.

Workgroup on hypoglycemia, american Diabetes association. Defning and reporting hypoglycemia in diabetes: a report from the american Diabetes association workgroup on hypoglycemia. Diabetes Care, 2005; Vol. 28: pp. 1245–9.
Comments: Important discussion on defning and classifcation of hypoglycemic episodes.

Allen KV, Frier Bm. nocturnal hypoglycemia: clinical manifestations and therapeutic strategies toward preven- tion. endocr Pract, 2004; Vol. 9: pp. 530–43.
Comments: almost 50% of all episodes of severe hypoglycemia occur at night during sleep. Recurrent exposure to nocturnal hypoglycemia may impair cognitive function; other substantial long-term morbidity includes the development of acquired hypoglycemia syndromes, such as impaired awareness of hypoglycemia.

Gabriely I, Shamoon h. hypoglycemia in diabetes: common, often unrecognized. Cleve Clin J med, 2004; Vol. 71: pp. 335–42.
Comments: hypoglycemic episodes often go unrecognized, and over time, patients with diabetes may lose ability to sense hypoglycemia, increasing their risk.

Yale JF. nocturnal hypoglycemia in patients with insulin-treated diabetes. Diabetes Res Clin Pract, 2004; Vol 65 Suppl 1: pp. S41–6.
Comments: nocturnal hypoglycemia is a frequent event among patients with type 1 diabetes, while severe hypoglycemic episodes are approximately three times more likely in patients on intensive insulin therapy than in those on conventional therapy.

Cryer PE. Hypoglycemia: Pathophysiology, Diagnosis and Treatment. New York: Oxford University Press; 1997.
Comments: Textbook describing the diagnosis and treatment of hypoglycemia.

Tattersall RB, Gill GV. Unexplained deaths of type 1 diabetic patients. Diabet Med, 1991; Vol. 8: pp. 49–58.
Comments: A report from the UK indicating that about half of unexpected deaths in type 1 diabetes were compatible with nocturnal hypoglycemia.

The DCCT Research Group. Epidemiology of severe hypoglycemia in the diabetes control and complications trial. Am J Med, 1991; Vol. 90: pp. 450–9.
Comments: In the DCCT, intensive treatment of IDDM increased the frequency of severe hypoglycemia relative to conventional therapy. Severe hypoglycemia occurred more often during sleep (55%); 43% of all episodes occurred between midnight and 8 am.

Hirsch IB, Smith LJ, Havlin CE, et al. Failure of nocturnal hypoglycemia to cause daytime hyperglycemia in patients with IDDM. Diabetes Care, 1990; Vol. 13: pp. 133–42.
Comments: Demonstration that induced nocturnal hypoglycemia does not increase hyperglycemia throughout the following day.

Tordjman KM, Havlin CE, Levandoski LA, et al. Failure of nocturnal hypoglycemia to cause fasting hyperglycemia in patients with insulin-dependent diabetes mellitus. NEJM, 1987; Vol. 317: pp. 1552–9.
Comments: Demonstration that induced nocturnal hypoglycemia does not increase fasting blood glucose.

餐后低血糖

Ari Eckman, MD, and Christopher D. Saudek, MD

定义
- 在没有使用降糖药的情况下,餐后 2~5 小时出现低血糖(≤ 70mg/dl)及低血糖症状。
- 也称反应性低血糖。
- 高度争议和有争议的实体。

流行病学
- 口服葡萄糖耐量后 4~6 小时有 10% 的正常人血葡萄糖浓度 < 50mg/dl。
- 一个没有证实的观察显示,对于糖尿病前期或者早期糖尿病轻度 2 型糖尿病患者,由于胰岛素过多的胰岛素分泌延迟,可能导致餐后低血糖。
- 餐后低血糖通常出现在消瘦的人中,或者在极度体重下降的患者。
- 由于症状非特异而且在症状发生时很少测量血糖,所以很难确定患病率和发病率。
- 在减肥手术后可以见到这种现象,由于倾倒综合征或者 β – 细胞增生。

诊断
- Whipple 三联征:低血糖相关症状,证实的血葡萄糖降低,治疗低血糖后症状改善。
- 整夜禁食,然后进食(尽管引起低血糖),备好非必需药物,通过写 log 观察病人低血糖的症状和体征,如果不是必需,在实验完成前禁止给予治疗。
- 进食后的 300 分钟内每隔 30 分钟测量一次血浆葡萄糖。一些专家还建议如果血浆葡萄糖 < 60mg/dl(3.3mmol/L)测量分析胰岛素、C 肽和胰岛素前体。
- 混合餐实验(10 千卡 / 千克热量,45% 碳水化合物,15% 蛋白质,40% 脂肪)已经由于诊断,但是目前解释标准尚未建立。
- 通常不推荐口服葡萄糖耐量实验(Cryer),但是在糖尿病前期和早期糖尿病患者中是有帮助的。
- 要考虑人为低血糖的可能,通过仔细的用药史和在尿中筛查磺脲类药物排除。
- 胰岛素自身抗体在这些抗体更易出现的人群中有助于选择人群(例如亚洲)症状和体征。
- 自主神经症状:出汗、心悸、颤抖、饥饿、焦虑、虚弱、震颤、或大汗。
- 极少情况下会引起精神状态改变或死亡。
- 神经低血糖症状:混乱、嗜睡、讲话困难可能不是由于餐后低血糖引起的。

临床治疗
- 饮食是主要的治疗方法,可以成为诊断和治疗的一个简单方法。
- 预计症状出现的时间(例如上午晚些时候或者下午快到晚上),患者应该摄取含有少量碳水化合物的零食（15~30mg）。这样有助于避免血糖降低，而且如果有效，易于操作而且与餐后低血糖的诊断相符（Brun）
- 避免服用含糖过高的饮食，快速吸收的糖类，富含葡萄糖或者蔗糖的饮料。
- 避免含糖饮料与酒同饮，尤其是空腹状态。
- 一些专家建议，虽然目前仍然没有证实确切有效，在饮食中增加蛋白质或者可溶性膳食纤维可以减慢胃排空，降低胰岛素反应。
- 如果症状持续存在，可以试用一些药物：（1）α-葡萄糖苷酶抑制剂（阿卡波糖，米格列醇）延缓淀粉和蔗糖的消化；（2）二甲双胍，500~850mg 口服，与饭同服。
- 在特殊情况下，生长抑素类似物奥曲肽已被使用。
- 二氮嗪由于其水钠潴留、多毛症和消化功能紊乱等副作用不推荐使用。

随访
- 鼓励症状患者长期进行饮食管理。
- 不是前进的障碍。
- 尽管少见，也可以引起精神状态改变或者死亡。
- 通常能很好的响应饮食改变。
- 在一些极端病例中，需要使用药物。

专家意见
- 如前所述，餐后低血糖是个有争议的实体，由于机制不明，很难被证明。大多数专家在质疑它是否是个真正的疾病。
- 由于肾上腺能症状与简单焦虑症状相似，都是由相同激素引起的（儿茶酚胺），潜在的焦虑、抑郁或者精神疾病有可能被误诊为低血糖。
- 必须除外空腹低血糖，这是确定诊断的一个重要诊断（见60页）。
- 血糖经常低于基线水平，正常拮抗激素（肾上腺素、胰高血糖素）可以将血糖恢复到基线。争论是否是或者这个过程如何导致症状。
- 对大多数患者，简单的饮食治疗就足够了。

参考文献

Cryer Pe, Axelrod L, Grossman AB, et al. evaluation and management of adult hypoglycemic disorders: an endocrine Society Clinical Practice Guideline. J Clin endocrinol metab, 2009; Vol. 94: pp. 709–28.
Comments: Recent guidelines provided for evaluation of reactive hypoglycemia.

Brun JF, Fedou C, mercier J. Postprandial reactive hypoglycemia. Diabetes metab, 2000; Vol. 26: pp. 337–51.
Comments: Important to add small meals at the middle of morning and afternoon, when glycemia would start to decrease. If composition of the meal is adequate, fall in blood glucose can be prevented.

Ozgen aG, hamulu F, Bayraktar F, et al. Long-term treatment with acarbose for the treatment of reactive hypoglycemia. eat weight Disord, 1998; Vol. 3: pp. 136–40.

Comments: Study showing that acarbose may be of value in preventing and treating reactive hypoglycemia by reducing early hyperglycemic stimulus to insulin secretion.

Hofeldt FD. Reactive hypoglycemia. endocrinol metab Clin north am, 1989; Vol. 18: pp. 185–201.

Comments: most patients with symptoms following meals have another diagnosis other than reactive hypogly-cemia, including neuropsychiatric disease.

Lev-Ran a, anderson Rw. The diagnosis of postprandial hypoglycemia. Diabetes, 1981; Vol. 30: pp. 996–9.

Comments: many patients with postprandial adrenergic symptoms had similar symptoms following placebo administration in place of glucose.

糖尿病和急性疾病的院外管理

Nisa M. Maruthur, MD, MHS

定义
- 医疗条件的急性改变可以引起高血糖[包括糖尿病酮症酸中毒（DKA）和糖尿病高渗状态（HHS）]或者低血糖。
- 由于疾病的压力，胰岛素或者其他糖尿病药物治疗不充分，脱水或者甜的饮品摄入过多会导致高血糖。
- 低血糖可能是由于热量摄入减少，内源性生糖激素减少（例如肾上腺危象或者肝功能衰竭），葡萄糖利用增加（例如感染）或者胰岛素清除率减少（例如肾功能衰竭）等原因导致的。

流行病学
- 感染是引起DKA和HHS最常见的原因。
- 其他疾病的重要急性改变可以引起高血糖，包括外伤、中风、心肌梗死、酗酒和胰腺炎。
- 糖尿病患者因为感染等急性疾病需要经常住院。

诊断
- 任何急性疾病情况下都需要更频繁的监测血糖。
- 对DKA高危患者，需要监测尿或者血中的酮体。
- 用于治疗急性疾病的药物（糖皮质激素、噻嗪类利尿剂、交感神经能拟似药和非典型抗精神病药物）也可以导致高血糖。
- 某些抗生素（如喹诺酮类）可能会导致高血糖和低血糖。

症状和体征
- 评估DKA（见45页），HHS（见51页），低血糖（见60页）的体征。

临床治疗
- 明显的高血糖可能需要改变门诊治疗方案，例如增加短效胰岛素。
- 如果无法进食，呕吐或者精神状态改变：推荐去急诊评估是否有DKA和HHS。
- 总之，治疗糖尿病的药物（包括胰岛素）应该在急性疾病时继续使用，但是应该调整剂量。
- 急性疾病期间需要每4个小时监测一次血糖，并根据血糖结果调整药物剂量。
- 鼓励患者疾病的早期联系他们的医疗服务提供者，而不是到后期再联系。
- 在急性疾病期间应该用短效或者速效胰岛素代替长效胰岛素。
- 推荐永远使用退烧药。
- 尽量自己进食补充高热量饮料和盐。
- 在急性疾病期间频繁监测血糖的同时可以配合自行监测尿中和血中酮体。

糖尿病和急性疾病的院外管理

专家意见
- 由于患者高血糖或者低血糖需要改变门诊患者治疗方案是需要给予患者既往对不同疾病的反应的病史（例如有酮症病史）和现在的治疗方案进行个体化调节。
- 及时的门诊或者急诊室随访是在急性疾病后稳定血糖控制，避免酮症酸中毒必须的解决步骤。
- 医生对伴有急性疾病的糖尿病患者，尽量早期就转诊到急诊或收入院进行观察和治疗。

参考文献

American Diabetes Association. Standards of medical care in diabetes—2011. Diabetes Care, 2011; Vol. 34 Suppl 1: pp. S11–61.
Comments: Standards of medical care recommended by the American Diabetes Association.

Aspinall SL, Good CB, Jiang R, et al. Severe dysglycemia with the fluoroquinolones: a class effect? Clin Infect Dis, 2009; Vol. 49: pp. 402–8.
Comments: VA study of over 1.2 million patients evaluating the effect of quinolone antibiotics on hyper- and hypoglycemia.

Weber C, Kocher S, Neeser K, et al. Prevention of diabetic ketoacidosis and self-monitoring of ketone bodies: an overview. Curr Med Res Opin, 2009; Vol. 25: pp. 1197–207.
Comments: Review of self-monitoring of ketones for preventing ketoacidosis in insulin-dependent diabetes.

Kitabchi AE, Umpierrez GE, Miles JM, et al. Hyperglycemic crises in adult patients with diabetes. Diabetes Care, 2009; Vol. 32: pp. 1335–43.
Comments: American Diabetes Association consensus statement, which includes discussion of sick day management.

Kitabchi AE, Umpierrez GE, Murphy MB, et al. Hyperglycemic crises in diabetes. Diabetes Care, 2004; Vol. 27 Suppl 1: pp. S94–102.
Comments: American Diabetes Association position statement on the management of diabetic ketoacidosis and hyperosmolar hyperglycemic state.

American Diabetes Association, American Psychiatric Association, American Association of Clinical Endocrinologists, et al. Consensus development conference on antipsychotic drugs and obesity and diabetes. Diabetes Care, 2004; Vol. 27: pp. 596–601.
Comments: Consensus statement concluding that clozapine and olanzapine increase risk of diabetes.

Cryer PE, Davis SN, Shamoon H. Hypoglycemia in diabetes. Diabetes Care, 2003; Vol. 26: pp. 1902–12.
Comments: Unstructured review of hypoglycemia including detailed description of pathophysiology.

日常预防保健

Nisa M.Maruthur, MD, MHS

定义
- 预防干预糖尿病的并发症,包括微血管并发症(糖尿病视网膜病变、糖尿病肾病、神经病变),大血管并发症(心血管疾病),感染性疾病,牙周疾病和癌症。

流行病学
- 相对于常规治疗的糖尿病患者,控制多种危险因素(控制血糖、高血压、高脂血症,使用阿司匹林治疗,戒烟)可以使死亡率下降46%,心血管死亡和事件分别下降57%和59%,微血管并发症下降55%(Gaede)。
- 流感和肺炎链球菌性肺炎与糖尿病高死亡率相关。
- 糖尿病易频繁并发牙周疾病,从而恶化血糖控制。
- 糖尿病增加癌症风险,包括乳腺癌(RR=1.2),结肠癌(RR=1.3),并增加癌症病人的全因死亡率(RR=1.4)。

诊断
- 糖化血红蛋白:如果改变治疗方案或者患者血糖尚未达标,每3个月查一次,对于血糖控制稳定的患者每6个月查一次。
- 自我血糖监测:对于每天多次注射胰岛素或者使用胰岛素泵的患者每天至少监测3次血糖,对于其他需要治疗指导的患者可以监测频率少些。
- 连续血糖监测:对于血糖比较脆的糖尿病患者非常有用。
- 血压:每个糖尿病患者日常随访的项目。
- 空腹血脂:至少每年测一次。
- 尿白蛋白排泄率:自糖尿病确诊后,对于1型糖尿病患者,每年监测一次(例如尿白蛋白肌酐比),对于2型糖尿病患者每5年监测一次。
- 血肌酐:每年监测评估肾小球率过滤。
- 眼科评估:1型糖尿病确诊5年后开始评估,2型糖尿病确诊后开始评估。
- 足部检查:每年检查(1)远端对称性多发性神经病变:针刺感觉,震动感,跟腱反射,单丝测试;(2)外周动脉疾病:间歇性跛行评估,远端脉搏检查(例如足背动脉和胫后动脉)。
- 自主神经评估:每年提供病史并且进行体格检查。
- 抑郁、焦虑和老年痴呆:在糖尿病患者日常随访过程中进行筛查,有且是对于坚持或者自我管理比较担心的患者。
- 根据年龄适当进行肿瘤筛查:美国预防服务工作组(http://WWW.ahrq.gov/CLINIC/uspstfix.htm)。
- 评估10年心血管疾病(CVD)风险:在常规糖尿病随访时评估(见心血管疾病的筛查和管理,203页)。

症状和体征

- 眼耳鼻喉症状:听力丧失,视敏度下降,复视,暗点,视物模糊,头晕,轻度头痛。
- 心血管症状:胸痛,运动受限,心悸,麻木,刺痛感,乏力,间歇性跛行。
- 肺部症状:气短,端坐呼吸,白天嗜睡或者疲劳。
- 胃肠道:便秘,恶心,腹痛。
- 泌尿系统:勃起功能障碍,膀胱功能障碍,尿路感染,小便失禁,泡沫尿。
- 四肢:足部溃疡,手部/足部疼痛,麻木,刺痛。
- 体位性低血压:从坐位到站位,收缩压下降大于20mmHg,舒张压下降大于10mmHg,这可能表明植物神经功能紊乱,但也可能与用药有关(例如利尿剂)(JNC7)。
- 精神方面:情绪变化,能量水平变化。

临床治疗

- 血糖控制(ADA规定糖化血红蛋白目标<7%,IDF是<6.5%):为了减少糖尿病微血管和大血管并发症。应该强化给予药物以达到糖化血红蛋白的目标值(见2型糖尿病:序贯疗法,194页,1型糖尿病:胰岛素治疗,177页)。
- 生活方式建议:(1)体力活动(见体力活动和锻炼,119页;高血压或者低血糖,糖尿病肾病,糖尿病神经病变可能限制体力活动);(2)饮食。建议减少体重的7%~10%(见营养:关于糖尿病的综述,102页)。
- 血脂控制(目标值LDL-C<100mg/dl,对于冠脉事件高危并认可<70mg/dl):如果患者有已知的心血管疾病或者40岁以上,有1个心血管疾病的危险因素,不管血脂水平如何,建议使用HMG辅酶A还原酶抑制剂(他汀类)。
- 高血压(血压目标<130/80mmHg):测量高于这个值应该进行进一步的评估和管理。
- ACEI:推荐用于以下患者:(1)已知的心血管疾病;(2)微量或大量蛋白尿(使用ACEI或ARB)。
- β受体阻滞剂:建议用于有既往心肌梗死至少2年的病人。
- 戒烟:对于心血管疾病预防,提供戒烟治疗,以5A模式咨询患者:询问(ask),建议(advise),评估(assess),帮助(assist),安排(arrange)。治疗药物包括尼古丁替代治疗,安非他酮,瓦伦尼克林(www.surgeongeneral.gov/tobacco)。
- 阿司匹林(75~162mg/d):用于心血管疾病的一级或二级预防。一级预防指征:在没有高出血风险的情况下(尤其是男性50岁,女性60岁)有一个危险因素(高血压,家族史,血脂异常,微量蛋白尿,早发CVD家族史或吸烟),10年心血管疾病(CVD)风险10%。对没有CVD但是10年风险中危(5%~10%)考虑使用阿司匹林。对没有CVD的低危患者不推荐一级预防使用阿司匹林(例如没有危险因素,10年风险5%)。二级预防的指征:有CVD的患者,如果对阿司匹林过敏可考虑使用氯吡格雷。

- 足部护理：如果患者吸烟，有神经功能障碍或者事先有脚病，建议转诊到足科医生。
- 疫苗：推荐使用肺炎和流感疫苗。

随访
- 患者需要至少3个月进行一次糖尿病专科随访。如果血糖控制稳定，可以延长随访间期（尤其对饮食控制良好的2型糖尿病患者）。

专家意见
- 糖尿病患者的日常管理是多方面的，管理计划中包括患者本人、家人、医生、护士、营养师和其他健康护理专家。
- 如果执行有效，日常预防管理可以延缓糖尿病患者并发症的发生并保持患者生命质量。
- 根据估计CVD风险，指南已经更新，推荐阿司匹林用于CVD一级预防。美国糖尿病协会发布会描述了多种心血管疾病的风险预测(1.http://www.dtu.ox.ac.uk/riskengine/index.php, 2. http://www.aricnews.net/riskcalc/html/RC1.html, 3. http://www.diabetes.org/living-with-diabetes/complications/diabetes-phd/)。

参考文献

American Diabetes Association. Standards of medical care in diabetes—2011. Diabetes Care, 2011; Vol. 34 Suppl 1: pp. S11–61.
Comments: Standards of medical care recommended by the American Diabetes Association.

Pignone M, Alberts MJ, Colwell JA, et al. Aspirin for primary prevention of cardiovascular events in people with diabetes: a position statement of the American Diabetes Association, a scientific statement of the American Heart Association, and an expert consensus document of the American College of Cardiology Foundation. Diabetes Care, 2010; Vol. 33: pp. 1395–402.
Comments: Statement from American Diabetes Association, American Heart Association, and American College of Cardiology Foundation on the use of aspirin for primary prevention in diabetes.

Gaede P, Lund-Andersen H, Parving HH, et al. Effect of a multifactorial intervention on mortality in type 2 diabetes. NEJM, 2008; Vol. 358: pp. 580–91.
Comments: Observational follow-up of the Steno-2 Trial participants (patients with diabetes and microalbuminuria) showing benefit of control of multiple risk factors in preventing death, cardiovascular morbidity, and mortality and microvascular complications.

Demmer RT, Jacobs DR, Desvarieux M. Periodontal disease and incident type 2 diabetes: results from the First National Health and Nutrition Examination Survey and its epidemiologic follow-up study. Diabetes Care, 2008; Vol. 31: pp. 1373–9.
Comments: Study based on National Health and Nutritional Examination Survey evaluating the relationship between periodontal disease and diabetes risk.

Barone BB, Yeh HC, Snyder CF, et al. Long-term all-cause mortality in cancer patients with preexisting diabetes mellitus: a systematic review and meta-analysis. JAMA, 2008; Vol.

300: pp. 2754–64.
Comments: Meta-analysis establishing link between diabetes and all-cause mortality in cancer patients.

Mealey BL, Oates TW, American Academy of Periodontology. Diabetes mellitus and periodontal diseases. J Periodontol, 2006; Vol. 77: pp. 1289–303.
Comments: Review (unstructured) commissioned by the American Academy of Periodontology describing the bidirectional relationship between periodontal disease and diabetes.

Larsson SC, Orsini N, Wolk A. Diabetes mellitus and risk of colorectal cancer: a meta-analysis. J Natl Cancer Inst, 2005; Vol. 97: pp. 1679–87.
Comments: Meta-analysis of observational studies evaluating the relationship between obesity and colon cancer risk.

US Dept of Health and Human Services. The seventh report of the Joint National Committee on Prevention, Detection, Evaluation, and Treatment of High Blood Pressure. NIH Publication No. 04-5230, August 2004.
Comments: Report of epidemiology, diagnosis, and management of hypertension.

Gaede P, Vedel P, Larsen N, et al. Multifactorial intervention and cardiovascular disease in patients with type 2 diabetes. NEJM, 2003; Vol. 348: pp. 383–93.
Comments: Main results of Steno-2 Trial in which modification of multiple risk factors reduced risk of macroand microvascular complications in patients with type 2 diabetes and microalbuminuria.

Smith SA, Poland GA. Use of influenza and pneumococcal vaccines in people with diabetes. Diabetes Care, 2000; Vol. 23: pp. 95–108.
Comments: Technical review from the American Diabetes Association reviewing the epidemiology and response to vaccinations for influenza and pneumococcal pneumonia in diabetes.

UK Prospective Diabetes Study Group. Tight blood pressure control and risk of macrovascular and microvascular complications in type 2 diabetes: UKPDS 38. BMJ, 1998; Vol. 317: pp. 703–13.
Comments: Randomized trial (UK Prospective Diabetes Study Group 38) showing benefit of tight compared to less tight blood pressure control on diabetes complications.

Patel A, ADVANCE Collaborative Group, MacMahon S, et al. Effects of a fixed combination of perindopril and indapamide on macrovascular and microvascular outcomes in patients with type 2 diabetes mellitus (the ADVANCE trial): a randomised controlled trial. Lancet, 2007; Vol. 370: pp. 829–40.
Comments: Results of blood-pressure lowering regimen (perindopril + indapamide) from the ADVANCE Trial, a factorial trial, which evaluated the effect of blood pressure-lowering and glycemic control on vascular disease in diabetes.

Larsson SC, Mantzoros CS, Wolk A. Diabetes mellitus and risk of breast cancer: a meta-analysis. Int J Cancer, 2007; Vol. 121: pp. 856–62.
Comments: Meta-analysis of observational studies evaluating the relationship between obesity and breast cancer risk.

糖尿病疫苗指导

Nisa M. Maruthur, MD, MHS

定义
- 根据免疫实践咨询委员会（ACIP）指南，建议可以通过接种疫苗预防的传染病控制。

流行病学
- 糖尿病患者合并如感染或者其他慢性疾病等因素增加其感染的风险和死亡率。
- 糖尿病患者伴随流感和肺炎球菌感染与高死亡风险相关（Smith）。
- 对于糖尿病患者，流感疫苗使住院风险减少54%，死亡风险减少58%（Looijmans-Van）。但是肺炎球菌疫苗遗憾的没有得出这项临床结果。
- 每年接种流感疫苗可能减少心血管疾病发病率和死亡率(Davis)。
- 糖尿病患者肺炎球菌疫苗的使用率在美国可能低于38%（Resnick），在总人群中估计的流感疫苗使用率波动在33%~75%（Kilmer）。

临床治疗

治疗
- 疾病控制和预防建议每个中心使用年龄特异性成人免疫接种时间表（特异性时间表见于：http://www.cdc.gov/mmwr/PDF/wk/mm5753-Immunization.pdf）。

流感——糖尿病的具体治疗建议
- 每年接种疫苗。
- 两个版本的流感疫苗：注射（灭活）疫苗和吸入（存活）疫苗，两种类型对糖尿病患者来说都是安全的。每种类型都可以引起轻微的症状，但是不是流感染。灭活疫苗注射的副作用：红斑、肿胀、注射部位疼痛。两种疫苗都可以上呼吸道感染症状(例如发热、肌痛)，更严重(但是罕见)的风险包括危及生命的过敏反应和格林-巴利综合症（在20世纪70年代的灭活猪疫苗中发生）(http://www.cdc.gov/vaccines/vac-gen/side-efects.htm#fu)。
- 每年10月份左右可以注射流感疫苗。

链球菌性肺炎——糖尿病特殊的治疗建议
- 65岁以前，接种一次肺炎球菌多糖疫苗。
- 65岁以后，没有接种肺炎球菌疫苗病史的，单次接种肺炎球菌多糖疫苗（没有必要重复接种疫苗）。
- 如果65岁以前接种过疫苗，每隔5年后再次接种一次。

专家建议
- 初级保健诊所应考虑疫苗接种策略，以确保适当坚持接种时间。
- 应当指出，肺炎疫苗只能预防肺炎链球菌引起的肺炎。

糖尿病疫苗指导

- 糖尿病患者应当常规接受如前所述的季节性流感疫苗和肺炎疫苗。
- 疾病预防控制中心在其网站提供了疫苗的具体目标建议。

参考文献

MMWR Adult Schedule, CDC 2009 Centers for Disease Control and Prevention. Recommended adult immunization schedule—United States, 2009. MMWR, 2009; Vol. 57: pp. Q1–4.
Comments: Centers for Disease Control and Prevention vaccination guidelines, 2009. Approved by Advisory Committee on Immunization Practices, the American Academy of Family Physicians, the American College of Obstetricians and Gynecologists, and the American College of Physicians.

Fiore AE, Shay DK, Broder K, et al. Prevention and control of seasonal influenza with vaccines: recommendations of the Advisory Committee on Immunization Practices (ACIP), 2009 MMWR Recomm Rep, 2009; Vol. 58: pp. 1–52.
Comments: Updated review of influenza vaccination from Centers for Disease Control and Prevention.

Kilmer G, Roberts H, Hughes E, et al. Surveillance of certain health behaviors and conditions among states and selected local areas—Behavioral Risk Factor Surveillance System (BRFSS), United States, 2006. MMWR Surveill Summ, 2008; Vol. 57: pp. 1–188.
Comments: Provides national estimates of influenza vaccination in the general population (in addition to other health behaviors).

Looijmans-Van den Akker I, Verheij TJ, Buskens E, et al. Clinical effectiveness of first and repeat influenza vaccination in adult and elderly diabetic patients. Diabetes Care, 2006; Vol. 29: pp. 1771–6.
Comments: Nested-case control study from PRISMA (Prospective, Randomized Trial on Intensive Self-Monitoring Blood Glucose Management Added Value in Non-Insulin Treated Type 2 Diabetes Mellitus Patients) conducted in the Netherlands to evaluate the effect of influenza vaccination on hospitalization and death in patients with diabetes.

Davis MM, Taubert K, Benin AL, et al. Influenza vaccination as secondary prevention for cardiovascular disease: a science advisory from the American Heart Association and the American College of Cardiology. J Am Coll Cardiol, 2006; Vol. 48: pp. 1498–502.
Comments: Science advisory from AHA/ACC regarding influenza vaccination for secondary prevention of CVD.

Resnick HE, Foster GL, Bardsley J, et al. Achievement of American Diabetes Association clinical practice recommendations among U.S. adults with diabetes, 1999–2002: the National Health and Nutrition Examination Survey. Diabetes Care, 2006; Vol. 29: pp. 531–7.
Comments: Study of patients with diabetes meeting general clinical recommendations (from 1999–2002: The National Health and Nutrition Examination Survey).

Smith SA, Poland GA. Use of influenza and pneumococcal vaccines in people with diabetes. Diabetes Care, 2000; Vol. 23: pp. 95–108.
Comments: Technical review from the American Diabetes Association of influenza and pneumococcal pneumonia epidemiology and response to vaccination in diabetes.

医院管理和外科手术

医院糖尿病管理

Joanne Dintzis, CRNP, CDE, and Sherita Hill Golden, MD, MHS

概述
- 住院病人的管理目标:控制血糖水平,提高糖尿病患者的预后,减少低血糖和医源性的高血糖血症(如糖尿病酮症酸中毒)。
- 对于危重患者,2009 年 AACE/ADA 推荐:使用静脉注射(IV)胰岛素控制血糖水平在 140~180mg/dl(不再推荐目标血糖水平低于 110mg/dl)(Moghissi)。
- 对于非危重患者,2009 年 AACE/ADA 推荐:餐前血糖控制在 140mg/dl 以下,随机血糖低于 180mg/dl;若随机血糖高于 100mg/dl 需重新考虑胰岛素治疗方案;若随机血糖低于 70mg/dl,降糖方案不必强化。

流行病学
- 可以引起血糖升高的因素有:感染,伤口愈合受损,肾功能衰竭,器官功能衰竭移植的风险以及整体死亡率。
- 导致血糖不稳定的医疗因素有:感染,肾功能衰竭,营养不良,高龄,类固醇和其他药物,损害糖代谢。
- 碳水化合物饲管,肠外营养,静脉给药等补充葡萄糖的方案常常会引起血糖升高。
- 绝食、厌食或喂养困难,是营养中断的常见原因,使患者处于低血糖风险状态。

临床治疗
- 口服降糖药物。
- 合并某些急性疾病时,使用口服药物有许多禁忌(图 2-1)。
- 一般建议患者在住院期间停止口服制剂。

图 2-1 口服降糖药物的禁忌证

住院病人口服降糖药的使用禁忌/注意事项：请注意许多禁忌证，会使得病情向不可预料的方向发展，因此一般推荐在住院期间停止口服降糖药物。

二甲双胍：禁忌证：（1）血清肌酐大于 1.5 mg/dl（男），大于 1.4mg/dl（女）；（2）需要药物控制的充血性心力衰竭；（3）代谢性酸中毒，包括酮症酸中毒；（4）低灌注；（5）涉及使用碘造影剂的研究，因停止使用或者在术前 48 小时停止使用。在肾功能重新评估正常后才能继续使用。警告：老年人。

磺脲类药物：禁忌证：酮症酸中毒；禁食状态。警告：有持续或者严重低血糖风险。禁忌时间的长短因人而异，尤其是肝肾功能受损的老年人。

噻唑烷二酮类：禁忌证：慢性心力衰竭。警告：会引起血容量增加，造成慢性心力衰竭的。与骨折有一定关联。罗格列酮与心肌梗死的风险相关，但吡格列酮可能不会。如果 ALT 大于正常值的上限 2.5。起效慢（6 星期）。

由 Joanne Dintzis 和 Sherita Hill Golden 提供

静脉滴注胰岛素

- 使用静脉滴注胰岛素控制危重患者的高血糖，以及所有糖尿病酮症酸中毒（diabetic ketoacidosis, DKA）患者或高渗高血糖状态（hyperglycemic hyperosmolar status, HHS）。
- 围手术期患者推荐使用静脉滴注胰岛素制剂控制血糖，尤其是需要高剂量激素冲击治疗的患者或皮下注射胰岛素治疗无反应的患者。
- 管理静脉滴注胰岛素的书面或电脑方案，根据血糖波动情况和胰岛素的使用剂量调节胰岛素的输注速率（通常按每小时计算）。

皮下注射胰岛素制剂

- 非危重患者：推荐根据血糖浮动调节皮下胰岛素注射的剂量，疗效明确，降低高血糖和低血糖的风险。
- 根据每日总剂量胰岛素（total daily dose, TDD）的概念，生理性胰岛素给药建议包括基础胰岛素剂量，餐时胰岛素剂量和校正胰岛素剂量（图 2-2 和 2-3）。
- 胰岛素缺乏患者（1 型糖尿病，胰腺切除术后，或在家中接受胰岛素 5 年的 2 型糖尿病患者）：在任何时候都使用基础胰岛素，即使不接受营养，也需防止酮症酸中毒的发生。
- 胰岛素的基础剂量通常是 40%~50% 的 TDD；若患者禁食，饮食不佳，或低血糖，需考虑减少 20%~40% 的基础剂量。
- 胰岛素缺乏的患者，如果正常饮食，需要餐时胰岛素剂量，通常为 10%~20% TDD；如果患者禁食或摄入少于 50% 的碳水化合物，停止使用餐时胰岛素剂量。
- 对于新发高血糖，或在家通过饮食或者口服降糖药控制血糖的 2 型糖尿病患者：给予最初的校正胰岛素剂量（按比例快速计算，参见图 2-4），然而，不建议长期单独使用按比例增减胰岛素剂量的方法控制血糖。

图 2-2. 胰岛素每天总剂量的计算方法*

家庭方案	入院前 24 小时总的皮下胰岛素注射剂量总和	推测 24 小时静脉输入胰岛素的剂量总和	按体重计算（若是住院患者，只用于初次使用胰岛素的 1 型糖尿病患者）
家庭常用的胰岛素类型的剂量总和，例如： • 所有中效胰岛素和常规胰岛素剂量。 • 所有混合型胰岛素剂量（70/30，75/25）。 • 所有长效（甘精胰岛素或地特胰岛素）和所有速效胰岛素（诺和锐或优泌乐）。	可以从患者的病历里得到	通过稳定的 6 小时静脉输入剂量来推算	0.3~0.5（病人体重按千克计算）

*指南推荐使用每天总剂量（total daily dose, TDD）。每天总剂量包括 24 小时内输入的基础-餐时胰岛素和校正胰岛素的总和。
由 Joanne Dintzis 和 Sherita Hill Golden 提供。

图 2-3. 生理性胰岛素剂量的组成

基础胰岛素	餐时胰岛素 (正餐或者用餐时间)	校正胰岛素
定时 预设剂量：满足胰岛素的持续需求并抑制肝糖原的分解。	预设剂量：满足碳水化合物的吸收。 · 速效胰岛素。 · 短效胰岛素。	PRN：当血糖大于 150 mg/dl 给予。 · 速效胰岛素。 · 短效胰岛素。 · 根据胰岛素的活跃程度制定分级量表。
类型 · 长效胰岛素，每天使用。 · 中效胰岛素，注射两次。	TDD 减去基础胰岛素的剂量： · 每餐分开使用。 · 如果病人食用的食物中包含至少 50% 的碳水化合物，可以在早餐、午餐和晚餐时给予。	当病人在进餐时，结合餐时胰岛素决定剂量。 如果患者规律的需要校正胰岛素，调整基础胰岛素和餐前胰岛素的剂量。
计算 TDD 的 40%~50%。		

由 Joanne Dintzis 和 Sherita Hill Golden 提供。

- 如果患者每 24 小时需要校正后的胰岛素剂量 20 个单位，或者校正后血糖仍持续升高，建议患者加入基础胰岛素剂量和 / 或餐时胰岛素。
- 如果高血糖持续不下，总校正后的胰岛素量超过过去 24 小时内估算的胰岛素总量，那么基础剂量增加校正后胰岛素总量的 50%；餐时胰岛素剂量增加校正后胰岛素总量的 15%。如果发生低血糖，TDD 减少 20%。考虑切换到一个不太激进的校正方案。

皮下外源性胰岛素泵
- 在家中使用胰岛素泵的患者可能有精神状态的变化，由于止痛药的使用，剥夺睡眠，医源性谵妄，严重的生理应激可以阻碍胰岛素泵的安全自我管理。
- 为了确保住院期间胰岛素泵的安全使用，需要建立系统化的方法筛选患者的禁忌证，对医护人员进行明确和详细的指引，以确保在泵发生故障的情况下能有效的处理。
- 机构的政策应明确安全措施以及患者、护士、处方者和药房的职责。
- 由护士观察患者的自我血糖监测，胰岛素的使用以及相关文档，并在病历做记录。

图 2-4 校正胰岛素的剂量方案

	低剂量算法（每天使用胰岛素少于 40 单位的患者）		中等剂量算法（每天使用胰岛素 40 至 80 单位的患者）		高剂量算法（每天使用胰岛素大于 80 单位的患者）	
	血糖	校正胰岛素 按低血糖治疗	血糖	校正胰岛素 按低血糖治疗	血糖	校正胰岛素 按低血糖治疗
餐后	0~60 mg/dl	0 单位	0~60 mg/dl	0 单位	0~60 mg/dl	0 单位
	61~120 mg/dl	1 单位	61~120 mg/dl	1 单位	61~120 mg/dl	2 单位
	121~170 mg/dl	2 单位	121~150 mg/dl	2 单位	121~160 mg/dl	4 单位
	171~220 mg/dl	3 单位	151~180 mg/dl	3 单位	161~200 mg/dl	6 单位
	221~270 mg/dl	4 单位	181~210 mg/dl	4 单位	201~240 mg/dl	8 单位
	271~320 mg/dl	5 单位并且 NHO	211~240 mg/dl	5 单位	241~280 mg/dl	10 单位
	>320 mg/dl		241~270 mg/dl	6 单位	281~320 mg/dl	12 单位并且 NHO*
			271~300 mg/dl	7 单位	>320 mg/dl	
			301~330 mg/dl	8 单位并且 NHO		
			>330 mg/dl			
睡前	0~60 mg/dl	0 单位	0~60 mg/dl	0 单位	0~60 mg/dl	0 单位
	61~250 mg/dl	1 单位	61~250 mg/dl	2 单位	61~250 mg/dl	4 单位
	251~300 mg/dl	2 单位	251~280 mg/dl	3 单位	251~290 mg/dl	5 单位
	301~350 mg/dl	3 单位并且 NHO	281~310 mg/dl	4 单位	291~350 mg/dl	6 单位并且 NHO
	>350 mg/dl		311~350 mg/dl	5 单位并且 NHO	>350 mg/dl	
			>350 mg/dl			

注意：睡前校正胰岛素的方案比较保守（也就是说，目标血糖为 250 mg/dl 或者更高）

营养注意事项

- 住院经常以意想不到的方式破坏营养：例如意想不到的禁食，喂养管的故障，提供肠外营养的线路故障。对于这些事件，基础/营养/校正的胰岛素剂量可以提高病人的安全性。
- 制定餐时胰岛素治疗的计划书，在碳水化合物摄入的同时，维持血糖正常，如果中断碳水化合物的摄入，则停止餐时胰岛素的给予，从而减少低血糖的危险。
- 患者进食或胃管喂养：速效胰岛素类似物比普通胰岛素更好的控制碳水化合物方面的吸收，改善血糖控制和减少早餐和午餐剂量之间胰岛素"堆积"的风险，从而减少下午低血糖的风险（图2-5）。
- 禁食状态：如果病人处在禁食状态，则考虑减少基础胰岛素剂量（例如20%~40%）；中断餐时胰岛素的供应，继续给予餐时胰岛素剂量。
- 持续性管饲营养：与不连续的进餐相比，持续肠内营养的血糖反应是相当大的；每隔4~6小时给予固定剂量的短期或速效餐时胰岛素治疗，从而达到血糖目标。如果管饲营养结束，中断餐时胰岛素的供应，减少低血糖的危险。胰岛素缺乏的患者还需继续接受皮下基础胰岛素和校正胰岛素治疗（Gottschlich）。
- 持续性肠外营养：与不连续的进餐相比，持续肠外营养的血糖反应是相当大的。可以将胰岛素加入肠外营养配方中，提供与碳水化合物混合的餐时胰岛素。如果停止肠外营养，餐时胰岛素也自动停止，从而减少低血糖的危险。胰岛素缺乏的患者还需继续接受皮下基础胰岛素和校正胰岛素治疗（Gottschlich）
- 循环的营养方案（肠内或肠外）：可以从内分泌专家或肠外/肠内营养专家获得有效的个性化治疗。

患者宣教

- 由于住院期间血糖控制方案变化显著，出院时需详细书写出院说明，内容包括后续1个月内，通过血糖仪监测血糖，使用血糖日志，并要求患者当血糖低于70mg/dl，高于300mg/dl，或4个连续的读数高达200mg/dl时，需立即联系血糖医疗服务者。
  - 诊断糖尿病的相关血糖水平；
  - 血糖监测：血糖检测仪，何时测试血糖，随机血糖的目标范围，如何得到帮助；
  - 低血糖意识：症状体征，治疗，安全转移，通知家属；
  - 一贯的饮食习惯，基本的膳食计划；
  - 何时以及如何采取降糖药物：口服药物，胰岛素；
  - 病态的日常管理；
  - 正确使用和处置针头和注射器。

图 2-5 进食或饲管营养患者的皮下胰岛素使用

例子	糖尿病类型	推荐胰岛素使用组合	基础胰岛素	餐时胰岛素	校正胰岛素
胰岛素缺乏的患者	• 1型糖尿病 • 胰腺全切术后 • 2型糖尿病使用家庭胰岛素大于5年 • 使用餐时胰岛素治疗（包括bid混合胰岛素或者bid中效胰岛素/速效胰岛素制剂）	• 基础胰岛素 • 餐时胰岛素 • 校正胰岛素	• 如果使用长效胰岛素，每天同一时间每隔4小时给予TDD的40%胰岛素。 • 如果使用中效胰岛素，早餐时给予20%的TDD胰岛素剂量，睡前给予20%TDD胰岛素剂量。	使用TDD的60%胰岛素剂量。根据餐次分量以满足不同剂量以满足餐后血糖控制。每餐给予速效胰岛素。 或者 如果患者在家里使用这种方法，可以使用碳水化合物比例来决定餐时胰岛素的剂量。	制定用餐时和睡前的速效校正胰岛素方案。睡前方案比较保守（也就是说，目标血糖水平250 mg/dl 根据TDD选择方案: 小于40单位TDD=低剂量 41~80单位TDD=中剂量 大于80单位TDD=高剂量

图 2-5 进食或饲管营养患者的皮下胰岛素使用（续）

例子	糖尿病类型	推荐胰岛素使用组合	基础胰岛素	餐时胰岛素	校正胰岛素
非胰岛素缺乏的患者	• 在家不需要胰岛素治疗的 2 型糖尿病 • 糖尿病患者的急性高血糖	• 早期治疗：校正胰岛素剂量 • 每日评估血糖水平后，根据需要加用基础和餐时胰岛素治疗	每天检测以下项目以决定是否使用： • 血糖水平（坚持一如既往的评估） • 24 小时内要求的校正胰岛素剂量 • 如果患者 24 小时内给予 20 单位校正胰岛素，血糖仍居高不下，可以加用 40% 的 TDD 基础胰岛素剂量	每天检测血糖水平以决定是否使用。如果加用基础胰岛素之后，血糖仍居高不下，可以考虑加用餐时胰岛素。	起初在用餐时给予低剂量胰岛素，睡前给予诺和锐的治疗方案，如果 24 小时后检测血糖仍居高不下，则考虑： • 以 TDD 为指南，换用更为强效的校正剂量 • 加用基础胰岛素

由 Joanne Dintzis 和 Sherita Hill Golden 提供.

- 以下几个方面应在出院前（图 2-6）进行审查和处理：

图 2-6 出院前需要回顾和注意的各项条目

1. 糖尿病诊断的理解程度
2. 血糖监测
a. 方法
b. 监测时间
c. 血糖监测目标
d. 获取供应
3. 警惕低血糖
a. 症状
b. 治疗
c. 安全驾驶
d. 通知卫生保健人员
4. 出院后糖尿病的护理，需与提供糖尿病护理相关反馈信息的卫生保健人员约定好
a. 何时通知卫生保健人员（例如：告知血糖参数的设置）
b. 如何参加糖尿病教育项目
5. 一贯的饮食方式 / 基础饮食计划的信息
6. 何时和如何使用降糖药物
a. 口服降糖药物
b. 胰岛素
7. 病假管理
8. 合理使用和处理胰岛素注射器和注射针
由 Joanne Dintzis 和 Sherita Hill Golden 提供.

随访

- 出院后的血糖方案：对住院期间使用胰岛素的患者出院后使用的降糖方案（图 2-7）。
- 为确保安全成功地过渡到门诊血糖管理，与门诊医生清晰的沟通是非常必要的。

专家意见

- 胰岛素治疗具有非常好的灵活性，同时也存在非常高的潜在风险，药物使用错误或者不良反应，如低血糖。
- 住院病人的胰岛素治疗需要不断的评估和校正。需要考虑影响胰岛素剂量的因素如类固醇激素药物剂量的改变，营养状态，肾功能的改变，发热和退热，感染和术前应激状态，活动量的改变。
- 因为急性疾病或者不可预料的营养中断而需要迅速改变胰岛素的剂量，是个挑战。
- 对于危重病人或者合并严重并发症的患者，或者不能频繁的调整血糖的患者，较高的血糖范围更易被接受。在临床研究中，血糖范围控制在 80～110mg/dl 之间的方案能否有利于降低死亡率，仍存在异议。而有些研究报道血糖水平控制在 80～110mg/dl 范围内会增加死亡率（Finfer；Grigesdale）。

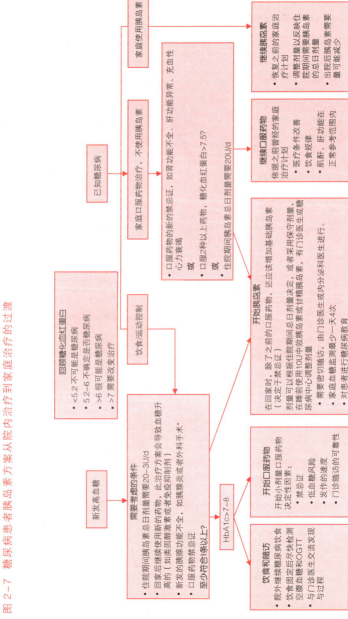

图 2-7 糖尿病患者胰岛素方案从院内治疗到家庭治疗的过渡

如果患者回家后治疗方案有任何改变：

1. 必须考虑个人和家庭的能动力。他们能理解衔接受训练吗？
2. 患者/家属必须早期参与。
3. 治疗原理需要共享。
4. 家庭治疗方案变化所带来的困惑需要通过额外的教育来消除，提高药物依从性。
5. 两周内找初级保健医生和/或预约的内分泌科医生做充分的随访。
6. 与门诊医生交流是必需的。

*注意：任何全胰腺切除术后患者，或新诊断的 1 型 DM 患者，出院后总是需要基础/餐时/矫正胰岛素。由 Joanne Dintzis 和 Sherita Hill Golden 提供。

- 在最近更新的住院病人目标血糖结果显示，反复低血糖可能会提高死亡率和远期认识的缺乏。
- 最新的指南推荐住院病人不使用强效的胰岛素治疗（Qaseem）。
- 需要教育和监控一个大的多学科交叉的团队使用新的复杂的胰岛素治疗模式，为了安全的达到这些目标，需要政府持续的、系统的支持和多学科之间的努力。

参考文献

Qaseem A, Humphrey LL, Chou R, et al. Use of intensive insulin therapy for the management of glycemic control in hospitalized patients: a clinical practice guideline from the american College of physicians. Ann Intern Med, 2011; 154: pp. 260–7.
Comments: Recently released guidelines from the ACP.

Moghissi ES, Korytkowski MT, Dinardi M, et al. American association of Clinical endocrinologists and american Diabetes associationcon sensus statement on inpatient glycemic control. Endocrine practice, 2009; Vol. 15(4): pp. 1–17.
Comments: guidelines from the AACE and ADA.

Griesdale DE, De Souza RJ, Van Dam RM, et al. Intensive insulin therapy and mortality among critically ill patients: a meta-analysis including niCe-SUgaR study data. CMAJ, 2009; Vol. 180: pp. 799–800.
Comments: Meta-analysis of randomized trials demonstrating differential effects of tight glucose control between medical vs surgical iCUs.

NICE-SUGAR Study investigators, Finfer S, Chittock DR, et al. intensive versus conventional glucose control in critically ill patients. NEJM, 2009; Vol. 360: pp. 1283–97.
Comments: Results of a large, international, randomized trial demonstrating increased mortality with intensive glucose control in iCU settings.

Michele M, Gottschlich, editor in chief. The A.S.P.E.N. Nutritional Support Core Curriculum. American Society for parenteral and enteral nutrition (A.S.P.E.N.): Silver Spring, MD; 2007.
Comments: Recommendations related to glycemic control during parenteral and enteral nutrition.

Combes JR, Cousins D, Kercherll, Rich V, et al. American Society of Health-Systemp harmacists'professional prac tice recommendations for safe use of insulin in hospitals, 2004. Available at American Society of Health-System pharmacists web site: http://www.ashp.org/s_ashp/docs/files/Safe_Use_of_insulin.pdf (accessed1/12/2010).
Comments: a comprehensive and systematic list of best practice recommendations for safe and effective insulin use in hospitals.

Clement S, Braithwaite SS, Magee MF, et al. Management of diabetes and hyperglycemia in hospitals. Diabetes Care, 2004; Vol. 27: pp. 553–91.
Comments: A comprehensive review of evidence related to management of hyperglycemia in hospitals, including focus on approaches to subcutaneous insulin use as well as iV insulin infusion.

Van Den Berghe G, Wouters P, Weekers F, et al. Intensive insulin therapy in the critically ill patients. NEJM, 2001; Vol. 345: pp. 1359–67.
Comments: landmark study demonstrating reduced mortality with improved glycemic control in a SICU.

糖尿病患者围手术期护理

Mary Huizinga, MD, MPH

概述
- 糖尿病患者围手术期的护理包括术前评估、降糖药物的调整以及术中术后的处理。

流行病学
- 大约有50%的糖尿病患者可能会手术。
- 糖尿病患者护理的复杂性，会增加感染、并发症和无症状冠状动脉疾病的风险。

临床治疗

术前评估
- 糖尿病患者的术前评估包括：目前使用的降糖药物；血糖控制水平（血糖的范围，过去3个月的糖化血红蛋白水平）；糖尿病酮症酸中毒的病史；远期并发症（糖尿病视网膜病变、糖尿病肾病、糖尿病周围神经病变）；低血糖病史（意识、频率、严重程度）。
- 如果血糖控制比较差，择期手术需延迟进行。
- 如果需要在围手术期和术后调整药物，那么术前是计划这些药物调整的最佳时机。
- 心血管：全面地了解病史和体格检查、心电图检查。如果有冠心病的症状，在行择期手术之前做心脏负荷试验。
- 肺：考虑合并阻塞性睡眠呼吸暂停（obstructive sleep apnea, OSA）的肥胖患者，为减少手术风险需治疗OSA两周以上。如果确诊OSA，那么需要持续正压通气治疗。其他还需考虑的肺疾病有慢性阻塞性肺疾病和哮喘。
- 肾脏：如果根据肾小球滤过率（glomerular filtration rate, GFR）分级存在慢性肾脏病，则会影响降糖药物的使用剂量。
- 高血压：明确术前的用药。术前早晨不要停用β受体阻滞剂，但要停用其他降血压的药物。
- 抗血小板药物治疗：术前7天开始停用阿司匹林。远期抗血栓治疗方案根据患者血栓形成的风险和外科手术的方式来决定。美国大学胸科医生建议高风险血栓形成的患者（如人工心脏瓣膜）应该使用华法林和肝素来过渡，而那些低风险患者可以在术前5天开始停用抗血栓形成的药物。若停药后，INR仍然较高，则需口服维生素K使INR正常。术后12~24小时需恢复抗血栓形成治疗。

围手术期的处理
- 有证据表明良好的基线血糖控制，可以降低术后的感染。
- ADA建议，对于非危重住院患者，快速血糖应小于140mg/dl，随机血糖应小于180mg/dl。
- 仅通过饮食控制血糖的2型糖尿病患者，通常术前不需要药物控制血糖。

然而，在围手术期的高血糖患者，应该按比例增减给予速效胰岛素控制血糖。
- 口服降糖药物的患者应该继续他们的常规药物治疗，直到术前的早上停止药物。大多数患者不需要附加治疗，但是很多患者在围手术期给予了按比例增减的胰岛素治疗。
- 胰岛素依赖的患者可以继续他们的皮下胰岛素注射，通常在术前的晚上长效胰岛素剂量减半，以预防低血糖的发生。手术的当天早上，停用短效胰岛素，给予 1/2 或者 2/3 的基础胰岛素剂量。1 型糖尿病患者必须使用基础胰岛素剂量以预防酮症酸中毒的发生。速效胰岛素可以用于术中控制血糖水平。同时按 75~125ml/h 的速度输注 5% 右旋糖酐，以避免代谢能源的耗竭和低血糖。此外，在术中可以静脉滴注胰岛素。
- 肾功能正常和术前血钾正常的患者，还需补充 10~20mEq/L 钾静脉滴注。
- 持续时间较长，复杂的手术要求更积极的处理，通常给予静脉滴注葡萄糖 – 胰岛素 – 钾补液。

术后处理
- 根据医院糖尿病管理（见第 78 页），尤其是患者术后胰岛素和住院血糖指标。
- 手术后立即监测血糖，每天四次（三餐前和睡前），如果是胰岛素输注则需要加频繁的监测。
- 一旦患者正常饮食，可以恢复口服降糖药物。如果肝功能、肾功能、心功能正常，则可以用二甲双胍降糖。同时，充血性心衰竭和肝功能受损的患者应避免使用噻唑烷二酮类药物，严重的肾衰竭应避免使用磺脲类药物。如果患者摄入的卡路里减少，则应相应地减少磺脲类药物的剂量，以免发生低血糖。

临床治疗
- 手术和全身麻醉相关的神经内分泌反应会引起低血糖和酮症。
- 首要目标是保持水、电解质平衡，防止明显的高血糖、酮症酸中毒、高渗性高血糖状态和低血糖。
- 次要目标是促进创伤愈合和保持适宜的血糖控制以减少手术后的分解代谢。

专家意见
- 立即代谢状态（高血糖、酮症），以及已存在的糖尿病并发症会增加手术风险。
- 择期手术比急诊手术有更多的时间做全面的术前评估和处理。
- 急诊手术时，使用静脉滴注和皮下注射速效胰岛素处理高血糖，5% 或 10% 的右旋糖酐补液应对低血糖。注意停用抗凝药物或使用抗溶血药物；停止使用二甲双胍；使用之前准备好的长效胰岛素。
- 择期手术，充分准备术前评估直到最佳手术时机。

参考文献
Moghissi ES, Korytkowski MT, Dinardo M, et al. American association of Clinical endocrinologists and American Diabetes association consensus statement on inpatient glycemic control. Diabetes Care, 2009; Vol. 32: pp. 1119–31.

Comments: Consensus statement from AACE and ADA of inpatient glycemic control with review of epidemiology of diabetes and hospitalizations.

Griesdale De, De Souza RJ, Van Dam RM, et al. Intensive insulin therapy and mortality among critically ill patients: a meta-analysis including NICE-SUGAR study data. CMAJ, 2009; Vol. 180: pp. 821–7.
Comments: Systematic review and meta-analysis of intensive insulin therapy and mortality among critically ill patients; shows significantly increased risk of hypoglycemia and no mortality benefit, however, may be beneficial in patients in surgical ICU.

NICE-SUGAR Study investigators, Finfer S, Chittock DR, et al. Intensive versus conventional glucose control in critically ill patients. NEJM, 2009; Vol. 360: pp. 1283–97.
Comments: NICE-SUGAR is the largest randomized controlled trial of intensive glucose management in ICU patients; intensive glucose management was found to increase mortality.

Douketis JD, Berger PB, Dunn AS, et al. The perioperative management of antithrombotic therapy: American College of Chest physicians evidence-based clinical practice guidelines (8th edition). Chest, 2008; Vol. 133: pp. 299S–339S.
Comments: American College of Chest physicians guidelines for the perioperative management of antithrombotic therapy.

Rodbard HW, Blonde L, Braithwaite SS, et al. American association of Clinical endocrinologists medical guidelines for clinical practice for the management of diabetes mellitus. Endocr Pract, 2007; Vol. 13 Suppl 1: pp. 1–68.
Comments: AACE medical guidelines for clinical management of diabetes.

Fleisher LA, Beckman JA, Brown KA, et al. ACC/AHA 2007 guidelines on perioperative cardiovascular evaluation and care for noncardiac surgery: a report of the american College of Cardiology/american Heart association task force on practice guidelines (Writing Committee to Revise the 2002 guidelines on perioperative Cardiovascular evaluation for noncardiac Surgery). Developed in collaboration with the American Society of echocardiography, American Society of nuclear Cardiology, Heart Rhythm Society, Society of Cardiovascular anesthesiologists, Society for Cardiovascular angiography and interventions, Society for Vascular Medicine and biology, and Society for Vascular Surgery. Circulation, 2007; Vol. 116: pp. e418–99.
Comments: ACC and AHA guidelines on perioperative cardiac evaluation for noncardiac surgery.

Dronge AS, Perkal MF, Kancir S, et al. Long-term glycemic control and postoperative infectious complications. Arch Surg, 2006; Vol. 141: pp. 375–80; discussion 380.
Comments: Retrospective cohort from the Va national Surgical Quality improvement program; found that A1c level was significantly associated with postoperative infections.

Van Den Berghe G, Wilmer A, Hermans G, et al. Intensive insulin therapy in the medical ICU. NEJM, 2006; Vol. 354: pp. 449–61.
Comments: Randomized controlled trial of intensive glycemic management in medical ICU patients found intensive management reduced morbidity but not mortality.

Gross JB, Bachenberg KL, Benumof JL, et al. Practice guidelines for the perioperative management of patients with obstructive sleep apnea: a report by the american Society of anesthesiologists task force on perioperative management of patients with obstructive sleep apnea. Anesthesiology, 2006; Vol. 104: pp. 1081–93; quiz 1117–8.
Comments: American Society of anesthesiologists statement on perioperative management of obstructive sleep apnea.

Clement S, Braithwaite SS, Magee MF, et al. Management of diabetes and hyperglycemia in hospitals. Diabetes Care, 2004; Vol. 27: pp. 553–91.
Comments: Review article written by ADA professional practice Committee.

Marks JB. Perioperative management of diabetes. Am Fam Physician, 2003; Vol. 67: pp. 93–100.
Comments: Clinically oriented review of perioperative management of diabetes.

Van Den Berghe G, Wouters P, Weekers F, et al. Intensive insulin therapy in the critically ill patients. NEJM, 2001; Vol. 345: pp. 1359–67.
Comments: Randomized controlled trial of intensive glycemic management in surgical ICU patients found that intensive management reduced morbidity and mortality.

胰腺切除术后糖尿病

Joanne Dintzis, CRNP, CDE, and Sherita Golden, MD, MHS

概述
- 胰腺切除后会引起胰腺内分泌功能缺失。
- 导致新发糖尿病的进展,糖尿病病情恶化,或者糖耐量异常的患者转变成糖尿病。
- 重要的影响因素有:大量的胰腺薄壁组织被移除,为邻近器官提供空间而被切除,术前胰岛功能,外围胰岛素抵抗,术前糖尿病和术后营养的改变。

流行病学
- 在美国过去的 20 年里,胰腺切除率增加了 15%。其中有 27% 切除的是良性胰腺疾病。
- 胰腺切除的手术指征包括:恶性肿瘤(根治性或者姑息性切除)、慢性胰腺炎(姑息性手术,假性囊肿切开引流,或者瘘道、梗阻的修复)和急性坏死性胰腺炎(清除坏死灶或假性囊肿切开引流、灌洗)。

临床治疗
一般原则
- 术后出现的肠梗阻、胰漏或淋巴漏,打乱了患者的营养方式,影响胰岛素的所需剂量,同时还要考虑术前的营养不良,还有因肠道和胰腺休息而要求给予的肠外营养。
- 胰腺恶性肿瘤患者血糖目标的设定,需要考虑总的预后和因化放疗引起的营养不均衡。可能需要设定较高的目标血糖。

全胰腺切除术
- 全胰腺切除术后将导致完全胰岛素缺乏且几乎失去胰高血糖素的保护作用。
- 所有全胰腺切除术患者需使用额外的基础和校正的胰岛素降低血糖。坚持在餐前使用速效或短效胰岛素来应对消化吸收的糖水化合物。
- 术后早期的胰岛素需求量常常比较低,这可能是因为缺乏胰高血糖素的保护作用,肝糖原分解减少引起的。
- 静脉滴注胰岛素合并低剂量的右旋糖酐,可以为禁食的患者提供最大的灵活性。
- 由于术后对胰岛素的敏感性非常大,因此静脉滴注转变为皮下注射常规剂量的胰岛素。

局部胰腺切除术
- 胰腺次全切除术:切除大约 95% 的胰腺组织,可用于缓解胰腺炎引起的难治性疼痛。术后 60%~75% 的患者需要胰岛素治疗。
- 近端胰腺切除术:大部分是经典的"Whipple"手术或者胰十二指肠切除术;切除胰头、十二指肠、远端胃(经常)、胆总管和胆囊。最新改进的手术方式认为可以保留幽门或/和十二指肠,可能会出现胰腺空肠吻合瘘,其他围手术期并发症,或者延迟胃排空。20%~50% 出现新发的糖尿病。

- 远端胰腺切除术：常用于发生在胰尾的疾病。脾脏可能需要被切除，而胰液的流动通道不能被中断。糖尿病发生率为3%~30%。
- 中段胰腺切除术：保留胰腺实质，减少外分泌和内分泌功能不全的风险。减少糖尿病，但瘘和胰漏的发生率较高。
- 在住院期间，进食则需密切血糖监测，必要时给予胰岛素治疗。
- 胰腺手术后，先前的降糖药物剂量似乎需要加强，通常需要给予胰岛素治疗。
- 坏死组织的切除，以及随后炎症的减少，很少能改善血糖控制。

随访

- 胃肠功能紊乱比较常见，有时持续较长时间，往往需要胰腺酶治疗。胃排空延迟，可能会出现恶心、腹泻。
- 在术后几个月口服药物的不规律和零散，是胰岛素管理面临的挑战。
- 在癌症患者的化疗过程中，附加的营养改变和胰岛素治疗常可发生。
- 在胰腺全切和远端切除术后，由于缺乏分泌胰高血糖素的细胞，患者常常伴有快速低血糖的风险。
- 胰腺全切术的患者，使用基础和校正胰岛素剂量，如果食物摄入比较稳定和统一，合用餐时胰岛素剂量。
- 胰腺次全切术后的患者对胰岛素的要求因人而异。术后糖化血红蛋白超过6%的患者需要胰岛素治疗。
- 术后的开始几个月，胰岛素的需求量可能会不稳定，直到身体逐渐恢复，围手术期炎症消失，营养摄入规律之后才逐渐稳定。在血糖不稳定的这个阶段，更多的是推荐保守的血糖目标。
- 需要胰岛素治疗的患者，出院后一个月内需要内分泌专家或者糖尿病教育者随访。
- 胰岛素的治疗包括胰岛素注射器/胰岛素瓶，胰岛素笔/针和紧急胰高血糖素试剂盒。
- 术后血糖升高的所有患者，在术后一个月内均需要使用血糖仪，血糖试纸和说明书来检测他们的血糖情况。
- 出院指征包括健康护理者提供的血糖在70mg/dl和300mg/dl之间，或者连续3次血糖检测低于250mg/dl。

专家建议

- 住院患者在胰腺切除术后应尽早地向营养专家或者糖尿病护理团队咨询。
- 患者应注意的是，在住院期间，应尽早地亲自体验胰岛素的自我管理和血糖检测，并坚持规律的强制性训练。
- 胰腺切除术后，患者常常伴有精神上和情绪上的压力，这可能会影响他们理解和坚持自我安全条例的能力。
- 胰腺全切术后的患者，尤其是需要门诊糖尿病宣教随访的患者，成为迅速的完全的胰岛素缺乏同时胰高血糖素缺乏，往往导致脆性糖尿病。

参考文献

Teh SH, Diggs BS, Deveney CW, and Sheppard BC. Patient and hospital characteristics on the variance of perioperative outcomes for pancreatic resection in the United States.

Arch of Surg, 2009; Vol. 144(8): pp. 713–21.

Comments: This article describes the effect of patient and hospital characteristics on perioperative outcomes (in-hospital mortality, perioperative complications, and mortality following a major complication) for pancreatic resection in the United States.

Irani JL, Ashley SW, Brooks DC, Osteen RT, et al. Distal pancreatectomy is not associated with increased perioperative morbidity when performed as part of a multivisceral resection. J gastointest Surg, 2008; Vol. 12: pp. 2177–2182.

Comments: This article evaluates the indications for and the outcomes from distal pancreatectomy.

King J, Kazanjian K, Matsumoto J, Reber Ha, et al. Distal pancreatectomy: incidence of postoperative diabetes. J. gastrointest Surg, 2008; Vol. 12(9): pp. 1548–1553.

Comments: This article describes the rate of clinically apparent new-onset diabetes in 125 patients after distal pancreatectomy.

Riediger H, Adam U, Fischeer E, Keck T, et al. Long-term outcome after resection for chronic pancreatitis in 224 patients. Gastoinest Surg, 2007; Vol. 11(8): pp. 949–59.

Comments: The focus of this article is on long-term outcome after pancreatic surgery for chronic pancreatitis. Morbidities examined include pain, exocrine/endocrine pancreatic function, and control of organ complications in 224 patients with a median follow-up period of 54 months.

Hamilton L, Jeyarajah DR. Hemoglobin A1c can be helpful in predicting progression to diabetes after Whipple procedure. Hbp (oxford, UK), 2007; Vol. 9(1): pp. 26–8.

Comments: This article from the official journal of the Hepato pancreato biliary association reports results of a small-scale study that utilizes preoperative A1c levels to predict progression to diabetes post pancreatic surgery.

Crippa S, Bassi C, Warshaw AL, Falconi M, et al. Middle pancreatectomy: indications, short- and long-term operative outcomes. Ann of Surg, 2007; Vol. 246(1): pp. 69–76.

Comments: This article evaluates the indications, perioperative and long-term outcomes of a large cohort of patients who underwent middle pancreatectomy.

Jethwa P, Sodergren M, Lala A, Webber JAC, et al. Diabetic control after total pancreatectomy. Digest liver Dis, 2006; Vol. 38(6): pp. 415–419.

Comments: This article describes a retrospective analysis of patients undergoing total pancreatectomy from a single institution over a 15-year time frame, comparing data of diabetic control.

Kahl S, Malfertheiner P. Exocrine and endocrine pancreatic insufficiency after pancreatic surgery. Best Pract Res Clin Gastroenterol, 2004; Vol. 18(5): pp. 947–955.

Comments: This article provides an overview of indications for pancreatic surgery and effects on exocrine and endocrine function following surgery.

Hutchins RR, Hart RS, pacifico M, bradley NJ, Williamson RC. Long-term results of distal pancreatectomy for chronic pancreatitis in 90 patients. Ann Surg, 2002; Vol. 236(5): pp. 612–8.

Comments: This article describes the indications for total pancreatectomy for chronic pancreatitis, and evaluates the risks, functional loss, and outcome of the procedure in 90 patients.

Slezak LA, Anderson DK. Pancreatic resection: effects on glucose metabolism. World J Surg, 2001; Vol. 25: pp. 452–460.

Comments: This article describes the characteristics of the endocrine abnormalities that develop postsurgical resection of the pancreas.

减肥手术

Octavia Pickett-Blakely, MD, MHS, and Mary Huizinga, MD, MPH

概述
- 为降低体重和减少因肥胖而引起的合并症如糖尿病,减肥手术是一种常见的、对肥胖患者有效的外科干预手段。体重的降低可以通过限制总的营养摄入,营养吸收不良和/或限制吸收与吸收不良的结合。
- 腹腔镜下可调式胃束带手术:在胃近端限制性地插入连接带,连接带用来调整限制胃容量的皮下端口。
- 腹腔镜下袖套式胃切除术:沿着胃小弯,限制性切除大部分胃大弯的大部分胃组织,留下一个袖套式的胃。这可以作为十二指肠转位手术的第一步,或者作为一个独立的步骤。
- Roux-en-Y胃旁路术:结合限制性和吸收不良性手术,通过分离远端胃和远端胃产生一个小的胃囊;胃囊近端与空肠吻合(Roux端),旁路的远端胃和近端小肠(Y端)分别与远侧的空肠吻合。
- 十二指肠转位或非十二指肠转位的胆胰分流术:联合限制性和吸收不良型手术,腹腔镜下袖套式胃切除术。留下的残余胃连接小肠下段或者小肠上段,从而形成独立的胆环。两者都与下段小肠吻合(十二指肠转位手术)。

流行病学
- 高达55%的糖尿病患者是肥胖患者(CDC)。
- 每年大约225 000患者施行肥胖手术治疗,其中15%~30%的患者伴有糖尿病(CDC)。
- 根据肥胖治疗手术方式的不同,48%~98%的糖尿病患者在手术后血糖得到控制(Segal; Vetter)。
- 胃旁路手术后,糖尿病相关的死亡率和全因死亡率显著降低(Christou; Segal)。

诊断
- 根据国家健康研究所(national institutes of health, NIH)治疗指南,肥胖手术治疗的指征:BMI>40kg/m^{2}或者BMI>35kg/m^{2}合并肥胖引起的相关疾病,如糖尿病、高血压、阻塞性呼吸暂停、肥胖型肺换气不足综合征、匹克威克综合征、严重的尿失禁、高血脂、渐进性的骨关节炎、非酒精性脂肪肝、冠心病、胃食管反流和假性脑瘤(NIH共识会议)。
- 2011年2月,腹腔镜下可调式胃束带手术通过了FDA的批准,用于BMI>30kg/m^{2}合并有一种肥胖相关的疾病。这项决定回应了制造商的研究结果,他们发现对于中等肥胖的患者在术后体重明显下降。
- 由保险公司决定各种手术治疗指南的覆盖范围(例如:在美国社会肥胖手术制定卓越中心登记的饮食和运动治疗失败的文件)。

减肥手术

临床治疗

术后早期的血糖控制（0~3天）

- 胰岛素依赖的患者，在围手术期因为口服药物的减少，经常需要低剂量的胰岛素和口服降糖药物。
- Roux-en-Y或者胆胰分流术的患者，在术后几天内高血糖会加重，尤其在体重明显下降之前。
- 根据机构或供应商特定的协议，然后进食。大多数饮食刚开始是透明液体，然后是全液体或泥状食物的高蛋白质、低脂肪和碳水化合物。
- 基础和速效胰岛素的结合是控制快速血糖在80~110mg/dl，餐后血糖低于180mg/dl范围内的首选方案。
- 因为饮食摄入的不规律和对胰岛素的要求降低，有些患者只需用餐时使用胰岛素。
- 非胰岛素依赖的患者必须停止或者调整口服降糖药物的剂量。特别地，胰岛素促分泌剂在围手术期应立即停止使用。

出院患者的血糖控制

- 口服摄入食物先从全液体和泥状食物开始，最后到规律饮食（少食多餐）包括高蛋白、低脂低糖饮食。
- 2型糖尿病的患者，在家里的餐前血糖和快速血糖应该定期检测。
- 肥胖治疗手术之后，根据患者的家中血糖检测来调整胰岛素和口服降糖药物的剂量，其中约有76%患者一年内可以减少剂量。
- 大部分患者手术3个月后可以不使用胰岛素和口服降糖药。

微量元素的缺乏

- 肥胖手术治疗之后的患者存在各种各样微量元素缺乏的风险：维生素B_{12}、铁、钙、维生素D、叶酸、维生素B_1或者其他。
- 所有接受肥胖治疗手术的患者在术后都应该补充多种维生素，包括铁、柠檬酸钙以及维生素D。
- 患者应该规律地检测微量元素，检测的周期根据手术类型来决定。腹腔镜下可调式束带手术每年检测一次，胃旁路手术需每隔3~6个月检测一次，胆胰分流术也是3~6个月检测一次。
- 虽然钙的吸收贯穿整个小肠和结肠，肥胖手术治疗后摄入富含钙的食物（如牛奶、奶酪）可能会引起腹胀、腹部绞痛和腹泻，从而存在缺乏的风险。推荐使用柠檬酸钙、维生素D补充钙，因为有利于吸收。
- 口服维生素B_{12}往往不能改善维生素B_{12}的缺乏。维生素B_{12}的补充应该给予舌下含服、鼻内营养或者肌内注射。因为解剖学上吸收破坏和胃旁路手术和营养吸收不良手术（胆胰分流术或十二指肠转位术）的内在因素，口服维生素B_{12}不易被吸收。
- 铁的吸收被破坏是因为胃旁路手术和其他营养吸收不良手术的十二指肠旁路（铁吸收位点）。有些患者需要静脉内铁剂治疗。
- 叶酸缺乏的发生可能是因为维生素B_{12}缺乏，口服摄入不足或者小肠吸收破坏。肥胖手术治疗后的患者常规推荐补充叶酸。
- 口服摄入不足或者小肠吸收的破坏会引起维生素B_1的缺乏，并且可能导致韦尼克科尔萨科夫综合征。维生素 B₁ 是大部分复合维生素的组成部分，但是缺乏的患者需要给予肌内注射治疗。
- 维生素 D 缺乏常常因为口服摄入的减少，维生素 D 和胆盐的复合物贫乏导致吸收破坏引起的。推荐每天口服补充。

并发症
- 内科的：电解质紊乱。
- 倾倒综合征（餐后 30 分钟左右因胃排空快，出现高胰岛素性低血糖）。阿卡波糖治疗效果较好。
- 胰岛母细胞增生症（高胰岛素性低血糖在餐后 1 小时左右更为严重，因为胰岛 β 细胞功能亢进）仍然存在争议 (Service)。
- 体重反弹。
- 胆结石。
- 减肥后的皮肤松弛。
- 腹腔镜下可调式束带手术：呕吐、疼痛、吞咽困难、反流。
- 外科的：Roux-en-Y 胃旁路手术或胆胰分流术：吻合口漏，边缘性溃疡，吻合口狭窄。
- 腹腔镜下可调式束带手术或袖套式胃切除术：束带功能障碍（束带滑移、侵蚀、感染），吻合口漏，出血，瘘道形成。

随访
- 根据手术的方式和合并症决定肥胖手术治疗后的随访时间。先前就要注意潜在的并发症。
- Roux-en-Y 胃旁路手术后糖尿病复发率高达 43%（与低 BMI 与围术期，减肥失败，体重反弹，围手术期高血糖相关）(Vetter)。
- 在围手术期应坚持检测糖化血红蛋白。
- 手术方式的不同决定体重的降低。Roux-en-Y 手术术后和腹腔镜下可调式束带手术术后的期望的平均下降体重在第 1~2 年分别为 45%~85% 和 29%~87%(Buchwald)。

专家意见
- 为提高术后胰岛素敏感性，术后的胰岛素和口服降糖药物的剂量明显减少。糖耐量可能正常化。
- 高度重视微量元素缺乏的可能。
- 肥胖治疗手术由一些保险公司担任（例如医疗补助计划），但是特定的治疗指南由这个保险公司决定。
- 肥胖治疗手术需要一种新的饮食方式：患者不能再像之前那样进食大量的食物。
- 近期发现围手术期和远期高胰岛素性低血糖发生率与胰腺 β 细胞增生（胰岛母细胞增生症）有关，然而，这些发现仍存在争议。

参考文献

Segal JB, Clark JM, Shore AD, et al. Prompt reduction in use of medications for comorbid conditions after bariatric surgery. Obes Surg, 2009; Vol. 19: pp. 1646–56.
Comments: Bariatric surgery can resolve type 2 diabetes.

Vetter ML, Cardillo S, Rickels MR, et al. Narrative review: Effect of bariatric surgery on type 2 diabetes mellitus. Ann Intern Med, 2009; Vol. 150: pp. 94–103.
Comments: This systematic review reports on the effect of bariatric surgery on T2DM.

Christou NV. Impact of obesity and bariatric surgery on survival. World J Surg, 2009; Vol. 33: pp. 2022–7.
Comments: Bariatric surgery reduces the relative risk of death in morbidly obese patients.

Mechanick JI, Kushner RF, Sugerman HJ, et al. American association of Clinical endocrinologists, the obesity Society, and American Society for Metabolic and bariatric Surgery medical guidelines for clinical practice for the perioperative nutritional, metabolic, and nonsurgical support of the bariatric surgery patient. Obesity (Silver Spring, MD), 2009; Vol. 17 Suppl 1: pp. S1–70.
Comments: Guidelines published for the perioperative management of bariatric surgery patients.

Dixon JB, O'brien PE, Playfair J, et al. Adjustable gastric banding and conventional therapy for type 2 diabetes: a randomized controlled trial. JaMa, 2008; Vol. 299: pp. 316–23.
Comments: Laparoscopic adjustable band surgery is superior to conventional diabetes therapy for the remission of diabetes and weight loss.

Adams TD, Gress RE, Smith SC, et al. Long-term mortality after gastric bypass surgery. NEJM, 2007; Vol. 357: pp. 753–61.
Comments: This article reviews how mortality is decreased after gastric bypass surgery.

Service GJ, Thompson GB, Service FJ, et al. Hyperinsulinemic hypoglycemia with nesidioblastosis after gastricbypass surgery. NEJM, 2005; Vol. 353: pp. 249–54.
Comments: Nesidioblastosis is an uncommon phenomenon in bariatric surgery patients associated with hyperinsulinemic hypoglycemia.

Centers for Disease Control and prevention (CDC) prevalence of overweight and obesity among adults with diagnosed diabetes—United States, 1988–1994 and 1999–2002. MMWR, 2004; Vol. 53: pp. 1066–8.
Comments: This article reports on the epidemiology of obesity in the diabetic population.

Buchwald H, Avidor Y, Braunwald E, et al. Bariatric surgery: a systematic review and meta-analysis. JAMA, 2004; Vol. 292: pp. 1724–37.
Comments: This systematic review reports on the efficacy of bariatric surgery for weight loss.

Consensus Development Conference Panel. NIH conference. Gastrointestinal surgery for severe obesity. Ann Intern Med, 1991; Vol. 115: pp. 956–61.
Comments: NIH consensus panel recommendations that bariatric surgery be considered for carefully selected, morbidly obese patients with acceptable operative risks.

生活方式和健康教育

营养：关于糖尿病的综述

Christopher D. Saudek, MD, and Emily Loghmani, MS, RD, LDN, CDE

定义
- 一份个人膳食计划，并结合口服降糖药以及胰岛素的使用，这是治疗糖尿病的基础。
- 专家们避免使用"配餐(diet)"这个术语，因为这个词会带来负面的含义，他们更愿意促进形成健康的饮食计划和规律的体力活动。
- 完善的膳食计划并不是标准统一的,不同患者的膳食计划是不完全相同的。
- 合理的膳食计划能够促进患者达到健康体重的要求，在避免出现低血糖的同时使糖化血红蛋白值达标，改善血脂及血压水平，从而提供好的生活质量。
- 膳食计划根据营养治疗（MNT）的过程来制定。包括对饮食习惯、糖尿病知识的评估，营养治疗目标的确认和协商，营养教育和干预，对结果进行持续的监测和评价。

临床治疗

总则
- 应根据患者的年龄、糖尿病类型、是否有合并症、心血管疾病危险因素、患者的意愿、文化以及个人情况为患者制定个性化的膳食计划。
- 综合考虑能量的需求量，营养素（碳水化合物、脂肪和蛋白质），维生素以及矿物质。
- 尽可能参考熟悉糖尿病的营养师的意见，最好与其进行多次交流。
- 选择一种患者既需要又能够完成的膳食计划方式：健康食物的选择，部分控制，对碳水化合物的认识，碳水化合物的计数以及转换。

糖尿病营养的目标（美国糖尿病协会）
- 达到目标血糖值的同时最大程度上减少高血糖和低血糖的发生。
- 控制血脂和血压水平以减少心血管疾病的危险因素。
- 满足儿童及青少年正常的生长发育的要求，成年人保持健康的体重。
- 预防、延缓或减少糖尿病的并发症。

具体的营养建议（美国糖尿病协会）
- 从五谷杂粮、水果、蔬菜、低脂牛奶和酸奶中获取碳水化合物。
- 追踪所有碳水化合物，但是要注意碳水化合物的来源和类型也会影响餐后血糖水平。
- 减少总脂肪、饱和脂肪酸以及胆固醇的摄入量，避免摄入反式脂肪酸。尽量多摄入单不饱和脂肪酸和多不饱和脂肪酸。
- 选择食用瘦肉、禽类、鱼以及其他低脂蛋白。

营养：关于糖尿病的综述

- 从五谷杂粮、干豌豆和豆类中增加纤维素的摄入，多吃水果蔬菜。
- 如果患者患有高血压，低钠饮食。
- 可以使用 FDA 批准的糖的替代品。

糖尿病前期患者的营养（空腹血糖受损或糖耐量受损）
- 如果患者超重，通过增加体力活动（碳水化合物 50 分钟/周）进行生活方式干预，减少 5%~10% 的碳水化合物体重（糖尿病预防计划）。
- 制定一份体重管理计划，帮助减少热量的摄入，增加体力活动，增加随访的次数。
- 减少额外的碳水化合物的摄入。
- 了解糖尿病前期或增加患糖尿病的危险因素类别，详见 134 页。

妊娠期糖尿病的营养
- 调整能量和碳水化合物的摄入使病人达到适度的体重增加和目标血糖值，避免发生酮症。
- 为孕产妇和胎儿提供必要的营养素。
- 监测空腹及餐后 1~2 小时的血糖水平。
- 如果饮食控制不能达到目标血糖值，加用外源性胰岛素。
- 鼓励孕妇进行体力活动以改善糖耐量。
- 鼓励母乳喂养。
- 促进生活方式的改变以避免 2 型糖尿病的进展。
- 详见 138 页妊娠期糖尿病。

随访
- 初始：包括营养评估以及根据膳食计划指南进行基本的营养教育，进行相关的关于预防和处理低血糖的教育。
- 随访：根据病例病情的复杂性及治疗效果决定随访的频率和时间长短。

专家意见
- 不能过分强调良好的营养是糖尿病管理不可分割的一部分的重要性。
- 个性化是关键。
- 总的来说，2 型糖尿病的治疗目标包括控制体重（Klein），而 1 型糖尿病的治疗目标包括严格的碳水化合物的摄入量来匹配胰岛素剂量和活性（美国糖尿病协会 2010）。
- 可持续发展的膳食计划是成功的关键；对饮食的极端的限制永远不会像比较适度、健康和可持续化的膳食计划那样有效。

参考文献
American Diabetes Association. Standards of medical care in diabetes—2011. Diabetes Care, 2011; Vol. 34 Suppl 1: pp. S11–61.

Comments: Discusses standards of care for prevention, treatment, and management of diabetes, with a section on type 1 diabetes.

American Dietetic Association. International Dietetics and Nutrition Terminology (IDNT) Reference Manual, Standardized Language for the Nutrition Care Process, 2nd edition. Chicago: American

Dietetic Association;2009.

Comments: Provides listings of standardized language to be used at each stage of the nutrition care process after critical evaluation of nutrition assessment data and information; helps with provision of more focused nutrition care and evaluation of outcomes by a registered dietician.

American Diabetes Association, Bantle JP, Wylie-Rosett J, et al. Nutrition recommendations and interventions for diabetes: a position statement of the American Diabetes Association. Diabetes Care, 2008; Vol. 31 Suppl 1: pp. S61–78.

Comments: Summarizes nutritional management for the prevention and treatment of diabetes.

Klein S, Sheard NF, Pi-Sunyer X, et al. Weight management through lifestyle modification for the prevention and management of type 2 diabetes: rationale and strategies. A statement of the American Diabetes Association, the North American Association for the Study of Obesity, and the American Society for Clinical Nutrition. Am J Clin Nutr, 2004; Vol. 80: pp. 257–63.

Comments: Reviews the use of lifestyle modifications to reduce energy intake and increase physical activity in overweight/obese patients with type 2 diabetes.

Franz MJ, Bantle JP, Beebe CA, Brunzell JD, et al. Evidence-based nutrition principles and recommendations for the treatment and prevention of diabetes and related complications. Diabetes Care, 2002; Vol. 25: pp. 148–198.

Comments: Summarizes the research and clinical evidence to support nutrition recommendations for diabetes;also defines medical nutrition therapy.

The Diabetes Prevention Program Research Group, Knowler WC, Barrett-Connor E, Fowler SE, et al. Reduction in the incidence of type 2 diabetes with lifestyle intervention or metformin. NEJM, 2002; Vol. 346: pp. 393–403.

Comments: Documents the safety and effectiveness of three treatment groups for the prevention of diabetes in a diverse population of high-risk individuals.

1 型糖尿病的营养

Emily Loghmani, MS, RD, LDN, CDE, and Christopher D. Saudek, MD

定义

- 1 型糖尿病（T1DM）的营养计划包括食物选择和体力活动，使用胰岛素治疗达到正常的生长、合适的体重、血糖水平和其他危险因素的最佳控制，同时避免低血糖。
- 根据年龄、性别、生长阶段、饮食喜好、平时的饮食、活动量以及学习工作的计划计算相应的食物摄入量。
- 使用食物摄入指南帮助达到和维持健康的血糖、血脂、血压水平以预防、减少或延缓并发症的发生。
- 提供注重年龄和生长发育原则的营养治疗（MNT）(Silverstein)。

临床治疗

营养治疗

- 评估与年龄、性别和活动量相关的生长与体质指数，计算能量的需要量。
- 提供充足的营养，保证儿童、青少年正常的生长发育。
- 成年人达到和/或保持健康的体重。
- 教患者学会碳水化合物计数，或者增强患者对碳水化合物的认识，以配合患者自己可以处理的情况。
- 为使用固定量胰岛素治疗的患者选择固定的碳水化合物摄入量，或者根据胰岛素和碳水化合物的比例，为进行胰岛素强化治疗以及胰岛素泵治疗的患者选择可变的碳水化合物的摄入量。
- 患者会通过自我监测根据饮食的量估计自己的血糖水平。
- 患者应该根据自己的运动量调整能量摄入。例如：每增加 1 小时额外的运动，需要增加 10~15g 碳水化合物摄入，或者活动增加时减少胰岛素用量。运动之前的能量摄入量需要根据运动的强度和时间来决定。
- 为避免症状性低血糖，当血糖水平低于 70mg/dl 时或血糖快速下降时应该摄入 15g 快速起效的碳水化合物，并于 15~20min 后再次监测血糖水平。对于 5 岁的孩子，如果血糖水平低于 100mg/dl 应该立即给予治疗。
- 为了进一步减少低血糖发生的危险，要限制酒精和含酒精食物的摄入。

1 型糖尿病的关键营养建议

- 进行胰岛素强化治疗的患者应该根据胰岛素 - 热量比通过计算食物的热量调整速效胰岛素的用量。例如，是用 1U 胰岛素中和 15g（平均水平）、10g（胰岛素低度敏感）还是 20g（胰岛素较敏感）碳水化合物。
- 可以用 500 为尺度：500/ 每日胰岛素用量（TDD）= 胰岛素热量比。例如：TDD 为 50U，500/50=1U 胰岛素中和 10g 碳水化合物。
- 胰岛素强化治疗的患者，除了日常饮食应用胰岛素中和外，需要根据血糖监测值追加相应剂量的胰岛素。例如血糖在 120mg/dl 以上时，每超过 40mg/dl，追加 1U 胰岛素；每超过 50mg，增加 1U（胰岛素较敏感）；

或每超过 30mg，增加 1U（胰岛素不敏感）。
- 可以以 1 800 为尺度追加胰岛素：1 800/每日胰岛素用量 = 校正比值。例如：每日胰岛素用量为 30U，1 800/30=1U/每超过目标血糖值 60mg/dl。
- 对于估计食物热量较困难的患者，可以采用固定量胰岛素注射，他们应该学会建立食物热量的概念，以 15g 碳水化合物为估测的单位。在这些病例应该每餐固定食物的热量，不要根据血糖变化调整胰岛素用量。
- 随着年龄的增长和减少低血糖目标（美国糖尿病协会）的变化，目标血糖值也会随之增加。
- 高脂饮食会延长碳水化合物的吸收，从而导致迟发高血糖。
- "智能泵"会根据上述的计算方法推荐胰岛素的使用量。注意要由专业医护人员调整"智能泵"的使用程序。

膳食计划
- 基于营养评估的碳水化合物、蛋白质、脂肪的分配。
- 监测饮食或点心中碳水化合物总量比监测其来源更重要。
- 根据患者的年龄、日常饮食、活动量、学习或工作量提供一日三餐和 1~3 次点心。
- 控制蛋白质和脂肪的摄入量，以及维持健康体重和控制血脂水平的碳水化合物的量。
- 坚持膳食计划及进食零食的类型和方式并及时调整以防出现高血糖，适当的处理低血糖，这些措施联合可更好地控制血糖 (Delahanty, 1993)。

随访
- 初始阶段：一旦确诊糖尿病，就应该对患者进行营养评估，教会其进行食物热量计算，或对食物热量建立概念，并能够对低血糖进行预防和简单处理。
- 进行阶段：定期审查和评估，通常每 3 个月进行一次。
- 针对特殊情况的强化：对于某些特殊情况，如强化胰岛素治疗方案的改变，开始胰岛素泵治疗，因糖尿病酮症酸中毒、严重的低血糖或怀孕住院后的出院饮食。

专家意见
- 对于治疗 1 型糖尿病，碳水化合物的认识是很有必要的，让患者知道饮食对于血糖的影响，使他们更好地调整食物入量以配合胰岛素治疗。
- 从另一方面来讲，不提倡限制碳水化合物。较好的血糖控制是建立在由碳水化合物提供总热量的 40%~55% 上的，调整胰岛素的用量来"对抗"这部分碳水化合物 (Delahanty, 2009)。
- 准确的碳水化合物计数能够根据碳水化合物的摄入量以及血糖值灵活的调整胰岛素的用量，从而促进更好地控制血糖，增加生活方式的灵活性。
- 含糖饮食能够直接导致血糖升高，应该尽量用复合碳水化合物代替糖的直接摄入，尽量不要在食物中直接加糖，如果偶尔需要，也要用足够的胰岛素进行中和。

- 血糖指数有时对于那些复杂的患者是有帮助的,但更多的时候,我们建议患者应该了解哪些食物能够使他们的血糖升的过高,并避免食用它们。

参考文献

American Diabetes Association. Standards of medical care in diabetes—2011. Diabetes Care, 2011; Vol. 34 Suppl1: pp. S11–61.
Comments: This American Diabetes Association statement addresses how medical nutrition therapy is in an integral component of care with a section devoted to type 1 diabetes.

American Diabetes Association Diabetes. Care in the school and day care setting. Diabetes Care, 2009; Vol. 32 Suppl 1: pp. S68–72.
Comments: This American Diabetes Association statement provides practical advice on the management of type 1 diabetes at school and in day care.

Delahanty LM, Nathan DM, Lachin JM, et al. Association of diet with glycated hemoglobin during intensive treatment of type 1 diabetes in the Diabetes Control and Complications Trial. Am J Clin Nutr, 2009; Vol. 89: pp. 518–24.
Comments: The paper reports how dietary composition is related to subsequent A1c levels in DCCT in the intensive treatment group. Poorer control perhaps due to insulin resistance was related to higher saturatedfat intake but not the amount of carbohydrate intake.

Silverstein J, Klingensmith G, Copeland K, et al. Care of children and adolescents with type 1 diabetes: a statement of the American Diabetes Association. Diabetes Care, 2005; Vol. 28: pp. 186–212.
Comments: This American Diabetes Association statement provides age-appropriate recommendations for the management of children and adolescents with type 1 diabetes.

Brand-Miller J, Hayne S, Petocz P, et al. Low-glycemic index diets in the management of diabetes: a meta-analysis of randomized controlled trials. Diabetes Care, 2003; Vol. 26: pp. 2261–7.
Comments: This research suggests that the use of foods with a low glycemic index may help promote a small reduction in glycemic control.

Gillespie SJ, Kulkarni KD, Daly AE. Using carbohydrate counting in diabetes clinical practice. J Am Diet Assoc,1998; Vol. 98: pp. 897–905.
Comments: This paper discusses carbohydrate counting as a meal planning approach with practical suggestions for teaching different levels of complexity (i.e., basic, intermediate, and advanced) to match what the patient can handle.

Delahanty LM, Halford BN. The role of diet behaviors in achieving improved glycemic control in intensively treated patients in the Diabetes Control and Complications Trial. Diabetes Care, 1993; Vol. 16:pp. 1453–8.
Comments: This paper reports how dietary behaviors (e.g., treatment of hypoglycemia, consistency of meals),were related to glycemic control (A1c levels) in the DCCT.

Loghmani E, Rickard K, Washburne L, et al. Glycemic response to sucrose-containing mixed meals in diets of children of with insulin-dependent diabetes mellitus. J Pediatr, 1991; Vol. 119: pp. 531–7.
Comments: This study reports no additional hyperglycemia when sucrose-containing foods are substituted for complex carbohydrates in healthy meals for children with type 1 diabetes. Sucrose-free diet contained 2% of total calories from sucrose versus 10% for the sucrose-containing diet.

营养：碳水化合物计数

Emily Loghmani, MS, RD, LDN, CDE, and Christopher D. Saudek, MD

定义
- 是一种估计碳水化合物摄入量的方法，对总量或是以 15 克为单位计算。
- 因为碳水化合物是影响餐后血糖的主要营养素，因此碳水化合物计数对于病人来说很重要 (Sheard)。
- 对于使用口服降糖药或固定胰岛素用量的糖尿病患者，碳水化合物计数能够促进一致的碳水化合物摄入量；对于减肥的人，碳水化合物计数能够帮助控制总热量；对于那些使用胰岛素的人：碳水化合物的比例，有助于其匹配餐前胰岛素用量。
- 碳水化合物计数使患者在选择食物时有更大的灵活性，而且有助于促进血糖控制 (Chiesa)。
- 其他估计碳水化合物摄入量的方法有：换算系统和以经验为基础的估计法 (Wheeler 2008a)。

临床治疗

碳水化合物计数的实用技巧
- 碳水化合物包括淀粉，纤维，糖醇（如山梨醇），和/或单糖（如蔗糖或果糖，无论是自然的或合成的）(Wheeler 2008b)。
- 15 克碳水化合物被定义为 1 份碳水化合物。
- 换算，淀粉/粮食、水果、乳制品中都含有碳水化合物。
- 1 份碳水化合物 =1 份淀粉/粮食类，或 1 个水果，或 1 份乳制品，每种都含有 15 克的碳水化合物。
- 健康膳食包括全谷物、干豆和豆类、低脂肪奶制品、水果等食物中的碳水化合物。
- 对于成人和儿童，推荐碳水化合物补充量至少 130 克/天（8~9 份），提供 45%~65% 的能量 (IOM, 2005)。
- 对于减肥的人：女性需要 30~45g/餐（2~3 份），15g/点心；男性需要 45~60g/餐（3~4 份），15~30g/点心。
- 阅读食物标签，了解制造商的产品规格和碳水化合物的总克数/份数，调整食用量。标注在营养标签上的"份"反映正常进食量的碳水化合物的量，1"份"不一定是 15g 碳水化合物的量。
- 食物标签上列举的"份"不一定等于 1 份碳水化合物（15g）（1 份碳水化合物）。
- 标签可能产生误导。通常一次吃的一包食物，会被标注"2 份"，比如标注每块含 150 卡热量的糖果，每份包含 2 块，其实一块就含 300 卡热量。

含 15 克碳水化合物的食品（选择您的食物：糖尿病患者的换算表）
- 淀粉/谷物：1/4 个大面包圈，1 片面包， 6 英寸的玉米饼，3/4 杯不加糖的冷麦片，1/2 杯煮熟的谷物，1/3 杯面食， 1/3 杯米饭，1 杯汤，1/2

营养：碳水化合物计数

杯玉米，1/2 杯土豆泥，5 块饼干，3 杯爆米花，3/4 盎司马铃薯/玉米片，1/2 杯煮熟的豆类或扁豆。
- 水果：1 个小的新鲜水果，1/2 个香蕉，1/2 罐低糖水果罐头，2 汤匙水果干，17 个小葡萄，1 杯冬瓜，3/4~1 杯浆果。
- 奶制品：1 杯牛奶，1/2 杯巧克力牛奶，1 杯豆浆，1 杯纯酸奶。
- 甜食：1 块 2 英寸方形蛋糕或无冰布朗尼，2 块小饼干，5 块香草薄饼，1/2 杯无糖布丁，1 汤匙糖或蜂蜜，1/2 杯普通的冰淇淋，1/4 杯果汁牛奶冻/果汁冰糕。
- 组合食物: 1/2 杯砂锅，1/2 块三明治，1 杯蔬菜炖肉，1 小块墨西哥玉米卷。

碳水化合物计数水平（(Gillespie)
- 从总的碳水化合物意识到碳水化合物计数，甚至考虑血糖指数，不同的患者可能有不同的知识层次和经验。
- 碳水化合物意识：
  1. 知道哪些食物含有碳水化合物。
  2. 选择健康的、一致的食物量。
  3. 拒绝甜食和含糖饮料。

- 基本的碳水化合物计数：
  4. 促进碳水化合物的摄入量的一致性。
  5. 了解食品、药品和体力活动对血糖水平的影响。

- 以及识别方式
  6. 使用食品标签和碳水化合物的计算资源，以获得碳水化合物的信息。
  7. 估计被摄入食物中的数份（或半份）。

- 高级碳水化合物计数：
  8. 除了以上内容，增加了对实际摄入克数的精确计算。
  9. 计算碳水化合物的克数比计算份数更精确（如 ±5 g）。
  10. 知道并定量不太明显的碳水化合物来源（非淀粉含量高的蔬菜、奶制品等）。
  11. 使用胰岛素对碳水化合物的比例来计算速效胰岛素的剂量。
  12. 调整高脂肪或纤维的食物。
  13. 调整个人的血糖指数（GI）。
  14. 注意摄入高脂肪食物能够减缓碳水化合物的吸收。

临床治疗
- 血糖指数比计算食物总能量更加优越，但是研究结果却不尽相同 (Sheard)。

专家意见
- 监测碳水化合物摄入量是达到目标血糖值的关键步骤（美国糖尿病协会）。
- 对于 1 型糖尿病，目标是根据碳水化合物摄入量、餐前血糖值和活动量匹配餐前胰岛素用量。
- 对于 1 型糖尿病，目标是将碳水化合物摄入量融入健康、低热量的膳食计划。
- 碳水化合物计数，可以帮助患者监测食物的摄入量以同时满足每日能量需求及减肥的要求。
- 对于各种食物的碳水化合物含量，许多出版物和网上有可信的信息。例如：选择你的食物：糖尿病的换算列表，糖尿病碳水化合物和脂肪克数指南，http://www.calorieking.com,http://www.acaloriecounter.com.
- 碳水化合物计数的学习必须具有个性化，要考虑到病人是否愿意去学习，是否具有数字（数学）能力以及其他的因素。
- 对于不愿意或不能够学习高级碳水化合物计数的人，向他们教授这些知识是无用的。
- 碳水化合物计数的水平可逐步改善。
- 许多人错误地认为，限制碳水化合物是管理糖尿病的推荐方法。
- 在实践中，我们很少涉及血糖指数。虽然有其科学道理，但是很多因素能够影响餐后碳水化合物的吸收，如吸收的数量（血糖负荷），碳水化合物的类型，吸收的速度，食物中的脂肪和蛋白质，加工程度，烹饪方法等等。通常情况下，经验的方法更为实用。个人测餐后 2 小时血糖，并了解哪些食物能把自己的血糖升高到惊人的水平。

参考文献

Holzmeister, LA. Diabetes Carbohydrate and Fat Gram Guide, 4th edition. Alexandria, VA: American Diabetes Association; 2010.

Comments: Provides complete nutrition information, including grams of carb, for over 8000 foods and menu items.

American Diabetes Association. Standards of medical care in diabetes—2011. Diabetes Care, 2011; Vol. 34 Suppl1: pp. S11–61.

Comments: Reviews recommended medical nutrition therapy for type 1 and type 2 diabetes, including carbohydrate intake.

Wheeler ML, Daly A, Evert A, Franz MJ, et al. Choose your foods: exchange lists for diabetes, 6th edition, 2008:Description and guidelines for use. J Am Diet Assoc, 2008a; Vol. 108: pp. 883–888.

Comments: Provides evidence base for nutrition recommendations and revisions in the basic nutrition education booklet for diabetes.

Wheeler ML, Pi-Sunyer FX. Carbohydrate issues: type and amount. J Am Diet Assoc, 2008b; Vol. 108: pp. S34–9.

Comments: Reviews how type and amount of different carbohydrates influence postprandial glucose levels and overall glycemic control.

American Diabetes Association and American Dietetic Association. Choose Your Foods: Exchange Lists for Diabetes,6th edition. Alexandria, VA: American Diabetes Association and American Dietetic Association; 2008.

Comments: Basic nutrition education booklet for healthy eating for people with diabetes; provides information and portion sizes for foods that contain carbohydrate, protein, and fat.

Chiesa G, Piscopo MA, Rigamonti A, et al. Insulin therapy and carbohydrate counting. Acta Biomed, 2005; Vol. 76 Suppl 3: pp. 44–8.

Comments: Reviews data on how carb counting benefits diabetes management.

Institute of Medicine, Food, and Nutrition Board. Dietary reference intakes for energy, carbohydrate, fiber, fat,fatty acids, cholesterol, protein, and amino acids. Washington, DC: The National Academies Press; 2005.
Comments: A series of reports that presents dietary reference values for the intake of nutrients by Americans and Canadians, including the role of various nutrients in the body and dietary intake data.

Sheard NF, Clark NG, Brand-Miller JC, et al. Dietary carbohydrate (amount and type) in the prevention and management of diabetes: a statement by the American Diabetes Association. Diabetes Care, 2004; Vol. 27: pp. 2266–71.
Comments: Discusses the role of carbohydrates on blood glucose levels, including influence of type and amount, glycemic index, and glycemic load.

Gillespie SJ, Kulkarni KD, Daly AE. Using carbohydrate counting in diabetes clinical practice. J Am Diet Assoc,1998; Vol. 98: pp. 897–905.
Comments: Provides historical background and information about the use of carbohydrate counting for planning meals and snacks, with description of step-wise approach to developing skills.

2 型糖尿病的营养

Emily Loghmani, MS, RD, LDN, CDE, and Christopher D. Saudek, MD

定义
- 良好的营养方案是预防和管理 2 型糖尿病的基础（T2DM）。
- 2 型糖尿病的营养计划通常强调体重控制和冠心病危险因素的控制。
- 营养治疗包括由合格的营养师制订的具体的有发展性的营养方案。

流行病学
- 美国 80%~90% 的 2 型糖尿病患者都超重或者肥胖。
- 在美国，16% 的 2 型糖尿病患者进行非药物干预治疗（如饮食控制），57% 的患者仅口服降糖药，14% 的患者仅使用胰岛素，13% 的病人联合使用口服降糖药和胰岛素。
- 在美国，2 型糖尿病患者从发病到明确诊断的平均滞后时间大约为 7 年。

临床治疗

营养治疗
- 评估与年龄、性别和活动量相关的体重与体质指数，计算能量的需要量。
- 对于超重或者肥胖的患者，促使其减肥以减少胰岛素抵抗（表 2-4）。
- 个性化的分配碳水化合物、蛋白质和脂肪的摄入，促使改善血糖、血脂水平和血压。
- 减少总脂肪和饱和脂肪酸的摄入，避免摄入反式脂肪酸。
- 教会病人健康饮食、对碳水化合物的认识或者碳水化合物计数来配合降糖药/胰岛素治疗和病人可以处理的情况。
- 根据患者的社会和文化、饮食习惯和改变的意愿制定个性化的膳食计划。
- 促使患者进行规律的体力活动。

配合营养治疗的药物治疗
- 一定量的药物治疗（胰岛素、磺脲类，metaglinides、艾塞那肽、pramlintide）可能引起低血糖，营养计划应该包括规律的饮食计划以及低血糖的治疗计划。
- 二甲双胍、艾塞那肽和 pramlintide 能够引起恶心，如果餐时服用要减少剂量。
- 葡萄糖苷酶抑制剂、艾塞那肽和 pramlintide 通过减慢碳水化合物的吸收和胃排空，可用于干预治疗低血糖。如果需要，可以使用含糖饮料。
- 使用噻唑类药物和胰岛素的一个常见的副作用就是体重增加，而使用磺脲类药物没有这么明显的作用。推荐认真坚持低热量的膳食计划。

2 型糖尿病的营养

表 2-4. 糖尿病预防计划推荐的减肥每日所需热量和脂肪量

初始体重（磅）	推荐热量（卡）	脂肪（克）
120~170	1 200	33
175~215	1 500	42
220~245	1 800	50
250 磅以上	2 000	55

改编自 Wing R, Gillis B. 糖尿病预防计划之改变生活方式：第五章：达到减肥目的方法概述。PittsPittsburgh,PA: University of Pittsburgh; 1996:5-3.

临床治疗

- 热量计数：每餐摄入热量应量出为入，在下餐之前应该耗尽。(Bravata)。
- 在任何时间，摄入比维持体重所需的热量少 3 500 卡以上的热量，将会减轻大约 1 磅的体重。但是，因为存在一些影响长期体重变化的因素，3 500 卡热量的赤字能减轻 1 磅体重的作用在长期控制体重的过程中会逐渐减弱（Katen）。
- 医学专家对于限制碳水化合物或脂肪的摄入是否是最有效的减肥方式还没有达成共识(Sacks；Gardner)。但是一些证据显示地中海饮食能够有效减肥并且促进血糖水平的控制(Shai)。（参见营养：流行的糖尿病食疗法，第 116 页）。
- 严格限制摄入碳水化合物(Atkins diet and others) 能够引起早期利尿作用(体重快速减轻但是并非减肥)，而且轻度酮症可以降低食欲(Hession)。
- 严格限制脂肪的摄入(Pritikin diet and others) 能够减少热量最高的营养物质的摄入。
- 可持续的膳食计划是很重要的，特别是对于一个从低热量饮食过渡到维持体重饮食的患者来说，尽量避免体重反弹。
- 饮食不均衡（极低的碳水化合物或脂肪）是最难以持续的。
- 通过还有较低饱和脂肪酸和反式脂肪酸，较高纤维素的饮食，可以促进患者血脂水平。
- 血压可以通过低钠饮食控制。
- 中等程度的减肥（减轻 7% 的体重）对于预防和治疗 2 型糖尿病都是非常有效的。

随访

- 营养治疗患者的需要多次随访，以便反复进行指导和巩固。
- 随访的频率因人而异。
- 有同伴支持和同伴压力的集体治疗，通常很有效。

专家意见

- 因人而异的营养治疗是关键。
- 虽然有些人能够很好地做到极端严格的限制碳水化合物或脂肪的摄入，但是我们还是推荐均衡的营养摄入（脂肪、碳水化合物和蛋白质）。
- 低热量饮食几乎可以立刻改善血糖水平。

- 胰岛素抵抗能够随体重降低而减轻。
- 尽管无营养（0热量）饮料是否会影响食欲还存在争议，但是却不会影响体重，而高果糖玉米糖浆饮料却是摄入大量热量的来源。
- 我们建议严重肥胖的患者（BMI>40）考虑进行减肥手术，因为这样的患者对营养管理没有反应而且存在明显的合并症（Buchwald）。
- 营养计划不仅要考虑到糖尿病的治疗，还要兼顾到常见的合并症以及冠心病危险因素——肥胖、心脏病、高血压。
- 浓缩甜食（蛋糕、糖果、饼干等）几乎没有营养却含有很高的热量。

参考文献

Katan MB, Ludwig DS. Extra calories cause weight gain—but how much? JAMA, 2010; Vol. 303: pp. 65–6.

Comments: A carefully reasoned consideration of the factors that regulate body weight gain in addition to the starting figure that 3500-calorie deficit equals about 1 pound.

Sacks FM, Bray GA, Carey VJ, et al. Comparison of weight-loss diets with different compositions of fat, protein, and carbohydrates. NEJM, 2009; Vol. 360: pp. 859–73.

Comments: 811 overweight adults assigned to one of four reduced-calorie diets that varied in fat, protein, and carbohydrate for 2 years. All diets promoted weight loss regardless of macronutrient composition.

Hession M, Rolland C, Kulkarni U, et al. Systematic review of randomized controlled trials of low-carbohydrate vs.low-fat/low-calorie diets in the management of obesity and its comorbidities. Obes Rev, 2009; Vol. 10: pp. 36–50.

Comments: Review of 13 studies that compared low-carbohydrate/high-protein and low-fat/high-carbohydrate diets. Data suggest that low-carbohydrate diets promote more weight loss at 6 months and similar weight loss at 12 months compared to low-fat diets.

Mattes RD, Popkin BM. Nonnutritive sweetener consumption in humans: effects on appetite and food intake and their putative mechanisms. Am J Clin Nutr, 2009; Vol. 89: pp. 1–14.

Comments: Comprehensive review of nonnutritive sweeteners including safety and influence on appetite, energy intake, and body weight.

Ludwig DS. Artificially sweetened beverages: cause for concern. JAMA, 2009; Vol. 302: pp. 2477–8.

Comments: A discussion of the contribution of high fructose corn syrup (HFCS) to caloric intake, and the argument for taxing sweetened beverages.

Buchwald H, Estok R, Fahrback K, et al. Weight and type 2 diabetes after bariatric surgery: systematic review and meta-analysis. Am J Med, 2009; Vol. 122: pp. 248–256.

Comments: Systematic review of 621 studies from 1990 to 2006 that document resolution of type 2 diabetes in 78% and improvement in 87% of patients undergoing bariatric surgery.

American Diabetes Association. Standards of medical care in diabetes—2011. Diabetes Care, 2011; Vol. 34 Suppl1: pp. S11–61.

Comments: This statement by the American Diabetes Association discusses medical nutrition therapy and its role in preventing and managing diabetes complications.

Shai I, Schwarzfuchs D, Henkin Y, et al. Weight loss with a low-carbohydrate, Mediterranean, or low-fat diet.NEJM, 2008; Vol. 359: pp. 229–41.

Comments: 322 obese subjects, randomized to low-fat calorie restricted, Mediterranean calorie restricted, or low-carbohydrate unrestricted diets. Concluded that Mediterranean was most effective in glycemic control, and low-carb diets more effective in lipid control. Both more effective than low-fat in weight control.

Gardner CD, Kiazand A, Alhassan S, et al. Comparison of the Atkins, Zone, Ornish, and LEARN diets for change in weight and related risk factors among overweight premenopausal women: the A TO Z Weight Loss Study: a randomized trial. JAMA, 2007; Vol. 297: pp. 969–77.

Comments: 311 obese women randomized to Atkins, Zone, Ornish and LEARN diets for 12 months. Authors concluded that the Atkins diet promoted greater weight loss and more favorable metabolic effects.

Bravata DM, Sanders L, Huang J, et al. Efficacy and safety of low-carbohydrate diets: a systematic review. JAMA,2003; Vol. 289: pp. 1837–50.

Comments: Review of 107 reduced carbohydrate diets of varying content and duration. Authors concluded that main determinants of weight loss were duration of diet and decreased caloric intake, not carbohydrate content.

Diabetes Prevention Program (DPP) Research Group. The Diabetes Prevention Program (DPP): description of lifestyle intervention. Diabetes Care, 2002; Vol. 25: pp. 2165–71.

Comments: Description of the successful lifestyle intervention for participants in the Diabetes Prevention Program. Goals of weight loss and physical activity were achieved with lifestyle coaches, frequent follow-up,behavioral strategies, supervised activity, individualization, and support.

营养：流行的糖尿病食疗法

Simeon Margolis, MD, PhD

定义
- 这些年出现了很多的减肥饮食而且通常只流行很短一段时间。
- 一些饮食特别限制热量，但是大多数是通过限制饮食中碳水化合物、脂肪以及蛋白质比例间接地达到限制热量摄入的目的。
- 其他一些流行的旨在控制血糖水平和/或降低冠心病危险的食品，通常含有药物成分。

临床治疗

减肥饮食
- 新的减肥食品层出不穷，有些有很好的销量。
- 最近的减肥时尚饮食本身不限制热量的摄入，但是却限制食品的种类。
- Atkins（阿特金斯）：20% 碳水化合物，50% 脂肪，30% 蛋白质。
- South Beach and Zone（南海滩和地区）：40% 碳水化合物，30% 脂肪，30% 蛋白质。
- 体重监控：40% 碳水化合物，40% 脂肪，20% 蛋白质，限制热量摄入。

控制血糖和/或冠心病危险因素饮食
- 美国糖尿病协会（ADA）饮食目标要达到和维持：（1）血糖水平越接近正常水平越安全；（2）血脂和蛋白的分布减少冠心病；（3）血压正常或尽可能接近正常水平 (American Diabetes Association)。
- 美国糖尿病协会营养推荐：（1）如果要达到正常体重，限制热量摄入；（2）50% 碳水化合物，30% 脂肪，20% 蛋白质（7% 的饱和脂肪酸、200mg 胆固醇/天）的均衡饮食 (American Diabetes Association)。
- Pritink 减肥突破：从脂肪中摄取大约 10% 的热量。非常低脂饮食能够提高甘油三酯水平，降低高密度脂蛋白水平。
- Ornish（欧尼斯）饮食：70% 碳水化合物，10% 脂肪，20% 蛋白质和回归冠状动脉粥样硬化的其他生活方式。
- Mediterranean（地中海）饮食：进食大量的水果、蔬菜、面包、小麦、谷物、土豆、豆类、坚果、种子和橄榄油，限制食用红色肉类和鸡蛋；摄入产生较多不饱和脂肪酸的食物。
- DASH 饮食：强调水果、蔬菜和低脂奶制品。这种饮食包括全谷物、家禽、鱼和坚果；也有很少量的红色肉类、甜食和含糖饮料；减少饱和脂肪酸和胆固醇的数量。
- 国家胆固醇教育计划（NCEP）和美国心脏病协会（AHA）饮食和美国糖尿病协会（ADA）饮食类似。
- 美国心脏病协会（AHA）饮食和美国糖尿病协会（ADA）推荐每周至少吃 2 次鱼或者尽可能吃鱼油补充（wang）。
- 低血糖指数（GI）和低血糖负荷饮食：食物的血糖指数（GI）是指与一

营养：糖尿病的热门饮食

定量参照食物（葡萄糖或白面包）摄入后血糖变化的程度相比，摄入相似量的某种食物使血糖水平相对升高的能力。低血糖指数食品：芸豆；高血糖指数食品：土豆泥。血糖负荷计算是食物组成部分的血糖指数乘以该部分实际可利用的碳水化合物的数量（Brand-Miller）。

- 慢性肾病的患者需低蛋白质饮食（Robertson）。

随访

- 对于长期减肥的人来说，Atkins（阿特金斯）、South Beach（南海滩）、Zone（地区）、Ornish（欧尼斯）饮食和大多数传统饮食都相似：大约是 6 个月 6kg，2 年 3.3kg（Sacks）。
- 非常低脂饮食并不比那些含有 25% 热量的脂肪饮食更能降低胆固醇水平，但是却能降低高密度脂蛋白水平，提高甘油三酯水平。
- DASH 饮食可降低血压（Appel），预防 2 型糖尿病的发展。
- 地中海饮食可以改善血脂的脂质格局，预防 2 型糖尿病（Martinez）。
- 国家胆固醇教育计划（NCEP）可以改善低密度脂蛋白水平。
- 低血糖指数饮食可以改善餐后血糖，长远来说好处不确定（Brand-Miller）。
- 低蛋白饮食可以预防肾病的进程（Robertson）。

专家意见

- 即使是相对少量的减肥，如减少 7% 的体重，也可以显著改善血糖控制水平。
- 热量计数。限制一种主要的食物成分（如阿特金斯限制碳水化合物）也可以减轻体重，这是因为总的热量摄入也减少了。
- 不同的饮食影响短期体重减轻的速度，但是最终减肥的结果是一样的；总之，尚未证实哪种单一的饮食是特别有利的（Sacks）。
- 不均衡饮食和严格限制热量的饮食是很难被病人坚持下去的，随着时间的推移，大多数患者即使食用减肥饮食，体重仍然会恢复。
- 专家的选择：采纳美国糖尿病协会（ADA）饮食，同时限制额外的纳的摄取，[如不额外添加盐（<3~4g/d）]。

参考文献

Sacks FM, Bray GA, Carey VJ, et al. Comparison of weight-loss diets with different compositions of fat, protein, and carbohydrates. NEJM, 2009; Vol. 360: pp. 859–73.
Comments: Over a 2-year period, overweight adults lost similar amounts of weight whether they followed lowfat, low-carbohydrate, or high-protein diets.

Liese AD, Nichols M, Sun X, et al. Adherence to the DASH Diet is inversely associated with incidence of type 2 diabetes: the insulin resistance atherosclerosis study. Diabetes Care, 2009; Vol. 32: pp. 1434–6.
Comments: Adherence to a DASH-like diet was associated with a decrease in the development of type 2 diabetes among whites but not blacks or Hispanics.

American Diabetes Association, Bantle JP, Wylie-Rosett J, et al. Nutrition recommendations and interventions for diabetes:a position statement of the American Diabetes Association. Diabetes Care, 2008; Vol. 31 Suppl 1: pp. S61–78.
Comments: Nutritional recommendations by American Diabetes Association.

Martinez-Gonzalez MA, de la Fuente-Arrillaga C, Nunez-Cordoba JM, et al. Adherence to Mediterranean diet and risk of developing diabetes: prospective cohort study. BMJ, 2008; Vol. 336: pp. 1348–51.

Comments: Adherence to a Mediterranean diet was associated with a lower risk of developing type 2 diabetes.

Tinker LF, Bonds DE, Margolis KL, et al. Low-fat dietary pattern and risk of treated diabetes mellitus in postmenopausal women: the Women's Health Initiative randomized controlled dietary modification trial. Arch Intern Med, 2008; Vol. 168: pp. 1500–11.

Comments: A low-fat dietary pattern among generally healthy postmenopausal women showed no evidence of reducing diabetes risk after 8.1 years.

Robertson L, Waugh N, Robertson A. Protein restriction for diabetic renal disease. Cochrane Database Syst Rev, 2007; CD002181.

Comments: Reducing protein intake appears to slightly slow progression to renal failure but the differences were not statistically significant.

Appel LJ, Brands MW, Daniels SR, et al. Dietary approaches to prevent and treat hypertension: a scientific statement from the American Heart Association. Hypertension, 2006; Vol. 47: pp. 296–308.

Comments: DASH diet recommended to control hypertension.

Wang C, Harris WS, Chung M, et al. Fatty acids from fish or fish-oil supplements, but not alpha-linolenic acid, benefit cardiovascular disease outcomes in primary- and secondary-prevention studies: a systematic review. Am J Clin Nutr, 2006; Vol. 84: pp. 5–17.

Comments: Omega-3 fatty acids from fish or fish oil supplements, but not from alpha-linolenic acid, are beneficial for cardiovascular disease outcomes.

Dansinger ML, Gleason JA, Griffith JL, et al. Comparison of the Atkins, Ornish, Weight Watchers, and Zone diets for weight loss and heart disease risk reduction: a randomized trial. JAMA, 2005; Vol. 293: pp. 43–53.

Comments: Each popular weight-loss diet modestly reduced body weight and several cardiac risk factors at 1year. Overall dietary adherence rates were similar and low for all diets.

Brand-Miller J, Hayne S, Petocz P, et al. Low-glycemic index diets in the management of diabetes: a meta-analysis of randomized controlled trials. Diabetes Care, 2003; Vol. 26: pp. 2261–7.

Comments: Choosing low glycemic index (GI) foods in place of conventional or high GI foods has a small but clinically useful effect on medium-term glycemic control in patients with diabetes.

Lichtenstein AH, Van Horn L. Very low fat diets. Circulation, 1998; Vol. 98: pp. 935–9.

Comments: Very low-fat diets do not lower cholesterol more than diets containing 25% fat. They also raise triglycerides and lower HDL cholesterol.

体力活动和锻炼

Mariana Lazo, MD, ScM, PhD, and Mary Huizinga, MD, MPH

定义
- 体力活动和锻炼：由骨骼肌收缩产生的身体活动，这种活动需要的能量比身体静息时消耗的能量更多，并且能够改善身体素质。
- 身体素质：包括呼吸功能，肌肉功能和灵活性（见下文）。
- 体力活动强度的分类：轻度（达到最大心率的35%~54%）；中度（达到最大心率的55%~69%）；高度（达到最大心率的70%~89%）。
- 最大心率=220−年龄，最好由分级运动试验来确定（GXT）

流行病学
- 体力活动是预防和管理2型糖尿病的重要组成部分。
- 无论是单纯锻炼还是联合饮食控制，都对糖尿病患者有益处(Thomas；Wasserman)。
- 血糖控制：体育锻炼6个月后，糖化血红蛋白A1c降低0.3%~0.8%(Snowling；Church；Balducci)，在这个范围内显著减少微血管、大血管以及非血管并发症（UKPDS）。
- 身体组成：运动降低体重（平均为5%），减小腰围（2~3cm）和减少身体脂肪（平均15%）。无论带不带有氧运动，抗组训练都能增加瘦体重。
- 危险因素控制：改善血压（平均降低收缩压4~6mmHg，舒张压2~6mmHg），降低高血脂（甘油三酯平均降低26.6mg/dl，低密度脂蛋白降低9.6mg/dl，高密度脂蛋白平均升高3.7~5.0mg/dl），减轻肥胖。
- 心血管获益：最大耗氧量（VO_2max），血管结构和功能（内皮功能障碍和血管扩张性），心肌功能和CAD（冠状动脉疾病）风险和死亡率。
- 心理影响：改善生活质量和抑郁症的症状。

临床治疗

推荐锻炼计划前的病人需求评价
- 心脏风险：美国糖尿病协会建议考虑个人心电图负荷试验，40岁以上或30岁以上且有（1）患有1型或2型糖尿病10年以上；（2）伴有其他冠心病危险因素（高血压、抽烟和血脂异常）；或（3）存在微血管并发症（视网膜病变或肾病）的冠心病高风险者需要中−高强度锻炼。此外，有以下任何情况者：（1）已知或怀疑患有冠心病、中风、和/或周围血管疾病；（2）自主神经病变；或（3）晚期肾病，肾功能衰竭。不论年龄，都需要中−高强度锻炼。
- 如果存在以下情况，AHA/ACC推荐进行GXT试验：（1）患冠心病且在近2年内未进行过负荷试验；（2）胸部不适或呼吸困难的症状；（3）外周动脉疾病（PAD）或脑血管疾病的临床或实验室证据；（4）梗死或缺血的心电图证据；（5）剧烈运动的意愿。
- 非心脏因素：低血糖危险因素包括反复出现血糖测量值偏低，长期持续的糖尿病，低体重指数，未意识的低血糖损害，胰岛素治疗和降糖药（如磺脲类药物和 meglitinides）。在推荐锻炼前应考虑低血糖的预防措施（详见低血糖：预防和治疗，60 页）。
- 外周动脉疾病和足部护理：患有外周动脉疾病者需要个性化的监督锻炼计划，和预防足部损伤的措施如限速步行，水上运动或卧位踏车运动，适合的鞋子以及定期的足部检查。
- 微血管疾病：增殖性视网膜病变是进行有氧运动或活动（需要做 Valsalva 动作）的禁忌。
- 严重的周围神经病变：增加运动导致足部损伤的风险。
- Charcot 关节皮肤溃烂和发展的风险。

ADA/AHA 对于制订锻炼计划的指南

- 总则：中年患者力量和灵活性有限，以及其他一些合并症（如肥胖、骨关节炎）阻碍其进行各种运动。选择一个可以达到的目标 – 耗时少、周期短的轻快的活动来代替耗时 30 分钟的专门的运动。有氧运动结合抗阻训练能够增加耐力。
- 进增量：久坐不动的话，开始时应该处于较低水平，并逐步增加。
- 频率：每周最少 3 天。
- 强度：中等强度的锻炼有积极地影响。对应 40%~60% 的最大有氧能力。如果身体能够耐受并且没有禁忌证的话，推荐高强度的运动。
- 教育：指导患者辨别症状不典型的缺血，在自我监测血糖的基础上调整药物。进行锻炼之前进行适当的足部护理及合理营养。必要情况下准备糖尿病识别手镯或鞋子。
- 热身：5~19 分钟低强度有氧运动和 5~10 分钟肌肉伸展和降温期。
- 补水：开始锻炼前和锻炼的过程中，频繁的、足量的补充丢失的水分。
- 运动时间：每周 150 分钟中强度锻炼或 90 分钟高强度锻炼。每次活动至少 10 分钟。因为对于一些人来说，想要改善耐力和达到相似的效果，3 个 10 分钟的活动比 1 个 30 分钟的活动效果要好。
- 计划持续时间：通过体力活动，胰岛素抵抗会有急性或慢性的改善。身体成分的改变通常需要更长时间。理想的情况下，改变生活方式应该是永久性的。
- 类型：有氧运动：大的肌肉群以相同的节奏，进行重复、持续动作，每次至少 10 分钟（如步行、骑车、慢跑和游泳）。增加心肺功能和能量消耗。抗阻运动：使用肌肉的力量去移动重物或对抗阻性负荷做功的活动（如举重，使用重的器械锻炼）。增加肌肉力量以及身体对葡萄糖的利用。包括锻炼全身主要肌肉群（上半身、下半身和核心）的 5~10 组动作，完成 1~4 套这样的动作，重复做 10~15 次，直到力竭为止；可以随着时间的推移使用更重的重量，但是只能举 8~10 次。这两种锻炼的方式对于糖尿病来说都很重要，即便是联合较温和的锻炼方式（如瑜伽），组合锻炼也可以提供最大的健康益处。

胰岛素治疗的患者的特别注意事项

- 锻炼之前进行代谢控制：如果空腹血糖超过 250mg/dl 并且尿中出现酮体，应避免进行体力活动；如果只是血糖高还没有酮体时，也应该多加注意。如果血糖水平超过 100mg/dl，应该摄入格外的碳水化合物。

体力活动和锻炼

- 锻炼前后都要监测血糖：能够区分什么时候需要改变胰岛素的量或者食物的摄入量，这对于糖尿患者来说是很必要的。要了解进行不同锻炼的血糖反应。这一点对于不同的患者也是不尽相同的。
- 减少胰岛素用量：锻炼前通常要减少速效或短效胰岛素的用量。一般减少50%的量。针对不同的患者和不同的锻炼方式减少滴定胰岛素（Titrate insulin）用量。进行剧烈的有氧运动时减少胰岛素的用量通常比抗阻运动时减少的更多。使用胰岛素和胰岛素促分泌素治疗的患者，发生低血糖的风险更高，建议必要时应补充一些碳水化合物。
- 食物摄取：对于无计划的运动，应增加碳水化合物的消耗以避免出现低血糖。要随身携带一些碳水化合物食物，在体力活动过程中以及活动后可以及时补充。对于有计划的运动来说，减少速效或短效胰岛素的用量比摄入额外的碳水化合物效果更好。
- 低血糖：如果在锻炼过程中出现低血糖的症状，立即停止运动。警惕锻炼后6~12小时出现的低血糖延迟作用。
- 高血糖：有些患者在进行抗阻运动或剧烈的有氧运动时，因为体内儿茶酚胺的增加而引起血糖升高，但这种情况并不常见。

2型糖尿病的预防

- 对于有糖尿病危险因素的成年人，应该坚持每周至少2.5小时的中度－剧烈的体力活动以预防2型糖尿病。
- 较大量的体力活动也可以降低妊娠糖尿病的发展的风险。
- 糖尿病预防计划显示：那些坚持强化生活方式计划的糖尿病前期患者能够降低58%的糖尿病进展风险。（详见"糖尿病照顾的关键研究：预防和血糖控制，第15页）。

随访

- 影响坚持的因素：认知障碍和利益，自我效能，动机，社会支持，访问，提供者的支持，存在抑郁或焦虑。
- 有效的促进长期坚持的因素：进行个人或团体辅导，活动咨询，团队支持和电话咨询。

专家意见

- 锻炼对糖尿病的益处是有据可查的，包括对代谢的影响，危险因素控制，心血管益处和心理上的影响。
- 运动处方包括运动前心脏风险评估、非心脏风险评估以及详细的运动方案（如运动持续的时间、频率、强度以及运动的类型等）。
- 鼓励患者进行有氧运动和抗阻运动相结合的运动方式。
- 目标达到至少3个不连续天/周的训练，最低为150分钟/周中等强度的运动或90分钟/周高强度的运动，持续10分钟以上的个人运动或有氧运动。建议抗阻运动每周2~3次。
- 存在已知的冠心病不是体育锻炼的绝对禁忌证，但是需要进行有监督的心脏康复计划。
- 透析的患者也可进行运动。

- 未控制的增殖性视网膜病变的患者不要进行那些能够增高眼压和出血风险的运动。
- 对于患有外周神经病变的患者来说,中等强度的步行运动不会增加其溃疡性病变的风险。
- 要重点发挥体力活动方案中的自我效能。
- 鼓励长期锻炼计划以获得最大利益。

建议的基础

Colberg SR, Sigal RJ, Fernhall B, et al. Exercise and type 2 diabetes: the American College of Sports Medicine and the American Diabetes Association: joint position statement executive summary. Diabetes Care, 2010; Vol. 33: pp. 2692–6.

Comments: American Diabetes Association and American College of Sports Medicine joint position statement on exercise and type 2 diabetes.

Marwick TH, Hordern MD, Miller T, et al. Exercise training for type 2 diabetes mellitus: impact on cardiovascular risk: a scientific statement from the American Heart Association. Circulation, 2009; Vol. 119: pp. 3244–62.

Comments: Most recent scientific statement of this topic from the American Heart Association.

其他参考文献

Balducci S, Zanuso S, Nicolucci A, et al. Effect of an intensive exercise intervention strategy on modifiable cardiovascular risk factors in subjects with type 2 diabetes mellitus: a randomized controlled trial: the Italian Diabetes and Exercise Study (IDES). Arch Intern Med, 2010; Vol. 170: pp. 1794–>803.

Comments: Describes the metabolic benefits of supervised combination exercise training versus control group over 1 year in diabetes.

Church TS, Blair SN, Cocreham S, et al. Effects of aerobic and resistance training on hemoglobin A1c levels in patients with type 2 diabetes: a randomized controlled trial. JAMA, 2010; Vol. 304: pp. 2253–62.

Comments: This randomized controlled study found that combination aerobic and resistance training over 9 months was more beneficial than either alone in reducing HbA1c (-0.3%, p=0.03).

Weltman NY, Saliba SA, Barrett EJ, et al. The use of exercise in the management of type 1 and type 2 diabetes. Clin Sports Med, 2009; Vol. 28: pp. 423–39.

Comments: Provides a summary of the recommendations from the American College of Sport Medicine.

Williamson DA, Rejeski J, Lang W, et al. Impact of a weight management program on health-related quality of life in overweight adults with type 2 diabetes. Arch Intern Med, 2009; Vol. 169: pp. 163–71.

Comments: Describes improvements in quality of life and depression scores in the Look AHEAD study that were mediated by enhanced physical fitness.

Snowling NJ, Hopkins WG, Effects of different modes of exercise training on glucose control and risk factors for complications in type 2 diabetic patients: a meta-analysis. Diabetes Care, 2006; Vol. 29: pp. 2518–27.

Comments: Meta-analysis demonstrating the effects of exercise on A1c and other measures of glucose control and risk factors.

Thomas DE, Elliott EJ, Naughton GA. Exercise for type 2 diabetes mellitus. Cochrane Database Syst Rev, 2006;Vol. 3: CD002968.

Comments: Systematic review of trials testing the effects of exercise in people with T2DM.

Zinman B, Ruderman N, Campaigne BN, et al. Physical activity/exercise and diabetes. Diabetes Care, 2004; Vol. 27 Suppl 1: pp. S58–62.

Comments: Summary of ADA recommendations of Physical Activity and Diabetes based on technical reviews. Covers type 1 and type 2 diabetes recommendations.

Sigal RJ, Kenny GP, Wasserman DH, et al. Physical activity/exercise and type 2 diabetes. Diabetes Care, 2004;Vol. 27: pp. 2518–39.

Comments: Most comprehensive review of the literature on the role of exercise and Type 2 diabetes.

Desai MY, Nasir K, Rumberger JA, et al. Relation of degree of physical activity to coronary artery calcium score in asymptomatic individuals with multiple metabolic risk factors. Am J Cardiol, 2004; Vol. 94:pp. 729–32.

Comments: Large observational study demonstrating that individuals who engage in physical activity are less likely to present with atherosclerosis.

Stewart KJ. Exercise training and the cardiovascular consequences of type 2 diabetes and hypertension: plausible mechanisms for improving cardiovascular health. JAMA, 2002; Vol. 288: pp. 1622–31.

Comments: Well-conducted narrative review of the current evidence of the benefits of exercise training beyond the glycemic control and blood pressure reduction.

UK Prospective Diabetes Study (UKPDS) Group. Intensive blood-glucose control with sulphonylureas or insulin compared with conventional treatment and risk of complications in patients with type 2 diabetes (UKPDS 33).Lancet, 1998; Vol. 352: pp. 837–53.

Comments: This study helped to determine clinically meaningful reductions in A1c, setting a reference value for RCT of therapies for T2DM.

Jakicic JM, Wing RR, Butler BA, et al. Prescribing exercise in multiple short bouts versus one continuous bout:effects on adherence, cardiorespiratory fitness, and weight loss in overweight women. Int J Obes Relat Metab Disord, 1995; Vol. 19: pp. 893–901.

Comments: Early RCT that supports the benefit of prescribing short bouts of exercise among people with obesity.

Wasserman DH, Zinman B. Exercise in individuals with IDDM. Diabetes Care, 1994; Vol. 17: pp. 924–37.

Comments: Evidence of effect of exercise in T1DM.

患者教育：糖尿病概述

Nancyellen Brennan, CRNP, CDE, and Rita Rastogi Kalyani, MD, MHS

定义
- 患者教育是一个持续不断的过程，糖尿病患者通过这个过程学习到关于糖尿病的知识、态度和必要的技能，以便他们决策用药、体力活动、饮食计划和应对那些影响他们血糖水平、冠心病危险因素和生活质量的心理社会挑战。
- 包括以证据为基础的临床知识、行为策略以及教育理论。

流行病学
- 糖尿病教育改善临床指标：糖化血红蛋白 A1c（4~6 个月后降低 1.9%），血压（4~6 个月后降低 5mmHg），体重减轻（12~14 个月后减轻 1.6kg）（Duke）。
- 主要由护士和营养师提供相关教育，也可由药剂师、临床医生和社区卫生工作者提供。

临床治疗

指导原则
- 下列一般原则就如何对待所有患者提供了一个框架，可根据需要使用。
- 赋权：促进和支持患者的能力，这种能力使他们做出明智的自我照顾的决策。这不是专制的教育方式，而是一种以患者为中心的教育方式。
- 成人学习：如果患者（1）相信这些信息对他们来说很重要；（2）解决了过去帮助或阻碍学习的经验的影响；（3）控制了学习经验，那么他们就会学习的很好。
- 关于糖尿病，确定患者知道什么，他们想学什么以及他们的学习类型。
- 健康行为改变的跨理论模式：患者在愿意改变的不同阶段，需要具体的干预措施进入行动阶段。帮助患者基于他们改变的愿意选择现实的目标。
- 健康信念模式：有助于预测或解释基于态度和个人的信仰的健康行为：（1）疾病的易感性的；（2）疾病的严重性及其并发症；（3）预期效益及成本；（4）对于自己能够做出改变的能力的信心（自我效能）。方法是：（1）了解病人对自己所患糖尿病的严重程度以及糖尿病对自己生活的影响的观点（2）确定自我保健的风险和利益；（3）评价他们的信心水平。

干预
- 设定目标：（1）定义与患者合作的目标；（2）计划具有特定性（您打算在什么步骤减肥？），可测量性（你会坚持多久？）和可实现性（1 到 10 这个范围内，您有可能坚持执行这个计划的程度是几？）。例如目标：我会步行 15 分钟，每周 3 次。我将停止饭后吃零食。
- 解决问题：集思广益设立方案，挑选最好的选择，并评估该选择的效果。这可以用来帮助患者树立自己的目标。
- 动机访谈：一种指令，是运用反映性倾听和探索矛盾心理的方法帮助病

患者教育：糖尿病概述

人改变困难行为的以病人为中心的咨询方式。（1）反映性倾听，帮助患者分清他们想改变的行为，并让他们知道你已经听到了他们的话；（2）识别关于改变的矛盾心理以帮助病人改变他们的行为；（3）以患者为中心的模式能够帮助病人确立一个更容易达到的目标。

- 前两种干预措施可以在门诊实施并且很容易培训，动机访谈需要花费较多的时间，而且需要多次培训。

随访

- 频率：糖尿病教育仅仅进行一次是无效的，它需要随访和巩固。随访的频率、时间和地点是可变化的。
- 即时随访：通过回答患者的问题进行教育：今天您对糖尿病有什么问题？今天您想学习那些关于糖尿病的知识？告诉我您今天想要解决的一件事。
- 评估目标：哪些可以做？哪些不可以做？你的计划中有哪些问题？谁可以帮助和支持你？你从哪里获得帮助？
- 设置新目标：下次随访您想做什么？
- 庆祝成功：无论实现多么小的目标，我们都要庆祝。

专家意见

- 健康教育者的责任不仅是提出建议，而且对于患者的糖尿病保健目标和达到这些目标的个性化方式，要确保他们获得最佳教育。
- 患者的责任是每天都要执行这些建议。
- 多听，少说：患者知道他们要怎么做。我们的任务是帮助患者拿出自己的解决方案，提供他们需要的信息以及支持他们的努力。
- 构建成功：过去您是怎么做的？上次您是怎么减肥的？

建议的基础

Anderson RM, Funnell MM. Patient empowerment: Myths and misconceptions. Patient Educ Couns, 2009; Vol. 79:pp. 277–82.

Comments: Excellent discussion of the use and misuse of empowerment.

Bodenheimer T, Handley MA. Goal-setting for behavior change in primary care: an exploration and status report.Patient Educ Couns, 2009; Vol. 76: pp. 174–80.

Comments: Review of the literature on goal setting. It does not look at outcomes. Goal setting was performed by clinicians during the visit, nonclinicians after a visit, or computer-based programs.

Duke SA, Colagiuri S, Colagiuri R. Individual patient education for people with type 2 diabetes mellitus. Cochrane Database Syst Rev, 2009.

Comments: This systematic review suggests a benefit of individual education on glycemic control when compared with usual care in a subgroup of those with a baseline HbA1c greater than 8%. In the small number of studies comparing group and individual education, there was an equal impact on HbA1c at 12–18 months.

Russell SS. An overview of adult-learning processes. Urol Nurs, 2006; Vol. 26: pp. 349–52, 370.

Comments: Description of the adult learning theory in clinical practice.

Deakin TA, McShane CE, Cade JE, Williams R. Group based training for self-management strategies in people with type 2 diabetes mellitus. Cochrane Database of Systematic Reviews, 2005.

Comments: Adults with type 2 diabetes who have participated in group based training programs show improved diabetes control (fasting blood glucose and glycated hemoglobin) and knowledge of diabetes in the short (4–6 months) and longer-term (12–14 months). There is some evidence that group based education programs may increase self-empowerment, quality of life, self-management skills, and treatment satisfaction.

Miller WR, Rollnick S. Motivational Interviewing: Preparing People to Change Addictive Behavior. New York:The Guilford Press; 2002.
Comments: This is the original publication on motivation interviewing—it describes the process in detail.

Prochaska JO, Velicer WF. The transtheoretical model of health behavior change. Am J Health Promot, 1997;Vol. 12: pp. 38–48.
Comments: Description and use of the transtheoretical model.

其他参考文献

Hill-Briggs F, Gemmell L. Problem solving in diabetes self-management and control: a systematic review of the literature. Diabetes Educ, 2007; Vol. 33: pp. 1032–50; discussion 1051–2.
Comments: Review of the literature of 52 studies on problem solving, individual and group sessions by nonclinicians.37% of the studies showed an improvement in A1c.

Hill-Briggs F. Problem solving. In: The Art and Science of Diabetes Self-Management Education: A Desk Reference for Healthcare Professionals. Chicago: American Associates of Diabetes Educators; 2006; pp. 731–759.
Comments: Good summary of how to do problem solving with patients.

Rosenstock IM. Understanding and enhancing patient compliance with diabetic regimens. Diabetes Care, 1985;Vol. 8: pp. 610–6.
Comments: Discussion of health belief model and self efficacy as a concept for supporting behavior change.

American Diabetes Association. http://www.diabetes.org/.
Comments: American Diabetes Association website has information for health professionals and patients,such as type 1, type 2, prediabetes, nutrition, and different age groups, and some information is available in Spanish. The site is somewhat difficult to navigate. You can cut and paste paragraphs to design your own patient handouts.

American Dietetic Association. http://www.eatright.org.
Comments: This website has one-page handouts on over 50 topics related to nutrition, which can be downloaded(not as PDF file). The handouts sponsored by food companies are biased; read carefully before using. The handouts authored by the association are better.

National Diabetes Education Program. http://www.ndep.nih.gov/.
Comments: This website has over 100 brochures and one-page handouts for patients and health professionals. The publications can be downloaded as PDF files or purchased from them for a low price. It covers a wide range of topics, including age, ethnicity, work place, and school issues, in 21 languages. Easy to navigate.

National Institute of Diabetes and Digestive and Kidney Diseases. http://www.diabetes.niddk.nih.gov.
Comments: This website has information on over 100 topics related to diabetes and complications. You can cut and paste to make your own handouts. They have an "easy-to-read" series. Easy to navigate.

患者教育：糖尿病的课程主题

Nancyellen Brennan, CRNP, CDE, and Rita Rastogi Kalyani, MD, MHS

定义
- 协调设置信息和教育经验，包括学习结果和教育方法的效果。
- DSME（糖尿病自我管理教育）是一种结构化和持续化的，学习糖尿病成功管理的必要知识和技能的过程。
- 在美国，获得认证的糖尿病教育者(CDE)是受过糖尿病教育的专业培训的医疗保健专业人员，其完成了1 000小时的糖尿病患者教育并且通过相关的考试。其他国家才刚刚开始自己的CDE计划。

流行病学
- 2007年，美国有57%的成年人参加了由门诊提供的DSME。
- 由护士、营养师、药剂师、医生和曾经指导过糖尿病管理的咨询师进行教育，获得认证的糖尿病教育者(CDE)进行教育更好。
- 强调实际问题解决技能，协作护理和维持自我管理的方式。

临床治疗

生存技能 – 新确诊患者需要了解的信息
- 改编自糖尿病患者管理指南的生存技能。
  - 如何以及何时服药：服药的时间（饭前或饭后），最常见的副作用；如果使用胰岛素，注射的技术，胰岛素的储存以及针头的处理。
  - 如何以及何时监测血糖和尿糖：如何使用血糖仪和尿液试纸并记录结果。
  - 膳食计划的基础："健康饮食"，碳水化合物的类别（图片示例很有帮助），强调碳水化合物摄入的规律性和一致性。
  - 如何处理低血糖：随时审查症状，管理，进行处理（如橘汁和糖块）。
  - 病态的日常管理: 高血糖(或低血糖)的风险,需要改变胰岛素的剂量,经常监测血糖,尿酮体检测。
  - 随访的日期和事件。
  - 如何获得进一步的糖尿病教育的信息。什么时候给医生打电话获得建议。

较晚期的糖尿病自我管理教育（美国糖尿病协会）
- 糖尿病：如何诊断，发病机制，危险因素的管理，治疗方案。
- 营养：描述含碳水化合物的食物，使用平板法了解碳水化合物的分布，阅读食品标签；如果使用胰岛素，则需要进行碳水化合物计数。
- 体力活动：有氧运动与抗阻运动，推荐活动的频率，如何适应体力限制。
- 药物：用药方式，不良反应，如何以及何时服药，适当的储存方式。
- 血糖监测：如何检测血糖和尿糖，记录结果，根据这些结果调整食物的摄入量和活动量，糖化血红蛋白检测的使用以及解释。
- 预防性筛查：包括特定检测的推荐和频率。
- 预防、检测和治疗急性并发症（糖尿病酮症酸中毒、低血糖、高血糖高渗综合征)：症状、治疗、何时就诊。
- 预防、发现和治疗慢性并发症(视网膜病变、肾病、神经病变、心血管疾病)：症状、治疗、何时就诊。
- 发展个人战略，以解决心理问题和疑虑：缺乏支持和抑郁症可以通过团体支持得到解决，这些团体包括家庭或教会成员，社会工作者或辅导员。
- 发展个人战略，以促进健康和行为的变化：目标设定以明确改变的愿望，同伴支持以及团体支持可以帮助维持改变，家庭通过健康膳食计划进行帮助，聚会交流和维持所需的药物。

随访

- 评估个人目标，如增加运动频率或限制进食不健康零食。如果没有实现，重新评估；如果实现，设置新的目标，但在同一时间段内设置目标不要超过两个。
- 学习内容,准备一页讲义,上面写上患者感兴趣的内容或者回答患者的问题。

专家意见

- 了解糖尿病相关知识能够帮助糖尿病患者及其家属学习如何成功管理糖尿病患者。
- 可以有大量的信息：在需要知道的知识基础上或1~2小时的较短的时间段内覆盖要了解关于糖尿病的知识。
- 使用直观教具(图片、模型)使患者教育具有互动性和趣味性，或进行小组活动(游戏、短剧)。
- 如果患者有独特的需求(身体、学习或社会限制)，可以提供个体教育。否则，群体教育对于患者支持和分享想法很有价值。支持团体也可以有教育组成部分。

建议的基础

Duke S-AS, Colagiuri S, Colagiuri R. Individual patient education for people with type 2 diabetes mellitus.Cochrane Database of Systematic Reviews, 2009; Vol. 21: CD005268.
Comments: Review of the value of individual education.

Funnell M, Brown T, Childs B, Haas L, et al. National Standards for Diabetes Self-Management Education. Diabetes Care, 2008; pp. S97–104.
Comments: Summary of ADA standards for education.

Centers for Disease Control and Prevention. Age-Adjusted Percentage of Ever Attended Diabetes Self-Management Class for Adults . 18 Years with Diabetes, United States, 2000–2007. Behavior Risk Factor Surveillance System; 2007. http://www.cdc.gov/diabetes/statistics/preventive/fY_class.htm,
Comments: Graph depicting adults attending DSMT.

Deakin TA, McShane CE, Cade JE, Williams R. Group-based training for self management strategies in people with Type 2 diabetes mellitus. Cochrane Database of Systematic Reviews, 2005; Vol. 18: CD003417.
Comments: Review of the value of group education.

American Healthways. Inpatient Management Guidelines for People with Diabetes; 2004. http://www.healthways. com/WorkArea/showcontent.aspx?id=322.

Comments: List of survival skills on p. 10.

International Diabetes Federation. Consultative Section on Education International Standards for Diabetes Education. Brussels: International Diabetes Federation; 2003.
Comments: Summary of International Diabetes Federation standard for diabetes education; very similar to ADA standards.

International Diabetes Federation Consultative Section on Education. http://www.idf.org/Diabetes_Education.

其他参考文献

American Diabetes Association. http://www.diabetes.org/living-with-diabetes/treatment-and-care/blood-glucose-control/blood-glucose-meters.html.
Comments: One-page patient handout on blood glucose meters.

American Diabetes Association. http://www.diabetes.org/living-with-diabetes/treatment-and-care/blood-glucose-control/hypoglycemia-low-blood.html.
Comments: Patient handout on hypoglycemia.

American Diabetes Association. http://www.diabetes.org/living-with-diabetes/treatment-and-care/who-is-on-your-healthcare-team/when-youre-sick.html.
Comments: Patient handout on sick day management.

American Diabetes Association. http://www.diabetes.org/living-with-diabetes/treatment-and-care/who-is-on-your-healthcare-team/visiting-your-health-care.html.
Comments: Patient handout on visiting the doctor.

患者教育：克服糖尿病障碍

Nancyellen Brennan, CRNP, CDE, and Rita Rastogi Kalyani, MD, MHS

定义
- 干扰患者学习或管理其糖尿病能力的任何情况。
- 障碍可能与患者、教育者或环境有关。

流行病学
- 健康素养不高的人，出现血糖控制不良和视网膜病变的概率是其他人的两倍 (Schillinger)。
- 根据糖尿病相关的计算能力能够预测 A1c 水平，并且能够解释血糖控制的种族差异 (Osborn；Cavanaugh)。
- 一半注射胰岛素的患者报告说如果有可以减轻疼痛的产品，他们就更能够坚持定期注射胰岛素 (Rubin)。
- 41% 的糖尿病患者报告心理素质欠佳，从而影响糖尿病护理 (Peyrot)。
- 抑郁症是一种糖尿病患者常见的合并症，其影响糖尿病护理。

临床治疗

克服病人障碍
- 素养：(1) 讲义以图片为基础，多次重复，短时间教学，一次覆盖一个主题，与识字的照顾者或家庭成员分享书面指导；(2) 询问病人其喜欢的学习方式（例如阅读、视频、音乐、游戏或短剧）。Vanderbilt 糖尿病识字和算术教育工具包 (DLNET) 是一个很好的资源。
- 文化：(1) 在其文化基础上了解健康信仰、食物以及补充和替代的药物很重要；(2) 包括计划中的目标文化的成员；(3) 为所有员工提供文化敏感性培训。
- 生理缺陷：(1) 视力：使用大字印刷或音频工具，电脑助手等；(2) 听力：使用书面材料，带上朋友或家庭成员，电脑辅助学习；(3) 身体灵活性：观察血糖仪的使用和胰岛素注射技术，选择更容易使用的血糖仪，使用胰岛素笔或预充式注射器。
- 疼痛：(1) 短痛，反复；(2) 止痛药可能干扰注意力；(3) 选择每次扎不同的手指可以减轻针刺式血糖仪带来的疼痛。
- 情绪：(1) 休克、愤怒、否认和感觉不堪重负很常见；在随访开始前让患者讲一会儿或采用反映性听听方式；(2) 筛查抑郁症患者；(3) 有压力的生活状况（如犯罪、经济问题、酒精、语言和性虐待或忽视）；这样的患者需考虑转到精神健康机构和/或社会工作机构。
- 健康信念：患者没有看到关于糖尿病学习的重要性是因为他们不理解与这种无症状的疾病相关的风险；随访期间与患者进行讨论或参考教育。
- 社会耻辱：患者可能会因为害怕被人歧视而不愿意与他人分享自己的病情，这阻碍他们发挥最佳的自我管理糖尿病能力。鼓励患者谈论他们关注的问题，支持团体可能会有所帮助。
- 缺乏社会支持：帮助患者识别他们的支持系统。家庭和朋友可能并不总

患者教育：糖尿病的课程主题

是有帮助的；其他形式的社会支持包括网络或电话同行支持和志愿者组织（如教会、糖尿病协会或服务团体）。
- 社会地位低下的：患者将从素养干预、参与式决策和社会支持中受益。

克服临床障碍
- 糖尿病教育者可能比医生有更多时间进行评估和教育。
- 将医生和糖尿病教育者之间，教育内容和哲学之间（如代谢控制目标）的感知和实际的差异缩小到最小化。教育者应作为一个团队为病人提供课程或和讲义。
- 如果医生推荐，患者更愿意参加教育会议。

克服健康体系障碍
- 缺乏获得认证的糖尿病教育者：不足以满足患者的需要。解决方案：培训诊所工作人员或教会教友，糖尿病协会成员，在候诊区张贴宣传海报或播放教育视频，发放有关患者问题和关注点的单一主题的书面材料，进行团队医疗访问，其中就包括教育(Deitrick)。
- 后勤：不方便的时间或地点和交通不便。解决方案：延长糖尿病门诊时间，方便患者在同一天内既能看医生，也能看糖尿病教育者；在社区内开展教育（如教会，妇女或男子团体，学校）。
- 社区资源不足：由于成本或交通问题无法获得药物；无人帮助管理胰岛素，无人帮助购买或准备食物导致的不良饮食。解决方案：帮助患者识别和招募可以帮助完成这些任务的志愿者，如邻居、亲属或教会的成员，并制作成名单。

开始使用胰岛素的障碍
- 害怕打针：展示注射技术，使用超细针和胰岛素注射笔。
- 害怕低血糖：强调如果管理得当，严重低血糖的发生率很低。
- 害怕体重增加：加强健康饮食和身体活动。
- 失败的感觉：强调疾病的自然进程，大多数糖尿病患者最后都需要胰岛素治疗。

随访
- 回顾知识和技能：你教的知识病人是否记得并执行？
- 继续寻找障碍：什么使您很难……服药？……监测您的血糖？

专家意见
- 对于那些药物治疗不能达到目标血糖值的患者来说，解决其教育的障碍很重要。
- 对于有明显障碍的患者，要考虑个性化的教育和频繁的随访。
- 患者经常听到关于糖尿病的相互矛盾的信息，协调您的团队给患者提供一致的信息。
- 教育者和患者之间支持性的关系是其成功学习和健康行为改变的关键。

建议的基础

American Association of Diabetes Educators. AADE position statement. Cultural sensitivity and diabetes education:recommendations for diabetes educators. Diabetes Educ, 2007; Vol. 33: pp. 41–44.

Comments: Position statement by American Association of Diabetes Educators, includes definition and ways to incorporate cultural sensitivity into your practice.

其他参考文献

Peyrot M, Rubin RR, Funnell MM, et al. Access to diabetes self-management education: results of national surveys of patients, educators, and physicians. Diabetes Educ, 2009; Vol. 35: pp. 246–8, 252–6, 258–63.

Comments: Interview of 1169 patients, 1871 diabetes educators, and 629 doctors to determine perceived barriers to receiving DSME.

Osborn CY, Cavanaugh K, Wallston KA, et al. Diabetes numeracy: an overlooked factor in understanding racial disparities in glycemic control. Diabetes Care, 2009; Vol. 32: pp. 1614–9.

Comments: Cross-sectional study examining the mediating effect of health literacy and numeracy on the relationship between African American race and glycemic control.

Cavanaugh K, Wallston KA, Gebretsadik T, et al. Addressing literacy and numeracy to improve diabetes care: two randomized controlled trials. Diabetes Care, 2009; Vol. 32: pp. 2149–55.

Comments: Randomized controlled trials evaluating the impact of providing literacy- and numeracy-sensitive teaching in a diabetes care program on A1c and other diabetes outcomes.

Rubin RR, Peyrot M, Kruger DF, et al. Barriers to insulin injection therapy: patient and health care provider perspectives. Diabetes Educ, 2009; Vol. 35: pp. 1014–22.

Comments: A survey of patient and provider perspectives on barriers to insulin injection therapy.

Funnell MM, Brown TL, Childs BP, et al. National standards for diabetes self-management education. Diabetes Care, 2009; Vol. 32 Suppl 1: pp. S87–94.

Comments: Guidelines designed to define quality diabetes self-management education and to assist diabetes educators to provide evidence-based education.

Brown AF. Patient, system and clinician level interventions to address disparities in diabetes care. Curr Diabetes Rev, 2007; Vol. 3: pp. 244–8.

Comments: Discusses evidence on interventions at the individual, provider, healthcare system, and community levels that have the potential to reduce diabetes disparities.

Marrero DG. Overcoming patient barriers to initiating insulin therapy in type 2 diabetes mellitus. Clin Cornerstone, 2007; Vol. 8: pp. 33–40, discussion 41-3.

Comments: Reviews the importance of starting insulin early and how to overcome patient's resistance to starting insulin.

Peyrot M, Rubin RR, Lauritzen T, et al. Psychosocial problems and barriers to improved diabetes management:results of the Cross-National Diabetes Attitudes, Wishes and Needs (DAWN) Study. Diabet Med, 2005; Vol. 22:pp. 1379–85.

Comments: Cross-sectional study looking at the patient- and provider-reported psychosocial problems and barriers to effective self-care.

Deitrick L, Swavely D, Merkle LN, et al. Group medical visits for patients with type 2 diabetes: patient and physician perspectives. Abstr Academy Health Meet, 2005; Vol. 22: abstract no. 4077.
Comments: Description of the successful use of group medical visits for diabetes education.

Schillinger D, Grumbach P, Piette J. Association of Health Literacy with Diabetes Outcomes. JAMA, 2002; Vol. 288:p. 475.
Comments: Cross-sectional study showing that inadequate health literacy is independently associated with poorer glycemic control and higher rates of retinopathy.

Vanderbilt University Diabetes Research and Training Center Diabetes Literacy and Numeracy Education Toolkit(DLNET). http://www.mc.vanderbilt.edu/diabetes/drtc/preventlonandcontrol/tools.php.
Comments: 24 modules covering diabetes topics for those with low health literacy. Can be used as needed over multiple visits.

糖尿病前期

糖尿病前期或增加患糖尿病的风险类别

Rachel Derr, MD, PhD

定义

- 空腹血糖受损(IFG)和糖耐量受损(IGT)是处于正常和显性糖尿病之间的糖代谢异常。
- 糖尿病前期,是指IFG或IGT,或两者兼而有之。
- 空腹血糖受损(IFG),只需要检测空腹血糖。糖耐量受损(IGT)需要行75克口服葡萄糖耐量试验。
- 糖化血红蛋白5.7%~6.4%可将该人视为"糖尿病高风险人群"(ADA糖尿病的医疗标准)。
- 确切的定义见表2-5。

表2-5. 糖耐量异常状态的诊断标准

状态	空腹血糖(mg/dl)	75克OGTT后两小时血糖(mg/dl)	A1c (%)
正常*	< 100	< 140	< 5.7
空腹血糖受损(IFG)	100~125	< 140	—
糖耐量受损(IGT)	< 100	140~199	—
IFG合并IGT	100~125	140~199	—
糖尿病前期或糖尿病高风险**	100~125	140~199	5.7~6.4
糖尿病**	≥ 126	≥ 200	> 6.5

*WHO和IDF建议,空腹血糖受损是110~125mg/dl
** 至少有一个条件满足诊断标准。
摘自Rachel Derr.

流行病学

- 在美国,2005-2006年期间20岁的人IFG的患病率为5.7%和IGT为13.8%,约30%的人患有IFG或IGT (Nathan; Cowie)。
- 10年来IFG发病率为14%,IGT为48%,平均年龄以57年为基线(Meigs)。
- 一个或两个异常增高了患2型糖尿病的风险(约25%在3~5年内发病,一生中患病多达70%)和增加了心血管疾病的风险(HR1.1~1.4)(Nathan)。

糖尿病前期或增加患糖尿病的风险类别

- 危险因素同糖尿病。

诊断

- 个人筛选，45岁或任何年龄的成人只要BMI达到$25mg/kg^2$和有其他糖尿病的危险因素（见2型糖尿病的遗传危险因素，第192页，见2型糖尿病环境危险因素与筛选，第188页），以确定未来患糖尿病的风险（糖尿病ADA标准）。
- 通常没有明显症状。
- 空腹血糖指空腹和不摄入碳水化合物至少8个小时。
- 75g OGTT后两小时血糖（mg/dl）：为诊断糖尿病前期的黄金标准，但比较消耗时间。
- 糖化血红蛋白："增加患糖尿病的风险类别"的新标准包括糖化血红蛋白5.7%~6.4%。
- 所有这些检测中，风险是连续。

临床治疗

护理标准（根据美国糖尿病协会）

- 中等强度的运动（每天30分钟），根据糖尿病预防计划（DPP）的协议减轻体重（体重的5%~10%），并戒烟。
- 二甲双胍，应用于有IFG和IGT个人和有以下情况者：年龄60岁，BMI $35mg/m^2$，糖尿病家族病史，高甘油三酯，降低高密度脂蛋白，高血压，糖化血红蛋白6.0%。
- 其他药物研究（噻唑、阿卡波糖），也可能有效地预防糖尿病，但因其继发的副作用，并不一致推荐。

治疗后的预后（随机对照试验）

- dPP（3 234例）：3年以上从IFG或IGT进展为糖尿病对照组有29%，而强化生活方式组有14%的（58%相对减少），二甲双胍组22%（31%相对减少）；二甲双胍在BMI达$35kg/m^2$年轻患者最有效（knowler）。
- 芬兰糖尿病预防研究（522例）：4年以上从IGT进展DM，在对照组有23%，而重量减少/运动组只有11%的（减少58%）（Tuomilehto）。
- 在大庆研究（557例）：6年以上从IGT向DM的进展，在对照组有67.7%，在饮食和运动组有46%（减少31%）（PAN）。
- dPPos发现生活方式干预有持续长远的利益，在10年后有减少34%糖尿病的发病率（knowler）。这些结果与其他用生活方式干预糖尿病患者的长期随访研究相似，包括芬兰糖尿病预防研究（7年内减少43%）(Lindstrom)和大庆的研究（在20年减少43%）（Li）。

随访

- 至少每年进行一次减肥咨询和测量空腹血糖和血脂。
- 如果服用二甲双胍，每年进行两次糖化随访测量。
- 糖尿病前期的患者视网膜病变和肾病的风险并没有增加，但神经病变和大血管并发症的危险性增高，所以考虑这些方面的筛查。

专家意见

- 单纯空腹血糖受损（IFG）主要表示肝脏胰岛素抵抗，糖耐量受损（IGT）主要提示（外周）肌肉胰岛素抵抗。
- 早期诊断糖尿病前期可允许患者有机会进行预防或延缓2型糖尿病的发病。
- 随机试验表明成功的生活方式改变和适度减肥比药物在防止糖尿病方面更有效，有利于成本效益和长期坚持。
- 生活方式干预是很难实现的，并且减轻体重是很难维持的。因此，如果6个月后没有观察到足够的减肥效果，可考虑二甲双胍。

参考文献

American diabetes Association. standards of medical care in diabetes—2011. diabetes Care, 2011; Vol. 34 suppl 1: pp. s11–61.
Comments: screening, diagnosing, and management recommendations for favorably affecting health outcomes of patients with diabetes.

International Expert Committee international Expert Committee report on the role of the A1c assay in the diag-nosis of diabetes. diabetes Care, 2009; Vol. 32: pp. 1327–34.
Comments: Consensus view from the 2008 committee that proposes the use of the A1c assay for the diagnosis of prediabetes and diabetes, suggests appropriate cut-points, and argues that A1c testing has many advantages over plasma glucose testing.

Nathan dM, davidson Mb, defronzo rA, et al. impaired fasting glucose and impaired glucose tolerance: implica-tions for care. diabetes Care, 2007; Vol. 30: pp. 753–9.
Comments: summary of the AdA consensus position on prediabetic states in 2006, addressing the definition, pathogenesis, natural history, consequences, and treatment of ifG and iGT.

Knowler WC, barrett-Connor E, fowler sE, et al. reduction in the incidence of type 2 diabetes with lifestyle intervention or metformin. NEJM, 2002; Vol. 346: pp. 393–403.
Comments: Landmark rCT showing the beneficial effects of lifestyle changes and metformin on prevention of type 2 diabetes among subjects with baseline ifG and iGT.

其他文献

Cowie CC, rust kf, ford Es, et al. full accounting of diabetes and pre-diabetes in the U.s. population in 1988–1994 and 2005–2006. diabetes Care, 2009; Vol. 32: pp. 287–94.
Comments: Using data from National Health and Nutrition Examination survey in 1988–2004 and 2005–2006, provides estimates for prevalence of diabetes and prediabetes in the Us using glucose criteria.

Knowler WC, fowler sE, Hamman rf, et al. 10-year follow-up of diabetes incidence and weight loss in the diabetes Prevention Program outcomes study. Lancet, 2009; Vol. 374: pp. 1677–86.
Comments: A summary of the results of the dPPos follow-up study.

Li G, Zhang P, Wang J, et al. The long-term effect of lifestyle interventions to prevent diabetes in the China da Qing diabetes Prevention study: a 20-year follow-up study. Lancet, 2008; Vol. 371: pp. 1783–9.
Comments: A summary of the results of the da Qing follow-up study.

Lindström J, ilanne-Parikka P, Peltonen M, et al. sustained reduction in the incidence of type 2 diabetes by lifestyle intervention: follow-up of the finnish diabetes Prevention study. Lancet, 2006; Vol. 368: pp. 1673–9.
Comments: A summary of the results of the finnish diabetes Prevention follow-up study.

World Health organization and international diabetes federation. definition and diagnosis of diabetes mellitus and intermediate hyperglycemia: report of WHo/idf consultation. World Health organization; 2006.
Comments: describes the WHo/idf criteria for diabetes, iGT, and ifG.

Meigs Jb, Muller dC, Nathan dM, et al. The natural history of progression from normal glucose tolerance to type 2 diabetes in the baltimore Longitudinal study of Aging. diabetes, 2003; Vol. 52: pp. 1475–84.
Comments: Characterizes the natural history of progression from normal glucose tolerance to ifG/iGT to type 2 diabetes using data from , 20 years of biennial oral glucose tolerance tests performed in a large cohort.

Tuomilehto J, Lindstrom J, Eriksson JG, et al. Prevention of type 2 diabetes mellitus by changes in lifestyle among subjects with impaired glucose tolerance. NEJM, 2001; Vol. 344: pp. 1343–50.
Comments: first large rCT showing that type 2 diabetes can be effectively prevented by changes in lifestyle among subjects with baseline iGT.

Pan Xr, Li GW, Hu YH, et al. Effects of diet and exercise in preventing NiddM in people with impaired glucose tolerance. The da Qing iGT and diabetes study. diabetes Care, 1997; Vol. 20: pp. 537–44.
Comments: A summary of the results of the da Qing iGT and diabetes study.

怀孕

妊娠糖尿病

Wanda K. Nicholson, MD, MPH, MBA

定义
- 妊娠糖尿病（GDM）指最先发现于妊娠期间的葡萄糖耐受异常，它不同于1型和2型糖尿病，后二者是于非孕期确诊的（糖尿病）。

流行病学
- GDM是妊娠期间最常见的代谢疾病。
- 每年，有大约170 000（1%~14%）美国孕妇被诊断为GDM，这（人数的浮动？）决定于诊断标准的不同和人口特征的差异（Jovanovic）。
- 在患有GDM的女性患者中，30%~50%会在下次妊娠中再次发病（Bellamy；kim）。
- 进一步区分可以发现，20%~50%的患过GDM的人，会在生产后的5~10年内得上2型糖尿病（Jovanovic）。
- 最近的meta分析指出：GDM会使患2型糖尿病的危险性增加7.4倍（bellamy）。

诊断
- 在第一次产前检查时，孕妇若有患上GDM高危因素的话（包括严重肥胖，先前有过生产巨大胎儿的历史，尿内出现葡萄糖，多囊卵巢综合征，患有GDM的个人史，或者是糖尿病家族史），则其应进行检测糖尿病的标准检查。
- 美国糖尿病协会（ADA）的最新指南建议进行75g的口服糖耐量检测（OGTT），并在空腹、1小时和2小时的时候进行血浆葡萄糖含量的检测，这一检查适用于孕期24~28周的所有未患有糖尿病的妇女。
- OGTT应在至少空腹8小时后的早晨进行。
- GDM的诊断应在血清葡萄糖的值超过下述指标的时候决定：空腹92mg/dl（5.1mmol/L），1小时180mg/dl（10mmol/L）或者2小时153mg/dl（8.5mmol/L）。
- 传统的GDM的诊断标准是建立在50克OGTT检查异常时，同时发现3小时100克OGTT有两项异常；而这种对GDM的两步筛选法已不再建议使用。

标志和症状
- 经典的高血糖症状（如多尿、烦渴、视物模糊、阴道真菌感染）要在血糖高于180mg/dl的时候才得以显现。而GDM常常是没有症状的。
- 怀孕期间的常见症状包括多尿，但这与高血糖症状并不一定相关。

妊娠糖尿病

临床治疗

葡萄糖控制
- 严格的血糖控制是主要目标，这与怀孕前有糖尿病史的孕妇的治疗目标相似。
- 大概可以接受的孕期血糖浓度已列在表 2-6 中。

表 2-56. 血糖控制的适当范围

空腹	60~90（或 95）mg/dl
餐前	60~100mg/dl
餐后 1 小时（餐后）	< 140mg/dl
餐后 2 小时	< 120mg/dl
睡前	< 120mg/dl
2:00-6:00（AM）	60~120mg/dl

来源：ACOG Committee on Practice Bulletin.ACOG Practice Bulletin.Clinical management guidelines obstetrician-gynecologists.Number 60,March 2005 Pregestational diabetes mellitus. Obstet Gynecol,2005;105(3):675-85
经 Lippincott Wiliams&Wilkins 许可复制。

非药物治疗
- 治疗 GDM 的最关键的目标在于将母亲血糖尽量控制在靠近正常血糖的水平，以此降低流产或者母亲和新生儿患病的概率。
- 诊断为 GDM 的肥胖妇女，需要开始 ADA 规定的 30kcal/(kg·d) 的食谱饮食。
- 碳水化合物应限制在总食量的 40%~50%。
- 建议进行日常轻中度的运动。

药物治疗
- 若饮食治疗无效，则应开始进行药物干预。胰岛素治疗应该作为首选。
- 目前，ADA 和美国妇产科医师协会并不支持在孕期常规使用抗高血糖药物，该治疗 GDM 的计划也尚未经过美国食品和药物管理局的同意。
  - 虽然胰岛素应为优选，但是格列苯脲和二甲双胍在实践中仍被使用着。
  - 二甲双胍在多囊卵巢综合征的患者，基本可使用 14 周，这在一项有效的临床试验中，被证明是安全的（Rowan）。
  - 在母亲或新生儿中，使用格列苯脲或者二甲双胍与使用胰岛素相比，并无差别（rowan, nicholson, langer, moore）。
- 参见第 142 页怀孕与糖尿病部分以获得胰岛素治疗的相关信息。

随访
- 一般在产后可以停止对 GDM 的药物治疗，因为产后胰岛素敏感性将显著增高。
- 约 75% 的 GDM 患者产后都可恢复葡萄糖耐量，但是他们日后获得 2 型糖尿病的危险性将增高。
- 美国妇产科协会（ACOG）和美国糖尿病协会(ADA)建议在产后 6~12

周对产后妇女进行糖尿病筛查。
- 如果正常,每三年对血糖状况进行一次评估。
- 最近的系统综述显示,空腹血糖作为 2 型糖尿病产后筛查指标,其敏感性较低。

专家建议
- 妊娠通常会导致胰岛素抵抗。胰岛素分泌功能正常的女性则会通过增加胰岛素分泌量来克服(胰岛素抵抗)。
- 如果一个女性患上了 GDM,则暗示其胰岛素储备异常。
- 在少数情况中,1 型糖尿病会在孕期出现,孕妇在产后依然依赖胰岛素且血糖水平不稳定则提示 1 型糖尿病。
- 据大型的随访型临床试验报道,围产期孕妇血糖轻微的升高(甚至在非糖尿病范围内)与新生儿的预后相关,这也促进了最近关于 GDM 诊断标准的改变(Metzger)。

建议依据
American Diabetes Association. standards of medical care in diabetes—2011. Diabetes Care, 2011; Vol. 34 suppl1: pp. s11–61.

Comments: Describes new America Diabetes Association guidelines on diagnosis and treatment of GDM.

其他参考
Bellamy l, Casas JP, Hingorani AD, et al. Type 2 diabetes mellitus after gestational diabetes: a systematic review and meta-analysis. lancet, 2009; Vol. 373: pp. 1773–9.

Comments: systematic review and pooled estimates of development of type 2 diabetes after gestational diabetes.

Nicholson W, bolen s, Witkop CT, et al. benefits and risks of oral diabetes agents compared with insulin in women with gestational diabetes: a systematic review. obstet Gynecol, 2009; Vol. 113: pp. 193–205.

Comments: systematic review of 4 RCTs and 5 observational studies on the effectiveness and safety of metfor-min and glyburide compared to insulin among women with gestational diabetes. bennett Wl, bolen s, Wilson lM, et al. Performance characteristics of postpartum screening tests for type 2 dia-betes mellitus in women with a history of gestational diabetes mellitus: a systematic review. J Womens Health (larchmont, NY), 2009; Vol. 18: pp. 979–87.

Comments: systematic review of 11 studies comparing sensitivity and specificity of fasting blood glucose to 75-g 2-hour oGTT.

Metzger bE, lowe IP, Dyer AR, et al. Hyperglycemia and adverse pregnancy outcomes. N Engl J Med, 2008; Vol. 358: pp. 1991–2002.

Comments: A large study (~25,000 pregnant women) that found a strong, continuous association of mater-nal glucose levels within the nondiabetic range with increased birth weight and increased cord-blood serum C-peptide levels. Prompted recent changes in ADA guidelines for diagnosis of GDM.

Rowan JA, Hague WM, Gao W, et al. Metformin versus insulin for the treatment of gestational diabetes. NEJM, 2008; Vol. 358: pp. 2003–15.

Comments: Randomized clinical trial of 754 women with gestational diabetes at

20–33 weeks gestation in Australia and New Zealand.

Kim C, berger DK, Chamany s. Recurrence of gestational diabetes mellitus: a systematic review. Diabetes Care, 2007; Vol. 30: pp. 1314–9.
Comments: systematic review and pooled estimates of development of recurrence of gestational diabetes.

Jovanovic l, Pettitt DJ. Gestational diabetes mellitus. JAMA, 2001; Vol. 286: pp. 2516–8.
Comments: Review article of epidemiology of gestational diabetes.

Langer o, Conway DI, berkus MD, et al. A comparison of glyburide and insulin in women with gestational diabetes mellitus. NEJM, 2000; Vol. 343: pp. 1134–8.
Comments: Randomized clinical trial of 404 women with gestational diabetes in the united states.

妊娠与糖尿病

Wanda K. Nicholson, MD, MPH, MBA

定义
- 糖尿病妊娠包括孕前和孕期糖尿病。
- 孕前糖尿病：在一个女性怀孕前诊断出的糖尿病。
- 妊娠糖尿病（GDM）：在妊娠开始后才诊断出的糖尿病。

流行病学
- 1%的怀孕女性患有孕前糖尿病（包括1型和2型）（Lawrence）。
- 其他出处描述的GDM流行病学（资料）。
- 在1型糖尿病中，糖尿病患病时间是早产的一项重要预测指标。慢性高血压与早产以及围产期死亡相关（Gonzalez）。
- 在2型糖尿病中，怀孕前三个月时较高的A1c强烈提示遗传畸形以及围产期死亡；在第三个月时较高的A1c与早产有关。巨大胎儿与早产率增高相关（Gonzales）。

诊断
- 关于孕前糖尿病的诊断，参见 第6页糖尿病的诊断和分级。
- 关于GDM的诊断，参见妊娠糖尿病，第138页。

临床治疗
糖尿病妊娠时的降糖目标
- 为了使新生儿遗传病（其发生与怀孕前三个月的高血糖相关）、巨大胎儿（与最后两个三月的高血糖相关）、早产和围产期死亡的风险降到最低，在孕期应制定一个极为严格的血糖控制目标。
- 降糖目标见表2-6（参见妊娠糖尿病，第139页）。（达到）使用自我监测（目标值），平均空腹血糖水平100mg/dl，目标血红蛋白A1c 6%。
- 虽然自我糖监测对于及时的护理更为有效，但是（也可以）每月检查HbA1c（代替）。

对于糖尿病妊娠的测评
- 实验室诊断性检查：确认怀孕后，对代谢指标进行全面检查，甲状腺功能检查以及心电图检查。
- 视网膜病变筛查：如果在一年内未做过评估，则求诊于眼科（医生）。
- 肾功能：通过瞬时或24小时尿蛋白含量和肌酸酐清除率进行评估。
- 超声检查：对预产期早期进行超声检查；解剖学超声检查（18~22周）；于孕期28~32周以及34~36周时进行连续的超声检查以测评胎儿生长百分数。
- 胎儿超声检查：于18~22周时进行以检测胎儿心脏结构；于34~36周时，用以评估室间隔的超声检查也建议进行。其尺寸的增加可以提示血糖控制不佳。

妊娠与糖尿病

- 胎儿检测：在孕期 32~34 周开始，应在维持适当的检查时间间隔并应将胎动计数和非压力实验、收缩力检测以及胎儿生理活动评估同时进行。32~34 孕周开始，广为推荐的是每两周一次胎儿检测，但是可以个体化调整。
- 脐动脉多普勒检测血流速：对于监测胎儿发育不良有效。

对孕期血糖的饮食和药物治疗

- 对 GDM 患者，采取对碳水化合物进行适当控制足以达到饮食控制的目的。建议总食谱中的碳水化合物含量在 40%~50%。营养学家则可以帮助计算卡路里和碳水化合物；正常体重的女性需要的热量可达 30~35kcal/(kg·d)。患有轻度孕期糖尿病的女性[例如 OGTT 检测异常，但是空腹血糖水平低于 95mg/dl（5.3mmol/L）]单独采取饮食治疗便足以达到效果。
- 口服降血糖药物，包括格列苯脲（美国药物及食品管理局 C 类）和二甲双胍（美国药物及食品管理局 B 类）可以考虑在 GDM 患者中使用，但是，胰岛素应作为首选治疗药物，尤其是当高血糖只发生在饮食后。
- 胰岛素可通过皮下注射或者胰岛素泵（对 1 型糖尿病而言）等给药方式。
- 普通胰岛素、优泌乐、诺和锐以及中效胰岛素都属于 FDA 分类中的 B 类药物；来得时、地特胰岛素、赖谷胰岛素都属于 FDA 分类 C 类胰岛素。
- 餐前给予短效或者速效胰岛素 (regular, lispro, and aspart) 以降低餐后高血糖。
- 餐前 30 分钟给予普通胰岛素。优泌乐、诺和锐在饭后马上服用。
- 优泌乐、诺和锐作用速度很快，所以，如若事物尚未消化吸收，则在注射后短期内就会出现低血糖。若果病人经常呕吐或者有"晨吐"则应特别小心使用。
- 长效和速效胰岛素（中效胰岛素、来得时、地特胰岛素）每天使用一次或两次。
- 孕期的胰岛素需求往往会增加，特别是在第三个三月，但是在产后会迅速降低；患者通常早产后或者哺乳期时需要更少的胰岛素量（如果先前需要的话）。
- 最好在腹部注射胰岛素，没有证据表明这样会伤害到胎儿。

糖尿病妊娠时的接产

- 在生育过程中，使用静脉注射胰岛素的方式将血糖控制在低于 120mg/dl 的水平。
- 对糖尿病导致的复杂妊娠的接产，在 39 孕周时会比较安全。
- 可以在经羊水穿刺确定胎肺成熟时提前终止妊娠，特别是由于糖尿病血管病变导致的复杂妊娠发生时。
- 虽然超声经常用于在产前评估胎儿体重以及排除巨大胎儿的可能性，但是其所达到的效果并不优于临床评估。
- 如果糖尿病孕妇的胎儿预计体重大于 4.5kg，则应考虑采取剖腹产。
- 可疑巨大胎儿时，引产并不能够降低胎儿产伤的可能性，并且会增加剖腹产的可能性。

糖尿病妊娠的并发症

- 糖尿病孕妇妊娠期间并发症发生的频率会增高，但是与非孕期糖尿病女性发生的概率相似。
- 糖尿病会增加剖腹产以及术后并发症的可能性。
- 肩部难产的概率是非糖尿病妊娠时的三倍。
- 糖尿病妊娠时，先兆子痫的风险增加了13%~14%。
- 糖尿病孕妇羊水过多者更为常见。
- 孕母高血糖可导致流产或者早产。
- 孕母高血糖还可导致血管性疾病，包括高血压、肾病、中风以及糖尿病视网膜病的恶化。
- 孕母高血糖会导致胎儿胎肺成熟不佳或延迟。
- 加速发育的胎儿在未控制孕母高血糖时会导致大龄产儿。巨大胎儿，定义为体重大于4.5kg的胎儿，出现于高达10%的糖尿病妊娠中。甚至，轻度的高血糖也会导致胎儿出生体重的增加（london）。
- 在胎儿：新生儿低血钾/癫痫、低血钙、高胆红素血症、红细胞增多症的出现概率更大；另外，遗传病、围产期死亡、宫内生长迟缓的几率都将增加（伴有同时存在的孕母血管疾病）。

随访

- 应告知患有妊娠糖尿病的女性其日后患有糖尿病的可能性，并对其进行适当的预防性筛查。

专家建议

- 预先安排的处理措施应包括：使A1c值尽可能接近7，评估用于治疗糖尿病及其并发症的药物，因其可能存在孕期禁忌，这些药物包括：他汀类药物、ACEI和ARB类降压药以及多数非胰岛素糖尿病治疗药物。
- 糖尿病眼病在孕期可能会恶化，因此需要在孕前和孕中由眼科医生进行评估。
- 有证据显示，胎儿期处于孕母高血糖环境中会使胎儿的代谢状况发生改变（"胎儿期编程"），这使新生儿倾向于在儿童期发生肥胖以及糖尿病。

参考文献

American Diabetes Association. Preconception care of women with diabetes. Diabetes Care, 2004; Vol. 27 Suppl 1: pp. S76–8.

Comments: Outlines the American Diabetes Association guidelines on preconception care in women with diabetes.

其他参考

Landon MB, Spong CY, Thom E, et al. A multicenter, randomized trial of treatment for mild gestational diabetes.NEJM, 2009; Vol. 361: pp. 1339–48.

Comments: A randomized clinical trial indicating that even mild elevation in mean glucose, within range of impaired glucose tolerance, is associated with larger birth weight. Study also found that treatment of mild gestational diabetes mellitus did not significantly reduce the frequency of a composite outcome (stillbirth,perinatal disease, neonatal complications).

Lawrence JM, Contreras R, Chen W, et al. Trends in the prevalence of preexisting diabetes and gestational diabetes mellitus among a racially/ethnically diverse population of pregnant women, 1999–2005. Diabetes Care, 2008; Vol. 31: pp. 899–904.

Comments: Epidemiology of pregestational and gestational diabetes.

Gonzalez-Gzonzalez NL, Ramirez O, Mozas J, et al. Factors influencing pregnancy outcome in women with type 2versus type 1 diabetes mellitus. Acta Obstet Gynecol Scand, 2008; Vol. 87: pp. 43–9.

Comments: Describes factors associated with adverse perinatal outcomes in women with type 1 and type 2diabetes.

社会／法律

糖尿病对驾驶的影响

Rita Rastogi Kalyani, MD, MHS

定义
- 多数糖尿病患者能安全正常驾驶。
- 但是,糖尿病患者在驾驶时,可能会对其产生影响的三个因素为:低血糖、糖尿病并发症以及高血糖症。
- 而低血糖时无明显感觉,这是对驾驶时更大的威胁。

流行病学
- 只有0.4%~3%的致死性机动车事故(MVAs)是由于疾病状态导致的(Grattan)。其中,癫痫是最常见的原因(38%),其次是胰岛素治疗阶段的糖尿病(18%),以及急性心肌梗死(8%);21%的情况中,未找到(明确)原因。
- 达胰岛素治疗阶段的糖尿病患者,根据人群的不同,其所占MVA比率与其他疾病状态诱因相比,或高或低或相似(Cox;Mathieson)。
- 在1型糖尿病的美国患者中,31%承认在过去的两年中有过在低血糖恍惚的情况下驾驶过;28%的患者在过去的六个月中,在驾驶时经历过低血糖。而2型糖尿病患者,该数字则相对较低(分别是8%和6%)(Cox)。
- 低血糖无知觉可能会导致在驾驶时的低血糖未引起注意,这种情况在1型糖尿病的患者中占到了25%;此发生率在2型糖尿病患者中则相对较低(Johnson;Zammit)。
- 在糖尿病患者中,需胰岛素治疗的糖尿病以及病程超5年这两个因素与更高的受伤发生率相关(Koepsell)。
- 与未患有糖尿病者相比,需要胰岛素治疗的糖尿病患者,其入院率略微增高(De Klerk;Kennedy)。
- 据美国高速交通安全局的一项涉及68 770人的调查显示,患有糖尿病(或者其他代谢病)且其驾驶证未被限制者,其事故发生率是因过失而发生事故者的1.44倍。
- 糖尿病眼病会导致视力下降,而激光凝固(Laser coagulation)治疗手段也会降低外围视力(Pearson)。周围神经病变也会影响驾驶。
- 认知失调可能会影响驾驶能力;其发生与急性或可能的慢性高血糖综合征、严格的血糖控制以及急性低血糖相关。
- 老年糖尿病患者可以说是MVAs中的更为危险的群体(McCoy),但是,老年女性糖尿病患者与无糖尿病的老年女性相比,更倾向于不开车。(Forrest)

症状和表现
- 驾驶会导致糖尿病患者的代谢水平升高,表现为心率加快、自主神经活动加强以及分泌更多肾上腺素的趋势(Cox)。

糖尿病对驾驶的影响

临床治疗

低血糖以及血糖状态感受训练
- 对于1型糖尿病患者而言,他们的血糖过低与否是很难正确判断的;在一项研究中,受试者反映,他们的血糖在40mg/dl(2.2mmol/L)时,他们38%~47%仍会继续驾驶(Clarke)。
- 不知觉性低血糖使驾驶时低血糖症发生记得可能性提高(Stork)。
- 对于1型糖尿病患者,已在驱动模拟研究中通过高胰岛素钳夹技术诱导出低血糖症以检验对效能的影响。
- 轻度低血糖(50mg/dl; 2.6mmol/L)会导致驾驶能力下降(转弯、旋转、及时越过中间线、及时离开公路)并且会更多的采取慢速行驶;他们中只有50%承认在现实生活中遇到类似情况时不会进行驾驶。
- 在类似实验中,当受试者被给予自我处理症状或者停止驾驶的选择时,虽然他们中79%的人察觉到了轻度的低血糖,但只有32%的患者采取了正确的措施。
- 但是,在现实生活中,情况会更加复杂,而且这些实验中并未涉及对照组。
- 血糖感知训练计划教育患者更加准确的估计其血糖水平;受到相应教育的糖尿病患者,其MVA比率明显低于未受教育的患者。(Cox; Broers)

避免驾驶中的低血糖的发生
- 在车中常备碳水化合物食品。
- 车中备有血糖自我检测设备(如血糖仪)。
- 考虑驾驶前进行血糖测量,特别是低血糖无知觉的患者。
- 一经发现有可能的低血糖症状便停止驾驶,在确保血糖水平处于正常范围前不要恢复驾驶。
- 教育患者当血糖低于70mg/dl(4mmol/L)时驾驶水平会有变差的可能性。
- 驾驶证审批部门以及机动车保险公司应当被告知患者在驾驶时发生了低血糖综合征;患者对于法律条款的依从性应总体上良好。(Graveling)

法律限制
- 先行的对于糖尿病患者驾驶的法律限制以及驾驶权利的规定差别很大;多数的法律条规是基于低血糖症可能会带来的风险而设定的,但很不幸的是,有些法律是在对糖尿病及其并发症知之甚少的情况下制定的。
- 法律条规应该权衡患者的个人利益与公共交通安全。
- 在美国,许多州制定了对于糖尿病患者的限制驾驶计划。
- 在加州,强制要求医生报道可能会源于低血糖症的意识丧失,通常会使该患者的驾驶证受到吊销。
- 在其他的多数州,这种上报是自愿的。
- 许胰岛素治疗的患者自动取消其州际商业性驾驶执照,没有例外;但是,在过去的十年间,50个州中的39个州颁发了豁免许可(Stork)。
- 在欧洲,对糖尿病患者的驾驶限制,从加大医疗检查频率到取消驾驶执照不等。

专家意见

- 直接由糖尿病导致的 MVAs 占少数。
- 许多糖尿病患者仍能也确实做到了安全驾驶,但是也有少数不能做到者。
- 在过去三年中无低血糖症(随精神状态而定)以及可感知低血糖症表明安全驾驶的可能性较高。
- 糖尿病患者,特别是使用胰岛素治疗的糖尿病患者,其在驾驶中低血糖症确实会出现,并会导致 MVAs 发生的可能性轻度上升。
- MVA 的危险因素包括,近期出现的低血糖症(视精神状态而定),低血糖不知觉以及老龄(其认知功能会迅速下降)。
- 我们建议对每个患者进行个体化评估,而不是设置一个总体的政策进而导致对糖尿病患者的不公平歧视。
- 关于 MVAs 与糖尿病的关系需要进一步的实验以更好地解释其相关性。

参考文献

Stork AD, van Haeften TW , Veneman TF. Diabetes and driving: desired data, research methods and their pitfalls, current knowledge, and future research. Diabetes Care, 2006; Vol. 29: pp. 1942–9.

Comments: Most up-to-date review on the current knowledge regarding diabetes and driving, along with recommendations for future research directions.

其他参考

Stork AD, van Haeften TW , Veneman TF. The decision not to drive during hypoglycemia in patients with type 1 and type 2 diabetes according to hypoglycemia awareness. Diabetes Care, 2007; Vol. 30: pp. 2822–6.

Comments: Individuals with hypoglycemia unawareness are more likely to drive.

Zammitt NN , Frier BM. Hypoglycemia in type 2 diabetes: pathophysiology, frequency, and effects of different treatment modalities. Diabetes Care, 2005; Vol. 28: pp. 2948–61.

Comments: Describes epidemiology of hypoglycemia in type 2 diabetes.

Broers S, van Vliet KP, le Cessie S, et al. Blood glucose awareness training in Dutch type 1 diabetes patients: oneyear follow-up. Neth J Med, 2005; Vol. 63: pp. 164–9.

Comments: Dutch study describing beneficial effects of blood glucose awareness training; educated versus uneducated patients less likely to be involved in accidents (0.6 vs 0.2 accidents per patient per year, p = 0.04).

Cox DJ, Kovatchev BP, Gonder-Frederick LA, et al. Relationships between hyperglycemia and cognitive performance among adults with type 1 and type 2 diabetes. Diabetes Care, 2005; Vol. 28: pp. 71–7.

Comments: Cognitive dysfunction associated with hyperglycemia in adults with diabetes.

Graveling AJ, Warren RE , Frier BM. Hypoglycaemia and driving in people with insulin-treated diabetes: adherence to recommendations for avoidance. Diabet Med, 2004; Vol. 21: pp. 1014–9.

Comments: Describes how well individuals with diabetes adhere to guidelines for avoiding hypoglycemia while driving.

Cox DJ, Penberthy JK, Zrebiec J, et al. Diabetes and driving mishaps: frequency and correlations from a multinational survey. Diabetes Care, 2003; Vol. 26: pp. 2329–34.

Comments: Describes the frequency of driving injury in persons with diabetes using data from a large, multinational survey. In US, 31% admitted to driving in hypoglycemic stupor in past 2 years and 28% experienced hypoglycemia while driving in past 6 months. Type 1 diabetic drivers reported more crashes than type 2 diabetic drivers and nondiabetic spouses (19% vs 12% vs 8%, p , 0.001).

Johnson ES, Koepsell TD, Reiber G, et al. Increasing incidence of serious hypoglycemia in insulin users. J Clin Epidemiol, 2002; Vol. 55: pp. 253–9.
Comments: Describes epidemiology of hypoglycemia in insulin-treated diabetes.

Kennedy RL, Henry J, Chapman AJ, et al. Accidents in patients with insulin-treated diabetes: increased risk of lowimpact falls but not motor vehicle crashes—a prospective register-based study. J Trauma, 2002; Vol. 52: pp. 660–6.
Comments: Suggests that accident rates not significantly different between adults with insulin-treated diabetes (44.4 per 100,000 people per year) compared to the general population (34.4); relative risk = 1.29, nonsignificant.

Cox DJ, Gonder-Frederick LA, Kovatchev BP, et al. The metabolic demands of driving for drivers with type 1 diabetes mellitus. Diabetes Metab Res Rev, 2002; Vol. 18: pp. 381–5.
Comments: Patients with type 1 diabetes divided into 2 groups: watching a driving video or actually driving a simulator during constant insulin/dextrose infusion to maintain euglycemia. Actual driving associated with significantly higher dextrose infusion rate, more autonomic symptoms, increased heart rate, trend toward greater epinephrine release, and significantly more frequent hypoglycemic self-treatment.

Cox DJ, Gonder-Frederick L, Polonsky W, et al. Blood glucose awareness training (BGAT -2): long-term benefits. Diabetes Care, 2001; Vol. 24: pp. 637–42.
Comments: Describes beneficial impact of blood glucose awareness training on accident rates. After 4 years, 6.8 accidents/million miles driven in educated group versus 29.8 in control group.

National Highway Traffic Safety Administration. Medical conditions and driver crash risk: do license restrictions affect public safety? Ann Emerg Med, 2000; Vol. 36: pp. 164–5.
Comments: National Highway Traffic Safety Administration's investigation on impact of restricted driving licenses on accident rate in persons with different medical conditions, including diabetes.

Cox DJ, Gonder-Frederick LA, Kovatchev BP, et al. Progressive hypoglycemia's impact on driving simulation performance. Occurrence, awareness and correction. Diabetes Care, 2000; Vol. 23: pp. 163–70.
Comments: In driving simulation study, the authors examined the impact of progressive hypoglycemia on driving performance. Diminished driving performance was seen at all glucose levels (4.0–3.3, 3.3–2.8, ,2.8 mmol/L). Only 32% took corrective action, although 79% detecthypoglycemia ,2.8 mmol/L.

Clarke WL, Cox DJ, Gonder-Frederick LA, et al. Hypoglycemia and the decision to drive a motor vehicle by persons with diabetes. JAMA, 1999; Vol. 282: pp. 750–4.
Comments: Persons with diabetes may not accurately judge when they are hypoglycemic.

Pearson AR, Tanner V, Keightley SJ, et al. What effect does laser photocoagulation have on driving visual fields in diabetics? Eye (London), 1998; Vol. 12 (Pt 1): pp. 64–8.
Comments: Summary of laser treatment's effects on peripheral vision in patients with diabetic retinopathy.

Mathiesen B, Borch-Johnsen K. Diabetes and accident insurance. A 3-year follow-up of 7599 insured diabetic individuals. Diabetes Care, 1997; Vol. 20: pp. 1781–4.
Comments: Danish Diabetes Association reported that risk of any accident significantly lower in those with diabetes (0.7 per 1000 persons) compared with two control groups (4.5 and 5.5, respectively).

Forrest KY, Bunker CH, Songer TJ, et al. Driving patterns and medical conditions in older women. J Am Geriatr Soc, 1997; Vol. 45: pp. 1214–8.
Comments: Older women with diabetes are significantly more likely to give up driving compared to those without diabetes (odds ratio 2.53, 95% CI 1.57–4.07).

Koepsell TD, Wolf ME, McCloskey L, et al. Medical conditions and motor vehicle collision injuries in older adults. J Am Geriatr Soc, 1994; Vol. 42: pp. 695–700.
Comments: Authors reported a 2.6-fold increased risk of driving injury in older drivers with diabetes, especially for insulin-treated patients and diabetes duration .5 years.

McCoy GF, Johnston RA, Duthie RB. Injury to the elderly in road traffic accidents. J Trauma, 1989; Vol. 29: pp. 494–7.
Comments: In general, older adults are more likely to sustain driving injuries than younger adults.

De Klerk NH, Armstrong BK. Admission to hospital for road trauma in patients with diabetes mellitus. J Epidemiol Community Health, 1983; Vol. 37: pp. 232–7.
Comments: Describes higher rate of hospital admissions for driving-related trauma among persons with diabetes in men ,55 years, both as pedestrians and drivers.

Grattan E, Jeffcoate GO. Medical factors and road accidents. BMJ, 1968; Vol. 1: pp. 75–9.
Comments: Describes relatively low frequency of accidents caused by medical conditions.

就业和歧视

Christopher D. Saudek, MD

定义
- 就业歧视是指由于其医疗状况，一个人不合情理地被拒绝一份工作、终止雇佣或者不能得到晋升。
- 一个糖尿病患者可能由于其不能很好地胜任一项工作而受到就业歧视。
- 对于就业歧视的法律定义，不同州或者不同国家之间是有差别的，因而其情况可能会很复杂。
- 若要评估某个案例是否涉及就业歧视，则需要一个经验丰富的律师。

流行病学
- 目前尚无可靠的关于糖尿病患者就业歧视现状的统计学证据。
- 这种歧视可能会不显著，因为雇主可能不会特别指出糖尿病是某个人未被雇佣、未能晋升或者被中止雇佣的原因；它也可以很明显，如果雇主已经针对糖尿病患者或者服用胰岛素者制定了相应的政策。
- 这种歧视可能会发生在某个个体身上、独立情况或者作为一项广泛采取的雇佣政策。
- 由于雇主对于糖尿病（包括其治疗）的误解，就业不公平或者潜在的就业歧视行为会发生。

诊断
- 在美国，美国残疾人法案（ADA）保护残疾人的合法权益。由于始于2009年成功的修正法案，基本上所有的糖尿病患者都被认为带有"残疾"因而得到 AD 的保护。
- ADA 要求雇主制定"合理的调整措施"以帮助残疾人。
- 对于糖尿病患者，合理的调整措施包括，例如：允许患者携带零食或者在工作期间测量血糖水平。
- 如前所述，可能会需要一个有经验的律师来确定到底哪些确实属于就业歧视。

症状
- 任何设立不雇佣糖尿病患者的总括性政策的雇主都应被认定为就业歧视。
- 一个潜在的雇主在给予录用信前不得询问一个求职者的健康状况，包括其是否患有糖尿病，但是一个工作录用信中可以包括要求提交一份医疗史或者对求职者进行体检。
- 未能对糖尿病患者雇员作出合理的调整措施者，可被归为就业歧视。

临床治疗
- 经常性的邀请卫生保健专业人员对受雇糖尿病患者进行健康评估。
- 医学评估需要考虑：该求职者是否有可能会严重影响其胜任该工作的长

期并发症？他/她近期有无低血糖史？工作要求有哪些？该个体是否能在有糖尿病的前提下独立完成该工作？
- 卫生保健专业人员应致力于向雇主说明其公平对待糖尿病患者的益处。
- 当如此建议雇主时，一些关键点可以包括：（1）糖尿病患者可以并且已经成功的完成了基本上所有工种；（2）糖尿病患者通常更关心其健康和安全，从个人角度其谨慎的程度高于雇员的平均水平；（3）最主要的风险——严重的低血糖症——只是发生在那些采取某些本身易引起低血糖症的患者身上。
- 有时，卫生保健专业人员需要致力于鼓励糖尿病患者积极寻找工作。
- 给予此类建议时，很重要的一点在于不能太悲观或者预设重重限制。因为除了某些特种行业（如军队）强制要求不能雇用糖尿病患者外，多数的职业愿意也应该雇用。
- 糖尿病患者不需要在得到工作邀请函前告诉潜在的雇主其健康史（包括患有糖尿病），但在之后需要进行入职前体检。
- 在一些特殊情况下，如果有就业歧视现象的发生，卫生保健专业人员可能会需要帮助糖尿病患者采取进一步的法律措施。诸如美国糖尿病协会等糖尿病相关组织经常会起到帮助作用。

专家意见

- 卫生保健专业人员的第一职责是保护患者。这与保障公共安全以及雇主的法律利益是相适应的。
- 卫生保健专业人员应保障工作场所的安全并确保劳动力的效率。
- 当雇主知道糖尿病的实际情况时，他们往往乐于接受糖尿病教育并愿意雇用以及晋升糖尿病患者。
- 为了保护糖尿病患者免遭就业歧视，首要原则是要做到对每个患者进行个体化评估。不是所有的患者都能做所有的工作（例如糖尿病视网膜病变会使该患者不能从事对视力要求较高的工作）；但是对糖尿病患者的一概性的拒绝政策则可能会涉及歧视并且是违法的。
- 帮助雇主制定针对糖尿病雇员的合理的适应性工作调整，以及帮助糖尿病患者建立合理的工作预期，这些是卫生保健专业人员的理想的职责。
- 严重的低血糖症（需要他人帮助）是某些高压力工作的真正的潜在威胁，而低血糖症是否得到控制则不是。
- 总之，在众多的就业岗位中，糖尿病患者亦能成为一个出众的雇员。

参考文献

American Diabetes Association. Diabetes and employment. Diabetes Care, 2009; Vol. 32, Suppl 1: pp. S80–4.

Comments: The American Diabetes Association's policy statement, with good advice for healthcare professionals on all aspects of evaluating individuals.

特殊人群或亚型

儿童及 2 型糖尿病

Ali Mohamadi, MD, and David W. Cooke, MD

定义
- 2 型糖尿病过去被认为只在成年人中发病，因此曾被称为"成人糖尿病"。
- 然而，现在我们更清楚地认识到 2 型糖尿病可以发生在低于 19 岁的儿童身上，并且发病率在不断上升。
- 儿童的 2 型糖尿病的病理生理过程同成人的 2 型糖尿病相似。

流行病学特征
- 在近几十年，2 型糖尿病在儿童中的发病率明显上升，较 1982 年到 1994 年发病率增长了十倍。
- 在 9 岁以下非西班牙白人儿童中，2 型糖尿病占新发糖尿病的 15%，少数民族儿童，2 型糖尿病占新发糖尿病的一半以上。
- 在青春期前的儿童 2 型糖尿病的发病率很低，但在 10~19 岁的儿童中 2 型糖尿病的发病率高达 11.8/100 000。
- 肥胖，可引起胰岛素抵抗，也是 10~19 岁 2 型糖尿病儿童中可塑性最强的危险因素。2 型糖尿病的发病率增高和儿童群体中肥胖率增高相关。
- 越来越多的儿童出现胰岛素抵抗，青春期内源性性激素的产生会加速青少年的 2 型糖尿病的进程。
- 遗传因素是 2 型糖尿病儿童的危险因素之一，患儿有多个家族成员患有 2 型糖尿病。

诊断
- 美国儿科学会和美国糖尿病协会建议对肥胖且有多种其他 2 型糖尿病的危险因素，如有阳性家族史、非白人儿童、黑棘皮症的儿童进行体检。
- 儿童 2 型糖尿病的诊断标准同成人。
- 因为 2 型糖尿病在青春期儿童发生较少，在儿童达到青春期或 10 岁后才进行相关检查。

症状和体征
- 通过常规对高危儿童进行尿糖和血糖的检查以鉴别出无症状的 2 型糖尿病，其中血糖更为敏感。
- 阴道或阴茎念珠菌病或是夜尿症提示 2 型糖尿病。
- 部分儿童表现出经典的糖尿病症状：现象包括多饮、多食、易激惹、体重下降。
- 高达 33% 的儿童在诊断糖尿病时发现有酮症，5%~25% 的 2 型糖尿病患儿表现为酮症酸中毒（包括昏迷）。
- 虽然很少，2 型糖尿病患儿仍有表现为高渗状态的。

- 对那些表型和家族史都不是典型的 1 型糖尿病、2 型糖尿病或 MODY，检查自身抗体和筛查基因突变来区分亚型。

临床治疗
- 治疗 2 型糖尿病包括三个方面：(1) 改变生活方式；(2) 口服降糖药；(3) 胰岛素治疗。
- 在诊断时无酮症、酮症酸中毒和高渗状态者，改变生活方式（饮食和锻炼）应该是治疗青年 2 型糖尿病的最初方法。
- 减肥的目标是 5%~7% 的体重，运动的目标是一天 20~30 分钟的剧烈运动。
- 2 型糖尿病患儿通过改变生活方式在 3~6 个月后仍达不到正常的血糖，或者糖化血红蛋白在诊断时达到 8%，应该应用药物治疗。
- 尚缺乏足够的证据指导用药，2 型糖尿病患儿的发病史并不被完全了解。
- 只有胰岛素和二甲双胍是被 FDA 批准可用于儿童的药物。
- 如果一个孩子出现酮症酸中毒或在诊断时其糖化血红蛋白达到 9%，应采用胰岛素治疗。
- 治疗目标：使血糖水平达到正常并将长期并发症的风险降到最小。
- 糖化血红蛋白的控制目标是 7%~8% 且在没有明显的低血糖的情况下，尽量使糖化血红蛋白的值接近于正常。
- 二甲双胍最小剂量是 500mg，一天两次，最高达 1 000mg，一天两次；二甲双胍应在进餐时服用，开始 500 毫克每天一次，连续 5~7 天，然后增加至 500mg 每天两次以减少胃肠道不良反应。

随访
- 每三个月测量一次糖化血红蛋白，糖化血红蛋白达到 7%~8% 表明需要加强治疗。
- 每 2 年筛查一次血脂。对于青春期后的儿童，低密度脂蛋白（LDL）达 160mg/dl 提示需要药物治疗。
- 经常监测血压，积极治疗高血压（收缩压和/或舒张压超过其所在年龄、性别的第 95 百分位）。
- 每年进行尿微白蛋白测试（微量白蛋白/肌酐），对于持续性微量白蛋白尿服用血管紧张素转换酶抑制剂（ACEI）或血管紧张素受体阻断剂（ARB）处理。
- 诊断糖尿病后由眼科专家进行视网膜的检查，其后每年检查一次。

专家意见
- 尽管正式 ADA 指南提出了 1 型糖尿病患儿 HbA1c 的目标 (6~12 岁 HbA1c 控制在 8%，年龄 13~18 岁 HbA1c 控制在 7.5%)，2 型糖尿病患儿 HbA1c 水平的目标并不明确。
- 患儿采用类似成年人的糖化血红蛋白的控制目标有其合理性。一项研究发现，T2DM 的患儿未能达到成人 ADA 目标（Valent）。
- 因此，HbA1c 目标需要个性化：有些孩子可以安全达到 6.5%~7%；其他孩子为达到这些目标可能会引起严重的低血糖。
- 小儿初级保健提供者必须熟悉 T2DM，必须随时准备好诊断和治疗 T2DM。

儿童及 2 型糖尿病

- 医师在 2 型糖尿病的患儿的发病史的知识和选择患儿最佳治疗方法的方面仍然存在差距。
- 鉴于可能存在终身风险积累,治疗应根据现有的最佳数据,寻求证据,发现最佳治疗方案。

参考文献

American Academy of Pediatrics and American diabetes Association. Type 2 diabetes in children and adolescents. Pediatrics, 2000; Vol. 105: pp. 671–80.

Comments: Consensus statement of AAP and AdA providing guidelines for screening for T2dM in children.

其他参考文献

American diabetes Association. Standards of medical care in diabetes—2011. diabetes Care, 2011; Vol. 34 Suppl 1: pp. S11–61.

Comments: Outlines standards of medical care for adults and children with diabetes.

Valent d, Pestak K, Otis M, et al. Type 2 diabetes in the pediatric population: are we meeting AdA clinical guide-lines in Ohio? Clin Pediatr (Philadelphia), 2010; Vol. 49: pp. 316–22.

Comments: Suggests that adherence to AdA clinical guidelines for pediatric patients with type 2 diabetes is not good. Authors recommend that specific evidence-based guidelines be developed for children with type 2 diabetes.

Grant rW, Moore AF, Florez JC. Genetic architecture of type 2 diabetes: recent progress and clinical implications. diabetes Care, 2009; Vol. 32: pp. 1107–14.

Comments: 2009 review of recently identified genes implicated in T2dM and potential clinical applications of new genetic knowledge to risk prediction, pharmacologic management, and patient behavior.

Writing Group for the SEArCh for diabetes in youth Study Group, dabelea d, bell rA, et al. incidence of diabetes in youth in the United States. JAMA, 2007; Vol. 297: pp. 2716–24.

Comments: landmark population-based study providing data on the incidence of dM among US youth accord-ing to racial/ethnic background and dM type.

Fourtner Sh, Weinzimer SA, levitt Katz IE. hyperglycemic hyperosmolar non-ketotic syndrome in children with type 2 diabetes. Pediatr diabetes, 2005; Vol. 6: pp. 129–35.

Comments: large retrospective chart review providing information on typical clinical course and sequelae of hyperglycemic hyperosmolar nonketotic syndrome in children with T2dM.

Expert Committee on the diagnosis and Classification of diabetes Mellitus. report of the expert committee on the diagnosis and classification of diabetes mellitus. diabetes Care, 2003; Vol. 26 Suppl 1: pp. S5–20.

Comments: report of international expert committee establishing current standards for definition and description of diabetes, classification of the disease, diagnostic criteria, and testing for diabetes.

青年人中的成年发病型糖尿病（MODY）

Ali Mohamadi, MD, and David W. Cooke, MD

定义
- 青年人中的成年发病型糖尿病（MODY）是一种单基因形式的早发性糖尿病（DM），通常在儿童期、青春期或青年期发病。
- 它的特点是常染色体显性遗传性非酮症糖尿病，发病年龄在25岁之前，并且有胰腺β-细胞功能障碍。

流行病学
- 高达5%抗体阴性的DM患者已发现有MOYD基因缺陷(Owen)。
- 对MOYD家族进行分子遗传研究发现，它不是一个单一的表现，而是一个临床和遗传异质性疾病。
- 八个基因的突变被确定可导致MOYD。
- MODY2是由一个基因编码的酶激酶（GCK）的缺陷造成的，而MODY8是由于羧基酯脂肪酶（CEL）的基因突变引起的。
- MODY1和MODY3-7转录因子的基因缺陷引起的：肝细胞核因子-4α（HNF-4 alpha/MODY1），肝细胞因子-1α（HNF-1 alpha/MODY3-最常见，早MODY中占20%~75%）；胰十二指肠的同源盒1（PdX1/MODY4），肝细胞核因子1β（HNF-1β/MODY5），神经分化因子1（神经D1-β2/MODY6），Krüppel样因子11（KIF11/MODY7）。

诊断
- 被公认的MODY诊断条件有至少5条。包括：
  - 至少有一个，最好两个家族成员在25岁之前被诊断为高血糖。
  - 常染色体显性遗传模式，垂直传播至少连续三代，糖尿病患者的家庭成员有类似的糖尿病表型表现。
  - 在诊断至少5年后可不用胰岛素治疗或者对于用胰岛素治疗的患者亦没有显著C-肽水平的改变。
  - 虽然胰岛素水平往往在正常范围内，但存在低程度的高血糖，提示β细胞功能存在缺陷。
  - 为正常体型、超重或肥胖的比例偏低。
- 值得注意的是，虽然轻度高血糖可能导致DM的典型症状，但在成年前，不能做出诊断。

症状和体征
- MODY常见的临床表现通常较轻，患者常常非肥胖体型，表现为无症状的高血糖。
- 影响胰岛素的敏感性因素可能诱导发作，如急性疾病或感染，往往在青春期或怀孕期间发病。
- 各种亚型之间的临床表现不同，这取决于受突变的基因。

青年人中的成年发病型糖尿病（MODY）

- MODY1（HNF-4α）和 MODY3（HNF-1α）：随着胰岛素的分泌的减少，空腹和餐后血糖（PG）的浓度轻、中度的增加。
- MODY2（葡萄糖激酶）：由于糖耐量受损，出现轻度空腹高血糖。少于50%的携带者表现为明显的糖尿病，与糖尿病相关的并发症是罕见的。
- MODY4（PDX1）：表现从糖耐量异常到糖尿病各异，PDX1纯合或复合杂合突变与胰腺发育不全相关。
- MODY5（HNF-1β）：显性 DM 与肾囊肿相关。
- MODY6（NEUROD1β-2）：少见，表型特点是肥胖和胰岛素抵抗。
- MODY7（KFl11）：非常罕见，表型从糖耐量受损或空腹血糖受损到 DM 表现各异。
- MODY8（CEL）：非常罕见，与胰腺外、内分泌缺陷相关与脱髓鞘性周围神经病变有关。

临床治疗

- 治疗方式决定于 MODY 的基因型和潜在基因缺陷。
  - MODY1（hNF-4 alpha）和 MODY3（hNF-1 alpha）：口服降糖药物在疾病的早期可能有效，随着内生胰岛素分泌减少，患者通常需要胰岛素治疗。
  - MODY4（PdX1）：口服降糖药物，可考虑口服降糖药物，虽然大部分人将需要胰岛素治疗。
  - MODY5（hNF-1 beta）：胰岛素治疗
  - MODY6（Neurod1-beta 2）：口服降糖药物或胰岛素治疗。
  - MODY7（KFl11）：口服降糖药物或胰岛素治疗。
  - MODY8（CEl）：胰酶替代和胰岛素治疗。

随访

- 由于其他原因可引起的 DM，应该定期随访并对糖尿病进行日常管理。
- 对于所有 DM 患者，预防、筛查和管理 DM 并发症。
- 由于某些 MODY 亚型随着时间的推移高血糖会加重，应警惕根据血糖控制需要改变相关治疗。

专家意见

- 利用 MODY 基因筛查，可以在他们的家族成员出现高血糖之前，识别出家庭成员中携带有特定的基因突变者。
- 如果儿童携带突变，建议定期检测碳水化合物的代谢情况。
- 我们需要较大规模的遗传和流行病学研究以确定单基因糖尿病的基因也会增加其他 DM 的遗传风险（如2型糖尿病）。

参考文献

Vaxillaire M, d P, bonnefond A, Froguel P. breakthroughs in monogenic diabetes genetics: from pediatric forms to young adulthood diabetes. Pediatr Endocrinol rev, 2009; Vol. 6: pp. 405–17.

Comments: review describing genetic and molecular mechanisms underlying the clinical features of MOdy, and how new genetic and biological insights led to novel pharmacogenomic approaches.

Vaxillaire M, Froguel P. Monogenic diabetes in the young, pharmacogenetics and relevance to multifactorial forms of type 2 diabetes. Endocr rev, 2008; Vol. 29: pp. 254–64.
Comments: review of updating advances in research on genetics of MOdy and explaining how these genes may play a role in multifactorial forms of T2dM.

Winckler W, Weedon MN, Graham rr, et al. Evaluation of common variants in the six known maturity-onset dia-betes of the young (MOdy) genes for association with type 2 diabetes. diabetes, 2007; Vol. 56: pp. 685–93.
Comments: Study determining patterns of common sequence variation in the genes encoding MOdy subtypes; concluded common variants contribute modestly to T2dM.

Slingerland AS. Monogenic diabetes in children and young adults: challenges for researcher, clinician and patient. rev Endocr Metab disord, 2006; Vol. 7: pp. 171–85.
Comments: Article detailing genes and mutations involved in insulin synthesis, secretion, and resistance. Provides guidance for genetic testing for MOdy and other forms of monogenic diabetes.

Owen Kr, Stride A, Ellard S, et al. Etiological investigation of diabetes in young adults presenting with apparent type 2 diabetes. diabetes Care, 2003; Vol. 26: pp. 2088–93.
Comments: describes the changing diagnostic approach to the growing population of youth and young adults who present with hyperglycemia but lack clinical and biochemical findings pathognomonic of type 1 diabetes.

Fajans SS, bell Gi, Polonsky KS. Molecular mechanisms and clinical pathophysiology of maturity-onset diabetes of the young. NEJM, 2001; Vol. 345: pp. 971–80.
Comments: Key review of genetics, pathophysiology, and treatment of MOdy subtypes.

线粒体糖尿病

Ali Mohamadi, MD, and David W. Cooke, MD

定义
- 线粒体基因组（mtDNA）的特定，已知突变可导致糖尿病（DM）。
- 区分线粒体的临床特征为糖尿病协会和其他的症状，包括耳聋、神经病变、心力衰竭和肾功能衰竭。
- 这些突变可以是大片段的缺失、重复或点突变。

流行病学
- 线粒体突变占糖尿病患者的 0.5%~2.8%。
- 线粒体基因是母系遗传，因此线粒体糖尿病的重要特征是有母系遗传家族史。
- 自发（非遗传）mtDNA 突变也进行了描述。
- 亚洲人的线粒体糖尿病的发病率较高（在整个日本的人口中高达 1.5%）。
- 线粒体疾病可以只表现为 DM，但更常见的是同其他的特征性的表现一起出现（见下文）。

诊断
- DM 患者伴有耳聋、肌病、小脑性共济失调或其他不寻常的神经功能，应考虑线粒体糖尿病。
- 有家族聚集性糖尿病或是母系遗传史更支持线粒体糖尿病。
- 在 40 岁之前发病和消瘦体质是线粒体糖尿病的发病特点（类似于比较常见的 1 型糖尿病）。
- 线粒体糖尿病与 MODY 不同的是它表现为母系遗传和表型。
- 听力检测发现听觉受损，且听觉感知下降 5 千赫以上的频率。
- 确诊是遗传分析发现 mtDNA 突变。
- 在核苷酸位置 3243 点替换（A 至 G）在线粒体 DNA 编码 trNAleu(UUR) 基因是最常见的与 DM 相关线粒体 DNA 突变。
- A3243G 突变的结果造成的表型与 1 型糖尿病类似，包括胰岛素分泌受损，肌肉中的糖代谢改变和由于糖异生的增加生产过剩乳酸。
- 线粒体 A3243G 突变引起的糖尿病平均发病年龄约 38 岁，外显率为 100%。

症状和体征
- 虽然只有母亲能将线粒体传给孩子，但男孩或女孩都可能会受到影响。
- 表型类似于 1 型（T1DM）或 2 型糖尿病（T2DM），这取决于胰岛细胞破坏的严重程度。
- A3243G 携带者中大部分将表现为 1 型的表型。
- 在过程中，胰岛的破坏是快速的，大部分患者在糖尿病发病后不久便需要注射胰岛素治疗。
- 听力障碍一般出现在 DM 发病之前数年。

- 许多 A3243G 突变携带者也出现视网膜色素的变化。
- 其他的合并症包括胃肠道异常（吞咽困难、运动功能障碍、胃食管反流），心肌病，肾功能不全。
- 其他相关综合征：MELAS（线粒体脑肌病、乳酸性酸中毒和卒中样发作）、Kearns-Sayre 综合征（眼外肌麻痹、视网膜病变、心脏传导异常）、MERRF 综合征（肌阵挛，癫痫，衣衫褴褛的红纤维）。

临床治疗

- 由于渐进式胰岛素缺乏，外源性胰岛素是治疗的重要支柱。
- 不太常见的 2 型糖尿病样表型，可以将改变饮食结构或磺酰脲类药物作为初步治疗。
- 禁用二甲双胍，因为乳酸性酸中毒的危险。
- 辅酶 Q10 和肉碱已被用于治疗合并线粒体肌病的患者（Maassen）。

随访

- 对 T1DM 或 T2DM 患者进行后续治疗和 DM 并发症的筛查。
- 由于大量的线粒体糖尿病患者中很大比例的患者合并了其他的合并症，后续随访应与相关的专家合作。

专家意见

- 研究表明，T2DM 在有母亲患病的病人中更为常见，其中，有些患者被发现可能携带 mtDNA 突变。
- 线粒体糖尿病的准确诊断需要检查与 mtDNA 突变相关的其他合并症。
- 表型的多样性增加了遗传咨询的难度，诊断线粒体糖尿病患者时若发现有其他高风险的母系亲属，应对那些有临床症状提示线粒体病的家属进行检查。

参考文献

Pagel-langenickel i, bao J, Pang l, et al. The role of mitochondria in the pathophysiology of skeletal muscle insulin resistance. Endocr rev, 2010; Vol. 31: pp. 25–51.

Comments: Analyzes the data regarding skeletal muscle mitochondrial biology in the pathogenesis of insulin resistance.

Ma y, Fang F, yang y, et al. The study of mitochondrial A3243G mutation in different samples. Mitochondrion, 2009; Vol. 9: pp. 139–43.

Comments: Comparison of the mutation ratio of A3243G in blood, urine, hair follicle, and saliva samples in patients with A3243G mutations and their maternal relatives to determine which sample type (urine) is most appropriate for detection of the patients and carriers.Scaglia F, hsu Ch, Kwon h, et al.

Molecular bases of hearing loss in multi-systemic mitochondrial cytopathy. Genet Med, 2006; Vol. 8: pp. 641–52.

Comments: Evaluation of the clinical features and molecular bases of hearing loss associated with multisys-temic mitochondrial cytopathyFinsterer J. Genetic, pathogenetic, and phenotypic implications of the mitochondrial A3243G trNAleu(UUr) mutation. Acta Neurol Scand, 2007; Vol. 116: pp. 1–14.

Comments: Comprehensive review of the mitochondrial A3243G trNAleu(UUr) mutation, the most common cause of mitochondrial dM.

Maassen JA, T hart IM, Van Essen E, et al. Mitochondrial diabetes: molecular mechanisms and clinical presenta-tion. diabetes, 2004; Vol. 53 Suppl 1: pp. S103–9.

Comments: review of clinical characteristics of mitochondrial diabetes and its molecular diagnosis, also discussing recent developments in the pathophysiological and molecular mechanisms leading to diabetes.

成人隐匿性自身免疫糖尿病（LADA）

Ari Eckman, MD, and Christopher D. Saudek, MD

定义
- 成人隐匿糖尿病（LADA）是一个缓慢发展的 1 型糖尿病，通常被误诊为 2 型糖尿病。LADA 通常进展相对较快，较快发展为胰岛 β–细胞功能衰竭并形成胰岛素依赖。
- 也称为"缓慢的胰岛素依赖型糖尿病"，"2 型糖尿病与胰岛自身抗体"和"1.5 型糖尿病"。

流行病学
- 在英国前瞻性糖尿病研究（UKPDS），约 10% 的患者似乎有 2 型糖尿病谷氨酸抗体脱羧酶（GAD）和进展胰岛素依赖（Turner；Stenström）。
- 在患者 35 岁的年龄，抗体阳性的频率提高到 25%（Turner; Stenström）。
- 与经典的 1 型糖尿病相似，患者可能有自身免疫性疾病个人或家族历史等（如自身免疫性甲状腺疾病、恶性贫血、腹腔疾病、白癜风）。
- 往往没有糖尿病家族史。
- 血糖控制强 LADA 患者心血管疾病的风险系数比与 2 型糖尿病可能与代谢的患病率较低，可能与 LADA 患者的代谢综合征的低发生率相关（isomaa）。
- HLA–DR4-DQ8 抗原：与对 β 细胞的破坏进展相关，尤其在经典的 1 型糖尿病比 LADA 中更为多见。

诊断
- 基于三个标准：诊断时已经成年，存在糖尿病相关的自身抗体，由于需要胰岛素控制高血糖延误诊断（至少 6 个月）。
- 谷氨酸脱羧酶自身抗体（抗–GAD）、胰岛细胞的自身抗体（抗 ICA）、酪氨酸磷酸酶抗体（抗–IA2 或反 CA512）检测呈阳性，预测在 3 年之内的胰岛素依赖（Turner）。
- 最敏感的抗体标记抗–GAD：灵敏度 85%。
- 抗胰岛细胞自身抗体在经典 1 型糖尿病患者比 LADA 患者更为常见
- 相关的频率增加 HLADR3（28%）、DR4（27%）和 dr3/dr4（22%）（OLA）。
- HLA–DR4-DQ8 抗原：与 β 细胞的破坏性进展关联，与 LADA 相比，HLA–DR4-DQ8 抗原在经典 1 型糖尿病患者中更普遍。

症状和体征
- 高血糖起病隐匿。
- 缺乏急性高血糖危症（如糖尿病酮症酸中毒 DKA）。
- 体型通常为正常或稍微超重。
- 通常缺乏明显的在传统的 2 型糖尿病人中存在的胰岛素抵抗的迹象，如棘皮病（在身体皱褶的皮肤变黑）或 acrochordons（皮肤标签）。

成人隐匿性自身免疫糖尿病（LADA）

- 与 2 型糖尿病相比，代谢综合征的频率减少。
- C – 肽水平可能低 / 正常 (Fielding)。

临床治疗

- 选择胰岛素治疗，治疗参照 1 型糖尿病。
- 控制高血糖和其他并发症的风险因素。
- 肥胖的 LADA 患者会从限制消耗的热量和增加体力活动水平中收益。
- 如果超重，考虑二甲双胍治疗胰岛素抵抗。
- 噻唑烷二酮类药物可改善 β 细胞分泌功能。
- 磺脲类药物，可能会耗尽内源性胰岛素的储备应避免使用 (Maruyama)。
- 对于早期使用胰岛素治疗是否有助于保护 β 细胞功能仍不清楚(Maruyama)。
- 早期胰岛素治疗能更好地控制血糖和减少并发症。

随访

- 在诊断后六年，大多数患者出现胰岛素依赖（Fourlanos）。
- 在 LADA 中发生视网膜病变和肾病的频率类似于 2 型糖尿病，它们取决于相同的风险因素，特别是高血糖。神经病最初罕见，但随着病程而增加。
- 视网膜病变的患病率、冠状动脉心脏病（CHD）和心血管疾病的死亡率 LADA 和 2 型糖尿病相似。

专家意见

- LADA 一种自身免疫性糖尿病，在遗传和免疫方面与 1 型糖尿病相似，但往往呈渐进性发作，到成人时发病。
- 由于自体免疫导致的胰岛 β 细胞的破坏速度远远慢于经典的 1 型糖尿病。
- LADA 是成年起病的糖尿病，缺乏 2 型糖尿病的常见的特征，如体型肥胖和对口服药物反应良好。
- 漏诊 LADA 可能导致是没有尽早期使用足够量的胰岛素。

参考文献

Appel SJ, Wadas TM, rosenthal rS, et al. latent autoimmune diabetes of adulthood (IAdA): an often misdiag-nosed type of diabetes mellitus. J Am Acad Nurse Pract, 2009; Vol. 21: pp. 156–9.

Comments: IAdA is a common and often underrecognized form of diabetes whose clinical presentation falls somewhere between that of type 1 dM and type 2 dM. From a pathophysiological perspective, it is more closely related to type 1 dM. Often misdiagnosed and treated as type 2 dM.

Fielding AM, brophy S, davies h, et al. latent autoimmune diabetes in adults: increased awareness will aid diag-nosis. Ann Clin biochem, 2007; Vol. 44: pp. 321–3.

Comments: high titres of serum glutamic acid decarboxylase (GAd) antibodies act as a marker for IAdA. Serum C-peptide concentrations are also lower in autoimmune diabetic patients. Early insulin treatment may prevent pancreatic beta-cell failure.

Ola TO, Gigante A, leslie rd. latent autoimmune diabetes of adults (IAdA). Nutr Metab Cardiovasc dis, 2006; Vol. 16: pp. 163–7.

Comments: Associated with increased frequency of hIA dr3 (28%), dr4 (27%), and dr3/dr4 (22%).

Fourlanos S, Perry C, Stein MS, et al. A clinical screening tool identifies autoimmune diabetes in adults. diabetes Care, 2006; Vol. 29: pp. 970–5.
Comments: Study aimed to develop clinical screening tool to identify adults at high risk of lAdA who require islet antibody testing.

Leslie rd, Williams r, Pozzilli P. Clinical review: Type 1 diabetes and latent autoimmune diabetes in adults: one end of the rainbow. J Clin Endocrinol Metab, 2006; Vol. 91: pp. 1654–9.
Comments: Explores pathogenic and clinical spectrum of type 1 diabetes, including a form of adult onset autoimmune diabetes referred to as lAdA.

Stenström G, Gottsäter A, bakhtadze E, et al. latent autoimmune diabetes in adults: definition, prevalence, beta-cell function, and treatment. diabetes, 2005; Vol. 54 Suppl 2: pp. S68–72.
Comments: lAdA occurs in 10% of individuals older than 35 years and in 25% below that age; proved impaired beta-cell function at diagnosis of diabetes, insulin is the treatment of choice.

Fourlanos S, dotta F, Greenbaum CJ, et al. latent autoimmune diabetes in adults (lAdA) should be less latent. diabetologia, 2005; Vol. 48: pp. 2206–12.
Comments: Majority of patients become insulin-dependent within 6 years of diagnosis.

Owen Kr, Stride A, Ellard S, et al. Etiological investigation of diabetes in young adults presenting with apparent type 2 diabetes. diabetes Care, 2003; Vol. 26: pp. 2088–93.
Comments: lAdA subjects can be identified by presence of pancreatic ß-cell antibodies, of which most useful is GAd. have a different disease profile from type 2 diabetes, being lean and insulin sensitive with a more rapid progression to insulin treatment.

Hosszúfalusi N, Vatay A, rajczy K, et al. Similar genetic features and different islet cell autoantibody pattern of latent autoimmune diabetes in adults (lAdA) compared with adult-onset type 1 diabetes with rapid progres-sion. diabetes Care, 2003; Vol. 26: pp. 452–7.
Comments: Compares clinical parameters, C-peptide levels, pattern of islet cell-specific autoantibodies, and prevalence of predisposing genotypes in subjects with lAdA and those with adult-onset type 1 diabetes with rapid progression.

Maruyama T, Shimada A, Kanatsuka A, et al. Multicenter prevention trial of slowly progressive type 1 diabetes with small dose of insulin (the Tokyo study): preliminary report. Ann Ny Acad Sci, 2003; Vol. 1005: pp. 362–9.
Comments: Small doses of insulin effectively prevent beta-cell failure in slowly progressive type 1 diabetes. recommend avoiding SU treatment, instead administering insulin to NiddM patients with high GAdA titer.

Schranz db, bekris I, landin-Olsson M, et al. Newly diagnosed latent autoimmune diabetes in adults (lAdA) is associated with low level glutamate decarboxylase (GAd65) and iA-2 autoantibodies. diabetes incidence Study in Sweden (diSS). horm Metab res, 2000; Vol. 32: pp. 133–8.
Comments: young adult new-onset lAdA patients have low-level GAd65Ab and iA-2Ab. The low-level autoan-tibodies may signify a less aggressive beta-cell

autoimmunity, possibly explaining why these patients are often classified with type 2 or non-insulin-dependent diabetes.

Isomaa b, Almgren P, henricsson M, et al. Chronic complications in patients with slowly progressing autoimmune type 1 diabetes (lAdA). diabetes Care, 1999; Vol. 22: pp.1347–53.
Comments: lAdA patients had lower bMi, waist-to-hip ratio, fasting C-peptide concentrations, and less hypertension than the type 2 diabetic patients. Glycemic control is a stronger risk factor for retinopathy and cardiovascular disease in lAdA patients than in patients with type 2 diabetes.

Turner r, Stratton i, horton V, et al. UKPdS 25: autoantibodies to islet-cell cytoplasm and glutamic acid decarbox-ylase for prediction of insulin requirement in type 2 diabetes. UK Prospective diabetes Study Group. lancet, 1997; Vol. 350: pp. 1288–93.
Comments: Among young adults with type 2 diabetes, phenotype of those with iCA or GAd antibodies was simi-lar to that of classic juvenile-onset insulin-dopondont diabetes, and either phenotype or antibodies predicted insulin requirement. in older adults, phenotype was closer to that of patients without antibodies and only the presence of antibodies predicted an increased likelihood of insulin requirement.

Zimmet PZ, Tuomi T, Mackay ir, et al. latent autoimmune diabetes mellitus in adults (lAdA): the role of antibodies to glutamic acid decarboxylase in diagnosis and prediction of insulin dependency. diabet Med, 1994; Vol. 11: pp. 299–303.
Comments: One of the earliest papers describing the role that testing for GAd antibodies has on detecting lAdA at earliest possible stage.

老年糖尿病

Ana Emiliano, MD, and Rita Rastogi Kalyani, MD, MHS

定义
- 在老年人中，2型糖尿病（T2DM）是一个重大的公共卫生问题。
- 正常老化可能导致胰岛素敏感性降低（roder；defronzo；Elahi），这可能是由于在肌肉中的葡萄糖载体GLUT4的密度降低导致胰岛素抵抗（houmard）。
- 与衰老相关的生理上的变化也可能加重对胰岛素敏感性降低，包括腹部脂肪量的增加，运动的减少，线粒体功能障碍，荷尔蒙的变化，氧化应激增加和炎症反应（Goulet）。
- 往往同时有合并症、认知功能障碍和功能障碍会影响糖尿病的管理，尤其是中老年人。

流行病学
- 三分之一65岁以上的老人患有糖尿病（Cowie），几乎有一半未确诊。养老院老人的发病率可能会更高。
- 另外有40%的老年人患有前期糖尿病（Cowie）。
- 随着个体寿命的延长和肥胖率的增加，T2DM中老年人患病率预计将增加。
- 在老人中，糖尿病相关并发症的发病率和死亡率较高（Bethel）。
- 与中年发病的糖尿病相比，老年发病型糖尿病某些并发症较少，如视网膜病（Selvin）。
- 老年人低血糖会增加心血管疾病的风险事件和痴呆症的风险（Whitmer）。
- 抑郁症和老年痴呆症在患有糖尿病的老年人中更常见，这导致自我管理的困难，以致血糖控制不佳。
- 老年人糖尿病病例中记录有病例出现肌力下降，肌肉萎缩，肌肉体积的减少，特别是在下肢（Park）。
- 老年糖尿病病人功能性残疾的发生率是普通糖尿病病人的2~3倍，包括行走四分之一公里以上的路程，提重物，做家务，参与休闲活动等方面（Kalyani）。

诊断
- 因为葡萄糖不耐受会随着年龄的增加而加重，有人建议，应对老年人糖尿病的诊断标准作出相应的修改，但目前仍使用与年轻的个人相同的标准（见糖尿病的诊断与分型，第6页）。

症状和体征
- 与年轻人类似，老年人血糖控制不佳可表现为多尿、多饮、体重减轻、视力模糊。然而，这些症状并非总能体现出来，这增加了发生严重高血糖的风险。
- 老年人严重高血糖时，更容易发生脱水。
- 视力下降包括继发于视网膜病变的失明，可能会出现并损害身体机能。
- 在患有糖尿病的老年人中，微量白蛋白尿转化为显性慢性肾脏病更经常发生。

老年糖尿病

- 由于长期的血管和神经系统疾病导致的足部问题更常见。老人糖尿病神经病变的患病率高达 40%（Young）。老年糖尿病患者因其身体和认知障碍，导致其无法发现其足部状况，这增加了足病继续发展的风险。
- 由于周围自主神经病变，低血糖、功能性残疾、视力障碍和服用多种药物，晕倒现象（Falls）在老年糖尿病患者中更为常见。
- 与没有糖尿病妇女相比，患有糖尿病老年妇女更易发生尿失禁（Jackson）。

临床治疗
生活方式干预
- 对于超重或肥胖的老年人建议减肥。衰弱养老院老人不建议减轻体重（Wedick）。
- 总的来说，锻炼可使后期生活受益，以防止向糖尿病发展和增加生存（Mozaffarian）。
- 推荐摄入低血糖指数的食物（Mozaffarian）。
- 停止吸烟。

药物治疗
- 如果没有其他禁忌证（如肌酐清除 60ml/min，血肌酐 1.5mg/L 或充血性心脏衰竭）。对于超重的老年患者首选二甲双胍。
- 与年轻人相比，在老年人中磺脲类更容易引起低血糖。格列吡嗪和格列美脲造成低血糖的可能性较低，优于格列本脲或氯磺丙脲。
- 噻唑可以使用，但在 III 级或 IV 级心脏衰竭的老年患者是绝对禁忌。
- α-葡萄糖苷酶抑制剂（阿卡波糖和米格列醇）对于中老年人应该安全，尽管其使用不广泛。
- 二肽基肽酶IV（DPP-IV）抑制剂对于衰弱的个人是比较有吸引力的选择，因为他们对体重没有影响。该药物在中老年人的使用有限。
- GLP-1 为基础的疗法，有着注射的限制，可能无法作为有功能残疾老年患者的首选。对于年老体弱、低体重的个人不是一个很好的选择，因为它会导致体重下降。
- 胰淀素类似物普兰林肽对于中老年人可能不是一个很好的选择，因为低血糖风险很大并需要每日多次注射。
- 大多数 2 型糖尿病患者最终需要注射胰岛素。在使用胰岛素之前，应先评估视力、活动能力、认知功能和照顾情况。
- 长效、每日一次的胰岛素疗法可能是更简单易行和最安全的选择。

治疗的目标
- 患有 T2DM 健康老年人和有 5 年的预期寿命患者，应将糖化血红蛋白控制在 7%（ADA 指引）。
- 合并多种并发症的老年患者，功能残疾或预期寿命有限的患者可能会受利于较宽松的糖化目标（即 8%），但需要更严谨的研究（Brown）。
- 患者需要对自己意识到和防治低血糖的能力进行定期评估，这可能是潜在的危险，可能会限制强化血糖带来的好处
- 低血糖是治疗糖尿病的严重并发症，尤其是中老年人，并应尽量减少。
- 可能引起低血糖情况，同时服用的胰岛素增敏剂或胰岛素，锻炼，控制

饮食，限制热量，最近住院，服用多种药物治疗，服用水杨酸盐类、磺胺类、纤维酸衍生物以及华法林（Neumiller）。

随访

- 应始终关注老年患者的肝和肾的功能变化并进行相应的药物调整。
- 终末期肾脏疾病老年患者对胰岛素的需求，会随着肾脏功能的损害和对胰岛素的代谢延迟而下降，低血糖可能会随之出现，胰岛素剂量应作相应的调整。
- 功能状态的变化也可能会影响治疗的目标。

专家意见

- 老人更容易发生糖耐量异常，可能由于衰老引起胰岛素敏感性受损的生理变化。
- 身体情况衰弱且合并多种并发症的老人与和预期寿命有限者更适合较宽松的糖化血红蛋白目标。
- 临床治疗应根据患者的个性化需求。

参考文献

Kalyani rr, Saudek Cd, brancati Fl, et al. Association of diabetes, comorbidities, and A1c with functional disabil-ity in older adults: results from the National health and Nutrition Examination Survey (NhANES), 1999–2006. diabetes Care, 2010; Vol. 33: pp. 1055–60.
Comments: diabetes was associated with 2–3 times increased odds of disability across many different functional groups (p <0.05).

American diabetes Association. Standards of medical care in diabetes—2011. diabetes Care, 2011; Vol. 34 Suppl 1: pp. S11–61.
Comments: Consensus guidelines on the management of diabetes by the American diabetes Association.

Goulet Ed, hassaine A, dionne iJ, et al. Frailty in the elderly is associated with insulin resistance of glucose metabolism in the postabsorptive state only in the presence of increased abdominal fat. Exp Gerontol, 2009; Vol. 44: pp. 740–4.
Comments: This study found that age, abdominal fat mass, and muscle mass index were significantly cor-related with insulin sensitivity.

Cowie CC, rust KF, Ford ES, et al. Full accounting of diabetes and pre-diabetes in the U.S. population in 1988–1994 and 2005–2006. diabetes Care, 2009; Vol. 32: pp. 287–94.
Comments: This national representative study found that one-third of the elderly population had diabetes and three-quarters had diabetes or prediabetes.

Whitmer rA, Karter AJ, yaffe K, et al. hypoglycemic episodes and risk of dementia in older patients with type 2 diabetes mellitus. JAMA, 2009; Vol. 301: pp. 1565–72.
Comments: This study examined dementia risk in relation to the frequency of severe hypoglycemic episodes, defined as episodes that required a hospital visit/admission. Patients with a single episode had a hazard ratio for dementia of 1.26 (Ci 1.10–1.49).

Mozaffarian d, Kamineni A, Carnethon M, et al. lifestyle risk factors and new-onset diabetes mellitus in older adults: the cardiovascular health study. Arch intern Med, 2009; Vol. 169: pp. 798–807.

Comments: Prospective study examining the incidence of diabetes among 4883 elderly men and women dur-ing a 10-year period. A low-risk lifestyle was associated with a significantly reduced incidence of new-onset diabetes.

Neumiller JJ, Setter SM. Pharmacologic management of the older patient with type 2 diabetes mellitus. Am J Geriatr Pharmacother, 2009; Vol. 7: pp. 324–42.
Comments: Comprehensive review of the use of pharmacologic agents to treat older adults with T2dM, with an emphasis on prevention of hypoglycemia and drug interactions.

Bethel MA, Sloan FA, belsky d, et al. longitudinal incidence and prevalence of adverse outcomes of diabetes mellitus in elderly patients. Arch intern Med, 2007; Vol. 167: pp. 921–7.
Comments: longitudinal analysis examining mortality and morbidity rates in 33,772 elderly patients newly diagnosed with diabetes compared to 25,563 elderly controls, followed from 1991–2004. The group with diabe-tes had an excess mortality of 9.2%.

Park SW, Goodpaster bh, Strotmeyer ES, et al. Accelerated loss of skeletal muscle strength in older adults with type 2 diabetes: the health, aging, and body composition study. diabetes Care, 2007; Vol. 30: pp. 1507–12.
Comments: This study found that patients with T2dM had a 13.5% loss in knee extensor strength compared to a 9% loss in individuals without diabetes ($p = 0.001$). in addition, patients with type 2 diabetes also lost greater amounts of lean leg mass ($p<0.05$).

Selvin E, Coresh J, brancati Fl. The burden and treatment of diabetes in elderly individuals in the US. diabetes Care, 2006; Vol. 29: pp. 2415–9.
Comments: Elderly patients with middle age onset diabetes had a much greater burden of microvascular disease compared to elderly onset diabetes.

Jackson Sl, Scholes d, boyko EJ, et al. Urinary incontinence and diabetes in postmenopausal women. diabetes Care, 2005; Vol. 28: pp. 1730–8.
Comments: in this study, women with diabetes reported more severe urinary incontinence, which correlated significantly with diabetes duration, peripheral neuropathy, and retinopathy.

Brown AF, Mangione CM, Saliba d, et al. Guidelines for improving the care of the older person with diabetes mel-litus. J Am Geriatr Soc, 2003; Vol. 51: pp. S265–80.
Comments: review article containing evidence-based recommendations to guide clinicians caring for elderly person with diabetes.

Wedick NM, barrett-Connor E, Knoke Jd, et al. The relationship between weight loss and all-cause mortality in older men and women with and without diabetes mellitus: the rancho bernardo study. J Am Geriatr Soc, 2002; Vol. 50: pp. 1810–5.
Comments: 1801 elderly men and women, with and without diabetes, were followed for 12 years. Weight loss of 10 pounds was associated with an increased hazard ratio for all-cause mortality in nondiabetic men (hr = 1.38; 95% Ci 1.06–1.80) and women (hr = 1.76; 95% Ci 1.33–2.34) and diabetic men (hr = 3.66; 95% Ci 2.15–6.24) and women (hr = 1.65; 95% Ci 0.70–3.87) after adjusting for age, smoking, and sedentary life style.

Elahi d, Muller dC, Egan JM, et al. Glucose tolerance, glucose utilization and insulin secretion in aging. Novartis Found Symp, 2002; Vol. 242: pp. 222–42, discussion 242-6.
Comments:review article exploring basic, epidemiological, and clinical data on the development of glucose intolerance and insulin resistance with aging.

Roder ME, Schwartz rS, Prigeon rl, et al. reduced pancreatic b cell compensation to the insulin resistance of aging: impact on proinsulin and insulin levels. J Clin Endocrinol Metab, 2000; Vol. 85: pp. 2275–80.
Comments: in this study, 26 older subjects (mean age 67 years) and 22 younger subjects (mean age 22 years) had their insulin sensitivity and beta-cell function assessed. The older subjects had a 50% reduction in insulin sensitivity and beta-cell function.

Houmard JA, Weidner MD, dolan Pl, et al. Skeletal muscle GlUT4 protein concentration and aging in humans. diabetes, 1995; Vol. 44: pp. 555–60.
Comments:in this study, GlUT4 protein levels were lower in older individuals, irrespective of sex (men r = -0.28, women r = -0.51). GlUT4 levels were positively correlated with insulin sensitivity (r = 0.42).

Young MJ, boulton AJ, Macleod AF, et al. A multicentre study of the prevalence of diabetic peripheral neuropathy in the United Kingdom hospital clinic population. diabetologia, 1993; Vol. 36: pp. 150–4.
Comments: A cross-sectional study of 6487 individuals with diabetes in 118 centers in the UK, ages ranging from 18–90 years. The prevalence of peripheral neuropathy in T2dM increased significantly with age, going from 5% in the 20–29 age group to 44.2% in the 70–79 age group.

deFronzo rA. Glucose intolerance and aging. diabetes Care, 1982; Vol. 4: pp. 493–501.
Comments: This article reviews the factors involved in the progressive decline of glucose tolerance seen with aging, primarily related to the intrinsic development of tissue unresponsiveness to insulin.

激素诱发糖尿病

Rachel Derr, MD, PhD

定义
- 糖皮质激素,如泼尼松、地塞米松和可的松(GC),是强有力的抗炎和免疫抑制剂,可以有效地治疗宽谱疾病。
- 高血糖是葡萄糖无法被肌肉运用的常见的不良作用(Pagano)。
- GC诱导的高血糖达到了糖尿病范围,但不使用GC时血糖正常。

流行病学
- 三级医院10%的住院患者和3%的60岁的门诊患者有开糖皮质激素的处方医院(Donihi; Choi)。
- 在既往无糖尿病史高剂量使用糖皮质激素的三级医院住院患者中(泼尼松每天至少40毫克,至少2天),糖皮质激素诱导的高血糖患病率约为54%~64%(Donihi)。
- 危重患者在加护病房后使用糖皮质激素,高血糖的风险增加五倍。
- 与未使用糖皮质激素的患者相比,使用糖皮质激素的慢性阻塞性肺病的门诊患者和住院患者,使用新的降糖药物的风险分别增加2倍和4倍(Gurwitz; Niewoehner)。
- 糖皮质激素的剂量与高血糖的程度呈正相关,需要降血糖药物治疗(Gurwitz)。

诊断
- 对于激素诱发的糖尿病没有正式的诊断标准,在使用激素后第一次发现糖尿病便可诊断。
- 糖尿病的诊断标准是不变的。
- 对预先存在糖尿病的患者以任何形式使用激素都会加重高血糖。

症状和体征
- 预期的高血糖的迹象和症状:多尿、烦渴恶化、多食、乏力。
- 由于高血糖和免疫抑制的联合作用,感染可能较为普遍。
- 其他的症状和体征可能与慢性外源性类固醇激素的使用有关:如水牛背、皮肤薄、高凝、近端肌肉无力、水肿。

临床治疗

治疗可能带来的好处
- 对于住院患者,能够改善高血糖有关的症状和减少医院住院时间。
- 减少感染:平均血糖较高的患者,在骨髓移植中的中性粒细胞减少相关感染率较高,尤其在中性粒细胞减少时使用激素的患者(Derr)。
- 一些证据表明,在癌症患者中能改善死亡率:在胶质母细胞瘤患者(许多接受激素以减轻脑水肿),平均血糖高的患者死亡率比平均血糖低的患者高57%以上(Derr)。

管理策略
- 如果激素引起的高血糖是轻度的,二甲双胍和噻唑可有效降低胰岛素抵抗。
- 对于中度或严重的高血糖,并在医院环境中,胰岛素是首选,因为它起效快,允许剂量灵活,更有效。
- 一些专家建议处方应加大基础胰岛素的比例,因为激素诱导的高血糖会在餐后恶化。(Clement)。

随访
- 胰岛素的需求会随着激素剂量的调整和以后注射的失效而发生巨大的变化。密切随访是必需的。
- 当停用激素时,应该估计降低胰岛素剂量的需要,以避免低血糖。
- 当激素停用时,对于糖耐量正常的患者,通常不再需要降血糖药物。
- 停用降血糖药物后仍有低血糖的症状,提示可能有继发性肾上腺皮质功能不全(AI)。为了预防继发性肾上腺皮质功能不全(AI),激素应该缓慢减量。
- 以前有激素诱导的糖尿病史的患者发展为显性糖尿病风险的相关资料很少,可假定它是以后发生糖尿病的危险因素。

专家意见
- 糖皮质激素,特别是在高剂量时,对糖耐量的作用可能是巨大的,可能引起的症状甚至高渗性非酮症状态,以及对住院患者造成负面影响。
- 患有糖尿病的患者打算使用糖皮质激素时(例如口服或注射),应警惕可能影响预期的高血糖。
- 住院患者使用糖皮质激素,至少每天一次监测血糖,糖尿病门诊患者使用糖皮质激素,应增加监测次数。
- 停用降血糖药物后仍有低血糖的症状,提示可能有继发性肾上腺皮质功能不全(AI)。为了预防继发性肾上腺皮质功能不全(AI),激素应该缓慢减量。

参考文献

Derr rl, ye X, islas MU, et al. Association between hyperglycemia and survival in patients with newly diagnosed glioblastoma. J Clin Oncol, 2009; Vol. 27: pp. 1082–6.

Comments:in patients with newly diagnosed glioblastoma, hyperglycemia was associated with shorter survival, after controlling for glucocorticoid dose and other confounders.

Derr rl, hsiao VC, Saudek Cd. Antecedent hyperglycemia is associated with an increased risk of neutropenic infections during bone marrow transplantation. diabetes Care, 2008; Vol. 31: pp. 1972–7.

Comments: in a bone marrow transplant population highly susceptible to infection, mean antecedent glycemia was associated with later infection risk, particularly in patients who received glucocorticoids while neutropenic.

Donihi AC, raval d, Saul M, et al. Prevalence and predictors of corticosteroid-related hyperglycemia in hospital-ized patients. Endocr Pract, 2006; Vol. 12: pp. 358–62.

Comments: Using a pharmacy database at a tertiary academic hospital, evaluates prevalence of and risk factors for hyperglycemia in patients receiving high-dose glucocorticoids.

Choi hK, Seeger Jd. Glucocorticoid use and serum lipid levels in US adults: the Third National health and Nutri-tion Examination Survey. Arthritis rheum, 2005; Vol. 53: pp. 528–35.

Comments: reports prevalence of glucocorticoid use in The Third National health and Nutrition Examination Survey (1988–1994), determined from household interview regarding prescription medication use.

Clement S, braithwaite SS, Magee MF, et al. Management of diabetes and hyperglycemia in hospitals. diabetesCare, 2004; Vol. 27: pp. 553–91.

Comments: reviews and evaluates the evidence relating to the management of hyperglycemia in hospitals, including management in special circumstances such as glucocorticoid use.

Niewoehner dE, Erbland Ml, deupree rh, et al. Effect of systemic glucocorticoids on exacerbations of chronic obstructive pulmonary disease. department of Veterans Affairs Cooperative Study Group. NEJM, 1999; Vol. 340: pp. 1941–7.

Comments: randomized controlled trial (rCT) that found that systemic glucocorticoids moderately improve outcomes in COPd, but hyperglycemia warranting treatment is the most frequent complication.

Gurwitz Jh, bohn rl, Glynn rJ, et al. Glucocorticoids and the risk for initiation of hypoglycemic therapy. Arch intern Med, 1994; Vol. 154: pp. 97–101.

Comments: Using a Medicaid database, quantifies the risk of developing hyperglycemia requiring hypoglycemic therapy after oral glucocorticoid use.

Pagano G, Cavallo-Perin P, Cassader M, et al. An in vivo and in vitro study of the mechanism of prednisone-induced insulin resistance in healthy subjects. J Clin invest, 1983; Vol. 72: pp. 1814–20.

Comments: landmark basic science study, which found that prednisone induces insulin resistance due to depressed peripheral glucose utilization from impaired glucose transport.

1 型糖尿病

1 型糖尿病：危险因素

Gregory O. Clark, MD

定义
- 遗传易感人群在某些环境的作用下可发展为 1 型糖尿病。
- 决定易感性的遗传危险因素反映了疾病与遗传的相关性。
- 环境危险因素与 1 型糖尿病易感性有关已得到流行病学研究的证实。

流行病学
- 1 型糖尿的发病率目前在全球每年增加 3%~4%，这反映了环境对疾病的影响（DIAMOND Project）。
- 其中发病率在 5 岁以下儿童中增长最快，Patterson 预计从 2005 年到 2020 年，新发病例将增加一倍。
- 发病高峰年龄出现在青春期，10~14 岁。
- 50% 的患者是成年人。
- 世界各个国家的 1 型糖尿病发病率相差可达 100 倍，最高的是芬兰和意大利的撒丁岛，最低的是中国和委内瑞拉（Borchers）。
- 一般情况下，欧洲高加索人群的患病率最高（20 例 / 年 · 100 000 人），尤其是在北欧的高加索人群，以及他们在北美、澳大利亚和新西兰的后裔。在科威特，1 型糖尿病患病率也高。
- 1 型糖尿病在亚洲患病率低（1 例 / 年 · 100 000 人）。
- 详见 1 型糖尿病的流行病学（第 9 页）。

诊断
- 由于利用基因检测或环境因素对 1 型糖尿病进行危险评估尚未应用于临床，因此目前还没有已知的预防措施。
- 基于研究目的，可将高风险个体（第一直系亲属）以基因型和循环自身抗体的出现为标准进行危险分层。这些自身抗体包括胰岛细胞胞浆抗体、胰岛素自身抗体、谷氨酸脱羧酶自身抗体以及胰岛瘤相关抗体 2，它们都是自身免疫早期阶段的标记。研究的目标是为了能更好的预测和预防对胰岛 β 细胞的自身免疫性破坏。
- 如果第一直系亲属患有 1 型糖尿病，那么发生该病的风险是 5%。
- 同卵双胞胎同时患病的概率是 40%~60%，这表明遗传风险由其他大概是环境因素显著调节。

临床治疗
遗传风险因素
- 针对遗传因素引起的 1 型糖尿病尚没有治疗方法。

1型糖尿病：危险因素

- 与免疫调节有关的人类白细胞分化抗原 2 基因，与 1 型糖尿病有极强的相关性。
- 特定的人白细胞 DR 抗原（human leukocyte antigenDR，HLA-DR）和人白细胞 DQ 抗原（human leukocyte antigenDQ，HLA-DQ）单倍型在该病的易感以及预防中同时起着作用。
- HLA DR3/DR4 杂合子使个体具有 1 型糖尿病易感性，但该表型只出现在最多 2% 的新生儿和 30% 的患 1 型糖尿病的儿童中。此基因型的绝对患 1 型糖尿病的风险概率为 1/20（Eisenbarth）。
- 其他与 1 型糖尿病有关的基因（非 HLA）：CTLA4（细胞毒性 T- 淋巴细胞相关蛋白 4），IFIH1（解螺旋酶 C 结构域 1 诱导干扰素），ITPR3（1，4，5 - 三磷酸肌醇受体 3），IL－2 受体，PTPN22（酪氨酸磷酸酶非受体型 22）。
- 超过 40 个基因位点已发现与 1 型糖尿病的发展有关（Barrett）。

相关的环境风险因素

- 没有环境因素已明确与 1 型糖尿病有关。如下述变异的证据。
- 病毒（肠病毒、柯萨奇病毒、先天性风疹）可能因为分子拟态（类似于 β 细胞蛋白的病毒蛋白）触发自身免疫程序。
- "卫生假说"表明，儿童期感染的缺乏可能有助于增加自身免疫性疾病和过敏症的发生。婴儿早期饮食：提前用牛奶喂养可能会导致对牛胰岛素（与人胰岛素类似并且是已知的 1 型糖尿病有关重要自身抗原）免疫反应，谷物蛋白或其他谷物衍生蛋白质也会导致相同的反应。
- 毒素：亚硝胺。
- 地理：随着离赤道距离增加，发病率增加。
- 维生素 D 缺乏：这可能涉及到在大部分北半球地区的发病率较高。相比之下，在这些地区有较少的紫外线照射。
- 肥胖/体重增加：该因素可能由于 β－细胞凋亡暴露 β－细胞抗原而启动免疫过程，或由于胰岛素抵抗使 β 细胞的需求增加而促进该过程，这就是所谓的"加速器假说"（Wilkn）。
- 高社会经济地位。

专家意见

- 事实上，遗传危险因素和环境危险因素是很难分辨的。例如，在撒丁岛的原住民有相似的遗传基因和暴露环境，但是并不是所有的人都患 1 型糖尿病。移民研究可帮助区分危险因素，并且表明遗传和环境对于 1 型糖尿病的地理区域流传都很重要。
- 新生儿糖尿病：必须分析 Kir6.2 基因（磺脲类药物受体）的突变，因为它与一半的新生儿糖尿病有关，并且单独口服高剂量磺脲类药物可以治疗新生儿糖尿病。

参考文献

Borchers AT, Uibo R, Gershwin ME. The geoepidemiology of type 1 diabetes. Autoimmun Rev, 2010; Vol. 9:pp. A355–65.

Comments: Detailed review of evidence related to both genetic and environmental risks of T1DM and how they interplay.

Patterson CC , Dahlquist GG, Gyurus E, et al. Incidence trends for childhood type 1 diabetes in Europe during 1989–2003 and predicted new cases 2005–20: a multicentre prospective registration study. Lancet, 2009; Vol. 373: pp. 2027–33.
Comments: Alarming results indicating a rapid increase in the incidence of T1DM in young children.

Barrett JC, Clayton DG, Concannon P, et al. Genome-wide association study and meta-analysis find that over 40 loci affect risk of type 1 diabetes. Nat Genet, 2009; Vol. 41: pp. 703–7.
Comments: Landmark study of genes associated with T1DM.

Eisenbarth GS. Update in type 1 diabetes. J Clin Endocrinol Metab, 2007; Vol. 92: pp. 2403–7.
Comments: Concise overview of the genetics of T1DM and emerging science and technology that might improve outcomes.

DIA MOND Project Group. Incidence and trends of childhood type 1 diabetes worldwide: 1990–1999. Diabet Med,2006; Vol. 23: pp. 857–66.
Comments: Demonstrates worldwide increases in the incidence of T1DM.

Wilkin TJ. The accelerator hypothesis: weight gain as the missing link between Type I and Type II diabetes. Diabetologia, 2001; Vol. 44: pp. 914–22.
Comments: Implicates weight gain and obesity in the increasing incidence of T1DM.

1 型糖尿病：胰岛素治疗

Gregory O. Clark, MD

定义
- 1 型糖尿病是一种自身免疫性疾病。
- 胰岛素 β 细胞的破坏导致患者的胰岛素缺乏。
- 外源性胰岛素可用于治疗 1 型糖尿病（DeWitt）。

流行病学
- 请参阅 1 型糖尿病流行病学，见第 9 页。

诊断
- 糖尿病的诊断标准不改变取决于糖尿病的分类。
- 循环自身抗体是 1 型糖尿病的特征，如：胰岛细胞胞浆自身抗体（islet cell cytoplasmicautoantibodies，ICA），胰岛素自身抗体，谷氨酸脱羧酶（GAD65）抗体以及胰岛素瘤相关抗体 2（见胰岛素抗体，第 648 页）。
- 酮症酸中毒表面胰岛素缺乏，通常意味着 1 型糖尿病，但在 2 型糖尿病中也会发生（Umpierrez）。
- 一些新发的 1 型糖尿病成年人患者（例如成人隐匿性免疫性糖尿病）发病时并没有出现酮症酸中毒，这归因于一个较缓慢的自身免疫过程。由于这种情况可能会误诊为 2 型糖尿病。

症状和体征
- 无论何种类型的糖尿病，不受控制的高血糖是共同的症状，其他症状还有：多尿、多饮、多食、消瘦和视力模糊。
- 1 型糖尿病的儿童患者往往首发表现为糖尿病酮症酸中毒，并需要住院治疗。
- 有时候，血糖升高不明显以至于没有症状表现出来，这种情况尤其在成年人 1 型糖尿病新发患者中常见。
- 其他自身免疫性疾病也可能存在，如甲状腺功能减退症。

临床治疗
1 型糖尿病胰岛素治疗的启动
- 胰岛素治疗应用于每一个诊断为 1 型糖尿病的患者。
- 目前的证据建议，即使血糖水平接近正常（"蜜月期"或成人隐匿性免疫性糖尿病），一旦诊断为 1 型糖尿病（通常以自身抗体阳性为诊断依据），都应立即使用胰岛素，无论 β 细胞功能已减弱还是力求保留一些 β 细胞功能。
- 由于 1 型糖尿病预期的不稳定性，通常开始时就同时使用长效和短效/速效胰岛素。
- 一个临床决策应该遵循它的确切方案，及如何强化胰岛素治疗。
- 胰岛素每日总剂量（TDD）单位 = 体重 (kg) × 0.5，对于肥胖患者，每日总剂量 = 体重 (kg) × 0.7。这仅仅是一个估算值，使用剂量应当根据个体反应以 10%~20% 的增量做进一步调整。
- 在不需要使用长效胰岛素强化治疗时，可通过胰岛素泵缓慢注射速效胰岛素以维持基础水平（Walsh）。

胰岛素强化治疗
- 根据糖尿病控制与并发症试验（Diabetes Control and Complications Trial,DCCT）结果，首选治疗以减少并发症为目的（DCCT 研究组）。
- 每天要求注射胰岛素 4 次以上。
- 通过进食次数和量计算碳水化合物量，可以允许一个灵活的生活方式；虽然膳食甚至可以忽略，但是不推荐。
- 胰岛素的剂量是灵活的，鼓励病人学习安全调整胰岛素剂量。
- 快速血糖检测指导治疗（Hirsch；Bode）：在有血糖升高或减少症状以及偶尔出现夜间血糖异常时，快速血糖检测至少在饭前进行（目标值：血糖 70~120mg/dl），也可以在饭后 2 小时检测（目标值：血糖 140~180mg/dl），以及睡前（目标值：血糖 100~140mg/dl）。
- 每日胰岛素总剂量的 50% 作为基础量，余下的 50% 作为餐前量。
- 理论上长效胰岛素类似物没有作用峰，但其可提供稳定的基础胰岛素。虽然一部分人在分剂量使用长效胰岛素时效果更好，但类似物降糖作用可持续达 24 小时。
- 速效胰岛素类似物被吸收进入全身血液循环比普通胰岛素更快。其作用峰在 1~2 小时后出现，3~5 小时后消失。

传统的胰岛素治疗方案
- 在患者缺乏条件或动力适应强化治疗时使用。
- 要求每天 2 次或 3 次的胰岛素注射。
- 胰岛素的剂量是固定的。
- 必须调整饮食和体育锻炼，以弥补固定的胰岛素剂量。
- 中性精蛋白锌胰岛素具有较广的作用峰，达 4~10 小时，其活性是不定的，可持续 10~16 小时。
- 普通胰岛素峰在 2~4 小时出现，活性 5~8 小时后削弱。
- 相比胰岛素强化治疗，尤其是在中性精蛋白锌胰岛素峰时，低血糖的风险增加。
- 午前胰岛素注射剂量：2/3 中性精蛋白锌胰岛素，1/3 普通胰岛素。二者可以在同一注射器中混合后使用，或者直接使用 70/30 预混胰岛素。早餐和午餐配额应当和胰岛素的剂量相匹配。出现午餐高血糖时，应当减少午餐进食量。延迟午餐常常会引起低血糖。
- 午后胰岛素注射剂量：2/3 中性精蛋白锌胰岛素，1/3 普通胰岛素或者直接使用 70/30 预混胰岛素。晚餐和睡前加餐的比例应该满足该胰岛素剂量。晨起低血糖可能由中性精蛋白锌胰岛素峰导致。在睡前减少中性精蛋白锌胰岛素剂量（每天分 3 次注射），以减少夜间低血糖。

基础胰岛素（长效胰岛素）
- 抑制两餐之间肝糖和酮体的生成以及脂肪分解。

1型糖尿病：胰岛素治疗

- 目标是在没有进食、体育锻炼或使用餐前胰岛素时，保持血糖稳定。
- 调整空腹血糖为70~120mg/dl。
- 甘精胰岛素（Lantus）：每日一次，通常在睡前给，不能与其他胰岛素混合同时皮下注射（pH值不同）。
- 地特胰岛素（Levemir）：通常每日两次，不能与其他胰岛素混合同时皮下注射。
- 中性精蛋白锌胰岛素：如上所述，1型糖尿病为每日两次。

餐前胰岛素（短效胰岛素或速效胰岛素）

- 确定餐前剂量以营养部分和修正部分为基础。
- 营养部分包括餐要消耗，即胰岛素碳水化合物比（insulin-to-carbohydrate ratio, I:C）。一个有用的计算I:C比方法为I:C=500/TDD。例如：如果TDD=50单位，每10克碳水化合物使用1单位胰岛素（500/50=10）。
- 修正部分用于纠正高血糖。有用的计算方法是校正因子（correctional factor, CF）=1 800/TDD。例如，当TDD=30单位时，每单位胰岛素降低血糖60mg/dl（1 800/30=60），以达到目标血糖（通常为120mg/dl）。有的人使用1 500来计算CF。
- 使用速效胰岛素包括赖脯人胰岛素、门冬胰岛素、格鲁辛胰岛素是等效的。
- 普通胰岛素同样可以使用，但是要求在饭前30分钟实施。

随访

- 在开始实施胰岛素治疗后的几周里，持续的沟通和精细的胰岛素剂量调整是重要的。
- 每次随访都应检查糖化血红蛋白（A1c）。
- 根据血糖异常程度，大部分胰岛素剂量调整都应有10%~20%的增量。

专家意见

- 避免胰岛素累积：指当餐后胰岛素增加和在餐前胰岛素提前起作用前，控制额外的胰岛素，否则可导致低血糖。
- 避免运动引起的低血糖症：患者认为在运动前进食和使用胰岛素可以预防血糖过低是不正确的。运动增加胰岛素敏感性，因此可以预防低血糖。相对平ીय（达到50%），饭前运动和增加进食或者使用较少胰岛素取决于运动强度和持续时间。
- 保持稳定的生活方式以使血糖变异最小化：1型糖尿病的特点是血糖变异大。鼓励患者保持小剂量、常规膳食和胰岛素剂量，以尽量减少血糖变异。
- 持有符合实际的期望：即使控制最好的1型糖尿病患者，每天都有数小时血糖达到200mg/dl。治疗的目标是使血糖正常的时间最大化。
- 日常疾病管理的负担重，心理和社会方面的问题都应考虑到管理计划中。
- 每3个月咨询医疗工作者通常是有益的，可根据患者情况调整胰岛素剂量，其中包括访问糖尿病教育专员、营养师和医生。

参考文献

Hirsch IB, Bode BW, Childs BP, et al. Self-Monitoring of Blood Glucose (SMBG) in insulin-and non-insulin-using adults with diabetes: consensus recommendations for improving SMBG accuracy, utilization, and research. Diabetes Technol Ther, 2008; Vol. 10: pp. 419–39.

Comments: Details the rationale for frequent self-monitoring of blood glucose to help guide therapy.

Hirsch IB. Insulin analogues. NEJM, 2005; Vol. 352: pp. 174–83.

Comments: A nice review of the utility of the newer insulin analogs compared to the older, less expensive forms of insulin.

DeWitt DE, Hirsch IB. Outpatient insulin therapy in type 1 and type 2 diabetes mellitus: scientific review. JAMA, 2003; Vol. 289: pp. 2254–64.

Comments: The most detailed review of scientific literature related to the use of insulin in the management of both type 1 and type 2 diabetes.

Walsh, J., Roberts, R. Pumping Insulin: Everything You Need for Success with an Insulin Pump, 3rd edition. San Diego: Torrey Pines Press; 2000.

Comments: A thorough guide for both patient and physician that covers all aspects of insulin pump therapy.

Umpierrez GE, Casals MM, Gebhart SP, et al. Diabetic ketoacidosis in obese African Americans. Diabetes, 1995; Vol. 44: pp. 790–5.

Comments: A characterization of 35 African Americans with type 2 diabetes admitted to Grady Memorial Hospital with ketoacidosis.

DCCT Research Group. The effect of intensive treatment of diabetes on the development and progression of longterm complications in insulin-dependent diabetes mellitus. The Diabetes Control and Complications Trial Research Group. NEJM, 1993; Vol. 329: pp. 977–86.

Comments: Landmark trial showing that intensive insulin therapy, compared to conventional insulin therapy,can be used to reduce HbA1c and prevent and slow the progression of diabetes microvascular complications.

胰岛素泵的管理

Christopher D. Saudek, MD

定义
- 胰岛素泵，专业称为持续皮下胰岛素注射（continuous subcutaneous insulin infusion, CSII），胰岛素泵通过一根尖端插入皮下的导管，以设定好的速度向体内输注胰岛素。大多数常用品牌都是戴在皮带上的，其导管和注射点每3天调整一次。某品牌的胰岛素泵是直接缝在皮肤上的，每3天更换一次。
- 由于与血糖检测仪连接，可显示实时血糖结果，但是胰岛素的释放不是由血糖结果驱动的，完全封闭的环状释放系统目前还没有。胰岛素的释放速率和剂量是由病人决定的。
- CSII适用于1型糖尿病患者，或者不稳定的，需要胰岛素治疗的2型糖尿病患者。
- 仅用于速效（如门冬胰岛素、赖脯人胰岛素或格鲁辛胰岛素）或普通胰岛素。

流行病学
- 胰岛素泵自20世纪80年代开始应用以来，每年售出超过400 000台。
- 胰岛素泵在各个国家使用情况差别很大：在美国，1型糖尿病患者中多达20%的人在使用胰岛素泵，在其他国家不超过1%。
- 虽然严重的低血糖发生频率似乎有减少，但各种报告对于CSII能否改善血糖控制是不一致的（Pickup）。
- 使用CSII时，酮症酸中毒的发生更常见，这是因为如果胰岛素泵停止，胰岛素的释放也会立即停止（Hanas）。
- 在美国，医疗保险对2型糖尿病患者使用CSII不是一定报销的，其要求一个C肽检测结果以证明内源性胰岛素的缺乏。

临床治疗

胰岛素泵的启动
- 患者的选择是至关重要的：如果患者能很好地了解其病情，每天能多次自我监测血糖和计算碳水化合物入量，有因大剂量胰岛素输注导致不可控制的或严重的低血糖，有多变和必要的生活方式，最好的情况是患者能接受该技术，并且愿意使用胰岛素泵。
- 在使用胰岛素泵之前，糖尿病教育专员应当复查潜在患者的碳水化合物计量，并向其演示如何使用胰岛素泵。
- 胰岛素输注量包括基础量和餐前量。计算起始剂量基于以前的每日总胰岛素需要量。
- 基础剂量约为每日总剂量的50%，按编好的程序，以小时为顺序依次释放，该过程每24小时重复。例如，如果每日总剂量为48U/d，则基础剂量为24U/d，或者1.0U/h，餐前剂量一共为24U/d。保守情况下，起始基础总量约为患者之前使用长效胰岛素剂量的80%。
- 一般情况下，最佳选择为2~4个不同的基础输注速率。如半夜选择速率

1,凌晨选择速率2,增加30%~50%,白天全天选择速率3,速率4可在晚上使用,也可以不用。

- 餐前胰岛素量在进餐前输注,通常是为了纠正两餐间的高血糖。
- 典型的餐前剂量包括"营养素部分"加上"校正部分"。营养素部分取决于食物中碳水化合物的量(1单位胰岛素/15克碳水化合物)。校正部分胰岛素是为了使血糖恢复到目标水平(当血糖超过120mg/dl时,1单位胰岛素可降低血糖30mg/dl)。这些剂量仅仅是假设,每一个患者应根据自己的具体情况选择适当的剂量。
- 对于先前没有计算碳水化合物量的患者,为了估算碳水化合物比例,可使用"500"原则,既:500/TDD=每单位胰岛素对应的碳水化合物量。举例说明:当TDD为500时,500/50=10,即每进食10克碳水化合物,餐前应输注1单位胰岛素。
- 为估算速效胰岛素校正剂量时使用"1 800"原则(普通胰岛素为1 500):1 800/TDD=每单位胰岛素可以降低的血糖水平。每个患者应以自己的病史个体化。比如说,当TDD为45,1 800/45=40,即在血糖高于目标水平时,每单位胰岛素可降低血糖40mg/dl。
- 检查紧急启动程序,尤其在任何情况下出现的胰岛素泵释放中断(如导管故障),其中应包括重启多剂量胰岛素注射程序。患者应备有长效胰岛素以备紧急情况下需要。

胰岛素泵的特殊选项

- 大剂量向导计算器:不同的胰岛素泵对此有不同的名称,但所有的餐前剂量都需要根据已设定好的碳水化合物比例,胰岛素敏感系数以及目标血糖水平来计算,患者应做的是输入已消耗的碳水化合物重量和餐前血糖水平。胰岛素持续作用的剂量是从计算好的大剂量中扣除的。虽然胰岛素泵会给出建议剂量,但仍需要患者自己输入所需剂量。
- 胰岛素的持续作用:是用于预防餐前胰岛素的过度补偿,其可自最后一次餐前胰岛素的时间算起,由于胰岛素存在效应时间,大量的胰岛素仍然在发挥作用。这部分胰岛素可以从日常饮食所需的胰岛素中扣除,以获得大量的额外餐前胰岛素用于注射。
- 方波大剂量:相对于常规大剂量的快速输注,随着时间缓慢输注一个大剂量。一般用于高脂肪、高蛋白食物的延迟吸收和由于胃轻瘫引起的延迟消化。
- 每日总剂量:计算每天总的基础和餐前给药剂量。
- 临时基础率:在某些条件如体育活动、疾病或月经期胰岛素需要量升高或降低时,由患者编程和激活。

随访

- 必须具备专业的医护知识,当患者开始启动胰岛素泵治疗后,要与患者保持密切联系。
- 基本的随访跟踪内容包括非连续的胰岛素输注紧急管理、病假、非常规体育运动、导管尖端过敏以及经常更改胰岛素泵设置。
- 一些患者会申请"泵假期"(例如由于美观原因),选择在短期内重新使用传统的胰岛素注射,即使这种间断使用并不被推荐。
- 讨论在进行体育锻炼时应做些什么。比如说,如果要进行30分钟的活动,

胰岛素泵的管理

就应该取下胰岛素泵，降低基础速率或提前进食一些点心。

专家意见

- 患者必须愿意并且渴望使用胰岛素泵，不应该强迫不愿意使用胰岛素泵的患者。此外，患者需要知道胰岛素泵是一个"开放环"，不是自动输注胰岛素，而需要患者输入相关程序。
- 不鼓励不切实际的期望；胰岛素泵可以给患者带来明显的益处，但要求患者本人必须参与其中。
- 许多人发现胰岛素泵可以有效控制血糖的明显波动，并且相比每日多次注射胰岛素更加灵活。通常情况下，既可以改善患者生活质量，又可以改善患者A1c糖化血红蛋白情况。
- 胰岛素泵治疗的不足有：需要一直戴着胰岛素泵并且价格昂贵。订购胰岛素泵之前应确定其花费包括在医疗保险里。
- 大多数基础速率（如6~10单位/天）是无效的，建议患者在不同餐间使用不同的基础速率，而不是为某一餐选择校正餐前剂量。
- 不推荐在进餐后给予餐前剂量胰岛素。同时，也不推荐在两餐间频繁给以校正剂量，建议进餐前的餐前剂量尽量少。一般情况下，不推荐在睡前给予餐前剂量，但若有进食点心除外，需考虑更加保守的剂量。
- 不要指望胰岛素泵能纠正不好的生活方式造成的血糖控制不佳，或逆转已出现长时间的糖尿病并发症。

参考文献

Hanas R, Lindgren F, Lindblad B. A 2-yr national population study of pediatric ketoacidosis in Sweden: predisposing conditions and insulin pump use. Pediatr Diabetes, 2009; Vol. 10: pp. 33–7.
Comments: A database review found more ketoacidosis in children using CSII.

Hirsch IB . Clinical review: realistic expectations and practical use of continuous glucose monitoring for the endocrinologist. J Clin Endocrinol Metab, 2009; Vol. 94: pp. 2232–8.
Comments: An excellent expert review of clinical use of CSII.

Olinder AL, Kernell A, Smide B. Missed bolus doses: devastating for metabolic control in CSII-treated adolescents with type 1 diabetes. Pediatr Diabetes, 2009; Vol. 10: pp. 142–8.
Comments: Emphasizes the need to use bolus doses for successful use of CSII.

Churchill JN, Ruppe RL, Smaldone A. Use of continuous insulin infusion pumps in young children with type 1 diabetes: a systematic review. J Pediatr Health Care, 2009; Vol. 23: pp. 173–9.
Comments: A review of CSII use in children.

Bailon RM, Partlow BJ, Miller-Cage V, et al. Continuous subcutaneous insulin infusion (insulin pump) therapy can be safely used in the hospital in select patients. Endocr Pract, 2009; Vol. 15: pp. 24–9.
Comments: A review of CSII use in hospitalized patients.

Noschese ML, DiNardo MM, Donihi AC , et al. Patient outcomes after implementation of a protocol for inpatient insulin pump therapy. Endocr Pract, 2009; Vol. 15: pp. 415–24.
Comments: A description of CSII use in hospitalized patients providing a protocol for use.

Bolli GB, Kerr D, Thomas R, et al. Comparison of a multiple daily insulin injection regimen (basal once-daily glargine plus mealtime lispro) and continuous subcutaneous insulin

infusion (lispro) in type 1 diabetes: a randomized open parallel multicenter study. Diabetes Care, 2009; Vol. 32: pp. 1170–6.
Comments: A clinical trial comparing CSII to multiple-dose insulin using glargine insulin, found no advantage to CSII.

Noschese ML, DiNardo MM, Donihi AC , et al. Patient outcomes after implementation of a protocol for inpatient insulin pump therapy. Endocr Pract, 2009; Vol. 15: pp. 415–24.
Comments: A description of CSII use in hospitalized patients providing a protocol for use.

Pickup JC, Renard E. Long-acting insulin analogs versus insulin pump therapy for the treatment of type 1 and type 2 diabetes. Diabetes Care, 2008; Vol. 31 Suppl 2: pp. S140–5.
Comments: A comparison of CSII with multiple dose insulin, finding that there was less severe hypoglycemia on CSII in comparison with NPH insulin, though no difference when compared to use of long-acting analog insulins.

Davidson PC , Hebblewhite HR, Steed RD, et al. Analysis of guidelines for basal-bolus insulin dosing: basal insulin, correction factor, and carbohydrate-to-insulin ratio. Endocr Pract, 2008; Vol. 14: pp. 1095–101.
Comments: Useful review of general guidelines for using CSII.

Jeandidier N, Riveline JP, Tubiana-Rufi N, et al. Treatment of diabetes mellitus using an external insulin pump in clinical practice. Diabetes Metab, 2008; Vol. 34: pp. 425–v38.
Comments: Useful review of guidelines for clinical use of CSII.

Zisser H, Robinson L, Bevier W, et al. Bolus calculator: a review of four "smart" insulin pumps. Diabetes Technol Ther, 2008; Vol. 10: pp. 441–.
Comments: Reviews bolus dose calculations.

Cope JU, Morrison AE , Samuels-Reid J. Adolescent use of insulin and patient-controlled analgesia pump technology: a 10-year Food and Drug Administration retrospective study of adverse events. Pediatrics, 2008; Vol. 121: pp. e1133–.
Comments: A recent FDA review of reported complications of insulin pump use; the review was uncontrolled and reached over-alarming conclusions.

Weinzimer SA , Steil GM, Swan KL, et al. Fully automated closed-loop insulin delivery versus semiautomated hybrid control in pediatric patients with type 1 diabetes using an artificial pancreas. Diabetes Care, 2008; Vol. 31: pp. 934–9.
Comments: Research into the future use of a "closed loop" insulin pump, with automatic insulin delivery based on continuous glucose monitoring.

Lee SW, Cao M, Sajid S, et al. The dual-wave bolus feature in continuous subcutaneous insulin infusion pumps controls prolonged post-prandial hyperglycaemia better than standard bolus in type 1 diabetes. Diabetes Nutr Metab, 2004; Vol. 17: pp. 211–.
Comments: Review of how to calculate basal rates.

Pickup J, Keen H. Continuous subcutaneous insulin infusion at 25 years: evidence base for the expanding use of insulin pump therapy in type 1 diabetes. Diabetes Care, 2002; Vol. 25: pp. 593–
Comments: Not recent, but a meta-analysis of articles evaluating outcomes of CSII use over 25 years. Generally, a benefit in reducing hypoglycemia, but variable effect on lowering HbA1c.

胰腺移植

Gregory O. Clark, MD

定义
- 胰腺移植（PTx）是指全胰腺的同种异体移植（人与人之间的移植），包括胰岛、腺泡组织、胰管及胰腺的血管。
- 单胰腺移植（PTA）是不包括肾脏移植的胰腺移植。
- 胰肾联合移植（SPK）包括胰腺和肾脏同时移植。
- 肾后胰腺移植是患者在已接受肾脏移植后再实施PTx。
- 胰岛自体移植是将从患者自身胰腺中分离出的胰岛重新植入其体内。
- 胰岛异体移植是从供体胰腺中获得胰岛（为1%~2%的胰腺组织块），通过门静脉将上述组织移植到受体体内。

流行病学
- 每年约有1 200例胰腺移植实施，其中900例为肾脏联合移植。
- 自1999年到2009年，37个CITR（Collaborative Islet Transplant Registry）注册点报道了631例胰岛异体移植受体和501例自体移植受体。
- 美国器官共享网络管理器官的获取，并将这些信息公布在网络上，它是一个非营利性的科教组织，拥有当前的关于移植流行病学方面的数据。

临床治疗
胰腺移植
- PTx的适应证：终末期肾脏疾病的1型糖尿病患者，需要联合肾脏移植。
- 更多争议性的适应证包括威胁生命的未察觉的低血糖症，合并终末期肾脏疾病的2型糖尿病或者正在迅速发展的并发症。
- 成功PTx的获益：改善生存质量，纠正胰岛素依赖，正常化糖代谢，终止低血糖，使约40%病例的动脉硬化复原。
- 风险：外科手术（心脏疾病、术后感染、合并胰腺外分泌物肠内引流的吻合口瘘），终身免疫抑制（肾毒性、感染和恶性肿瘤风险增加），急性排斥反应发生率为4%~15%，10年后慢性排斥反应发生率为33%~50%。（White）
- SPK移植后存活率和接受率都是最高的，尤其是早期，在透析前就进行手术。3年移植存活率为85%（White）。
- PAK除尸体胰腺移植外，允许活体肾脏捐赠，相对于SPK，PAK可减少等待时间，3年移植存活率为78%（White）。
- PTA具有较多的争议性，唯一的适应证是未被察觉的低血糖症。考虑到PTA治疗后的死亡率增加，目前PTA手术应用越来越少。（Venstrum）30%接受PTA手术的患者在10年后由于免疫抑制的毒性反应需要接受肾移植。

胰岛同种异体移植
- 只有在明确的研究背景下才能实施，目前还没有标准的临床护理。

- 微创,虽然免疫抑制的风险依然存在,但可避免大手术的风险。
- 把从胰腺中消化得到的胰岛细胞安放在肝脏上,这种方法的胰岛细胞更容易死亡,同时,预后也不如全器官移植。
- 通常需要一次以上的手术才能实现胰岛素脱离(胰岛来自2个及以上尸体供者)。
- 最近,Edmonton方案成功运用一例没有类固醇药物的免疫抑制治疗方案,使一年胰岛素脱离率从之前报道的10%增加到90%(Shapiro)。
- 大部分患者在5年内要求重新注射胰岛素,但即使存在少量有功能的β细胞仍能改善代谢调控,并且能保护患者免于严重的低血糖发作(Ryan)。

胰岛自体移植
- 目前,该手术只有专业的临床中心在开展,但其费用可由医疗保险和补助中心(CMS)报销。
- 该手术的作用是力图保存全胰腺切除患者的胰岛素分泌功能。
- 因此其适应证是全胰腺切除(比如说慢性胰腺炎引起的疼痛)。
- 不需要免疫抑制,因为不存在对移植自身组织的同种异体免疫,也不存在像1型糖尿病的那样的自身免疫。
- 尽管β细胞数量少,但是其延长胰岛功能和胰岛素脱离率优于胰岛同种异体移植。

专家意见
- 适当的患者应当移交给擅长于PTx或研究胰岛移植的专业中心。
- 对于无症状低血糖,首选考虑移植治疗,尽全力完善医学治疗,包括考虑持续的血糖检测技术。
- 即使1型糖尿病患者每年平均有一例需要救护的严重低血糖发作,但这没有必要构成PTx的适应证之一。
- 2型糖尿病只有患者没有功能性内源性胰岛素情况下考虑PTx(要求胰岛素治疗以及存在极不稳定的血糖水平)。
- 总的来说,在ESRD需要肾脏移植以及相应的免疫抑制情况下,我们考虑PTx的潜在益处超过其风险。

参考文献

White SA, Shaw JA, Sutherland DE. Pancreas transplantation. Lancet, 2009; Vol. 373: pp. 1808–17.
Comments: An excellent overview of the indications, categories, and outcomes of pancreas transplantation.

Mineo D, Pileggi A, Alejandro R, et al. Point: steady progress and current challenges in clinical islet transplantation. Diabetes Care, 2009; Vol. 32: pp. 1563–9.
Comments: Review that highlights the success and progress in the field of islet transplantation that warrants broader clinical application.

Khan MH, Harlan DM. Counterpoint: clinical islet transplantation: not ready for prime time. Diabetes Care, 2009; Vol. 32: pp. 1570–4.
Comments: Review that highlights remaining limitations of islet transplantation and argues for continued careful research.

Sutherland DE, Gruessner AC, Carlson AM, et al. Islet autotransplant outcomes after total pancreatectomy: a contrast to islet allograft outcomes. Transplantation, 2008; Vol. 86: pp. 1799–802.

Comments: Report of one leading center's experience with islet autotransplant, comparing to islet allograft outcomes.

Ryan EA, Paty BW, Senior PA, et al. Five-year follow-up after clinical islet transplantation. Diabetes, 2005; Vol. 54: pp. 2060–.

Comments: Disappointing follow-up study from the Edmonton Protocol reporting only ~10% insulin-independence at 5 years, although ~80% retain some beneficial beta-cell function.

Venstrom JM, McBride MA, Rother KI, et al. Survival after pancreas transplantation in patients with diabetes and preserved kidney function. JAMA, 2003; Vol. 290: pp. 2817–3.

Comments: Study that brings into question the utility of pancreas transplant alone in patients with preserved renal function.

Shapiro AM, Lakey JR, Ryan EA, et al. Islet transplantation in seven patients with type 1 diabetes mellitus using a glucocorticoid-free immunosuppressive regimen. NEJM, 2000; Vol. 343: pp. 230–.

Comments: Landmark study that propelled the field of islet transplantation by reporting insulin-Independence for an average of 1 year after islet transplantation in patients treated with an immunosuppressive regimen free of steroids (referred to as the Edmonton Protocol).

2 型糖尿病

2 型糖尿病：环境危险因素与筛查

Ari Eckman, MD, and Rita Rastogi Kalyani, MD, MHS

定义
- 与 2 型糖尿病（T2DM）相关的危险因素，遗传因素（常与阳性家族史有关）除外。
- 常用于筛查 2 型糖尿病。

流行病学
- 美国糖尿病协会（ADA）推荐在如下人群中进行糖尿病筛查：（1）年龄 ≥ 45 岁的无症状个体，肥胖（BMI ≥ 25kg/m²）同时伴有任何一个糖尿病高危因素（见诊断部分）；或（2）对年龄 ≥ 45 岁（特别是 BMI ≥ 25kg/m²）的个体每三年进行一次筛查，或根据其高危因素进行更频繁的糖尿病筛查（ADA 医疗保健标准）。
- 一项回顾性研究对过去 20 年中未患糖尿病的 46 000 名患者进行检查发现，66% 患者满足 ADA 糖尿病筛查标准，而这些患者中，45 岁以上并同时伴有多个危险因素的占 11%（sheehy）。
- 符合糖尿病筛查标准的人群中，完成一种或多种血糖测试的占 86%，其中诊断为糖尿病的占 5%。
- 高危因素的流行率：年龄 ≥ 45 岁（55%），超重（52%），高胆固醇血症（50%），高血压（26%），血管疾病（6%），糖尿病高风险种族（4%），糖尿病前期（0.4%），多囊卵巢疾病（0.4%）。
- 与新发糖尿病高度相关的危险因素有：糖尿病前期（16%），多囊卵巢综合征（13%），血管疾病（10%）。
- 2000 年起，美国预防医学工作组（USPSTF）推荐在高血压及高脂血症患者中进行糖尿病筛查。然而，从 2008 年更新指南后，仅推荐血压持续大于 135/80mmHg 的无症状患者进行糖尿病筛查（USPSTF 指南）。
- 同一研究中，仅有 26% 的患者符合 2008 年 USPSTF 糖尿病筛查标准（Sheehy）。

诊断
- ADA 糖尿病高危因素包括：体力运动不足（小于 3 次/周），高危种族（如非洲裔美国人、拉丁美洲人、美洲印第安人、亚裔美国人、某些太平洋岛上居民等），≥ 4kg 婴儿生产史或曾诊断妊娠糖尿病，高血压，高密度脂蛋白（HDL-c）≥ 35mg/dl(0.9mmol/L) 和/或甘油三酯 ≥ 250mg/dl(mmol/L)，多囊卵巢综合征，与胰岛素抵抗相关的临床表现（如重度肥胖、黑棘皮病等），心血管病史，一级亲属患有 T2DM（遗传风险因素）（ADA 医疗保健标准）。
- 腹型肥胖：男性腰围 ≥ 40 英寸（102cm），女性腰围 ≥ 35 英寸（88cm）或男性高加索人腰臀比 ≥ 0.95，女性高加索人腰臀比 ≥ 0.80 为高危因素，但界值随不同的种族而不同（Chan）。

2 型糖尿病：环境危险因素与筛查

- 其他风险因素：高龄（Cowie），趋同（Nicholson），少量（相比中等量）饮酒（Koppes），吸烟（Willi）；（暂时）戒烟（Yeh），压力或抑郁症（Golden），低社会经济状态特别是拉丁美洲人和非洲裔美国人（Aviel-curiel; Schootman），饮食（如高脂、低纤维、西式饮食）（Shai），低镁摄入（larsson），食用苏打（Nettleton）。
- 慢性环境暴露：饮用水中的无机砷（Navas-acien）、有机磷和有机氯农药（Montgomery）、双酚A（用来制作硬、聚碳酸酯塑料的单体）和一些环氧树脂（lang）。
- 城市化趋势：某些太平洋岛国居民如瑙鲁人、皮马印第安人，他们以西式生活方式为主，肥胖较多，糖尿病发病率几乎从0%到50%（Zimmet）。在印度，居住在农村的亚洲印度人糖尿病发病率为2%，当搬到城市环境后，糖尿病发病率增加到10%（Ramachandran）。

临床治疗

糖尿病危险因素的管理

- 减肥（5%~10%）(Knowler)。
- 增加体力活动（每周至少3~5次运动，每次持续30分钟）(Knowler)。
- 通过调节生活方式或必要时药物治疗以降低甘油三酯，升高HDL水平。
- 通过调节生活方式或必要时药物治疗高血压。
- 预防心血管疾病。
- 尽量不摄入软饮料或含糖食物。
- 高纤维饮食。
- 戒烟，但可能会暂时增加T2DM发病风险（Yeh）。
- 压力管理。

专家意见

- 降低危险因素：T2DM最强的环境危险因素如肥胖与缺少运动。
- 糖尿病预防项目中提到，改变生活方式能有效降低T2DM在高危人群中的发病率（发病风险降低60%）。
- 高危种族人群同时伴有其他糖尿病风险因素时，糖尿病发病率可能会增加。
- 糖尿病筛查方案可识别具有高危因素的个体。
- 早期危险因素的识别和早期干预是糖尿病预防的关键。

主要参考文献

american Diabetes association. standards of medical care in diabetes—2011. Diabetes care, 2011; vol. 34 suppl 1: pp. s11–61.

Comments: american Diabetes association consensus statement describing risk factors for diabetes and criteria for screening in asymptomatic individuals.

其他参考文献

eh Hc, Duncan bb, schmidt mi, et al. smoking, smoking cessation, and risk for type 2 diabetes mellitus: a cohort study. ann intern med, 2010; vol. 152: pp. 10–7.

Comments: analyzing a cohort study, smoking predicted T2Dm but cessation of smoking also caused a transient increase in T2Dm incidence.

sheehy am, Flood ge, Tuan WJ, et al. analysis of guidelines for screening diabetes mellitus in an ambulatory population. mayo clin proc, 2010; vol. 85: pp. 27–35.
Comments: retrospective analysis of 46,991 patients without diabetes 20 years seen at midwestern academic physician practice between years 2005–2007, investigating case-fnding ability of current guidelines to screen for diabetes and prevalence of high-risk factors.

cowie cc, rust kF, Ford es, et al. Full accounting of diabetes and pre-diabetes in the U.s population in 1988–1994 and 2005–2006. Diabetes care, 2009; vol. 32: pp. 287–94.
Comments: prevalence of diabetes and prediabetes in the United states using data from the national Health and nutrition examination surveys, stratifed by age, gender, and ethnicity.

nettleton Ja, lutsey pl, Wang y, et al. Diet soda intake and risk of incident metabolic syndrome and type 2 diabetes in the multi-ethnic study of atherosclerosis (mesa) Diabetes care, 2009; vol. 32: pp. 688–94.
Comments: observational study that reported a 67% greater risk of incident diabetes in adults who consumed diet soda at least daily.

navas-acien a, silbergeld ek, pastor-barriuso r, et al. arsenic exposure and prevalence of type 2 diabetes in Us adults. Jama, 2008; vol. 300: pp. 814–22.
Comments: after adjustment for biomarkers of seafood intake, total urine arsenic was associated with increased prevalence of type 2 diabetes.

lang ia, galloway Ts, scarlett a, et al. association of urinary bisphenol a concentration with medical disorders and laboratory abnormalities in adults. Jama, 2008; vol. 300: pp. 1303–10.
Comments: Higher bisphenol a concentrations were associated with diabetes.

montgomery mp, kamel F, saldana Tm, et al. incident diabetes and pesticide exposure among licensed pesticide applicators: agricultural Health study, 1993–2003. am J epidemiol, 2008 vol. 167: pp. 1235–46.
Comments: long-term exposure from handling certain pesticides, in particular organochlorine and organophosphate insecticides, may be associated with increased risk of diabetes.

U.s. preventive services Task Force. screening for type 2 diabetes mellitus in adults: U.s preventive services Task Force recommendation statement. ann intern med, 2008; vol 148: pp. 846–54.
Comments: most recent UspsTF recommendations for diabetes screening in adults.

avila-curiel a, shamah-levy T, galindo-gómez c, et al. Diabetes mellitus within low socioeconomic strata in mexico city: a relevant problem. rev invest clin, 2007; vol. 59 pp. 246–55.
Comments: Diabetes is highly prevalent among adults older than 30 years, mainly on the lower socioeconomic stratum in mexico city.

larsson sc, Wolk a. magnesium intake and risk of type 2 diabetes: a meta-analysis. J inter med, 2007; vol. 262: pp. 208–14.
Comments: study suggests that increased consumption of magnesium-rich foods such a whole grains, beans, nuts, and green leafy vegetables may reduce the risk of type 2 diabetes

schootman m, andresen em, Wolinsky FD, et al. The efect of adverse housing an neighborhood conditions on the development of diabetes mellitus among middle-aged african americans. am J epidemiol, 2007; vol. 166: pp. 379–87.

Comments: poor housing conditions appear to be an independent contributor to the risk of incident diabetes in urban, middle-aged african americans.

Willi c, bodenmann p, ghali Wa, et al. active smoking and the risk of type 2 diabetes: a systematic review and meta-analysis. Jama, 2007; vol. 298: pp. 2654–64.

Comments: active smoking is associated with an increased risk of type 2 diabetes.

golden sH a review of the evidence for a neuroendocrine link between stress, depression and diabetes mellitus. curr Diabetes rev, 2007; vol. 3: pp. 252–9.

Comments: reviews the evidence supporting an association between stress and diabetes.

shai i, Jiang r, manson Je, et al. ethnicity, obesity, and risk of type 2 diabetes in women: a 20-year follow-up study. Diabetes care, 2006; vol. 29: pp. 1585–90.

Comments: a diet high in cereal fiber and polyunsaturated fat and low in trans fat and glycemic load appears to have a stronger inverse association with diabetes risk among the minorities than among whites.

nicholson Wk, asao k, brancati F, et al. parity and risk of type 2 diabetes: the atherosclerosis risk in communities study. Diabetes care, 2006; vol. 29: pp. 2349–54.

Comments: increasing parity (particularly 5 or more live births) associated with 27% increased risk for diabetes after adjustment for confounders.

koppes ll, Dekker Jm, Hendriks HF, et al. moderate alcohol consumption lowers the risk of type 2 diabetes: a meta-analysis of prospective observational studies. Diabetes care, 2005; vol. 28: pp. 719–25.

Comments: moderate alcohol consumption (6–48 g/day) associated with an approximately 30% reduced risk of diabetes compared with alcohol 6 g/day in meta-analysis of 15 prospective, observational studies.

knowler Wc, barrett-connor e, Fowler se, et al. reduction in the incidence of type 2 diabetes with lifestyle intervention or metformin. neJm, 2002; vol. 346: pp. 393–403.

Comments: results of the Diabetes prevention program, demonstrating that the lifestyle intervention reduced the incidence of T2Dm by 58% and metformin by 31%, as compared with placebo.

zimmet p, alberti kg, shaw J. global and societal implications of the diabetes epidemic. nature, 2001; vol. 414: pp. 782–7.

Comments: in conjunction with genetic susceptibility, especially in certain ethnic groups, type 2 diabetes is brought on by environmental and behavioral factors such as a sedentary lifestyle, overly rich nutrition, and obesity.

ramachandran a, snehalatha c, latha e, et al. rising prevalence of niDDm in an urban population in india. Diabetologia, 1997; vol. 40: pp. 232–7.

Comments: increasing trend in the prevalence of type 2 diabetes in urban indians.

han Jm, rimm eb, colditz ga, et al. obesity, fat distribution, and weight gain as risk factors for clinical diabetes in men. Diabetes care, 1994; vol. 17: pp. 961–9.

Comments: Waist circumference was positively associated with the risk of diabetes among the top 20% of the cohort.

2 型糖尿病：遗传危险因素

Nisa M. Maruthur, MD, MHS

定义
- 决定 2 型糖尿病遗传易感性的因素。
- 单核苷酸多态性是指不同个体的特定 DAN 序列中单核苷酸的变异，同时也是目前研究糖尿病遗传变异的主要方向。

流行病学
- 如果父母一方患有 2 型糖尿病，其子女一生患 2 型糖尿病的危险可达 40%。
- 至少有 24 个单核苷酸多态性（包括 TCF712，FTO，PPARG 基因的 SNPs 位点）被确定与 2 型糖尿病发病相关，比数比从 1.1 到 1.4（见表 2-7）。
- 然而迄今为止发现的有致病风险变异似乎仅占 2 型糖尿病遗传因素的 5%~10%。

表 2-7. 与 2 型糖尿病相关的标记基因位点

基因	假定功能 *	风险等位基因比例 **	糖尿病比值比
PPARG	脂肪细胞转录因子	0.87	1.19
CDKAL1	胰岛葡萄糖毒性感受器	0.32	1.12
SLC30A8	胰岛素储存中重要的胰岛锌转运蛋白	0.69	1.12
CDKN2A/B	胰岛周期蛋白依赖性激酶抑制剂和肿瘤抑制因子	0.83	1.20
TCF7L2	调节胰岛素基因的转录因子	0.31	1.37
FTO	与体质指数有关	0.4	1.17

* 摘自 Flarez JC, Lablonski KA, Bayley N, et al. TCF7L2 polymorphisms and progression to diabetes in the Diabetes Prevention Program. NEJM, 2006;355:241-50
** 摘自 Perry JR, Frayling TM. New gene variants alter type 2 diabetes risk predominantly though reduced beta-cell function. Curr Opin Clin Nulr Metab Care, 2008;11(4):371-7

诊断
- 通过家族史评估遗传风险。
- 相对于 SNPs 检测，临床工作中常运用传统临床因素如体质指数和家族史对糖尿病进行风险评估。
- SNPs 检测在临床中很少见，但是患者可登录如下网站：www.23andme.com，www.decoDeme.com, and www.navigenics.com 申请基因检测。

临床治疗
- 目前还没有基因药物治疗的指南。

2 型糖尿病：遗传危险因素

专家意见

- 迄今为止发现的变异中，TCF7l2 基因变异与糖尿病发病风险增加的关系最密切，影响最大。
- 目前所了解的遗传风险变异并不比其他临床危险因素具有更好的糖尿病预测价值。
- 此外仍然存在很多影响作用小的单核苷酸多态性（基因变异）。
- 其他类型的遗传变异（如罕见变异、拷贝数变异、表观遗传学改变）可能会更多的解释糖尿病遗传易感性。
- 多个基因对糖尿病风险的影响，不仅与其导致的胰岛素分泌情况相关，同时也会影响个体的饮食行为或活动水平。
- 未来十年内，药物基因组学（药物制剂与基因间的相互关系）可能会在多种疾病治疗决策包括糖尿病的治疗中发挥作用。

参考文献

Stolerman es, Florez Jc. genomics of type 2 diabetes mellitus: implications for the clinician. nat rev endocrinol, 2009; vol. 5: pp. 429–36.
Comments: Unstructured review of clinical implications of diabetes genomics.

Meigs Jb, shrader p, sullivan lm, et al. genotype score in addition to common risk factors for prediction of type 2 diabetes. neJm, 2008; vol. 359: pp. 2208–19.
Comments: Framingham ofspring study participants; limited utility of genotype score over clinical factors in predicting diabetes.

Lyssenko v, Jonsson a, almgren p, et al. clinical risk factors, Dna variants, and the development of type 2 diabetes. neJm, 2008; vol. 359: pp. 2220–32.
Comments: illustrates limited value of genetic information of diabetes prediction over clinical factors in european subjects.

Perry Jr, Frayling Tm. new gene variants alter type 2 diabetes risk predominantly through reduced beta-cell function. curr opin clin nutr metab care, 2008; vol. 11: pp. 371–7.
Comments: Unstructured review of genetics of type 2 diabetes focused on efect of risk variants on insulin secretion.

Sladek r, rocheleau g, rung J, et al. a genome-wide association study identifes novel risk loci for type 2 diabetes. nature, 2007; vol. 445: pp. 881–5.
Comments: major genome-wide association study identifying snps associated with type 2 diabetes.

Florez Jc, Jablonski ka, bayley n, et al. TcF7l2 polymorphisms and progression to diabetes in the Diabetes prevention program. neJm, 2006; vol. 355: pp. 241–50.
Comments: Diabetes prevention program: confrmation that common variants in TcF7l2 are associated with type 2 diabetes risk.

Groop lc, Tuomi T. non-insulin-dependent diabetes mellitus—a collision between thrifty genes and an afuent society. ann med, 1997; vol. 29: pp. 37–53.
Comments: early review of genetic basis of diabetes incorporating thrifty gene hypothesis.

2 型糖尿病：序贯疗法

Christopher D. Saudek, MD

定义
- 控制糖尿病人的高血糖，应逐步强化治疗把血糖控制在正常范围内。
- 这要求首先明确血糖控制目标范围，特别是糖化血红蛋白值，同时避免低血糖的发生。其次，需要调整治疗来达到以上这些目标。

流行病学
- 糖尿病微血管并发症风险（视网膜病变、肾病、神经系统病变）与血糖控制程度密切相关。
- 大血管并发症是糖尿病发病率和死亡率的主要原因。
- 很多糖尿病患者血糖控制不达标（美国人平均的 HbA1c 为 7%），提示需要尽快改变治疗方案。
- 大血管并发症（心血管疾病）的预防与传统危险因素（血压、血脂、吸烟控制之间的关系密切。糖尿病患者更应该积极管理这些危险因素，同时控制血糖也很重要。

临床治疗
- 尽管调节饮食和增加体力运动比药物更能有效预防糖尿病，同时也是患者良好护理的基础，但并没有公认的统一治疗顺序(knowler)。
- 指南推荐，改变生活方式不能理想控制血糖时，需使用药物治疗。
- 二甲双胍：为治疗 2 型糖尿病的一线用药，除非有禁忌证或是不能耐受者才改换其他药物。开始用量为 500mg，每日两到三次（通常开始时的 2~4 周，每天一次，以减少胃肠道不良反应，然后快速代谢）。
- 服用二甲双胍最大化剂量（除非胃肠道不良反应不能耐受）。
- 目前 ADA 和美国临床内分泌学科学院（AACE）指南提供了二甲双胍启动治疗后的其他多种治疗方案。
- 如果血糖控制不理想，需联合用药，通常选用磺脲类药物，或是使用二甲双胍与磺脲类的复合制剂。值得注意的是，磺脲类可引起低血糖和轻度体重增加。
- 其他降糖药还包括噻唑烷二酮（对血脂有额外的益处）、metaglinide（用于餐后高血糖）、DPP-IV 抑制剂（很少引起低血糖）或早期使用胰岛素（如果 HbA1c>8%）。但在使用前应先了解以上药物的副作用和禁忌证。
- 一些特定情况下，可考虑注射肠促胰岛素类似物，如艾塞那肽（常导致体重减轻），或是服用 α-葡萄糖苷酶抑制剂（可引起胃轻瘫），或是减肥手术（对于重度肥胖患者）。使用前应先了解以上治疗的副作用和禁忌证。
- 患者被诊断为 1 型糖尿病后，应立即启用胰岛素治疗。
- 对于 2 型糖尿病患者，如果已经使用 2~3 种口服降糖药，而血糖控制仍不理想时，应考虑启用胰岛素治疗。

2 型糖尿病：序贯疗法

- 1 型糖尿病患者或 2 型糖尿病患者血糖控制不达标时应尽早使用强化胰岛素治疗。

随访
- 治疗方案的改变需要更加频繁的随访，并取决于患者的自身情况。
- 当决定治疗方案时应考虑患者的饮食结构及体力运动水平。

专家意见
- 血糖控制目标是使糖化血红蛋白达标，同时避免低血糖发生。
- 血糖管理中最常犯的错误是推进治疗方案太慢，使得血糖长期控制不佳。
- 提防"临床惯性"：临床医生通常不愿意改变治疗方案，即使这些治疗已经不起作用（Bolen）。
- 当启用胰岛素治疗后，应继续口服降糖药以利用人体的内源性胰岛素，直到胰岛素使用被强化，能够取代内源性胰岛素为止。
- 2 型糖尿病的治疗通常需要使用多种口服制剂和 / 或相对大剂量的胰岛素。
- 1 型糖尿病的治疗通常需要多种剂量的长效和短效胰岛素，但是所需胰岛素剂量常常低于 2 型糖尿病。
- 每个临床医生处方降糖药的先后顺序是不同的，而且目前也没有明确的证据支持先服用哪种降糖药会更好，但是二甲双胍一般是最先启用的，血糖控制不理想时，再加用其他降糖药。

主要参考文献
Nathan Dm, buse Jb, Davidson mb, et al. medical management of hyperglycemia in type 2 diabetes: a consensus algorithm for the initiation and adjustment of therapy: a consensus statement of the american Diabetes association and the european association for the study of Diabetes. Diabetes care, 2009; vol. 32: pp. 193–203.
Comments: a consensus committee's recommendation on sequencing of treatment of type 2 diabetes. quite nonspecifc after initiation of metformin.

其他参考文献
American Diabetes association. standards of medical care in diabetes—2011. Diabetes care, 2011; vol. 34 suppl 1: pp. s11–61.
Comments: The annually published standards of medical care published by the american Diabetes association.

Bolen sD, bricker e, samuels Ta, et al. Factors associated with intensifcation of oral diabetes medications in primary care provider-patient dyads: a cohort study. Diabetes care, 2009; vol. 32: pp. 25–31.
Comments: an interesting study of factors that contribute to "clinical inertia," the tendency not to adjust treatment even when it is not working.

Rodbard HW, blonde l, braithwaite ss, et al. american association of clinical endocrinologists' medical guidelines for clinical practice for the management of diabetes mellitus. endocr pract, 2007; vol. 13 suppl 1: pp. 1–68.
Comments: aace clinical guidelines for managing diabetes, describing in detail the available medications available, important characteristics, and a general statement

of choices for sequencing.

Jellinger ps, Davidson Ja, blonde I, et al. road maps to achieve glycemic control in type 2 diabetes mellitus: ace/aace Diabetes road map Task Force. endocr pract, 2007; vol. 13: pp. 260–8.
Comments: aace statement of recommended sequencing on treatments.

Mooradian aD, bernbaum m, albert sg narrative review: a rational approach to starting insulin therapy. ann intern med, 2006; vol. 145: pp. 125–34.
Comments: a useful review of available insulins and a practical consideration of how to start and then intensify insulin regimens.

Heine rJ, van gaal IF, Johns D, et al. exenatide versus insulin glargine in patients with suboptimally controlled type 2 diabetes: a randomized trial. ann intern med, 2005; vol. 143: pp. 559–69.
Comments: open label comparison of exenatide (an incretin mimetic) vs insulin glargine in type 2 diabetics who had failed oral agents. exenatide had similar glycemic efcacy, but more weight reduction, and higher incidence of gastrointestinal side efects.

Klein s, sheard nF, pi-sunyer X, et al. Weight management through lifestyle modifcation for the prevention and management of type 2 diabetes: rationale and strategies: a statement of the american Diabetes association, the north american association for the study of obesity, and the american society for clinical nutrition. Diabetes care, 2004; vol. 27: pp. 2067–73.
Comments: an expert committee statement of the rationale and approaches to weight control.

Yki-Järvinen H. Thiazolidinediones. neJm, 2004; vol. 351: pp. 1106–18.
Comments: an important review of the mechanisms of action, side efects, and clinical use of thiazolidinediones.

Miller ck, edwards l, kissling g, et al. nutrition education improves metabolic outcomes among older adults with diabetes mellitus: results from a randomized controlled trial. prev med, 2002; vol. 34: pp. 252–9.
Comments: a relatively small randomized trial in which patients were given nutrition education or not. Those educated in a sound nutrition plan showed better glycemic control.

Knowler Wc, barrett-connor e, Fowler se, et al. reduction in the incidence of type 2 diabetes with lifestyle intervention or metformin. neJm, 2002; vol. 346: pp. 393–403.
Comments: The Diabetes prevention program demonstrated that intensive lifestyle reduced incidence of diabetes by 58%, metformin by 31% in subjects with impaired glucose tolerance.

2 型糖尿病：胰岛素治疗

Sherita Hill Golden, MD, MHS

定义
- 胰岛素是治疗高血糖最古老也是最有效的方法。
- 胰岛素可任意程度地降低 HbA1c 水平，虽然没有限制胰岛素的最大剂量，但是 HbA1c 骤降可能有潜在危害性（Gerstein）。
- 现代采用 DNA 重组技术由酵母或细菌生产胰岛素。
- 人工生产胰岛素的氨基酸序列，可与天然胰岛素具有相同的结构，如人胰岛素，或对肽链进行修饰后改变胰岛素的药代动力学特征（如胰岛素类似物）。

流行病学
- 英国糖尿病前瞻性研究（UKPDS）数据显示 2 型糖尿病患者 β 细胞功能逐渐恶化，随着病程进展，多数患者最终都需胰岛素治疗达到良好的血糖控制。

症状和体征
- 2 型糖尿病胰岛素治疗的适应证包括（1）口服降糖药失效；（2）新发糖尿病重度高血糖（见下），或者（3）对口服降糖药有禁忌证，胰岛素作为初始治疗。
- 重度高血糖而立即使用胰岛素治疗的适应证包括：空腹血糖（FBG）> 250mg/dl；随机血糖 > 300mg/dl；糖化血红蛋白 > 10%；和/或有多尿、多饮、体重减轻症状。
- 综上所述，2 型糖尿病患者满足以上条件或是服用最大剂量降糖药后 HbA1c 仍持续升高（> 8%）即可开始胰岛素治疗。

临床治疗
- 睡前注射一次中效胰岛素（NPH-中性精蛋白锌胰岛素）或睡前或早上注射一次长效胰岛素（甘精胰岛素，Determir）。初始剂量为 10U 或 0.2U/kg。这是初始基础胰岛素治疗。
- 每天都应自我监测空腹血糖（FBG），根据监测结果，在初始剂量治疗的基础上，每隔 3 天增加胰岛素剂量 2U，直到 FBG 持续控制在目标范围内（70~130mg/dl）。
- 如果患者 FBG>180mg/dl，或为重度胰岛素抵抗（如肥胖），需加大胰岛素剂量，如每隔 3 天增加 4U。
- 如果发生夜间低血压或是 FBG < 70mg/dl，应减少睡前胰岛素 4 个单位或减少 10%（以较大者为准）。
- 使用基础胰岛素治疗后，应每 2~3 个月复查 HbA1c。如果 HbA1c < 7%，则维持目前治疗。
- 如果 HbA1c > 7%，FBG 在目标范围内（70~130mg/dl），需测午餐、晚餐前和睡前胰岛素，用来指导二次胰岛素的使用。

- 二次胰岛素注射如下：（1）如果午餐前血糖高，则在早餐时加用速效胰岛素（如赖脯胰岛素、门冬胰岛素、赖谷胰岛素）；（2）如果晚餐前血糖高，则在早餐时加用中效胰岛素（NPH）或是在午餐时加用速效胰岛素；（3）如果睡前血糖高，则在晚餐时加用速效胰岛素。当增加额外注射时，剂量从 4U 开始，以后每 3 天调整 2 个单位，直到餐前血糖控制在目标范围内（70~130 mg/dl）。这种速效胰岛素即营养补充后血糖升高之增加胰岛素。另外，对于配合的病人，见碳水化合物的计数（第 108 页）可用来计算营养补充后血糖升高之增加胰岛素的用量。
- 考虑到胰岛素抵抗情况，2 型糖尿病患者的平均胰岛素日用量为 1U/（kg·d）[而 1 型糖尿病患者的平均胰岛素日用量为 0.5 U/（kg·d）]。
- 在受过良好教育，自觉性高的患者中，根据患者餐前血糖水平，将校正或是可调量性快速胰岛素用于营养补充后血糖升高之增加胰岛素。图 2-4，第 83 页为低、中、高校正剂量胰岛素。
- 使用基础胰岛素的同时，可继续口服降糖药。若血糖水平仍未达标，则填加营养补充后血糖升高之胰岛素用量，停用磺脲类，继续使用胰岛素增敏剂。
- 使用胰岛素的同时加用胰岛素增敏剂，可减少胰岛素每日总需求量，并有助于防止体重增加。

随访

- 对于注射二次胰岛素的患者，应对其血糖水平进行持续评估；糖化血红蛋白应在加用二次胰岛素后三个月复查。
- 如果糖化血红蛋白仍大于 7% 时，应复查空腹血糖，以检测出较高的血糖为准（基于前面提到的算法）来计算胰岛素额外需求量。值得注意的是，国际糖尿病联盟（International Diabetes Federation）建议糖化血红蛋白控制目标值为 6.5%。
- 如果每日多次注射胰岛素，而糖化血红蛋白水平仍然持续上升时，需复查餐后 2 小时血糖，并调整餐前速效胰岛素的量，直到餐后血糖保持在 180mg/dl 以下。
- 经验丰富的医师应教授患者胰岛素注射技巧。

专家意见

- 新诊断的糖尿病患者，具有较高的糖化血红白水平（大于 10%）时，提示重度胰岛素缺乏，通常需要立即启用胰岛素治疗。
- 2 型糖尿病治疗中常见误区是很晚才使用胰岛素，导致患者在很长一段时间内血糖控制不佳。
- 对于没有内源性胰岛素生成的患者，理想的胰岛素治疗方案包括基础胰岛素治疗、弹丸治疗和改良的复合疗法。

主要参考文献

Nathan Dm, buse Jb, Davidson mb, et al. medical management of hyperglycemia in type 2 diabetes: a consensus algorithm for the initiation and adjustment of therapy: a consensus statement of the american Diabetes association and the european association for the study of Diabetes. Diabetes care, 2009; vol. 32: pp. 193–203.

Comments: This is a summary of the most up-to-date guidelines from the american

Diabetes association regarding medical management of hyperglycemia in patients with type 2 diabetes. it contains an insulin initiation and titration algorithm for patients with type 2 diabetes.

Rodbard HW, Jellinger ps, Davidson Ja, et al. statement by an american association of clinical endocrinologists/american college of endocrinology consensus panel on type 2 diabetes mellitus: an algorithm for glycemic control. endocr pract, 2009; vol. 15: pp. 540–59.

Comments: This is a summary of the most up-to-date guidelines from the american association of clinical endocrinologists.

其他参考文献

Action to control cardiovascular risk in Diabetes study group, gerstein Hc, miller me, et al. efects of intensive glucose lowering in type 2 diabetes. n engl J med, 2008; vol. 358: pp. 2545–59.

Comments: The accorD study demonstrated an increased risk of mortality with too intensive glucose lowering (a1c 6.0%) versus an Hba1c target of 7–7.9%.

Turner rc, cull ca, Frighi v, et al. glycemic control with diet, sulfonylurea, metformin, or insulin in patients with type 2 diabetes mellitus: progressive requirement for multiple therapies (UkpDs 49). Uk prospective Diabetes study (UkpDs) group. Jama, 1999; vol. 281: pp. 2005–12.

Comments: This UkpDs study describes the progression of type 2 diabetes such that patients ultimately require insulin.

Groop lc sulfonylureas in niDDm. Diabetes care, 1992; vol. 15: pp. 737–54.

Comments: This study had data showing that there is a progressive decline in beta-cell function over time in patients with type 2 diabetes (4%–5% declined in function/year).

第三部分

并发症和伴随疾病

心血管疾病、肥胖和危险因素	203
内分泌疾病	243
女性疾病	266
消化道疾病	275
血液系统疾病 / 恶性肿瘤	289
感染性疾病	297
男性疾病	330
肌肉、皮肤及骨骼病	336
神经系统疾病	359
眼科疾病	376
耳科疾病	386
精神疾病	389
肺疾病	398
肾和泌尿系统疾病	404

心血管疾病、肥胖和危险因素

心血管疾病的筛查和治疗

Sheldon H. Gottlieb, MD

定义
- 心血管疾病（Cardiovascular disease, CVD）包括冠状动脉性心脏病（Coronary heart disease, CHD）、充血性心脏衰竭（Congestive heart failure）、心脏瓣膜病和脑血管疾病（中风），冠状动脉性心脏病又包括无症状的疾病及心绞痛、心肌梗死或由于冠状动脉疾病导致的猝死。
- 冠状动脉疾病（Coronary artery disease, CAD）包括所有冠状动脉的病变：心外膜冠状动脉、分支动脉以及心内膜下血管。
- 美国糖尿病协会（American Diabetes Association, ADA）、美国心脏协会（the American Heart Association, AHA）和美国心脏病学会（American College of Cardiology, ACC）一致建议，糖尿病患者即使没有已知的心血管疾病，也应视为大血管疾病的高危状态。

流行病学
- 心血管疾病是全世界导致死亡的重要原因（Yusuf）。
- 40 岁以后心血管疾病风险开始增加，70 岁以上时明显增加；年龄是心血管疾病最强的危险因素（Vasan; Wald）。
- 其他心血管疾病的危险因素包括家族病史、男性、血脂异常、吸烟、高血压、糖尿病、腹型肥胖、心理社会因素、水果蔬菜的消费水平、酒精（过度饮酒）以及缺乏规律的体育活动（Yusuf）。
- 不良、中介和理想的心血管健康的定义，以及对 AHA 2020 目标所做的 NHANES 2005-2006 流行性分析，在 Lloyd–Jones 表 3 中列出。亦可见于 http://circ.ahajournals.org/cgi/content/full/106/25/3143。
- 80% 以上的 2 型糖尿病患者将会发展为 CVD（AHA/ADA 共识声明）。
- 糖尿病是 CVD 的一项主要危险因素（Yusuf）。糖尿病患者 CVD 的患病率较总体人群高 2~4 倍（Redberg）。
- 在有冠心病危险因素但无已知 CVD 的无症状人群中行冠脉 CT 检查以分析亚临床 CVD 的流行性，发现糖尿病人群较非糖尿病人群其流行性显著增高（例如，冠脉斑块在两组人群中的发现率分别是 91% 和 68%）（Iwaskaki）。
- 糖尿病传统上被认为是 CVD 的一项等危症 [例如，有糖尿病而无既往心梗病史的患者，与既往有心梗病史而无糖尿病的患者在 7 年内的主要心血管发生率相等（约 20%）]（Haffner）。
- CVD 是糖尿病患者的主要死亡原因；糖尿病患者与其他类似情况相比，因急性心肌梗死（MI）的死亡率较高（Grundy）。

诊断
- 临床疑诊：既往有冠心病、CHF 或卒中病史者有很高的发生心血管事件的风险。

- 病史：早发冠心病家族史（男性 < 55 岁，女性 < 65 岁）是一项重要危险因素，且当同时发生在一名父母和一名兄弟姐妹时危险性最强（Nasir）。初步评价时，完成糖尿病和心脏病的家系谱很重要。见 http://www.americanheart.org/downloadable/heart/1170790567218Family%20Tree%20Flyer%20b-w_2007.pdf

- 实验室检查：测定非空腹的总胆固醇和高密度脂蛋白及其比值。比值 > 3:1 与进展为颈动脉内膜增厚相关（新发危险因素协作组织）。超敏C反应蛋白（CRP）可能对评价CVD风险中危的患者有意义（Pearson）。

- 心电图（ECG）：在标准静息心电图中，可能发现左房扩大、左室肥厚（LVH）、校正QT间期延长、心房纤颤、频发房性期前收缩（PAC）或室性期前收缩（PVC）或呼吸时心率变异性消失（Pop-Busui）。

- 负荷试验：可能时建议行分级踏车运动负荷试验。如静息心电图难以解释（例如左束支传导阻滞或较大的ST-T改变），可行负荷成像。难以完成腿部活动的患者可行药物负荷成像。糖尿病患者基线危险分层为中危，故可能时建议行影像学检查。超声心动图和核素负荷成像对于左主干或严重三支血管病变的阴性预测值较高（Metz）。

- 成像技术：超声心动图是LVH、左心室（LV）形态和功能的有效检查，而颈动脉超声可有效评价颈动脉内膜增厚。

- 冠脉CT：可有效评价中危者的冠脉风险的一项影像学检查（包括所有年龄大于45岁的糖尿病患者）（Hecht）。冠状动脉钙化（CAC）积分直接评价冠状动脉负荷。大量糖尿病患者仅由危险因素评分为中危至高危时，可评估CAC积分以重新分组为低危（Hecht）或高危（Hadamitzky）。CAC在糖尿病患者中临床上有用且有成本效益（Hecht）。放射剂量为2mSv，相当于8个月的背景辐射剂量。

- 血管检查：见周围血管疾病，第236页。

- 胸部X线：主动脉结钙化常见于糖尿病患者，也是糖尿病病程的一项标志，提示冠状动脉多支病变的可能性。心胸比 > 0.5提示心脏扩大和心力衰竭。

- 基因检查：有关2型糖尿病和冠心病的基因已开始被识别、检出，但目前仍不推荐作为诊断性评估的常规检查。

症状与体征

- 症状：任何胸部不适的主诉（从中腹至下颌）并与劳力相关，任何步行受限或活动耐力减退，打鼾或睡眠障碍，中年或高龄人出现的进行性乏力。胸部不适的描述可能受年龄、性别、教育水平、种族和糖尿病病程的影响而不同。

- 警告：同时患糖尿病和CVD者常常无症状，尤其是女性患者。

- 体征和体格检查：血压（BP） > 130/80mmHg，静息时心率（HR） > 80bpm，呼吸频率 > 15 /min，角质弓，牙列不齐，牙周疾病，检查到的血管硬化，脉压增高（ > 50mmHg），主动脉狭窄的杂音、向颈动脉传播，响亮的S_4或任何S_3奔马律，任何神经病变体征，踝反射或膝反射减弱，足背动脉搏动减弱，任何足部溃疡或严重足部胼胝体。

- 认知功能检查，例如简易精神测验，应作为有逐渐出现认知功能减退风险的糖尿病和CVD患者初步评估的一部分。

心血管疾病的筛查和治疗

- 出现勃起功能障碍的较年轻男性有较大出现 CAD 可能性（Miner）。

临床治疗
- CVD 风险计算工具。
- 风险计算工具：以临床数据或临床、实验室及影像学数据为基础的计算机化风险模型。
- QRISK 风险计算工具（可访问 http://www.QRISK.org）当患者处于工作站时十分有效，其图表用处较多，而且它能计算在 10 年跨度中的"相对风险"和"心脏年龄"。该风险计算器能够识别处于冠心病中危的患者。然而所有年龄在 45~55 岁以上的糖尿病患者均为中危。冠状动脉钙化积分能够将这些患者中的很大一部分重新划分为较低或较高风险组。
- 弗雷明汉心脏研究风险计算工具可能低估糖尿病患者的 CVD 风险，因为该研究包含了相对较少的糖尿病人群（可访问 http://hin.nhlbi.nih.gov/atpiii/ calculator.asp?usertype=prot）。
- 其他专用于糖尿病患者的风险计算工具包括 UKPDS（http://www.dtu.ox.ac.uk/riskengine/index.php），ARIC 研究（http://www.aricnews.net/riskcalc/html/ RC1.html），以及 ADA's Diabetes PhD（http://www.diabetes.org/living-with-diabetes/complications/diabetes-phd/）。

预防性治疗
- 控制危险因素：戒烟；血压 < 130/80mmHg，而近期研究提示过度降压（例如收缩压 < 120mmHg）并不合理。血脂：总胆固醇与 HDL-c 比值 < 3:1，LDL < 100mg/dl（有已知 CVD 的患者控制目标应 < 70mg/dl），甘油三酯 < 150mg/dl（有已知疾病的患者目标应 < 100mg/dl）；A1c < 7.0%（当控制更小于此水平时，减低 CVD 风险的获益并不明确，而过度严格的控制，例如 A1c < 6% 时可能造成损害）（Yudkin；Pfeffer；Cushman；Gerstein）。
- 糖尿病：长期研究中对 2 型糖尿病患者显示出单纯心血管获益的两类降糖药物是二甲双胍和阿卡波糖。这两种药物都具有多方面作用。近期有研究显示控制血糖在预防 CVD 中的重要性（Selvin；Hanefeld；Zhou）。
- 高血压：控制血压是一项必要治疗；血管紧张素转换酶抑制剂对糖尿病患者常作为首选。推荐剂量半量、联合用药，可能获得更强药效且减少药物不良反应（Laws）。
- 卡维地洛在有糖尿病的美国黑色人种中有较强的降压效果。
- 利尿剂也能较好地控制血压；当半量使用时，其在血糖控制上的负反应轻微，例如氯噻酮 12.5mg/d。
- 脂代谢紊乱：口服他汀类药物的患者常出现不伴 CK 升高的肌肉疼痛。使用强效、持续时间长的他汀类药物，如瑞舒伐他汀 5~20mg/d，可获得有效的血脂控制。
- 由于糖尿病是 CVD 的重要危险因素，NHLBI 成人治疗小组 III（ATPIII）在制定 LDL 控制目标时将糖尿病列为 CVD 的等危症。
- 减轻体重：减肥手术在 2 型糖尿病治疗和预防 CVD 方面有重要作用，而患者必须对该手术可能的获益和风险有全面的了解，其获益包括改善高甘油三酯血症、低水平的 LDL、高血压和高尿酸血症（Sjöström）。

- 生活方式调整（饮食和运动）：见流行的糖尿病食疗法章节（第116页）和运动、锻炼章节（第119页）。
- 阿司匹林：有CVD病史的患者和近10年内出现CVD风险 > 10%且出血风险不高的糖尿病患者都具有应用阿司匹林的指征（见低血糖症：预防和治疗，第60页）。

随访
- 没有已知CVD患者的危险分层取决于年龄和其危险因素。若弗雷明汉危险评分或其他危险评分提示其10年风险 > 10%，患者需每4~5年被重新评分（Hecht；Warburton）。有已知CVD患者被重新评分的频率应个体化，并与其危险因素、症状和年龄有关。
- ADA/AHA/ACC近期发布的一项立场声明提出，许多大型临床研究合作发现过度严格控制血糖与心血管疾病发病风险有关，包括ACCORD、ADVANCE和VA糖尿病研究（Skyler）。
- CVD治疗目标在2010年美国糖尿病协会诊疗规范以及AHA/ADA的糖尿病患者CVD一级预防共识声明中都有详细体现。
- 关于治疗CVD和糖尿病的综合性指南可见美国医疗与公共服务部的医疗研究与质量机构（http://www.guideline.gov/search/search.aspx?term=diabetes+ cardiovascular）。

专家意见
- 多数糖尿病患者有不同程度的亚临床CVD；其发病率随病程延长而增加。应适当进行CVD的预防性筛查，尤其是对于有其他CVD危险因素者。
- 糖尿病被认为是CVD的"等危症"，但这一用语可能使CVD危险因素有较大变异，故仍存在争议（Grundy）。
- 只要患有糖尿病，患者即为CVD中危。吸烟、早发心脏病家族史、腹型肥胖、HDL减低、青年男性勃起功能障碍和踝肱比 < 0.9都提示风险增高。
- 心血管疾病死亡风险随年龄增加呈指数增长。
- 约15%糖尿病患者因其冠脉钙化积分为0而被再次划分为低危者（Hecht）。
- 我们对有症状的个体建议行负荷试验进行CVD危险分层，而对无症状的CVD高危患者首先建议行运动试验进行危险分层。
- 糖尿病患者无症状并不能除外CVD存在可能，多数患者为无症状。
- 控制可调整的CVD危险因素，包括戒烟、高血压、脂代谢紊乱和鼓励减轻体重。
- 对多数2型糖尿病合并CVD患者有效的药物举例：赖诺普利（ACE抑制剂）、卡维地洛（β受体阻滞剂）、氯噻酮（利尿剂）、阿司匹林、他汀类、二甲双胍和其他糖尿病药物。
- 糖尿病合并CVD患者的治疗目标是自我控制，同时辅助以适当的患者教育、反馈和小组治疗，如有需要可予个体管理。

推荐参考文献
American Diabetes Association. Standards of medical care in diabetes—2011. Diabetes Care, 2011; Vol. 34 Suppl 1: pp. S11–61.

Comments: Summary of American Diabetes Association recommendations for routine preventive care that offers specific authoritative recommendations and is evaluated and updated yearly.

Skyler JS, Bergenstal R, Bonow RO, et al. Intensive glycemic control and the prevention of cardiovascular events: implications of the ACCORD, ADVANCE, and VA diabetes trials: a position statement of the American Diabetes Association and a scientific statement of the American College of Cardiology Foundation and the American Heart Association. Diabetes Care, 2009; Vol. 32: pp. 187–92.
Comments: Joint statement ADA, AHA, ACC incorporating findings from ACCORD, ADVANCE, and VA-Diabetes studies.

Buse JB, Ginsberg HN, Bakris GL, et al. Primary prevention of cardiovascular diseases in people with diabetes mellitus: a scientific statement from the American Heart Association and the American Diabetes Association. Diabetes Care, 2007; Vol. 30: pp. 162–72.
Comments: Joint statement by AHA and ADA on recommendations for primary prevention of CVD.

Grundy SM, Benjamin IJ, Burke GL, et al. Diabetes and cardiovascular disease: a statement for healthcare professionals from the American Heart Association. Circulation, 1999; Vol. 100: pp. 1134–46.
Comments: The first description by the American Diabetes Association and the American Heart Associationof diabetes as a CVD equivalent.

其他参考文献

Miner MM. Erectile dysfunction: a harbinger or consequence: does its detection lead to a "window of curability?". J Androl, 2011; Vol. 32: pp. 125–34.
Comments: Review of data linking erectile dysfunction to risk for CAD, especially in young men.

Berger JS, Jordan CO, Lloyd-Jones D, et al. Screening for cardiovascular risk in asymptomatic patients. J Am Coll Cardiol, 2010; Vol. 55: pp. 1169–77.
Comments: Recent and thorough discussion of screening to determine CV risk.

Hadamitzky M, Hein F, Meyer T, et al. Prognostic value of coronary computed tomographic angiography in diabetic patients without known coronary artery disease. Diabetes Care, 2010; Vol. 33: pp. 1358–63.
Comments: Coronary artery calcium scoring identified diabetic patients at particularly high risk of major coronary events.

The ACCORD Study Group. Effects of combination lipid therapy in type 2 diabetes mellitus. NEJM, 2010; Vol. 362: pp. 1563–74.
Comments: In type 2 diabetic patients, adding a fibrate to a statin did not improve CV outcomes.

Hecht HS. A zero coronary artery calcium score: priceless. J Am Coll Cardiol, 2010; Vol. 55: pp. 1118–20.
Comments: Impact of coronary calcium screening in persons with diabetes: a significant number will have a low CAC score and be reclassified as "low risk" for CVD.

Collins F. Has the revolution arrived? Nature, 2010; Vol. 464: pp. 674–5.
Comments: Genes for type 2 diabetes and coronary heart disease have been identified. Personalized genomic analysis will soon be an important tool in cardiovascular medicine.

Pop-Busui R. Cardiac autonomic neuropathy in diabetes: a clinical perspective. Diabetes

Care, 2010; Vol. 33: pp. 434–41.
Comments: Excellent review of important and often ignored aspect of diabetes and heart disease.

Artinian NT, Fletcher GF, Mozaffarian D, et al. Interventions to promote physical activity and dietary lifestyle changes for cardiovascular risk factor reduction in adults: a scientific statement from the American Heart Association. Circulation, 2010; Vol. 122: pp. 406–41.
Comments: Recent review of nonpharmacologic treatment of CVD.

Pfeffer MA. ACCORD(ing) to a trialist. Circulation, 2010; Vol. 122: pp. 841–3.
Comments: A masterful introduction to the ACCORD trial.

Lloyd-Jones DM, Hong Y, Labarthe D, et al. Defining and setting national goals for cardiovascular health promotion and disease reduction: the American Heart Association's strategic Impact Goal through 2020 and beyond. Circulation, 2010; Vol. 121: pp. 586–613.
Comments: The statement from the American Heart Association regarding prevention and treatment of CVD. Section on behavioral medicine pp. 424–426 should be read by all medical practitioners.

ACCORD Study Group, Cushman WC, Evans GW, et al. Effects of intensive blood-pressure control in type 2 diabetes mellitus. NEJM, 2010; Vol. 362: pp. 1575–85.
Comments: A summary of the results of the ACCORD study on blood pressure.

Pencina MJ, D'Agostino RB, Larson MG, et al. Predicting the 30-year risk of cardiovascular disease: the Framingham Heart Study. Circulation, 2009; Vol. 119: pp. 3078–84.
Comments: Extends Framingham risk data to 30 years.

Petersson U, Ostgren CJ, Brudin L, et al. A consultation-based method is equal to SCORE and an extensive laboratory-based method in predicting risk of future cardiovascular disease. Eur J Cardiovasc Prev Rehabil, 2009; Vol. 16: pp. 536–40.
Comments: Clinical variables: age, sex, history of diabetes or hypertension, smoking, family history of CVD, measured hypertension, and waist/height ratio predicted 17-year history of major vascular events as well as models that included laboratory variables. The most effective estimation of CVD risk is obtained by the history and physical examination.

Shaw LJ, Min JK, Budoff M, et al. Induced cardiovascular procedural costs and resource consumption patterns after coronary artery calcium screening: results from the EISNER (Early Identification of Subclinical Atherosclerosis by Noninvasive Imaging Research) study. J Am Coll Cardiol, 2009; Vol. 54: pp. 1258–67.
Comments: Use of testing was appropriate in a large cohort after CAC screening.

Vasan RS, Kannel WB. Strategies for cardiovascular risk assessment and prevention over the life course: progress amid imperfections. Circulation, 2009; Vol. 120: pp. 360–3.
Comments: Summary of the Framingham risk assessment and advice regarding population, primary, and secondary prevention of coronary heart disease.

Emerging Risk Factors Collaboration, Di Angelantonio E, Sarwar N, et al. Major lipids, apolipoproteins, and risk of vascular disease. JAMA, 2009; Vol. 302: pp. 1993–2000.
Comments: Measuring nonfasting total cholesterol and HDL cholesterol without regard to triglycerides may be most practical way to evaluate and treat CV risk.

Lloyd-Jones D, Adams R, Carnethon M, et al. Heart disease and stroke statistics—2009 update: a report from the American Heart Association Statistics Committee and Stroke

Statistics Subcommittee. Circulation, 2009; Vol. 119: pp. e21–181.
Comments: Annual statistical update of heart disease and stroke from the American Heart Association.

Action to Control Cardiovascular Risk in Diabetes Study Group, Gerstein HC, Miller ME, et al. Effects of intensive glucose lowering in type 2 diabetes. NEJM, 2008; Vol. 358: pp. 2545–59.
Comments: A summary of the results of the ACCORD study on glucose lowering.

Gaede P, Lund-Andersen H, Parving HH, et al. Effect of a multifactorial intervention on mortality in type 2 diabetes. NEJM, 2008; Vol. 358: pp. 580–91.
Comments: The Steno-2 study demonstrated that a multifactorial intervention including multiple drug interventions and behavioral modification effectively reduced death from any cause and development of microvascular complications.

Waldstein SR, Rice SC, Thayer JF, et al. Pulse pressure and pulse wave velocity are related to cognitive decline in the Baltimore Longitudinal Study of Aging. Hypertension, 2008; Vol. 51: pp. 99–104.
Comments: Data suggest that treatment of risk factors for vascular stiffness may delay cognitive decline.

Stamler J. Population-wide adverse dietary patterns: a pivotal cause of epidemic coronary heart disease/cardiovascular disease. J Am Diet Assoc, 2008; Vol. 108: pp. 228–32.
Comments: Superb summary and analysis of data supporting title of his article. Important references.

Iwasaki K, Matsumoto T, Aono H, et al. Prevalence of subclinical atherosclerosis in asymptomatic diabetic patients by 64-slice computed tomography. Coron Artery Dis, 2008; Vol. 19: pp. 195–201.
Comments: This study used coronary CT to demonstrate that asymptomatic persons with diabetes and no known history of CVD had a much higher risk of coronary plaques and significant coronary stenosis compared to persons without diabetes.

Metz LD, Beattie M, Hom R, et al. The prognostic value of normal exercise myocardial perfusion imaging and exercise echocardiography: a meta-analysis. J Am Coll Cardiol, 2007; Vol. 49: pp. 227–37.
Comments: Distillation of extensive literature on use of two most commonly used types of exercise stress testing.

Grundy SM. Diabetes and coronary risk equivalency: what does it mean? Diabetes Care, 2006; Vol. 29: pp. 457–60.
Comments: Good discussion on whether the use of "coronary risk equivalent" is applicable for diabetes.

Law MR, Wald NJ, Morris JK. The performance of blood pressure and other cardiovascular risk factors as screening tests for ischaemic heart disease and stroke. J Med Screen, 2004; Vol. 11: pp. 3–7.
Comments: This paper is a classic and should be read carefully by all who provide medical care for persons with diabetes and especially by administrators and policy makers.

Gale EA. The Hawthorne studies—a fable for our times? QJM, 2004; Vol. 97: pp. 439–49.
Comments: Classic history of classic study that showed that close relationship and frequent review of process may improve outcomes. Should be read by all medical practitioners.

Selvin E, Marinopoulos S, Berkenblit G, et al. Meta-analysis: glycosylated hemoglobin and cardiovascular disease in diabetes mellitus. Ann Intern Med, 2004; Vol. 141: pp. 421–31.
Comments: This meta-analysis demonstrated that in pooled analysis, persons with type 2 diabetes had an 18% significantly higher risk of CVD with each 1% increase in HbA1c. In type 1 diabetes, the risk of CVD was 15% higher for each 1% increase in HbA1c but the results were not statistically significant.

Hanefeld M, Cagatay M, Petrowitsch T, et al. Acarbose reduces the risk for myocardial infarction in type 2 diabetic patients: meta-analysis of seven long-term studies. Eur Heart J, 2004; Vol. 25: pp. 10–6.
Comments: Meta-analysis of acarbose trials.

Sjöström L, Lindroos AK, Peltonen M, et al. Lifestyle, diabetes, and cardiovascular risk factors 10 years after bariatric surgery. NEJM, 2004; Vol. 351: pp. 2683–93.
Comments: In a large controlled trial of gastric bypass surgery in Sweden, cardiovascular risk factors were reduced in the bypass patients.

Yusuf S, Hawken S, Ounpuu S, et al. Effect of potentially modifiable risk factors associated with myocardial infarction in 52 countries (the INTERHEART study): case-control study. Lancet, 2004; Vol. 364: pp. 937–52.
Comments: The INTERHEART study reported that "Abnormal lipids, smoking, hypertension, diabetes, abdominal obesity, psychosocial factors, level of consumption of fruits, vegetables, and alcohol (lack of moderate consumption), and lack of regular physical activity account for most of the risk of myocardial infarction worldwide in both sexes and at all ages in all regions."

Pearson TA, Mensah GA, Alexander RW, et al. Markers of inflammation and cardiovascular disease: application to clinical and public health practice: a statement for healthcare professionals from the Centers for Disease Control and Prevention and the American Heart Association. Circulation, 2003; Vol. 107: pp. 499–511.
Comments: AHA/CDC guidelines on using hs-CRP to stratify CVD risk in practice.

Warburton RN. What do we gain from the sixth coronary heart disease drug? BMJ, 2003; Vol. 327: pp. 1237–8.
Comments: Editorial that reviews cost-effectiveness of drug therapy for prevention of CVD. Excellent introduction to the literature.

Redberg RF, Greenland P, Fuster V, et al. Prevention Conference VI: Diabetes and Cardiovascular Disease: Writing Group III: risk assessment in persons with diabetes. Circulation, 2002; Vol. 105: pp. e144–52.
Comments: Describes the increased risk of CVD in persons with diabetes.

Paffenbarger RS, Blair SN, Lee IM. A history of physical activity, cardiovascular health and longevity: the scientific contributions of Jeremy N Morris, DSc, DPH, FRCP. Int J Epidemiol, 2001; Vol. 30: pp. 1184–92.
Comments: Masterful review of exercise and CVD.

Zhou G, Myers R, Li Y, et al. Role of AMP-activated protein kinase in mechanism of metformin action. J Clin Invest, 2001; Vol. 108: pp. 1167–74.
Comments: Study of mechanism of metformin cardiovascular protection and pleiotropic effects.

Wald NJ, Hackshaw AK, Frost CD. When can a risk factor be used as a worthwhile screening test? BMJ, 1999; Vol. 319: pp. 1562–5.

Comments: Demonstration of when a risk factor may be useful as a screening test. Classic reference.

Haffner SM, Lehto S, Rmaa T, et al. Mortality from coronary heart disease in subjects with type 2 diabetes and in nondiabetic subjects with and without prior myocardial infarction. NEJM, 1998; Vol. 339: pp. 229–34.

Comments: This Finnish study demonstrated that persons with diabetes and no previous MI had as high a risk of incident MI over 7 years as persons without diabetes and history of previous MI.

Peabody FW. Landmark article March 19, 1927: the care of the patient. By Francis W. Peabody. JAMA, 1984; Vol. 252: pp. 813–8.

Comments: Classic essential article, written by Peabody as he was dying.

US Dept. of Health and Human Services, Centers for Medicare and Medicaid Services. http://www.cms.gov/CardiovasDiseaseScreening/. Accessed October 5, 2010.

Comments: CMS web site reviews cholesterol screening benefit for Medicare beneficiaries, who must have no signs or symptoms of CVD and must be fasting for 12 hours. There is no copay or deductible and the test may be ordered every 5 years.

脂代谢紊乱

Simeon Margolis, MD, PhD

定义

- 血脂（胆固醇和甘油三酯）水平升高和/或血中脂蛋白浓度异常，包括低密度脂蛋白胆固醇（LDL-C）升高，高密度脂蛋白胆固醇（HDL-C）减低和脂蛋白(a)[Lp(a)]升高。
- 空腹甘油三酯水平正常值应 < 150mg/dl。甘油三酯 > 500mg/dl 即为明显升高。
- 糖尿病患者 LDL-C 多应 < 100mg/dL，而 < 70mg/dl 时更为满意。
- HDL-C 水平在男性 < 40mg/dl、女性 < 50mg/dl 被认为过低。
- 非 HDL 胆固醇 = 总胆固醇 -HDL-C。
- Lp(a) 正常水平与所用的实验室测定方法相关。

流行病学

- 糖尿病患者的脂代谢紊乱：最常见的脂代谢紊乱为甘油三酯升高。而 HDL-C 水平减低几乎同样常见（Howard）。
- 糖尿病患者与非糖尿病患者相比，LDL-C 与 Lp(a) 平均水平并未升高。
- 糖尿病患者的脂代谢紊乱与致动脉粥样硬化的小而致密 LDL-C 水平升高相关。
- 严重胰岛素分泌不足可能与甘油三酯水平明显升高有关，同时急性胰腺炎风险升高。
- 心血管疾病是糖尿病最常见的死亡原因，在首诊为 2 型糖尿病时即有约一半患者存在心血管疾病，同样也是糖尿病患者存在未治疗的脂代谢紊乱时，可能出现的最重要的长期后遗疾病（Hoffman）。

诊断

- 诊断时检测空腹血脂（胆固醇、甘油三酯和 HDL-C），如正常应在随访时至少每年化验一次（见血脂，第 652 页）。
- 小而致密的 LDL-C 可通过测定载脂蛋白 B 或用 NMR 光谱法测定脂蛋白亚组分的方法分析其水平。
- 高甘油三酯血症的患者，可通过冰箱中过夜静置血清、观察上层脂类的方法，检测乳糜微粒的存在。
- 当患者甘油三酯水平大于 1 000mg/dl 时，可能诱发急性胰腺炎而血清淀粉酶及脂肪酶正常。
- 症状和体征
- 甘油三酯轻度升高或 LDL-C、HDL-C 或 Lp(a) 轻度异常时并无相关的症状、体征。
- 腱黄瘤和眼睑黄色瘤提示家族性高胆固醇血症可能，但约 50% 黄色瘤患者胆固醇水平正常。
- 黄色掌纹可见于异常 β 脂蛋白血症。

脂代谢紊乱

- 发疹性黄色瘤（带有含甘油三酯的白色顶部的斑丘疹），多见于肘部和膝部的结节性黄色瘤，以及视网膜脂血症见于严重高甘油三酯血症中。
- 甘油三酯极度升高可能引起胰腺炎，出现严重腹痛、恶心和呕吐。

临床治疗

- 目标：预防心血管疾病（Colhoun）。次要目标是预防急性胰腺炎。
- 控制脂代谢紊乱应首先调整生活方式。降低 LDL-C：饮食中脂肪应小于总热量的 35%，饱和脂肪应小于 7%，每日胆固醇摄入小于 200mg。
- 减轻体重和控制血糖在降低甘油三酯中尤其有效。
- 体育锻炼可以降低甘油三酯、升高 HDL-C，但在降低 LDL-C 中作用相对有限。
- 他汀类是降低 LDL-C 最有效的药物，常在合并糖尿病时启动治疗（见他汀类药物和联合药物，第 463 页）。
- 贝特类、Lovaza（omega-3-酸乙酯）和非处方鱼油胶囊是治疗甘油三酯异常升高的有效药物（见纤维酸衍生物，第 451 页）。
- 烟酸制剂能有效升高 HDL-C，且总体上并不显著影响血糖控制（见烟酸，第 456 页）。
- 吡格列酮与罗格列酮相比，能更有效地降低甘油三酯、升高 HDL-C 和降低 LDL-C（Goldberg）（见噻唑烷二酮类药物，第 503 页）。
- 胆汁酸螯合剂考来维伦可促进血糖控制，降低 LDL-C 约 15%，同时能减少小而致密的 LDL 含量（Fonseca）。
- 若甘油三酯水平在他汀治疗期间持续 > 200mg/dl，考虑加用贝特类或烟酸。
- 不同降脂方案的预期获益见表 3-1。

随访

- 若调整生活方式后 4~6 周仍不能达标，需加用降脂药物（Brunzell）。
- 加用药物治疗后 4~6 周应查血脂及肝酶以明确其有效性。
- 4~6 周后若 LDL-C 仍未达标而肝酶正常，应将他汀加量或加用依折麦布（见第 448 页）。
- 他汀治疗目标：LDL-C < 100mg/dl 或总胆固醇 /HDL-C < 2.0。
- 起始剂量以后，将他汀剂量进一步加倍可使 LDL-C 降低约 6%（与基线比较）。
- 如需加用贝特类药物降低甘油三酯，应选用纤维酸衍生物而非吉非罗齐，以减低肌炎风险。目标为非 HDL 胆固醇 < 100mg/dl。
- 高甘油三酯血症的二线用药为烟酸，可用于甘油三酯轻度升高，当甘油三酯 > 500mg/dl 时可同时加用非处方鱼油胶囊或处方药 Lovaza[见 Omega-3 脂肪酸（鱼油），第 460 页]。
- 许多专家建议当 HDL-C 在男性中持续小于 40mg/dl 或女性中持续小于 50mg/dl 时加用烟酸控释制剂（Grundy）。
- 若出现肌痛或乏力症状时需检测 CK（无须检测基线水平）。若肌肉不适症状出现，可停用或将他汀减量以观察肌肉症状是否消失。若

CK ≥ 1 000mg/dl 需停用他汀。若停药后 2 周内症状消失且 CK 小于 1 000，可再次加用小剂量的同种他汀或选择另一种他汀。若 CK ≥ 1 000mg/dl 时他汀应慎用。
- 若肝酶升高至正常上限 3 倍或以上，需停用他汀。
- 每次患者随访时需询问肌痛和乏力症状。

表 3-1. 不同降脂方案的预期获益

药物	总胆固醇和 LDL-C	甘油三酯	HDL	备注
他汀类	降低 25%~50%	降低 10%~20%	升高 6%~10%	若甘油三酯 > 500mg/dl，不建议加用他汀类药物
盐酸	降低 10%~25%	降低 15%~25%	升高 15%~30%	升高 HDL 的最有效药物
贝特类	降低 10%	降低 30%~50%	升高 6%~8%	初始甘油三酯 > 500mg/dl 时可能升高 LDL-C
胆汁酸螯合剂	降低 15%~25%	0 或升高	升高 6%~8%	不应用于甘油三酯升高的患者（> 200~300mg/dl），可能进一步升高甘油三酯水平
依折麦布	降低 10%~20%	0	0	有效降低总胆固醇及 LDL，常与他汀合用

由 Simeon Margolis 提供

专家意见
- 如随访结果仍未达标，需加大他汀药物剂量或加用其他药物。
- 对于有较高肌炎风险的患者（例如正在使用吉非罗齐、抗真菌药物或环孢素者），启动他汀治疗时需谨慎。
- 即使是轻度体重减轻（5%~19% 的体重）对于超重或肥胖的患者可见到明显的降低甘油三酯的效果。
- 需等到体重稳定时方可确定减轻体重对甘油三酯的降低作用，甘油三酯水平可能在减轻体重过程中假性减低。

推荐参考文献
Brunzell JD, Davidson M, Furberg CD, et al. Lipoprotein management in patients with cardiometabolic risk: consensus statement from the American Diabetes Association and the American College of Cardiology Foundation. Diabetes Care, 2008; Vol. 31: pp. 811–22.

Comments: Consensus statement from ADA and American College of Cardiology regarding lipoprotein management in patients with cardiometabolic risk.

其他参考文献
Colhoun HM, Betteridge DJ, Durrington PN, et al. Effects of atorvastatin on kidney outcomes and cardiovascular disease in patients with diabetes: an analysis from the

Collaborative Atorvastatin Diabetes Study (CARDS). Am J Kidney Dis, 2009; Vol. 54: pp. 810–9.
Comments: 2838 patients with type 2 diabetes and no prior history of cardiovascular disease were assigned to either 10 mg atorvastatin or placebo. During a median follow-up of 3.9 years, the treated group had about a 40% reduction in major cardiovascular events whether they had renal impairment or not.

Neeli H, Gadi R, Rader DJ. Managing diabetic dyslipidemia: beyond statin therapy. Curr Diab Rep, 2009; Vol. 9: pp. 11–7.
Comments: In the management of diabetic dyslipidemia, consideration should be given to lowering triglycerides and raising HDL-C in addition to lowering LDL-C with statins.

Mora S. Advanced lipoprotein testing and subfractionation are not (yet) ready for routine clinical use. Circulation, 2009; Vol. 119: pp. 2396–404.
Comments: It is not necessary to measure apoproteins or obtain particle number and size to determine risk of cardiovascular disease.

American Diabetes Association, Bantle JP, Wylie-Rosett J, et al. Nutrition recommendations and interventions for diabetes: a position statement of the American Diabetes Association. Diabetes Care, 2008; Vol. 31 Suppl 1: pp. S61–78.
Comments: ADA recommendations for nutritional management of diabetes.

Fonseca VA, Rosenstock J, Wang AC, et al. Colesevelam HCl improves glycemic control and reduces LDL cholesterol in patients with inadequately controlled type 2 diabetes on sulfonylurea-based therapy. Diabetes Care, 2008; Vol. 31: pp. 1479–84.
Comments: Colesevelam improves glycemic control and lowers LDL-C by about 15%.

El Harchaoui K, van der Steeg WA, Stroes ES, et al. Value of low-density lipoprotein particle number and size as predictors of coronary artery disease in apparently healthy men and women: the EPIC-Norfolk Prospective Population Study. J Am Coll Cardiol, 2007; Vol. 49: pp. 547–53.
Comments: LDL-C particle number and size are better predictors of cardiovascular disease risk than other measures of blood lipids and lipoproteins.

Goldberg RB, Kendall DM, Deeg MA, et al. A comparison of lipid and glycemic effects of pioglitazone and rosiglitazone in patients with type 2 diabetes and dyslipidemia. Diabetes Care, 2005; Vol. 28: pp. 1547–54.
Comments: Triglycerides fell significantly with pioglitazone but rose slightly with rosiglitazone. Pioglitazone also raised HDL-C more than rosiglitazone and was associated with a smaller rise in LDL-C.

Keech A, Simes RJ, Barter P, et al. Effects of long-term fenofibrate therapy on cardiovascular events in 9795 people with type 2 diabetes mellitus (the FIELD study): randomised controlled trial. Lancet, 2005; Vol. 366: pp. 1849–61.
Comments: The FIELD study randomized 9795 participants with type 2 diabetes to either fenofibrate or placebo for 5 years. Less than a third of the subjects had known cardiovascular disease. The effects on cardiovascular disease are difficult to interpret, but no dramatic benefits were observed.

Rubins HB, Robins SJ, Collins D, et al. Diabetes, plasma insulin, and cardiovascular disease: subgroup analysis from the Department of Veterans Affairs high-density lipoprotein intervention trial (VA-HIT). Arch Intern Med, 2002; Vol. 162: pp. 2597–604.

Comments: In the VA-HIT trial, gemfibrozil significantly reduced major cardiovascular events in men who had type 2 diabetes or insulin resistance and known coronary heart disease.

Grundy SM, Vega GL, McGovern ME, et al. Efficacy, safety, and tolerability of once-daily niacin for the treatment of dyslipidemia associated with type 2 diabetes: results of the assessment of diabetes control and evaluation of the efficacy of niaspan trial. Arch Intern Med, 2002; Vol. 162: pp. 1568–76.
Comments: Niacin (Niaspan) can be used to treat diabetic dyslipidemia with minimal adverse effects on glycemic control.

Huang ES, Meigs JB, Singer DE. The effect of interventions to prevent cardiovascular disease in patients with type 2 diabetes mellitus. Am J Med, 2001; Vol. 111: pp. 633–42.
Comments: This meta-analysis of 7 randomized trials in patients with type 2 diabetes found substantial cardiovascular benefits from lowering cholesterol levels.

Lemieux I, Lamarche B, Couillard C, et al. Total cholesterol/HDL cholesterol ratio vs LDL cholesterol/HDL cholesterol ratio as indices of ischemic heart disease risk in men: the Quebec Cardiovascular Study. Arch Intern Med, 2001; Vol. 161: pp. 2685–92.
Comments: Total cholesterol/HDL-C is a better predictor of cardiovascular risk than LDL-C/HDL-C.

Haffner SM, Lehto S, Rönnemaa T, et al. Mortality from coronary heart disease in subjects with type 2 diabetes and in nondiabetic subjects with and without prior myocardial infarction. NEJM, 1998; Vol. 339: pp. 229–34.
Comments: Individuals with diabetes but without a prior myocardial infarction have as high a risk of myocardial infarction as individuals without diabetes but with previous myocardial infarction.

Howard BV. Lipoprotein metabolism in diabetes mellitus. J Lipid Res,1987; Vol. 28: pp. 613–28.
Comments: A detailed description of the lipid abnormalities in diabetes and their underlying causes.

心力衰竭

Sheldon H. Gottlieb, MD

定义

- 心力衰竭：由于心功能失常，泵出的血量不能满足机体需要，导致机体发生的不良反应，包括容量过度负荷（充血），呼吸急促、疲劳、增加猝死风险。
- 充血性心力衰竭是心力衰竭的狭义定义，以充血的症状和体征为主。大多数心衰患者不出现充血的临床表现（尽管 BNP/Pro BNP 升高，参见症状与体征一节）。
- 收缩期心衰：射血分数达 45%。
- 舒张期心衰：也叫作比正常心衰。
- 慢性心衰：通常为门诊患者。
- 急性失代偿心衰：属急症需住院治疗。
- 晚期心衰：在适当治疗同时仍存在日常活动受限的症状。

流行病学

- 心衰的发生率和患病率随年龄成指数增长，60 岁患病率为 1%，80 岁可达 10%。40 岁的人群发生心衰的危险为 20%。
- 心衰是 65 岁以上人群入院和再入院最常见的病因，大多数心衰患者有 5 个共同问题。
- 在发达国家，每年处理心衰的费用占卫生保健预算总额的 1%~3%。在美国，每 10 000 人中约有 200 人因心衰住院，年住院率呈上升趋势，慢性心衰患者每年入院 1~2 次，甚至需要得到更好的照顾（更多住院机会）。
- 心衰 5 年死亡率高于乳腺癌和结肠癌。
- 糖尿病增加心衰发生风险 3~5 倍。
- 在发达国家，高血压和冠状动脉粥样硬化性心脏病常合并糖尿病和代谢综合征，是心衰最常见的病因。在发展中国家，由于传染、艾滋病毒或营养不良、缺乏维生素（脚气病）等导致的风湿性心脏病和心肌病是心衰的常见原因。
- 吸烟与心衰有高度关联。

诊断

- 心力衰竭是一组临床综合征，不是独立的疾病，所以明确心衰的原因，需要反复研究。
- 有呼吸急促、劳累及充血表现都提示心衰，但不是诊断心衰的必要条件。
- 实验室检查：ECG（心律不齐、LVH、局部缺血）、X 线检查（心脏大小、形状、心胸比、肺充血）、超声心动图（局部和整体心功能、心肌病、瓣膜病、心包疾病、肿瘤）和血液检查：利钠肽、BNP 和前 BNP。
- BNP 和前 BNP 有很高的负性预测值，正常值范围内可排除诊断心力衰竭。高值仍需与临床联系（见下文）；不能区分心衰是由于心脏收缩功能障碍还是舒张功能障碍造成。诊断心衰正常值和分割点依赖于年龄和肾脏功能（Arnold 2007）。
- 在急性代谢失调性心衰时肌钙蛋白 I 常常升高，甚至不伴有冠状动脉病变，这归因于左室舒张末压显著升高导致的心内膜下局部缺血。
- 心衰死亡率与糖化血红蛋白 A1C 之间的关系可能呈 U 形，当 HbA1c 水平控制在 7.1%~7.8% 时死亡率最低（Aguilar）。
- 当心衰不能归因于冠心病，或非侵袭性检查不能诊断病因时，应行冠脉介入检查。
- 临床鉴别诊断指南筛选出少见的心衰病因：血色沉着病，肉状瘤病，淀粉样变，HIV 感染，甲状腺疾病（功能亢进或低下），嗜铬细胞瘤，风湿病，营养不良，呼吸睡眠暂停综合征（Arnold 2006）。

症状和体征

- 心衰所表现的共同症状：呼吸困难，端坐呼吸，夜间阵发性呼吸困难，疲劳，无力，活动耐力降低，水肿，咳嗽，体重增加，腹胀，夜尿症，四肢发凉；少见症状：认知受损，精神状态改变或神经错乱，恶心，腹部不适，尿少，厌食，苍白病（Arnold 2006）。夜间咳嗽一般在心衰失代偿前 7~14 天发生。
- 波士顿标准，见表 3-2。
- 代偿期心衰患者常没有明显的充血表现（"暖干型"患者休息状态心输出量正常，"冷干型"患者休息状态心输出量降低。）（Nohria）。
- 诊断不明确时 BNP/ProBNP 水平是有意义的，尤其是连续测定的比值在一些晚期肺病和判定预后中有特殊价值。
- 机能分类：（1）非常兴奋，（2）中度兴奋，（3）抑制，（4）非常抑制或卧床休息。参见《退伍军人特定活动调查问卷（迈尔斯）》。纽约心脏协会分类：（1）无症状；（2）有症状，可正常活动；（3）有症状，低于正常的活动——洗澡或穿衣不能自理；（4）在休息时有症状。
- 患有严重代偿性慢性心衰的老年患者常可见精神错乱的症状；当发展至代偿期时，老年患者常有认知受损。
- 肺炎、败血症、心肌梗死或急性心律失常（房颤等）常引起老年患者心衰失代偿。心脏瓣膜病尤其是主动脉狭窄是老年患者心衰的常见诱因，这些老年同时患有冠心病和糖尿病。
- 慢性心衰的临床进程是一个缓慢的临床不易察觉的过程，中间可伴有严重的失代偿心衰。心衰患者会突然死亡或死于心脏衰竭的末期心衰。
- 虚弱的老年患者在心衰失代偿期可出现精神错乱，失代偿心衰可出现认知受损（arnold 2007）。

表 3-2. 波士顿充血性心力衰竭诊断评分

标准	分值
I 病史	
休息状态下呼吸困难	4
端坐呼吸	4
阵发性夜间呼吸困难	3
平地行走呼吸困难	2
上楼过程呼吸困难	1
II 体格检查	
心率异常（91~110 次 / 分，1 分；>110 次 / 分，2 分）	1-2
颈静脉压力升高（6cm H_2O，2 分；>6 cm H_2O 伴有肝脏肿大或水肿，3 分）	2-3
肺部湿啰音（仅限于肺底，1 分；肺底以外可闻及，2 分）	1-2
哮喘	3
出现第三心音	3
III 胸片	
肺泡肺水肿	4
肺间质水肿	3
双侧胸膜积液	3
心胸比 0.5（后前位）	3
上区流量再分配	2
每个分类下不多于 4 分，总分，每个分类的合计最高 12 分。心衰诊断：8~12 分确定诊断为心衰，4~7 可能诊断为心衰，4 分或小于 4 分，不太可能为心衰。	
Marantz pr, Tobin JN, Wassertheil-Smoller S, et al. The relationship between left ventricular systolic function and congestive heart failure diagnosed by clinical criteria. Circulation, 1998; vol. 77: pp. 607 - 12	

临床治疗

治疗

- 治疗充血引发的症状，寻找并治疗心衰的诱因和深层原因。
- 严重失代偿心衰治疗：利尿、吸氧、坐位、吗啡 IV 常用于缓解呼吸困难引起烦躁。
- 老年严重失代偿心衰常由心衰引起，年轻患者常由高血压或局部缺血引起。老年患者败血症可能引起心衰。
- 慢性心衰：常建议患者限制食盐和液体的摄入，但目前证据不足。适量限制食盐摄入（2g/d）是合理的。低钠血症患者（血钠 <135mmol/L）每日液体摄入小于 1 500ml；低钠血症本身是晚期心衰的主要征兆。大多数心衰患者过量的液体和盐不能被限制液体和盐的摄入减轻。推荐饮食：除食盐外食用高纤维、全谷物和蔬菜、多元不饱和脂肪酸、蛋白、

低饱和脂肪酸、调味品和适量酒精（地中海饮食）。
- 收缩功能障碍的心衰：局部缺血性心脏病应用利尿剂、ACEI、ARBs、β受体阻滞剂、醛固酮阻滞剂、洋地黄和他汀类降脂药。控制心率、血压。利尿剂、ACEI/ARBs、β受体阻滞剂是治疗的基础。
- 舒张功能障碍的心衰常见于肥胖同时患有2型糖尿病的患者，并常伴有呼吸睡眠暂停。治疗：应用利尿剂控制充血，控制血压、心率、血脂和血糖。
- 强烈的证据为基础的治疗可用于收缩功能障碍的心衰；较少证据支持舒张功能障碍心衰的治疗 – 利尿剂、肾素 – 血管紧张素抑制剂改善证据（Arnold 2006，见图3-1、表3-3）。
- 2型糖尿病患者，尤其是初始应用大量胰岛素的患者，胰岛素会导致钠潴留、容量负荷过重及失代偿心衰。应用胰岛素的心衰患者应限制食盐摄入，糖化血红蛋白控制目标为7%~8%。
- 二甲双胍往往中断心衰，这与乳酸酸中毒相关，但证据不足。一项前瞻性研究（Roberts）发现给予二甲双胍治疗的糖尿病患者死亡率下降。FDA已经解除心衰患者使用二甲双胍的警告。因此，肾功能正常（GFF 60ml/min）患者，二甲双胍可以继续使用。
- 噻唑烷二酮类与心衰相关的比率约2:1；有心衰病史患者禁用。

图 3-1. 心功能衰竭治疗

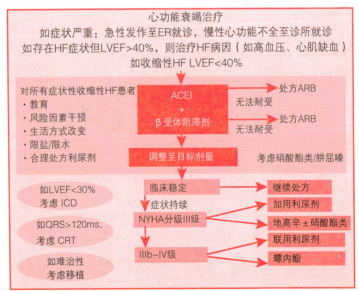

Source: Arnold JM, Liu P, Demers C, et al. Canadian Cardiovascular Society consensu conference recommendations on heart failure 2006: diagnosis and management. Can Cardiol, 2006; Vol. 22(1): 23 – 45. Reprinted with permission from Pulsus Group, Inc.

心力衰竭

表 3-3 大量临床实验研究中有依据的药物及口服剂量表

药物	起始剂量	目标剂量
ACEI		
卡托普利	6.25 mg~12.5 mg tid	25 mg~50 mg tid
依那普利	1.25 mg~2.5 mg bid	10 mg bid
雷米普利	1.25 mg~2.5 mg bid	5 mg bid*
赖诺普利	2.5 mg~5 mg qd	20 mg~35 mg qd
β 受体阻滞剂		
卡维地洛	3.125 mg bid	25 mg bid
比索洛尔	1.25 mg qd	10 mg qd
美托洛尔 CR/XL+	12.5 mg~25 mg qd	200 mg qd
ARB		
坎地沙坦	4 mg qd	32 mg qd
缬沙坦	40 mg bid	160 mg bid
醛固酮拮抗剂		
安体舒通	12.5 mg qd	50 mg qd
依普利酮	25 mg qd	50 mg qd
血管扩张剂		
硝酸异山梨酯	20 mg tid	40 mg tid
肼苯哒嗪	37.5 mg tid	75 mg tid

*HEART 试验显示 10mg/d 对缓解左室重构是有效的。
+加拿大无此药。

ACEI: 血管紧张素转换酶抑制剂; ARB: 血管紧张素受体抑制剂; bid: 每日两次; qd, 每日一次; CR/XL: 控释／长效; tid: 每日三次。

Arnold Jm, liu p, demers C, et al. Canadian Cardiovascular Society consensus conference recommendations on heart failure 2006: diagnosis and management. Can J Cardiol, 2006; vol. 22(1): 23 - 45. reprinted with permission from pulsus group Inc.

由于心脏瓣膜病引发的心衰需要外科手术修复病变瓣膜。手术时间需要临床经验和心脏内科专家会诊后决定。

心脏起搏器再同步对于收缩功能障碍的心衰及左束支传导阻滞或宽 QRS 波患者有益。最近研究提供证据支持中度心衰患者经起搏器再同步后预后更好。

应强烈建议吸烟患者戒烟。

过度饮酒患者心衰预后差。多数研究表明：适度饮酒（女性：1 杯／天；男性：1~2 杯／天）可降低心衰风险并改善预后。

随访

严重失代偿心衰属医疗急症需主要治疗。

慢性心衰患者需门诊随访；或由一个包含医生、护士、营养师、注册的糖尿病教育者及药剂师组成的医疗组跟进治疗。

- 判断及维持患者净重（weight at which signs of congestion have resolved but bp control and renal function are not impaired）是重要的。
- 每次随访都要观察颈静脉压：患者以45度角仰卧，颈静脉压应与锁骨持平，或垂直高于胸骨角12~15cm。
- 收缩期心衰患者明确的治疗目标：血钠135~145mmol/L，血钾4.5mmol/L，休息状态心率55~70bpm，血压140/90mmHg，静息状态有症状者理想血压为110/70mmHg，维持标准体重，血细胞比容34%。

专家意见

- 同时患有糖尿病和心衰的患者需要长期频繁随访，如果可能，心脏病学、内分泌学和内科学的护理不应中断。心衰患者经团队护理已多次被证实是有效的。如有任何症状进展的表现需要每月进行一次办公室随访。
- 对于因心衰症状有不适主诉的老年患者应详细检查并测定BNP/ProBNP。
- 保持患者标准体重是必要的，患者必须明确知道自己的标准体重并每天测量体重。
- 众多指南包括Arnold 2006指南均推荐糖化血红蛋白目标位7%，但对同时患有糖尿病和心衰的患者目标可能略高于7%（Aguilar）。
- 流感疫苗和肺炎疫苗的接种必须保持现状。
- 晚期心衰的治疗事实上是一种姑息治疗。临终问题必须和患者及家属或其他重要个人商量。

基于以下文献推荐

Hunt SA, Abraham WT, Chin MH, et al. 2009 focused update incorporated into the ACC/AHA 2005 Guidelines for the Diagnosis and Management of Heart Failure in Adults: a report of the American College of Cardiology Foundation/American Heart Association Task Force on Practice Guidelines Developed in Collaboration With the International Society for Heart and Lung Transplantation. J Am Coll Cardiol, 2009; Vol. 53: pp. e1–e90.
Comments: Authoritative review. Lengthy, not easy to read.

Howlett JG, McKelvie RS, Arnold JM, et al. Canadian Cardiovascular Society Consensus Conference guidelines on heart failure, update 2009: diagnosis and management of right-sided heart failure, myocarditis, device therapy and recent important clinical trials. Can J Cardiol, 2009; Vol. 25: pp. 85–105.
Comments: Part 3 of the Canadian Cardiovascular Society review of HF. All 3 are beautifully written, concise guides to the science and art of treating patients who have HF.

Arnold JM, Howlett JG, Dorian P, et al. Canadian Cardiovascular Society Consensus Conference recommendations on heart failure update 2007: prevention, management during intercurrent illness or acute decompensation, and use of biomarkers. Can J Cardiol, 2007; Vol. 23: pp. 21–45.
Comments: Concise and beautifully written, many clinical pearls; detailed advice regarding when and how to use biomarkers to diagnose and treat HF. Review of use of metformin in HF is outstanding. They recommend an A1c goal of ,7 for patients with diabetes and heart failure. See Expert Opinion section above for criticism of this goal.

Arnold JM, Liu P, Demers C, et al. Canadian Cardiovascular Society consensus conference recommendations on heart failure 2006: diagnosis and management. Can J Cardiol, 2006; Vol. 22: pp. 23–45.

Comments: Concise and beautifully written; the tables and figures are all well prepared and contain clinical pearls.

其他参考文献

Home PD, Pocock SJ, Beck-Nielsen H, et al. Rosiglitazone evaluated for cardiovascular outcomes in oral agent combination therapy for type 2 diabetes (RECORD): a multicentre, randomised, open-label trial. Lancet, 2009; Vol. 373: pp. 2125–35.

Comments: Thiazolidinediones must be used with great caution, if at all, in patients with HF. See also Arnold 2007.

Aguilar D, Bozkurt B, Ramasubbu K, et al. Relationship of hemoglobin A1C and mortality in heart failure patients with diabetes. J Am Coll Cardiol, 2009; Vol. 54: pp. 422–8.

Comments: Demonstration of "U-shaped curve" of A1c levels in HF.

Noyes K, Corona E, Veazie P, Dick AW, Zhao H, Moss AJ. Examination of the effect of implantable cardioverterdefibrillators on health-related quality of life: based on results from the Multicenter Automatic Defibrillator Trial-II. Am J Cardiovasc Drugs, 2009; Vol. 9(6): pp. 393–400.

Comments: Important review of use of device therapy in HF.

Roberts F, Ryan GJ. The safety of metformin in heart failure. Ann Pharmacother, 2007; Vol. 41: pp. 642–6.

Comments: Important review.

Doust JA, Pietrzak E, Dobson A, et al. How well does B-type natriuretic peptide predict death and cardiac events in patients with heart failure: systematic review. BMJ, 2005; Vol. 330: p. 625.

Comments: Biomarkers have become essential tools in the diagnosis and management of HF.

Nohria A, Tsang SW, Fang JC, et al. Clinical assessment identifies hemodynamic profiles that predict outcomes in patients admitted with heart failure. J Am Coll Cardiol, 2003; Vol. 41: pp. 1797–804.

Comments: Study of utility of clinical assessment of 4 different profiles of perfusion-congestion in HF patients.

Davis RC, Hobbs FD, Lip GY. ABC of heart failure. History and epidemiology. BMJ, 2000; Vol. 320: pp. 39–42.

Comments: First of a 10-part series on HF in the British Medical Journal. The presentation is outstanding; still a very useful series of articles.

Myers J, Do D, Herbert W, et al. A nomogram to predict exercise capacity from a specific activity questionnaire and clinical data. Am J Cardiol, 1994; Vol. 73: pp. 591–6.

Comments: The Veterans Specific Activity Scale quickly and accurately estimates exercise capacity.

Marantz PR, Tobin JN, Wassertheil-Smoller S, et al. The relationship between left ventricular systolic function and congestive heart failure diagnosed by clinical criteria. Circulation, 1988; Vol. 77: pp. 607–12.

Comments: Presentation of the "Boston Criteria" for diagnosis of heart failure.

高血压

Nisa M. Maruthur, MD, MHS

定义
- 糖尿病个体不同日两次测量血压，收缩压高于130mmHg或舒张压高于80mmHg。

流行病学
- 20%~60%糖尿病患者患有高血压。
- 1型糖尿病：高血压常由糖尿病肾病导致或糖尿病肾病发生在后。
- 2型糖尿病：高血压是一种常见的并发症，常发生于诊断糖尿病之前。
- 高血压与大血管并发症（如冠心病和脑卒中）、微血管并发症（糖尿病视网膜病变和糖尿病肾病）和死亡相关(UKPDS 36)。
- 降低血压可减少糖尿病并发症：大血管并发症、微血管并发症及死亡(UKPDS38，ADVANCE）。

诊断
- 糖尿病个体不同日两次测量血压，收缩压高于130mmHg或舒张压高于80mmHg，对于非糖尿病病患诊断标准为140/90mmHg。
- 实验室检查：尿常规、CBC、电解质、空腹血脂谱、心电图。
- 以下情况须检查高血压的继发原因：血压对3种及以上降压药物发生抵抗，严重高血压（180/110mmHg），明显高血压器官损害，20~50岁成年人患病者，无家族史及通过体检或实验室检查发现高血压的患者。
- 高血压继发因素包括：肾动脉狭窄，肾实质病变，主动脉缩窄，药物（如雌激素），饮食（如高盐高脂饮食），醛固酮增多症，嗜铬细胞瘤，Cushing综合征，睡眠呼吸暂停，促红细胞生成素副作用及其他内分泌紊乱（如甲状腺功能亢进）。

症状和体征
- 有头痛、胸痛及呼吸困难，但不一定都表现出来。
- 是慢性终末器官损害的预兆，包含动脉硬化、左室肥大、舒张功能障碍、慢性肾病、糖尿病视网膜病变。
- 高血压危象患者可能发生脑卒中或心肌梗死。
- 继发性高血压可出现腹部杂音，BUN/Cr升高，足部脉搏搏动延迟，电解质紊乱（如低钾血症、高钠血症），心动过速，多毛症，打鼾，嗜睡等。

临床治疗
- 收缩压130~139mmHg或舒张压80~89mmHg：坚持改变生活方式（控制饮食及适当锻炼），如3个月后血压仍高，则进行药物干预。
- 收缩压大于等于140mmHg或舒张压大于等于90mmHg：改变生活方式同时药物治疗。
- 改变饮食习惯降压：每日摄入食盐小于2.4g/d(JNC7)。

高血压

- 水果、蔬菜和低脂饮食为主的饮食途径阻止高血压,可以适度饮酒(女性:1杯/天;男性:1~2杯/天)。
- 中等或更强的身体活动(有氧的阻力训练),每周不少于150分钟。
- ACEI 和 ARB 类药物作为高血压的一线药物。
- 应用噻嗪类利尿剂 [GFR 高于 30ml/(min·1.73m^2)] 或袢利尿剂 [GFR 低于 30ml/(min·1.73m^2)] 作为血压达标(130/80mmHg)的辅助治疗。
- 血压达 150/90mmHg 推荐初始应用两药联合(INC7)。
- 无论初始血压状况如何,ADVANCE 试验建议应用 ACEI 和利尿剂的联合药物降压(培哚普利 + 吲达帕胺)对减少血管事件是有益的。
- 治疗高血压继发因素。

随访

- 家庭血压监测。
- 每次进行糖尿病随访时测量血压。
- 应用 ACEI、ARB 和利尿剂等类药物时定期检查血钾和 GFR,特别是在初始应用药物或改变剂量时。

专家建议

- 控制血压比实际的药理作用更重要。
- 对于降低糖尿病患者心血管发病率和死亡率,治疗高血压可能比控制血糖更重要。

基于以下文献推荐

American Diabetes Association. Standards of medical care in diabetes—2011. Diabetes Care, 2011; Vol. 34 Suppl 1: pp. S11–61.

Comments: American Diabetes Association recommendations for diabetes care including the management of hypertension in patients with diabetes.

Chobanian AV, Bakris GL, Black HR, et al. The seventh report of the Joint National Committee on Prevention, Detection, Evaluation, and Treatment of High Blood Pressure: the JNC 7 report. JAMA, 2003; Vol. 289: pp. 2560–72.

Comments: Widely accepted guideline for the treatment of hypertension with mention of special cases including diabetic hypertension; also describes use of DASH dietary pattern for reduction of hypertension.

Arauz-Pacheco C, Parrott MA, Raskin P. The treatment of hypertension in adult patients with diabetes. Diabetes Care, 2002; Vol. 25: pp. 134–47.

Comments: American Diabetes association technical review of the management of hypertension in patients with diabetes.

其他参考文献

US Dept of Health and Human Services. The seventh report of the Joint National Committee on Prevention, Detection, Evaluation, and Treatment of High Blood Pressure. NIH Publication No. 04-5230; August 2004.

Comments: Comprehensive report on the epidemiology, diagnosis, and management of hypertension.

Marwick TH, Hordern MD, Miller T, et al. Exercise training for type 2 diabetes mellitus: impact on cardiovascular risk: a scientific statement from the American Heart Association. Circulation,2009; Vol. 119: pp. 3244–62.

Comments: American Heart Association scientific statement to describe exercise recommendations for patients with diabetes in the context of cardiovascular disease and its risk factors.

Preis SR, Pencina MJ, Hwang SJ, et al. Trends in cardiovascular disease risk factors in individuals with and without diabetes mellitus in the Framingham Heart Study Circulation,2009; Vol. 120: pp. 212–20.

Comments Estimates trends in cardiovascular disease risk factors, including mean blood pressure, in the Framingham Heart Study.

Patel A, ADVANCE Collaborative Group, MacMahon S, et al. Effects of a fixed combination of perindopril and indapamide on macrovascular and microvascular outcomes in patients with type 2 diabetes mellitus (the ADVANCE trial): a randomised controlled trial Lancet,2007; Vol. 370: pp. 829–40.

Comments: Results of the blood pressure-lowering regimen (perindopril + indapamide vs placebo) of the ADVANCE trial, a factorial trial, evaluating the effects of blood pressure-lowering and glycemic control on vascular disease in diabetes.

American Heart Association Nutrition Committee, Lichtenstein AH, Appel LJ, et al. Diet and lifestyle recommendations revision 2006: a scientific statement from the American Heart Association Nutrition Committee. Circulation,2006; Vol. 114: pp. 82–96.

Comments American Heart Association dietary recommendations based on DASH diet.

Adler AI, Stratton IM, Neil HA, et al. Association of systolic blood pressure with macrovascular and microvascular complications of type 2 diabetes (UKPDS 36): prospective observational study. BMJ,2000; Vol. 321: pp. 412–9.

Comments UK Prospective Diabetes Study Group 36: Observational study of association between hypertension and macro- and microvascular complications and death.

[No authors listed]. Tight blood pressure control and risk of macrovascular and microvascular complications in type 2 diabetes: UKPDS 38. UK Prospective Diabetes Study Group. BMJ,1998; Vol. 317: pp. 703–13.

Comments Randomized trial (UK Prospective Diabetes Study Group 38) showing benefit of tight blood pressure control over less tight control on diabetes complications.

Appel LJ, Moore TJ, Obarzanek E, et al. A clinical trial of the effects of dietary patterns on blood pressure. DASH Collaborative Research Group. NEJM,1997; Vol. 336: pp. 1117–24.

Comments Original research article showing the blood pressure-lowering effect of the Dietary Approaches to Stop Hypertension (DASH) dietary pattern.

代谢综合征

Mary Huizinga, MD, MPH

定义
- 代谢综合征是多种代谢成分异常聚集的病理状态,是导致糖尿病和或心脑血管疾病的危险因素。
- 具体标准见诊断部分。
- 也称为"X 综合征"或"胰岛素抵抗综合征"。

流行病学
- 发病率增加,体现出肥胖症增加。
- 35%~40% 的美国人患有代谢综合征。
- 年龄的增长和拉丁裔族群与代谢综合征风险增加相关。在非洲裔美国人中,女人较男人患病风险高,但在欧洲人中并非如此。
- 至今尚无明确的病因,但胰岛素抵抗、缺乏运动、年龄和饮食不均都是危险因素。
- 年龄大于 50 岁的糖尿病患者,86% 存在代谢综合征 (Alexander)。
- 存在代谢综合征的患者发生糖尿病的风险较无代谢综合征人群增加 5 倍 (Grundy)。
- HDL、血压、糖尿病是代谢综合征患者发生冠心病(CHD)最重要的预测因素 (Alexander)。另外,这些因素与 CHD 的关联要大于与代谢综合征的关联 (Konstantinou)。
- 年龄大于 50 岁且没有糖尿病的代谢综合征患者,CHD 发病率为 14%;同时患有糖尿病和代谢综合征的患者 CHD 发病率为 19%。患有糖尿病但不患有代谢综合征的患者 CHD 发病率为 7.5% (Alexander)。

诊断
- 国际糖尿病联合会(IDF)和美国心脏协会(AHA)/国家心脏,肺和血液研究所(NHLBI)最近同意了以下定义;然而,腰围的标准随种族和组织而不同 (Alberti)。必须至少符合以下 5 项中的 3 项:
  1. 空腹甘油三酯升高:≥ 150mg/dl(1.7mmol/L) 或经药物治疗。
  2. HDL 下降:女性 <50mg/dl(1.3mmol/L),男性 <40mg/dl(1.03mmol/L)或经药物治疗。
  3. 空腹血糖升高:≥ 100mg/dl 或经药物治疗。
  4. 血压升高:收缩压 ≥ 130mmHg 或舒张压 ≥ 85mmHg,或经降压药物治疗。
  5. 腰围增加:随种族和组织不同(见表 3-4)。
- 血栓标志物升高(如 I 型纤溶酶原激活物抑制因子)与代谢综合征(MS)相关 (Appel)。

体征和症状

- 中心性肥胖。
- 胰岛素抵抗:黑棘皮病。
- 高血糖:多尿、烦渴、乏力、视物模糊。
- 高脂血症:疹性黄色瘤及脂血症性视网膜炎。
- 无法控制的高血压:头痛、头晕。
- 其他与胰岛素抵抗相关的情况(如睡眠呼吸暂停)。

临床治疗

- 初级目标是预防动脉粥样硬化疾病尤其是心血管疾病的发生,如戒烟。
- 生活方式改变:饮食和运动的效应可能是独立于体重下降之外的,如高血糖、高血压、高血脂的改善,鼓励患者在6~12个月之内减少7%~10%的体重(Alberti;Grundy)。
- 药物治疗的目标是减轻 MS 的单独成分,如高血压、血脂紊乱和高血糖。
- 药物治疗的目标是减少心血管危险因素(虽然其并不是MS的组成部分),如 LDL 水平的升高。
- Framingham 风险评分可以用来评估动脉粥样硬化性疾病发生的 10 年风险,可以用于指导药物治疗(见 http://hp2010.nhlbihin.net/atpiii CALCULATOR.asp?usertype=prof)。
- 在存在中度风险的人群可考虑预防性使用阿司匹林。

随访

- 每年监测 MS 患者是否发生糖尿病。
- 随访单纯糖尿病的患者是否出现了 MS 的其他表现。
- 在存在动脉粥样硬化相关疾病症状时考虑进行相关检查,如 CHD 症状的患者考虑进行冠心病相关检查(如憋气、胸痛)。

专家意见

- 同时存在糖尿病和代谢综合征的患者较只患有糖尿病或代谢综合征的患者有更高的心血管疾病的风险。
- 大部分糖尿病患者存在代谢综合征。
- MS 最重要风险因素为不健康的生活方式,生活方式改变被认为是初级治疗。
- 如患者为高危或生活方式治疗失败,可考虑对 MS 的不同组分进行药物治疗。
- 对 MS 组分的有效治疗,可以显著降低心血管事件风险。

表 3-4 目前各组织推荐的腹型肥胖腰围临界值

人群	组织（引用）	男性	女性
高加索人	IDF	≥ 94cm	≥ 80cm
白种人	WHO	≥ 94cm（风险增加）	≥ 80cm（风险增加）
		≥ 102cm（更高风险）	≥ 88cm（更高风险）
美国	AHA/NHLBI（ATP III）*	≥ 102cm	≥ 88cm
加拿大	加拿大卫生部	≥ 102cm	≥ 88cm
欧洲	欧洲心脏学会	≥ 102cm	≥ 88cm
亚洲（包括日本）	IDF	≥ 90cm	≥ 80cm
亚洲	WHO	≥ 90cm	≥ 80cm
日本	日本肥胖学会	≥ 85cm	≥ 90cm
中国	合作工作小组	≥ 85cm	≥ 80cm
中东，地中海	IDF	≥ 94cm	≥ 80cm
撒哈拉以南非洲	IDF	≥ 94cm	≥ 80cm
中美洲和南美洲的少数部落	IDF	≥ 90cm	≥ 80cm

* 新版 AHA/NHLBI 代谢综合征指南指出，腰围 ≥ 94cm 的男性和 ≥ 80cm 的女性发生 CVD 和糖尿病的风险增加，这两个指标作为个体增加胰岛素抵抗的切点。IDF：国际糖尿病联盟，WHO：世界卫生组织。

来　源：Alberti KG, Eckel RH, Grundy SM, et al. Harmonizing the metabolic syndrome: a joint interim statement of the International Diabetes Federation Task Force on Epidemiology and Prevention; National Heart, Lung, and Blood Institute; American Heart Association; World Heart Federation; International Atherosclerosis Society; and International Association for the Study of Obesity. Circulation, 2009; Vol. 120(16):p. 1640 (Table 2). Reprinted with permission of The American Heart Association.

基于以下文献推荐

Alberti KG, Eckel RH, Grundy SM, et al. Harmonizing the metabolic syndrome: a joint interim statement of the International Diabetes Federation Task Force on Epidemiology and Prevention; National Heart, Lung, and Blood Institute; American Heart Association; World Heart Federation; International Atherosclerosis Society; and International Association for the Study of Obesity. Circulation, 2009; Vol. 120: pp. 1640–5.

Comments:This article describes the latest criteria (2009) for defining the metabolic syndrome. It is a joint statement by the International Diabetes Federation and the American Heart Association/NHLBI.

Grundy SM, Cleeman JI, Daniels SR, et al. Diagnosis and management of the metabolic syndrome: an American Heart Association/National Heart, Lung, and Blood Institute Scientific Statement. Circulation, 2005; Vol. 112: pp. 2735–52.

Comments:Statement by the AHA/NHLBI for guidelines issued in 2005.

其他参考文献

Ogbera AO. Prevalence and gender distribution of the metabolic syndrome. Diabetol Metab Syndr, 2010; Vol. 2: p. 1.
Comments: Describes the prevalence of metabolic syndrome in patients with diabetes by age and gender.

Konstantinou DM, Chatzizisis YS, Louridas GE, et al. Metabolic syndrome and angiographic coronary artery disease prevalence in association with the Framingham risk score. Metab Syndr Relat Disord, 2010; Vol. 8: pp. 201–8.
Comments: Describes the utility of MS for predicting angiographically significant CAD.

Gardner M, Palmer J, Manrique C, et al. Utility of aspirin therapy in patients with the cardiometabolic syndrome and diabetes. J Cardiometab Syndr, 2009; Vol. 4: pp. 96–101.
Comments: This is a review of the mixed literature about aspirin use for the primary prevention of cardiac disease in patients with diabetes and metabolic syndrome.

Grundy SM, Cleeman JI, Daniels SR, et al. Diagnosis and management of the metabolic syndrome: an American Heart Association/National Heart, Lung, and Blood Institute Scientific Statement. Circulation, 2005; Vol. 112: pp. 2735–52.
Comments: Statement by the AHA/NHLBI for guidelines issued in 2005.

Appel SJ, Harrell JS, Davenport ML. Central obesity, the metabolic syndrome, and plasminogen activator inhibitor-1 in young adults. J Am Acad Nurse Pract, 2005; Vol. 17: pp. 535–41.
Comments: PAI-1 is associated with impaired fibrinolysis and was found to be correlated with waist circumference and metabolic syndrome in this study.

Alexander CM, Landsman PB, Teutsch SM, et al. NCEP-defined metabolic syndrome, diabetes, and prevalence of coronary heart disease among NHANES III participants age 50 years and older. Diabetes, 2003; Vol. 52: pp. 1210–4.
Comments: NHANES III study describing epidemiological features of metabolic syndrome using older NCEP metabolic syndrome definition. Limited to persons aged 50 years and older.

Ford ES, Giles WH, Dietz WH. Prevalence of the metabolic syndrome among US adults: findings from the third National Health and Nutrition Examination Survey. JAMA, 2002; Vol. 287: pp. 356–9.
Comments: Epidemiological description of metabolic syndrome from NHANES III (1988–1994).

Knowler WC, Barrett-Connor E, Fowler SE, et al. Reduction in the incidence of type 2 diabetes with lifestyle intervention or metformin. NEJB, 2002; Vol. 346: pp. 393–403.
Comments: Diabetes Prevention Program—a randomized controlled trial showing that ~7% weight loss significantly reduced the incidence of diabetes in persons with elevated fasting glucose.

肥胖

Jeanne M. Clark, MD, MPH

定义
- 多余的脂肪组织影响健康。
- 世界卫生组织(WHO)将肥胖临床定义为体重指数(BMI) ≥ 30kg/m^2。
- 进一步划分为：一级(BMI 30~34.9kg/m^2)、二级(BMI 35~39.9kg/m^2)、三级(BMI >40kg/m^2)。超重为BMI 25~29.9kg/m^2。
- 内脏型肥胖指腹腔内脂肪组织过多。
- 内脏型肥胖临床定义为一个腰围 >88cm/35英寸(女性)或 >102cm/40英寸(男性)(WHO)。

流行病学
- 2007-2008年度经年龄校正的肥胖总患病率：33.8%，其中男性32.2%、女性35.5%。超重(BMI ≥ 25kg/m^2)和肥胖的总体患病率估计为68%；其中男性72%和女性64%(Flegal)。
- 将近6%的成年美国人非常肥胖(三级)。
- 非西班牙裔黑人女性肥胖患病率最高(49.6%)。
- 在过去的10年中：女性的肥胖趋势不显著，但对于男性来说呈显著的线性趋势增加，最近几年逐渐平稳(Flegal)。
- 1999-2006年间，美国成人糖尿病患者的超重(体重指数 > 25kg/m^2)和肥胖(体重指数 >30kg/m^2)发病率分别是80%和49%。糖尿病患病率随着体重分级增加而增长，从8%(正常体重)到43%(三级)(Nguyen)。
- WHO评议会发现，在某些亚洲人群中，具有2型糖尿病(T2DM)和心血管疾病的高危因素病人的BMI低于目前WHO的超重临界值(>25kg/m^2)。然而，具有可见风险的临界值在22~25kg/m^{2}之间变化，但结果并不一致。在其他亚洲人群，高危人群的临界值变化在26~31 kg/m^{2}之间。因此，WHO的临界值没有因为种族不同重新定义(WHO专家评议会)。
- 其他组织，如国际糖尿病联合会，根据腰围为中央型肥胖提供民族特异性临界值(IDF共识声明)。

临床治疗

生活方式改变
- 包括减少饮食的热量、进行身体活动和采用行为技术(NIH实用指南)。
- 会导致在6个月内体重下降初始体重的5%~10%。
- 减少饮食热量：比适当热量饮食低500~1 000卡热量。适当热量饮食需求能够相当容易地计算出(IOM报告)。
- 简明指南规定的维持体重(适当热量)的热量要求：体重(磅)×12，或体重(磅)乘以10+25%(低体力劳动)、+50%(中体力劳动)、+75%(高体力劳动)。
- 男性平均减肥饮食：1 200~1 600kcal/d。

- 女性平均减肥饮食：1 000~1 200kcal/d。
- 饮食的类型（低脂肪、低碳水化合物或均衡）不如坚持和毅力重要（见营养：糖尿病概述 102 页和 2 型糖尿病的营养 112 页）。
- 适度的体力活动减少腹部脂肪，如快走，有助于适度减肥。
- 行为技术可以提高依从性，促进减轻体重，如自我监控、刺激控制和计划饮食。
- 自我监控（即检测记录饮食量、体力活动量和体重）是最有效的行为技术。

药物减肥

- 药物可能对体重指数 >30kg/m^2 或 27~29.9kg/m^2 有并发症的患者有效(Snow)。
- 目前 FDA 批准了一种可以长期使用(>2 年)的药物：奥利司他 orlistat(Xenical)（见 595 页）。
- 奥利司他（120 毫克）是胰脂肪酶抑制剂，餐前 30 分钟服用。
- 服用奥利司他 1 年减轻体重约 2.5~3.0 kg(6~6.5 磅)。
- 奥利司他的副作用：腹泻、松散的脂肪便，抽筋。
- 由于心血管风险，2010 年 10 月西布曲明撤出市场。
- 其他药物，如苯丁胺和二乙胺苯丙酮，被批准用于短期使用(<3 个月)，可以减轻体重 3.0~3.5 千克 (6.5~7.5 磅)。
- 许多非处方药物已被 FDA 禁止，因此一般情况下不应推荐。

减肥手术

- 体重指数 >40kg/m^2 或 >30~35kg/m^2 伴有并存疾病的患者可以考虑减肥手术(Snow)(见减肥手术 98 页)。
- 手术包括：Roux-en-Y 胃旁路术，胃束带手术（包括可调的），胆胰分流术（有或没有十二指肠开关）和胃袖状切除术。
- 许多保险公司需要在减肥手术前进行一段时间（通常是 6 个月）的减肥医学监督。
- 手术可以减轻体重 20~40 千克 (44~88 磅)，可以持续 15 年。
- 吸收不良型手术（胆胰分流术和 Roux-en-Y 胃旁路手术）的减肥效果较好，限制型手术（胃束带手术和胃袖状切除术）减肥效果较差。
- 围手术期死亡率约为 1%，经验丰富的外科医生所进行的手术最低。
- 其他所有不良事件，包括术后感染、内部损伤（如脾）、疝、需要再次手术等，发生率约 20%。
- 减肥手术是肥胖降低长期死亡率的唯一治疗(Sjostrom)。

体重维持

- 生活方式：持续的自我监控和每天 60 分钟的中度体力活动可以帮助维持体重减轻(Wing)。
- 药物：使用奥利司他可以有效的维持体重减轻。
- 手术：通常患者手术后大幅度的减肥效果可以保持 15 年。

随诊

- 生活方式改变:增加随访频率(每周)可以增加减肥效果。
- 进食 <800~1 000kcal/d 的患者应定期监测电解质,警惕电解质失衡。
- 药物:通常停止用药后体重会恢复,因此应预先考虑并商讨长期治疗 (Snow)。
- 如果 3 个月后体重没有下降,应该停止治疗。
- 奥利司他:患者应该在睡前服用复合维生素,防止脂溶性维生素缺乏症;车前草可以用来预防/治疗腹泻。
- 减肥手术:患者需要监测营养物质,警惕蛋白质营养不良(白蛋白、前白蛋白)以及电解质(钠、钾、磷)、维生素(维生素 B_{12}、维生素 D_{12}、维生素 E、维生素 K、叶酸、硫胺素)和矿物质(钙、铁、镁)的缺乏,必要时更换药物 (Mechanik)。

专家意见

- 适度减肥可以预防高危人群 2 型糖尿病 (T2DM) 的发生 (Knowler)。
- 大幅度的减肥可以减少或消除某些 2 型糖尿病患者药物治疗的必要性。
- 许多 2 型糖尿病患者在胃分流术后 3 个月内会被"治愈";因此,糖尿病治疗策略应在术前评估 (Mechanick)。
- 在几乎所有的研究中,维护体重降低远比最初减肥更难。成功的减肥手术可能是例外。

推荐依据

Snow V, Barry P, Fitterman N, et al. Pharmacologic and surgical management of obesity in primary care: a clinical practice guideline from the American College of Physicians. Ann Intern Med, 2005; Vol. 142: pp. 525–31.

Comments: This article summarizes the guidelines of the American College of Physicians on the use of pharmacologic and surgical treatments for obesity.

NIH/NHLBI. The Practical Guide: Identification, Evaluation and Treatment of Overweight and Obesity in Adults, 2000; NIH Publication Number 00-4084. http://www.nhlbi.nih.gov/guidelines/obesity/prctgd_c.pdf (accessed 3/1/2011).

Comments: This guide, available online, reviews the diagnosis and treatment of overweight and obesity.

其他参考文献

Nguyen NT, Nguyen XM, Lane J, et al. Relationship between obesity and diabetes in a US adult population: findings from the National Health and Nutrition Examination Survey, 1999–2006. Obes Surg, 2011; Vol. 21: 351–5.

Comments: Describes prevalence of overweight and obesity among nationally representative sample of US adults (NHANES).

Flegal KM, Carroll MD, Ogden CL, et al. Prevalence and trends in obesity among US adults, 1999–2008. JAMA, 2010; Vol. 303: pp. 235–41.

Comments: Reports obesity trends in the United States from 1999–2008 using data from the National Health and Nutrition Examination Surveys (NHANES).

Mechanick JI, Kushner RF, Sugerman HJ, et al. American Association of Clinical Endocrinologists, The Obesity Society, and American Society for Metabolic and Bariatric Surgery medical guidelines for clinical practice for the perioperative nutritional, metabolic, and nonsurgical support of the bariatric surgery patient. Obesity (Silver Spring), 2009; Vol. 17 Suppl 1: pp. S1-70, v.
Comments: These guidelines outline perioperative and postoperative medical care for bariatric surgery patients including management of diabetes and monitoring nutritional deficiencies.

Segal JB, Clark JM, Shore AD, et al. Prompt reduction in use of medications for comorbid conditions after bariatric surgery. Obes Surg, 2009; Vol. 19: pp. 1646–56.
Comments: This analysis of medical claims data in over 6000 people who underwent bariatric surgery demonstrated that by 12 months, medication use for diabetes had decreased by 76%, compared to 59% for hyperlipidemia, and 51% for hypertension. Use of thyroid replacement and antidepressant medications decreased by less than 10%.

Svetkey LP, Stevens VJ, Brantley PJ, et al. Comparison of strategies for sustaining weight loss: the weight loss maintenance randomized controlled trial. JAMA, 2008; Vol. 299: pp. 1139–48.
Comments: This trial demonstrates the difficulty in getting activated patients to maintain weight. After a mean weight loss of 8.5 kg in the first 6 months, participants in the trial regained more than half the weight (4.0-5.5 kg) by 2.5 years later, but regain was less in a group getting continued personal contact.

Sjöström L, Narbro K, Sjöström CD, et al. Effects of bariatric surgery on mortality in Swedish obese subjects. NEJM, 2007; Vol. 357: pp. 741-52.
Comments: The Swedish Obesity Study demonstrated that subjects undergoing bariatric surgery had a 25% lower mortality than a morbidly obese comparison group after up to 15 years of follow-up. The reduced mortality was mainly due to a reduction in deaths from cardiovascular disease and cancer.

Institute of Medicine (IOM) Food and Nutrition Board. Dietary reference intakes for energy, carbohydrate, fiber, fat, fatty acids, cholesterol, protein, and amino acids (macronutrients). Washington, DC: National Academy Press; 2005.
Comments: This report details the recommended energy intake for adults and references the use of the Harris-Benedict Equation. There is an easy-to-use calculator on the Mayo Clinic Website: http://www.mayoclinic.com/health/calorie-calculator/NU00598 (accessed 3/2/2011).

Li Z, Maglione M, Tu W, et al. Meta-analysis: pharmacologic treatment of obesity. Ann Intern Med, 2005; Vol. 142: pp. 532–46.
Comments: This meta-analysis found that on average at 12 months, orlistat use resulted in a weight loss of 2.9 kg and sibutramine 4.5 kg. After 6 months, phentermine reduced weight by 3.6 kg and diethylpropion 3.0 kg. Side effects can be significant and differ by medication.

Maggard MA, Shugarman LR, Suttorp M, et al. Meta-analysis: surgical treatment of obesity. Ann Intern Med, 2005; Vol. 142: pp. 547-59.
Comments: This meta-analysis found that bariatric surgery resulted in 20–30 kg weight loss, which can be sustained over 10 years. Overall mortality was 1% with about 20% of patients having a less serious adverse event.

WHO Expert Consultation Appropriate body-mass index for Asian populations and its implications for policy and intervention strategies. Lancet, 2004; Vol. 363: pp. 157-63.

Comments: A WHO consultation concluded that though risk for type 2 diabetes and cardiovascular disease may be higher at lower BMI cutoffs in Asian populations (i.e., 22–25 kg/m2), the cutoff for high risk varied between 26–31 kg/m2. No formal attempts were made to redefine cutoff points by ethnicity.

Knowler WC, Barrett-Connor E, Fowler SE, et al. Reduction in the incidence of type 2 diabetes with lifestyle intervention or metformin. NEJM, 2002; Vol. 346: pp. 393–403.
Comments: This randomized trial demonstrated that an average weight loss reduced the risk of diabetes development in an at-risk population by 58%, whereas metformin reduced the risk by 31% compared to placebo.

Wing RR, Hill JO. Successful weight loss maintenance. Annu Rev Nutr, 2001; Vol. 21: pp. 323–41.
Comments: Data from the National Weight Control Registry indicated that people who have successfully lost weight and maintained it over several years (average weight loss of 30 kg for an average of 5.5 years) have similar habits including eating a diet low in fat, frequent self-monitoring of body weight and food intake, and high levels of regular physical activity. Weight-loss maintenance may get easier over time. Once these successful maintainers have maintained a weight loss for 2–5 years, the chances of longer-term success greatly increase.

International Diabetes Federation. The IDF consensus worldwide definition of the metabolic syndrome. http://www.idf.org/webdata/docs/MetSyndrome_FINAL.pdf.
Comments: International Diabetes Federation consensus statement on definition of metabolic syndrome, which provides ethnicity-specific definitions of central obesity using different cutoffs for waist circumference.

周围血管疾病

Sheldon H. Gottlieb, MD

定义
- 周围血管疾病(PVD)包括心脏和大脑血管(动脉和静脉)的疾病。尤其是糖尿病患者患腿和脚动脉缺血的风险高,称为下肢周围动脉疾病(PAD)。
- 跛行是指活动时肢体疼痛。它是由于动脉供血不足导致肌肉缺血引起的。
- 严重肢体缺血(CLI)被定义为静止疼痛,溃疡或坏疽,预计6个月内有截肢的风险。
- "糖尿病足综合征"是血管和神经性损伤(足部溃疡)的综合结果,最终导致下肢截肢(Bild)。
- 周围动脉疾病(PAD)的主要原因不单单是动脉粥样硬化,此外还有多种情况,包括静脉功能不全、周围动脉疾病的模拟综合症——被称为"假跛行综合征";请参阅下面的鉴别诊断。

流行病学
- 在一般人群中,周围动脉疾病(PAD)的患病率随年龄增长呈指数增加,欧洲白种人85岁以上患病率高达60%,其他人群缺乏数据(Bennett 2009,QJM)。
- 在<50岁人群中,周围动脉疾病(PAD)几乎总是由于糖尿病联合一个其他动脉粥样硬化危险因素(吸烟、脂质、高血压)引起。
- 糖尿病患者中周围动脉疾病的患病率是20%~30%,糖尿病并且吸烟的患者中更高(Marso)。
- 糖尿病和周围动脉疾病(PAD)的风险比是15:1(即:糖尿病患者PAD的患病率是非糖尿病患者的15倍)(Bild)。(相比之下,吸烟与肺癌风险比约为10:1)。
- 鞋不合脚被认为是周围动脉疾病(PAD)患者截肢的主要原因(Hennis)。
- 周围动脉疾病(PAD)的死亡率高,下肢截肢后死亡率继续升高,5年内死亡率高达80%(Hambleton)。

诊断
- 病史:年龄<70岁伴有吸烟或糖尿病的危险因素或年龄>70岁,并有身体机能下降的症状。
- 鉴别诊断(DDX):包括机械性因素如神经根刺激、关节炎和炎症因素,动脉瘤或导致腿部疼痛的贝克囊肿,以及慢性间隔综合征。见表3-6的DDX和诊断依据。
- 踝肱指数(ABI):关键检查,对所有周围动脉疾病患者进行检查,来评估疾病严重程度,并建立一个基准。ABI<0.9诊断PAD具有95%敏感,几乎可以100%除外健康的人。ABI<0.5预示5年生存率极低。见Grenon介绍如何进行ABI检查以及Marso诊断算法。
- 由于侧支循环的建立,静息下ABI可能是正常的;运动时ABI也是一个重要检查(Grenon;Marso)。糖尿病患者ABI>1.0通常是由于血管钙化导致下肢血管不可压缩。
- 严重肢体缺血 (CLI) 存在时,必须确定血管病变的位置和严重程度,以及成功血管再生的血流动力学要求和血管内及手术修复的风险评估。
- 二维超声:确定阻塞的位置和严重程度。
- 对比造影:计划进行血管再生时考虑使用,谨慎考虑肾脏状态。

症状和体征
- 周围动脉疾病的症状和体征的分类包括:Fontaine 分期和 Rutherford 分级(见表 3-5),从无症状到溃疡或坏疽。

表 3-5. 周围动脉疾病的诊断分类

Fontaine 分期		Rutherford 分级		
分期	临床表现	分级	分类	临床表现
I	无症状	0	0	无症状
II a	轻度跛行	I	1	轻度跛行
II b	中-重度跛行	I	2	中度跛行
—	—	I	3	重度跛行
III	缺血性静息痛	II	4	缺血性疼痛
IV	溃疡或坏疽	III	5	小组织的损失
—	—	IV	6	溃疡或坏疽

来源:Bennett PC, Silverman SH, Gill PS, et al. Peripheral arterial disease and Virchow's triad. Thromb Haemost, 2009; Vol. 101: pp. 1032 - 1040. 由 Schattauer 股份有限公司及 Lip 教授授权转载。

- 跛行是间歇性的和可重复的，与活动（如散步）相关。用距离或时间来定量表示（走多少英寸或街区出现疼痛）。对于周围动脉疾病，跛行症状灵敏度低，但特异性高 (Marso)。
- 鉴别缺血性、神经性和下肢深静脉血栓和足部溃疡：缺血性溃疡有疼痛剧烈；神经性溃疡是无痛的，疼痛位于脚或踝关节按压点；静脉溃疡是中度疼痛。见表 3-6。

临床治疗
- 严重肢体缺血 (CLI) 是内科/外科急诊疾病，急诊评估和急诊血管再生治疗是必需的，可以避免 6 个月内进行高位截肢的可能性 (Hirsch)。
- 所有 PAD 的患者均需戒烟。
- 适当的足部护理至关重要，包括合适的鞋和足病护理 (Hirsch)。
- 指导运动治疗可以比药物治疗更有效，推荐最少 12 周，每周 3 次，每次 30~45 分钟 (Hirsch)。
- 糖尿病患者高血压的治疗目标是 <130/80mmHg。对于 PAD 患者，β 受体阻滞剂不是禁忌 (Hirsch)。
- 他汀类药物治疗的目标为低密度脂蛋白 <70mg/dl(Hirsch; McDermott)。他汀类药物改善功能的有益效果可能是独立于血脂降低 (McDermott)。
- 严重 PAD 和已知的心血管疾病使用抗血小板和其他抗血栓形成的药物治疗 (Sobel)。建议 PAD 患者每日口服 75~325mg 阿司匹林，以减少心脏事件和中风的发病率和死亡率。氯吡格雷可用于阿司匹林不耐受的患者。这些药物的主要好处是减少中风的发病率 (McDermott)。
- 在 PAD 患者管理中，控制血糖的获益证据不足。
- 西洛地唑只推荐使用在致残的跛行症状且不适合血管再生治疗患者中 (Sobel)。己酮可可碱无效 (Marso)。
- 外科治疗建议以下情况使用：PAD 症状导致残疾，对戒烟、锻炼和药物治疗反应不佳 (Hirsch)。

随访
- 管理患者达到戒烟的目标，调整降压调脂药物，提高行走能力，避免 CLI 和下肢截肢。
- 随访的频率进行个性化推荐。

表 3-6. 间歇性跛行的鉴别诊断

疾病	疼痛或不适的位置	疼痛特点	运动相关发作	休息的效果	改变体位的效果	其他特征
间歇性跛行	臀部、大腿或小腿肌肉,脚很少见	抽筋、疼痛、疲劳、虚弱、直接的疼痛	在相同程度的运动后	迅速缓解	没有	可自愈
神经根受压(如椎间盘突出)	通常从后部向腿放射	锋利,刺痛	很快,即使不是运动后立即发作	没有迅速缓解(也经常静息时发作)	可以通过调整后背体位帮助缓解	后背疾病史
脊髓狭窄	臀部、大腿、臀部(遵循皮片)	运动障碍比疼痛更突出	走路或站后变量的时间长度	只有体位改变后才能通过休息缓解	腰椎弯曲缓解(坐或向前弯腰)	反复后背疾病病史,由腹肉压增高诱发
关节炎、炎症过程	脚、足弓	酸痛	不同程度的运动后	没有迅速缓解(可能静息时发作)	不承重可以缓解	多变,可能与活动水平相关
髋关节炎	臀部、大腿、臀部	疼痛不适,通常局限在臀部	不同程度的运动后	没有迅速缓解(可能静息时发作)	坐着更舒服,腿不承重时	多变,可能与活动水平、天气变化相关
贝克囊肿症状	膝盖后部,沿小腿向下	肿胀、疼痛、压痛	运动时	休息时发作	没有	不是间歇性的
静脉跛行	整个腿,但通常在大腿和腹股沟	发紧、胀裂痛	走路后	慢慢消退	加速提升缓解	股深静脉血栓病史、静脉充血征象、水肿
慢性筋膜室综合征	小腿肌肉	发紧、胀裂痛	大量运动后(如慢跑)	非常慢地消退	加速提升缓解	通常出现在肌肉发达的运动员

表 3-6 间歇性跛行的鉴别诊断（续）

疾病	疼痛或不适的位置	疼痛特点	运动相关发作	休息的效果	改变体位的效果	其他特征
慢性筋膜室综合征	小腿肌肉	发紧，胀裂痛	大量运动后（如慢跑）	非常慢地消退	加速提升缓解	通常出现在肌肉发达的运动员

来源：Norgren L, Hiatt WR, Dormandy JA, et al. Inter-Society Consensus for the Management of Peripheral Arterial Disease (TASC II). Eur J Vasc Endovasc Surg. 2007; Vol. 33 Suppl 1: pp. S1–S70. 由允 Rightslink 授权转载。

专家意见
- 对于大多数糖尿病患者，足部检查脚将得出有用的信息，是体格检查的一个重要组成部分。
- 糖尿病患者必须学会如何检查他们的脚。
- 任何糖尿病和有吸烟史的患者都可能患有周围动脉疾病。在常规访问应对该症状进行评估。

推荐依据

Berger JS, Krantz MJ, Kittelson JM, et al. Aspirin for the prevention of cardiovascular events in patients with peripheral artery disease: a meta-analysis of randomized trials. JAMA, 2009; Vol. 301: pp. 1909–19.
Comments: Aspirin reduced nonfatal strokes but not cardiovascular events. Despite meta-analysis, statistical power remains lacking.

Momsen AH, Jensen MB, Norager CB, et al. Drug therapy for improving walking distance in intermittent claudication: a systematic review and meta-analysis of robust randomised controlled studies. Eur J Vasc Endovasc Surg, 2009; Vol. 38: pp. 463–74.
Comments: Excellent review of drug therapy for PAD symptoms.

Sobel M, Verhaeghe R, American College of Chest Physicians, et al. Antithrombotic therapy for peripheral artery occlusive disease: American College of Chest Physicians Evidence-Based Clinical Practice Guidelines (8th Edition). Chest, 2008; Vol. 133: pp. 815S–843S.
Comments: Evidence-based clinical practice guideline from the American College of Chest Physicians.

Hirsch AT, Haskal ZJ, Hertzer NR, et al. ACC/AHA 2005 Practice Guidelines for the management of patients with peripheral arterial disease (lower extremity, renal, mesenteric, and abdominal aortic): a collaborative report. Circulation, 2006; Vol. 113: pp. e463–654.
Comments: Complete online textbook of PAD.

其他参考文献

Grenon SM, Gagnon J, Hsiang Y. Video in clinical medicine. Ankle-brachial index for assessment of peripheral arterial disease. NEJM, 2009; Vol. 361: p. e40.
Comments: Outstanding and unique teaching guide.

Bennett PC, Silverman S, Gill PS, et al. Ethnicity and peripheral artery disease. QJM, 2009; Vol. 102: pp. 3–16.
Comments: Review of PAD among non-white European populations.

Bennett PC, Silverman SH, Gill PS, et al. Peripheral arterial disease and Virchow's triad. Thromb Haemost, 2009; Vol. 101: pp. 1032–40.
Comments: Historical review including development of Fontaine and Rutherford classifications of claudication. Highly recommended.

Hambleton IR, Jonnalagadda R, Davis CR, et al. All-cause mortality after diabetes-related amputation in Barbados: a prospective case-control study. Diabetes Care, 2009; Vol. 32: pp. 306–7.
Comments: This case-control study highlights the grave prognosis after a diabetes-related amputation.

Ankle Brachial Index Collaboration, Fowkes FG, Murray GD, et al. Ankle brachial index combined with Framingham Risk Score to predict cardiovascular events and mortality: a meta-analysis. JAMA, 2008; Vol. 300: pp. 197–208.
Comments: ABI improves Framingham Risk Score prediction of cardiovascular events.

Pearce L, Ghosh J, Counsell A, et al. Cilostazol and peripheral arterial disease. Expert Opin Pharmacother, 2008; Vol. 9: pp. 2683–90.
Comments: Review of the role of cilostazol in the management of PAD.

Marso SP, Hiatt WR. Peripheral arterial disease in patients with diabetes. J Am Coll Cardiol, 2006; Vol. 47: pp. 921–9.
Comments: Review of PAD in major cardiology journal.

Hennis AJ, Fraser HS, Jonnalagadda R, et al. Explanations for the high risk of diabetes-related amputation in a Caribbean population of black African descent and potential for prevention. Diabetes Care, 2004; Vol. 27: pp. 2636–41.
Comments: Ethnography of diabetes-related amputation.

McDermott MM, Guralnik JM, Greenland P, et al. Statin use and leg functioning in patients with and without lower-extremity peripheral arterial disease. Circulation, 2003; Vol. 107: pp. 757–61.
Comments: Statins but not aspirin, ACE inhibitors, vasodilators, or beta-blockers improved function in PVD. Non-randomized but well-conducted study, highly cited.

Bild DE, Selby JV, Sinnock P, et al. Lower-extremity amputation in people with diabetes. Epidemiology and prevention. Diabetes Care, 1989; Vol. 12: pp. 24–31.
Comments: Important reference, documents the evidence linking diabetes with PVD and lower-extremity amputation.

内分泌疾病

肢端肥大症

Nestoras Mathioudakis, MD, and Douglas Ball, MD

定义

- 生长激素（GH）分泌过多造成的一种临床综合征。
- 骨骺板闭合之前生长激素分泌过剩导致巨人症；骺板闭合之后生长激素分泌过剩导致肢端肥大症。
- 慢性生长激素分泌过多对机体及代谢的影响主要是高水平介导的胰岛素样生长因子1（IGF-1）。
- 肢端肥大症是糖尿病的一种罕见的次要原因。
- 过量生长激素（1）刺激糖原异生和脂肪分解，导致血糖和游离脂肪酸水平升高；（2）导致肝及外周胰岛素抵抗以及代偿性高胰岛素血症，相反，IGF-1可增加胰岛素灵敏性，然而，对于肢端肥大症患者，增加的IGF-1水平无法抵消生长激素过剩所造成的胰岛素抵抗状态。

流行病学

- 患病率为(40~130)/百万，尽管Chanson报道的患病率为(100~1 000)/百万人口。
- 病因几乎都是一个分泌生长激素的垂体腺瘤。
- 非常少见的原因包括下丘脑肿瘤分泌过多的生长激素释放激素，异位内分泌（神经源性肿瘤或者非内分泌肿瘤，如类癌和小细胞肺癌）。
- 也可能是某种遗传综合征的一部分，包括多发性骨纤维发育不良病，多发性内分泌肿瘤1型（MEN-1）综合征和Carney综合征。多发性骨纤维发育不良病的特点是由多发骨纤维异常增殖症，咖啡色斑点，性早熟，内分泌亢进（甲亢、巨人症、库欣氏症）。MEN-1主要导致垂体、甲状旁腺、胰腺的分泌亢进。Carney综合征导致粘液瘤，内分泌亢进、痣神经鞘瘤（Keil）。
- 由于症状和体征进展缓慢往往会导致诊断延迟，诊断时平均年龄为40岁。
- 这些患者心血管疾病、脑血管疾病、呼吸系统疾病的死亡率是普通人群的2倍；结肠肿瘤及其他肿瘤的风险增加。通过手术治疗，其死亡率降至正常人水平，视为手术治愈。
- 19%~56%的肢端肥大症患者有明显的糖尿病，16%~46%患者有糖耐量异常（Colao）。
- GH水平较高、老龄、病程较长都预测症状性糖尿病进展，家族史和高血压可能增加发病风险（Colao）。
- 糖尿病酮症酸中毒（DKA）是肢端肥大症的罕见症状。严重的糖尿病性视网膜病变也是一种罕见的并发症（Calao）。

肢端肥大症

诊断
- 最好的单一诊断测试是 IGF-1，在几乎所有的肢端肥大症患者升高。
- IGF-1 水平会随着年龄增长下降，因此对于老年人看似"正常"的值可能实际上较高。
- 对于 IGF-1 水平不确定的患者进行生长激素水平测定，对于高 IGF-1 水平的患者需要进一步作生化检查来验证。
- 生长激素因其分泌的波动性和昼夜差别而更难解释，影响因素包括如运动、压力、睡眠、和禁食。由于 GH 水平在一天中变异很大，所以最好不要取随机测量值（Bonert）。
- 未经控制的糖尿病可升高血清 GH 水平，还可导致肝脏疾病和营养不良。
- 确立诊断最具有特异性的检查是口服糖耐量试验（OGTT，口服 75g 葡萄糖两小时之内血清 GH 应该下降到 1ng/ml, 0.85% 的肢端肥大症患者这个值为 2ng/ml。随着放射免疫或免疫化学检测的敏感度越来越高，OGTT 之后，血清 GH 水平 0.3ng/ml 作为确立诊断。
- 一旦被证实为生长激素分泌过多，应作腺垂体 MRI 检查看是否有腺瘤，大多数患者在确立诊断时能发现大的腺瘤（1厘米）。

症状和体征
- 由于局部肿瘤和/或升高的 IGF-1 水平的系统性影响。
- 体征：视野赤字（俗称双颞侧偏盲），颅神经（3，4，5，6）麻痹，眼球震颤，视乳头水肿，肢端肥大（手和脚的软组织增厚），突颌，牙齿间距很大，前额骨肥大，颚咬合不正，关节炎，近端肌病，油性皮肤，皮垂，多毛症，结肠息肉，高血压，左心室肥厚，心肌病，巨舌症，甲状腺肿大，脏器增大（唾液腺、肝、脾、肾、前列腺），黑棘皮病，高尿钙和肾结石，甘油三酯，受损糖耐量和糖尿病，体重增加。
- 症状：头痛，视觉障碍（视力丧失、复视），关节痛，肢端感觉异常，腕管综合征，疲劳，怕热，多汗，睡眠障碍，阻塞性和中枢性睡眠呼吸暂停，月经异常，溢乳，性欲减退，阳痿。
- 指环、手套、鞋的大小改变提示肢端肥大。
- 其他实验室检查：由于生长激素对肾脏的直接影响导致高血磷和高钙尿症。
- 70%的患者血清胰岛素增加。
- 影像学检查：头颅平片显示颅骨增厚，上颌窦和额窦增大。手 X 线片显示软组织增加，关节软骨增宽，远端指骨"箭头簇绒"征，腕骨囊性改变。

临床治疗

手术
- 分泌生长激素的垂体腺瘤的主要治疗方法是经蝶手术。有经验的神经外科医生微腺瘤的治愈率高达 80%，大的腺瘤治愈率为 50%。
- 大的腺瘤患者需要辅助治疗（化疗与放疗）。为预防垂体功能低下的风险一般将放疗作为三线治疗。
- 最近的数据表明，术前应用生长抑素类似物可提高患者的手术治愈率。

肢端肥大症

药物治疗
- 生长抑素类似物（SSAS）抑制生长激素细胞增殖和GH分泌。主要疗效：实现生化达标率为50%~70%，肿瘤减小的有效率为50%。作为辅助治疗的有效性（术后）为20%。
- 生长抑素类似物（SSAS）包括奥曲肽，奥曲肽长效制剂，兰瑞肽Autogel（长效制剂）。奥曲肽给药方式通常皮下注射是每次100~250μg，每日3次。奥曲肽长效制剂给药方式为每月一次肌内注射，通常起始量为20mg，每次10mg递增，以达到临床和生化目标值。兰瑞肽Autogel每月90mg剂量皮下注射。
- 培维索孟是生长激素受体竞争性拮抗剂抑制生长激素作用。疗效：控制肢端肥大症的症状控制率为80%~90%，但不减少肿瘤的大小或GH水平。
- 多巴胺受体激动剂（如溴隐亭），卡麦角林也可以作为选择。

糖尿病治疗
- 对潜在疾病治疗后糖耐量异常和糖尿病通常会好转。
- SSA对葡萄糖平衡的影响仍存在争议，SSA可减少胰岛素抵抗，同时却也影响胰岛素的分泌。Calao研究证明对于既不应用SSA也不手术的患者，其葡萄糖耐量会恶化；BMI是血糖控制恶化的主要指标。
- 配位索孟治疗可降低空腹血糖水平和糖化血红蛋白水平（Barkan）。
- 肢端肥大症患者糖尿病的治疗与普通2型糖尿病的治疗类似。
- 从肢端肥大的患者其糖尿病病理角度考虑，口服促胰岛素分泌剂和/或胰岛素增敏剂是控制血糖的最好方法。
- 如果口服药物控制血糖不理想，应开始注射胰岛素。

随访
- 每6个月检测一次IGF-1水平。如果不正常，调整药物到最大量后，考虑联合治疗（SSA+多巴胺受体激动剂）。
- 术后MRI 3~4个月做MRI复查，药物治疗开始后每3~6个月做一次MRI。如果经手术已经治愈，MRI监测频率可以降低到每2~3年一次；如果疾病不能完全控制，MRI应每6~12个月一次。
- 手术或放疗后进行激素水平测试来评估前部和后部垂体功能（低下/尿崩症）。放射治疗10年之后可能发展为垂体功能缺陷。

专家意见
- 肢端肥大症是糖尿病的一种罕见的原因，特点是胰岛素抵抗。
- 通过对生长激素过剩的潜在疾病治疗，可更好地控制血糖。
- 肢端肥大症治疗（如SSAS）可能对血糖有潜在的不利影响，虽然文献对这点认识还存在争议。
- 如果经治疗后糖尿病仍存在，应根据2型糖尿病的标准治疗方案进行血糖控制。

推荐依据

Melmed S, Colao A, Barkan A, et al. Guidelines for acromegaly management: an update. J Clin Endocrinol Metab,2009; Vol. 94: pp. 1509–17.

Comments: This is an updated review of current management practices and guidelines.

Chanson P, Salenave S, Kamenicky P, et al. Pituitary tumours: acromegaly. Best Pract Res Clin Endocrinol Metab,2009; Vol. 23: pp. 555–74.

Comments: Detailed descriptions of clinical manifestations of acromegaly.

其他参考文献

Resmini E, Minuto F, Colao A, et al. Secondary diabetes associated with principal endocrinopathies: the impact of new treatment modalities. Acta Diabetol, 2009; Vol. 46: pp. 85–95.

Comments: Good review of diabetes in various endocrine conditions.

Aghi M, Blevins LS. Recent advances in the treatment of acromegaly. Curr Opin Endocrinol Diabetes Obes, 2009; Vol. 16: pp. 304–7.

Comments: Excellent review of the treatment modalities for acromegaly, particularly with respect to recurrent tumors.

Colao A, Auriemma RS, Galdiero M, et al. Impact of somatostatin analogs versus surgery on glucose metabolism in acromegaly: results of a 5-year observational, open, prospective study. J Clin Endocrinol Metab, 2009; Vol. 94: pp. 528–37.

Comments: One of very few studies looking directly at direct effects of SSAs on glucose metabolism.

Bonert V. Diagnostic challenges in acromegaly: a case-based review. Best Pract Res Clin Endocrinol Metab, 2009; Vol. 23 Suppl 1: pp. S23–30.

Comments: A case-based illustration of the diagnostic challenges of acromegaly, with emphasis on the laboratory evaluation.

Keil MF, Stratakis CA. Pituitary tumors in childhood: update of diagnosis, treatment and molecular genetics. Expert Rev Neurother, 2008; Vol. 8: pp. 563–74.

Comments: A good review of the familial pituitary tumor syndromes.

Carlsen SM, Lund-Johansen M, Schreiner T, et al. Preoperative octreotide treatment in newly diagnosed acromegalic patients with macroadenomas increases cure short-term postoperative rates: a prospective, randomized trial. J Clin Endocrinol Metab, 2008; Vol. 93: pp. 2984–90.

Comments: A recent study showing improved surgical cure rate with adjuvant medical therapy.

Barkan AL, Burman P, Clemmons DR, et al. Glucose homeostasis and safety in patients with acromegaly converted from long-acting octreotide to pegvisomant. J Clin Endocrinol Metab, 2005; Vol. 90: pp. 5684–91.

Comments: This study showed improved glucose homeostasis in acromegalic patients transitioned from octreotide to pegvisomant.

库欣综合征

Amin Sabet, MD

定义
- 长时期高浓度糖皮质激素引起的激素失调。
- 可能是由于外源性糖皮质激素（多见）或者内源性肾上腺皮质醇增多症。
- 由于分泌促肾上腺皮质激素（ACTH）垂体腺瘤引起的库欣综合征被称为库欣病。
- 过量的糖皮质激素，内源性或外源性，通过刺激糖原异生和抑制周边葡萄糖利用率（胰岛素抵抗）发挥强大的升高血糖效应。

流行病学
- 在西班牙，显性库欣综合征在一般人群中的发病率：2.4/(100万人·年)，标准化死亡率为3.8（Etxabe）。
- 隐匿Cushing在糖尿病患者中的发病率：超重、肥胖、2型糖尿病控制不佳的患者中发病率为2%~5%（Catargi）。
- 超重和2型糖尿病患者中约25%患者小剂量地塞米松抑制试验后清晨皮质醇抑制受损，但不一定是库欣综合征（Catargi）。
- 激素异常的最常见原因是肾上腺瘤患者。

诊断
- 详细询问外源性糖皮质激素（口服、外用、注射、吸入）使用史。
- CYP3A4抑制剂（特别是利托那韦）抑制糖皮质激素清除引起库欣综合征，并同时有吸入和注射类固醇的使用情况。
- 筛查：深夜唾液皮质醇浓度×2，24小时尿游离皮质醇（UFC）×2，小剂量地塞米松抑制试验（晚上11点后1毫克的地塞米松，上午8点皮质醇正常浓度为1.8 μg/L）。
- 使用不同的检查方法，至少有两次明显异常（如UFC实验有三次高于正常值）才能确立诊断。
- 皮质醇结合球蛋白浓度增加有可能使地塞米松抑制试验出现假阳性（例如，含有雌激素的口服避孕药）。
- 诊断为皮质醇增多症之后，如果血清中ACTH＜5pg/ml（1.1 pmol/L的）提示为ACTH依赖性疾病，下一步应该做肾上腺CT或者MRI检查。
- ACTH水平低或者受抑制提示非ACTH依赖性疾病：通常是肾上腺腺瘤、肾上腺癌、双侧肾上腺肥大。
- 正常或升高的ACTH提示的ACTH依赖性疾病：通常是由于垂体ACTH分泌瘤（库欣病），异位ACTH分泌肿瘤（例如支气管类癌）不常见。
- 垂体与异位促肾上腺皮质激素：垂体MRI成像（6mm，偶发瘤可能性小），高剂量8mg地塞米松测试（垂体瘤可被抑制），肾上腺皮质激素释放激素（CRH）刺激（垂体瘤更容易刺激），低血钾存在（更可能是异位内分泌），促肾上腺皮质激素升高程度（异位内分泌升高得更多），年龄（年轻患者可能异位的可能性小），岩下窦取材活检（最直接的检查）。

异位 ACTH 分泌肿瘤的检查可包括 CT、MRI、PET 或奥曲肽显像。
- 伪 Cushing 的患者：显著肥胖、糖耐量异常、严重抑郁症、酗酒的患者可能有库欣综合征非特异表现以及皮质醇轻微升高（正常值上限 1~3 倍）。

症状和体征
- 常见症状：向心性肥胖，面部充血，高血糖，高血压，情绪不稳，易青肿，月经稀少或闭经，多毛/痤疮（促肾上腺皮质激素依赖型）。
- 更特异的：宽紫纹（0.1 厘米），近端肌肉无力。
- 其他：骨质疏松，骨折，肾结石，多饮，多尿。
- 异位 ACTH：更严重的高血压，低血钾，色素沉着。
- 肾上腺癌：由于合并分泌雄激素，女性男性化（颞秃头，阴蒂增大，嗓音变粗）。
- 伪 Cushing：少有皮肤（易青肿，变薄）和肌肉（近段肌无力，肌肉萎缩）表现。

临床治疗
- 外源性库欣综合征：如果可能的话，停止激素治疗。
- 库欣病：一线治疗：经蝶骨垂体手术；二线治疗：垂体放疗；三线治疗：双侧肾上腺切除术后需要糖皮质激素和盐皮质激素终身替代治疗并监测尼尔森综合征（残余垂体腺瘤的迅速扩大）。
- 异位 ACTH：如果可能，手术切除肿瘤。不能手术切除的肿瘤，应用肾上腺酶抑制剂（如酮康唑、美替拉酮），药物性肾上腺切除（米托坦），或双侧肾上腺外科切除术。
- 非促肾上腺皮质激素依赖的肾上腺腺瘤：一般治疗是单侧肾上腺切除。
- 非 ACTH 依赖的双侧肾上腺增大：多数情况下治疗方案为双侧肾上腺切除。
- 肾上腺癌：手术可切除的应用外科手术或者米托坦治疗；进展期癌应用化疗，不可切除的疾病；皮质醇仍高的应用肾上腺酶抑制剂持续。
- 伪 Cushing 的治疗：治疗原发性疾病（例如抑郁症、糖尿病）。
- 库欣综合征的血糖控制可能与外源性激素诱导的高血糖治疗类似（见第 247 页）。

随访
- 糖皮质激素生理性替代治疗直到内源性肾上腺皮质功能恢复，这可能需要几个月时间。
- 连续监测皮质醇水平，而不是促肾上腺皮质激素水平，作为治疗的依据。
- 库欣病的手术治疗后期复发比较常见，需要长期对下丘脑 – 垂体 – 肾上腺轴进行定期评估。
- 对于库欣病患者，经有效治疗后高血糖、高血压、骨质疏松症会有所改善，但部分人这些症状仍存在。

专家意见
- 尽管不推荐对所有糖尿病患者进行库欣综合征筛查，建议有特异表现（肌病、皮薄、擦伤）或随着时间出现新的特征的患者进行筛查。

库欣综合征

- 伪库欣病患者中糖尿病比库欣综合征更常见,除了糖尿病一般治疗无须特殊处理。
- 偶发的垂体和肾上腺肿瘤在一般人群中比较常见,只有在高皮质醇血症确立之后才应该做影像检查。
- 深夜唾液皮质醇检测是一种使用广泛、易于执行、灵敏的库欣综合征的特异性筛查试验。
- 24小时尿游离皮质醇或1mg地塞米松抑制实验在提供初级保健机构是合理的替代筛检方法。
- 对于临床上疑似库欣综合征而筛选试验结果又模棱两可时,建议几个月后复查。

推荐依据

Nieman LK, Biller BM, Findling JW, et al. The diagnosis of Cushing's syndrome: an Endocrine Society Clinical Practice Guideline. J Clin Endocrinol Metab, 2008; Vol. 93: pp. 1526–40.

Comments: Most recent Endocrine Society consensus guidelines on diagnosis of Cushing's syndrome.

其他参考文献

Carroll T, Raff H, Findling JW. Late-night salivary cortisol measurement in the diagnosis of Cushing's syndrome. Nat Clin Pract Endocrinol Metab, 2008; Vol. 4: pp. 344–50.

Comments: Late night salivary cortisol testing has 92%–100% sensitivity and 93%–100% specificity for Cushing's syndrome.

Prevedello DM, Pouratian N, Sherman J, et al. Management of Cushing's disease: outcome in patients with microadenoma detected on pituitary magnetic resonance imaging. J Neurosurg, 2008; Vol. 109: pp. 751–9.

Comments: 13% of Cushing's disease patients in postoperative remission relapsed after average of 50 months.

Swearingen B, Katznelson L, Miller K, et al. Diagnostic errors after inferior petrosal sinus sampling. J Clin Endocrinol Metab, 2004; Vol. 89: pp. 3752–63.

Comments: Reported 90% sensitivity, 67% specificity, 99% positive predictive value (PPV), and 20% negative predictive value (NPV) using inferior petrosal sinus sampling after CRH for diagnosis of Cushing's disease.

Catargi B, Rigalleau V, Poussin A, et al. Occult Cushing's syndrome in type-2 diabetes. J Clin Endocrinol Metab, 2003; Vol. 88: pp. 5808–13.

Comments: Occult Cushing's syndrome seen in up to 5.5% of overweight or obese, type 2 diabetic patients.

Etxabe J, Vazquez JA. Morbidity and mortality in Cushing's disease: an epidemiological approach. Clin Endocrinol (Oxf), 1994; Vol. 40: pp. 479–84.

Comments: Established Cushing's incidence of 2.4 cases per million people per year with standardized mortality ratio of 3.8 for affected persons.

Oldfield EH, Doppman JL, Nieman LK, et al. Petrosal sinus sampling with and without corticotropin-releasing hormone for the differential diagnosis of Cushing's syndrome. NEJM, 1991; Vol. 325: pp. 897–905.

Comments: Reported 100% sensitivity and 100% specificity using inferior petrosal sinus sampling after CRH for diagnosis of Cushing's disease.

胰高血糖素瘤

Nestoras Mathioudakis, MD, and Douglas Ball, MD

定义
- 来源于胰脏 α 细胞的一种罕见肿瘤，导致胰高血糖素分泌增多。
- 轻度糖尿病是胰高血糖素瘤的典型特征。
- 高血糖症是胰高血糖素和胰岛素：胰高血糖素比例降低导致肝糖原分解和糖原异生的结果。

流行病学
- 胰高血糖素瘤发病率：13.5/2 千万人（Echenique-Elizondo）。
- 胰高血糖素瘤极为罕见，占所有胰腺内分泌肿瘤的 7%（Kindmark）。
- 此肿瘤对男性和女性影响相同。
- 大多数肿瘤（80%）是偶发的，剩余 20% 与多发内分泌肿瘤 1 型（MEN-1 综合征（垂体、胰岛细胞瘤、甲状旁腺肿瘤）有关。
- 发病年龄特征为 40~50 岁。
- 大多数胰高血糖素瘤（75%）是恶性的，确诊时已经转移。
- 胰高血糖素瘤患者中糖尿病患病率：38%~94%（Chastain）。
- 一般来说，糖尿病是轻度至中度，平均 HbA1c 9.8%（Wermers）。

诊断
- 坏死松解性游走性红斑（NME）：与胰高血糖素有关的特征性皮疹通常作为诊断的唯一线索。皮肤活检诊断 NME：病灶边缘是浅表性坏死、外皮层分离、血管周围淋巴细胞和组织细胞浸润（Chastain）。也可见于其他疾病。
- 如果考虑为此病，测量胰高血糖素。胰高血糖素 500pg/ml 强烈提示提示该病，1 000 则可确立诊断。
- 中度升高的胰高血糖素水平见于低血糖，空腹，败血症，肾衰竭或肝衰竭，急性胰腺炎。轻度胰高血糖素升高见于胰腺神经内分泌肿瘤（Zollinger-Ellison 症候群、胰岛素瘤、类癌）。
- 非特异表现：正常色素、正常细胞性贫血，低氨基酸血症（因氨基酸氧化和糖异生）。
- 如果患者有典型的临床表现和/或胰高血糖素水平升高，然后对胰脏进行影像学检查，首选腹部增强 CT 扫描胰腺肿瘤。不同于胰岛素瘤，高胰岛素瘤大多在确诊时已经很大并且在局部。
- 检测肿瘤大小 CT 无法检查出来的应用内镜超声（EUS，2~3mm 大小的肿瘤超声内镜都可检查到）。
- 超声内镜细针穿刺活检可确立诊断，通过免疫组织化学染色病理显示为胰高血糖素阳性的胰岛细胞瘤。
- 虽然奥曲肽扫描的诊断灵敏度很高，但由于大多胰高血糖素瘤都非常大，CT 就能很容易检测到，所以这个检查通常没必要做。

胰高血糖素瘤

- 肝脏病变提示转移瘤，应在 CT 引导下进行活检。

症状和体征

- 4DS：皮炎，糖尿病，深静脉血栓，抑郁症。
- 症状：消瘦，多尿，烦渴，腹痛，腹泻，便秘，情绪低落。
- 体征：口角炎，舌炎，口腔炎，眼睑炎，头发稀疏，指甲营养不良，贫血，共济失调，视神经萎缩，近端肌无力，老年痴呆症，抑郁症。
- NME 皮疹：红色丘疹或斑块，通常先出现在腹股沟和会阴处，然后延伸到臀部、四肢和脸部。1~2 个星期之后皮疹扩大融合，留下水疱，银屑病样病变，中央消退，皮损处瘙痒难忍。
- 与静脉血栓相关的症状：疼痛，肿胀，压痛，红肿/患肢皮肤颜色改变，浅表静脉可见。
- 扩张型心肌病（罕见）。

治疗

手术治疗

- 在诊断时以疾病的发展程度而定。最常见的转移：肝、区域淋巴结、骨、肾上腺、肾、肺。如果肿瘤局限在胰脏，胰腺切除术（简单摘除术，局灶性切除，Whipple）很有效，但只有 30% 的患者可以治愈（Morgan）。
- 对于奥曲肽扫描阳性、高胰高血糖素血症的转移性肿瘤，可选方案包括手术切除肝转移瘤，肝动脉栓塞化疗，射频或冷冻治疗，肝移植。

药物治疗

- 生长抑素类似物（如奥曲肽）可有效控制症状。奥曲肽皮下注射起始剂量 50 μg，每日 3 次，逐渐增加剂量控制症状（腹泻、NME、神经症状），然后过渡到长效制剂（Sandostatin LAR）。
- 对于肝外转移，可考虑全身化疗（链霉素、阿霉素），尽管反应率低（Chastain）。
- 干扰素（IFNa 的）对少数患者可能会有生化、放射学、临床疗效（Kindmark），由于疗效不确定和不良反应，所有使用受限。
- 由于支持长期高代谢状态导致的营养不良，所以需要营养支持，完全肠外营养、肠内营养或营养补充剂均可供选择。对于 NME，输注氨基酸和脂肪酸可能有效。
- 放射治疗可能会使症状减轻，无手术适应证的患者。。
- 糖尿病通常是轻度的，通过饮食、口服降糖药、胰岛素很容易控制。由于 β-细胞仍有功能，胰岛素分泌正常，所以糖尿病酮症酸中毒少见。
- 治疗潜在疾病是糖尿病血糖控制的最好方法（如肿瘤切除术）。
- 对于不能治愈的转移瘤患者，按照 2 型糖尿病标准治疗方案治疗高血糖。

随访

- 每年测量胰高血糖素和其他胃肠激素（如胃泌素）持续终身，可以早期发现复发和继发的内分泌失调，如 Zollinger-Ellison 综合征（可能会多年后发生）。
- 在确定 MEN 综合征时定期评估其他内分泌肿瘤的发展情况。

- 监测糖尿病的典型并发症（视网膜病变、蛋白尿、神经病变），通过治疗使血脂和血压达标。

专家意见
- 胰高血糖素是一种极为罕见的糖尿病的病因，诊断需要高度怀疑。
- 有糖尿病、体重下降和 NME 的典型皮疹的患者，应引起重视。
- 胰高血糖素患者的糖尿病症较轻但是比较普遍。
- 治疗潜在的胰高血糖素过多是控制血糖的最好办法，但是，如果没有成功，可以通过饮食，口服药物或胰岛素（很少）治疗。

推荐依据

Kindmark H, Sundin A, Granberg D, et al. Endocrine pancreatic tumors with glucagon hypersecretion: a retrospectivestudy of 23 cases during 20 years. Med Oncol, 2007; Vol. 24: pp. 330–7.
Comments: A more recent series of glucagonoma patients showing slightly lower prevalence of diabetes in this population than previously described.

Chastain MA. The glucagonoma syndrome: a review of its features and discussion of new perspectives. Am J Med Sci, 2001; Vol. 321: pp. 306–20.
Comments: An excellent clinically oriented review of the glucagonoma syndrome, with comprehensive differential diagnoses of both the NME rash and hyperglucagonemia in general.

Wermers RA, Fatourechi V, Wynne AG, et al. The glucagonoma syndrome. Clinical and pathologic features in 21 patients. Medicine (Baltimore), 1996; Vol. 75: pp. 53–63.
Comments: One of a few case series of glucagonoma patients.

其他参考文献

McGevna L, Tavakkol Z. Images in clinical medicine. Necrolytic migratory erythema NEJM, 2010; Vol. 362: p. e1.
Comments: Good images of NEM.

Morgan KA, Adams DB. Solid tumors of the body and tail of the pancreas. Surg Clin North Am, 2010; Vol. 90: pp. 287–307.
Comments: A good review on the surgical aspects of both endocrine and nonendocrine pancreatic tumors.

Fanelli CG, Porcellati F, Rossetti P, et al. Glucagon: the effects of its excess and deficiency on insulin action. Nutr Metab Cardiovasc Dis, 2006; Vol. 16 Suppl 1: pp. S28–34.
Comments: A good review of the physiologic relationship between glucagon and insulin, and of the pathophysiology of glucagon excess in glucagonoma and other metabolic conditions.

Echenique-Elizondo M, Tuneu Valls A, Elorza Orúe JL, et al. Glucagonoma and pseudoglucagonoma syndrome. JOP, 2004; Vol. 5: pp. 179–85.
Comments: A retrospective review showing a slightly higher prevalence o glucagonoma than previously reported. van Beek AP, de Haas ER,

Van Vloten WA, et al. The glucagonoma syndrome and necrolytic migratory erythema: a clinical review. Eur J Endocrinol, 2004; Vol. 151: pp. 531–7.
Comments: Good review of the pathophysiology of glucagonoma and the typica

rash of NEM. Also includes photo images of clinical features.

Oberg K, Kvols L, Caplin M, et al. Consensus report on the use of somatostatin analogs for the management of neuroendocrine tumors of the gastroenteropancreatic system. Ann Oncol, 2004; Vol. 15: pp. 966–73.

Comments: Excellent review of the mechanism of action, indications, and uses of somatostatin analogues in the management of neuroendocrine tumors. The review is not limited specifically to glucagonomas.

胰岛素瘤

Ana Emiliano, MD, and Douglas Ball, MD

定义
- 一种自主分泌胰岛素的胰腺神经内分泌肿瘤。
- 无限制的胰岛素分泌,导致肝糖原输出减少和低血糖(Rizza)。
- 高胰岛素性低血糖的内源性原因。

流行病学
- 罕见的肿瘤,发病率4/(100万人·年)。
- 一般都是孤立的、良性、有包膜的(约87%)。
- 可能起源于胰腺的任何位置,但很少起源于胰腺外(转移性肿瘤除外)。
- 10%是恶性的,恶性定义为出现转移、主要存在于肝脏和淋巴结,有时骨和腹膜组织。
- 在梅奥诊所20年中,所有胰岛素瘤患者年龄的中位数是50岁,范围是17~89岁(Placzkowski)。
- 各个种族均可发生此病。
- 90%病例是散发的。
- 6%~10%的病例为多发性内分泌肿瘤1型(MEN-1)或者或von-Hippel Lindau综合征(VHL)的一部分。
- MEN-1是一种常染色体显性遗传综合征,特点为原发性甲状旁腺功能亢进症、垂体前叶腺瘤和胃肠道胰脏神经内分泌肿瘤。约10% MEN-1患者会发生胰岛素瘤,MEN-1中最常见的诊断是胃肠道-胰腺神经内分泌肿瘤以及促胃液素瘤。90%胰岛素瘤是良性的,但通常是多发的,而非散发。
- VHL病是一种常染色体显性遗传综合征,包括中枢神经系统(CNS)、视网膜瘤、嗜铬细胞瘤、胰岛细胞瘤、肾细胞癌。与胰岛素瘤相关的VHL一般都是恶性的。

诊断
- Whipple's三联征:由低血糖引起的神经精神症状,发作时血糖低于60mg/dl,纠正低血糖之后症状缓解。
- 在低血糖(PG<60mg/L)时,血浆胰岛素水平升高(>3μU/ml)(Cryer)
- 此外低血糖的同时伴随血浆C肽水平升高(>0.6ng/ml),血浆胰岛素原水平升高(>5pmol/L的)和血浆β羟丁酸盐水平下降(<2.7mmol/L)提示内源性高胰岛素血症(Cryer)。
- 对于没有高胰岛素性低血糖记录的门诊患者,建议进行72小时空腹监测(具体说明,请参阅表3-7)。97%的胰岛素瘤患者在48~72小时内会发生低血糖症以及由此引起的神经精神症状(Hirschberg)。
- 排除低血糖假象:筛查尿中的磺脲类物质。测量血浆C-肽水平:如果胰岛素水平升高和低血糖的同时,C肽水平被抑制,提示有外源性的胰岛素注射。
- 高胰岛素性低血糖的其他原因：婴儿期的高胰岛素血症，倾倒综合征，胰岛素自身免疫综合征，等等。
- 临床症状和生化检查诊断为可疑胰岛素瘤的患者，应用超声、CT、介入放射学诊断胰脏肿瘤。
- 腹部超声和CT的检测率约70%（Mathur，Boukhman）。
- 内镜超声的敏感性因操作者而异40%~93%（Anderson;Nikfarjam）。
- 选择性动脉钙刺激试验，肝静脉采样（基于钙是胰岛素分泌的促分泌素）的敏感性约80%~94%（guettier;Mathur）。

表 3-7. 72小时快速监督

1. 记录患者最后一餐的时间。
2. 每小时用血糖仪监测血糖。
3. 血糖大于60mg/dl之前每6小时采一次血样，小于60mg/dl之后每1~2小时采集一次血样。
4. 把每次采样时间和血样送去检验（检验项目见表3-8）。
5. 血糖低于45mg/dl出现低血糖症状时应停止空腹。
6. 终止空腹时注射1mg葡萄糖，分别在10、20、30分钟后监测血糖浓度，血糖增加大于25mg/dl，提示胰岛素瘤，因为在空腹期间胰岛素不恰当地抑制了肝糖原分解，胰高血糖素则相反。

来源：Ana Emiliano and Douglas Ball 提供。

表 3-8. 实验结果解读：生化检验/胰岛素瘤的确认

生化指标	胰岛素瘤诊断值
血浆葡萄糖	<55mg/dl
胰岛素	> 3 μU/ml*
C-肽	>0.6ng/ml
胰岛素原	>5pmol/L
β 羟丁酸盐	<2.7mmol/L

* 使用 immunochemiluminescent 检测时
来源：Ana Emiliano and Douglas Ball 提供。

症状和体征

- 胰岛素瘤患者临床表现为空腹低血糖（<70mg/dl）（Service）。
- 约有6%的胰岛素，通常是男性，表现餐后低血糖（Placzkowski）。
- 约20%的胰岛素瘤患者表现为空腹低血糖和餐后低血糖。
- 经常出现低血糖症状提示神经源性低血糖以及肾上腺病态综合征。
- 转移性疾病，尤其是肝脏，可导致严重的、顽固性低血糖。
- 胰岛素瘤患者可能出现食欲及体重增加（Nikfarjam）。
- 估计有20%胰岛素瘤患者被误诊为精神或神经系统疾病。

临床治疗

手术治疗

- 胰岛素瘤切除术是治疗选择之一。
- 对83%~98%的患者在术中进行超声检查和胰腺触诊。
- 远端胰腺切除术，胰腺摘除术，胰十二指肠切除术最常见的术式（Nikfarjam）。
- 肿瘤切除通常可以治愈，因为大多数胰岛素瘤是良性的（Boukhman）。
- 对于小的、孤立的胰岛素瘤可采用腹腔镜手术。
- 对于可切除的肝转移，建议手术切除的转移灶和原发病灶。
- 对于不能手术切除的肝脏转移性肿瘤，治疗方案包括：化疗栓塞术、射频消融和冷冻。

药物治疗

- 指征：(1)由于无法切除的转移病灶导致严重，危及生命的低血糖；(2)不能进行手术的患者；(3)手术时不能确定为胰岛素瘤。
- 膳食富含碳水化合物是所有药物治疗的基础。
- 二氮嗪是一线药物，通过抑制胰岛素释放和刺激α-肾上腺受体发挥作用，初始剂量：150~200毫克，分2~3次给药，最大剂量每日1 200mg。
- 奥曲肽，生长抑素类似物，抑制胰岛素的分泌。临床效应取决于胰岛素瘤中生长抑素-2受体的密度，这个存在很大变异。
- 维拉帕米、普萘洛尔、苯妥英钠、胰高血糖素和糖皮质激素也用于缓解症状。
- 具体控制症状和不良反应请参阅表3-9。

胰岛素瘤

表 3-9 低血糖症状的药物治疗

药物	分类	症状控制	不良反应
二氮嗪	α-肾上腺受体拮抗剂	50%~60%	外周性水肿，恶心，多毛症
奥曲肽	生长抑素类似物	40%~60%	肿胀，腹部绞痛，营养吸收障碍，胆石病
维拉帕米	钙通道拮抗剂	未知	便秘，外周水肿，恶心
心得安	β受体阻滞剂	未知	心动过缓，抑郁，可能会加重低血糖症状
苯妥英钠	抗惊厥药	未知	多毛，齿龈肿胀，外周神经病变
胰高血糖素	胰高血糖素	减轻	低血糖反弹

来源：Ana Emiliano and Douglas Ball 提供。

随访

- 约6%的患者在初次手术后的6个月内复发低血糖症状，建议使病灶局限化和再次手术。
- 对于散发胰岛素瘤，在10年、20年的复发率分别为5%和7%（Service）。
- 对于 MEN-1 患者复发率较高：10年、20年复发率为20%（服务）。
- 在4年内复发的通常是由于未完全切除肿瘤的再生。
- 良性胰岛素瘤预后较好（Nikfarjam）。恶性胰岛素瘤患者的5年生存率为25%~35%。
- 恶性胰岛素瘤的随访包括密切监测病史、体格检查、神经内分泌肿瘤标志物（胰岛素、嗜铬素A）、首次切除3个月和6个月时进行影像学检查，之后每6~12个月做一次，至少持续3年。

专家意见

- 出现低血糖时应考虑胰岛素瘤，尤其是不明原因的空腹低血糖且内源性胰岛素水平升高（有别于糖尿病患者外源性胰岛素升高）。
- 医疗相关检验，有时也包括空腹监测，是诊断胰岛素瘤的重要环节。
- 定位或者手术前确定高胰岛素性低血糖。
- 进行高胰岛素性低血糖的生化检查以及术前肿瘤定位，避免盲目胰脏探查。
- 由有经验的外科医生小心切除肿瘤及包膜，防止局部复发。
- 由于胰岛素瘤可发生在整个胰腺，盲目胰腺部分切除术是不可取的。
- 对于不能手术切除的肝转移灶进行肝脏移植，目前经验有限，生存益处还存有问题。
- 传统的细胞毒作用化疗药对于恶性胰岛素瘤的疗效还不确切。新的疗法正在研究中，如小分子酪氨酸激酶抑制剂和以哺乳动物为抑制靶点的雷帕霉素（mTOR）。

- 根据胰腺切除程度的不同，胰岛素瘤切除术极少导致糖尿病（见胰腺切除术后糖尿病，第 95 页）。

推荐依据

Cryer PE, Axelrod L, Grossman AB, et al. Evaluation and management of adult hypoglycemic disorders: an Endocrine Society Clinical Practice Guideline. J Clin Endocrinol Metab, 2009; Vol. 94: pp. 709–28.

Comments: Expert Endocrine Society consensus on the evaluation and management of hypoglycemic disorders in adults.Chastain MA. The glucagonoma syndrome: a review of its features and discussion of new perspectives. Am J Med Sci, 2001; Vol. 321: pp. 306–20.

其他参考文献

Placzkowski KA, Vella A, Thompson GB, et al. Secular trends in the presentation and management of functioning insulinoma at the Mayo Clinic, 1987–2007. J Clin Endocrinol Metab, 2009; Vol. 94: pp. 1069–73.

Comments: A retrospective analysis of 237 insulinoma cases seen at the Mayo Clinic from 1987 through 2007, with an emphasis on the clinical presentation and trends in diagnostic and radiological evaluation during the 20-year period covered by the study.

Guettier JM, Kam A, Chang R, et al. Localization of insulinomas to regions of the pancreas by intraarterial calcium stimulation: the NIH experience. J Clin Endocrinol Metab, 2009; Vol. 94: pp. 1074–80.

Comments: Retrospective study assessing the accuracy of calcium stimulation in the preoperative localization of insulinoma in 45 patients, concluding that calcium stimulation was vastly superior to abdominal ultrasound, CT, or MRI.

Mathur A, Gorden P, Libutti SK. Insulinoma. Surg Clin North Am, 2009; Vol. 89: pp. 1105–21.

Comments: Comprehensive review of the clinical presentation, diagnosis radiographic evaluation, and medical and surgical treatment of insulinoma.

Nikfarjam M, Warshaw AL, Axelrod L, et al. Improved contemporary surgical management of insulinomas: a 25-year experience at the Massachusetts General Hospital. Ann Surg, 2008; Vol. 247: pp. 165–72.

Comments: Retrospective review of 61 patients with sporadic and MEN-1 associated insulinoma between 1983–2007, with a description of demographics, presentation, and diagnostic workup, including an assessment of the use of endoscopic ultrasound in the preoperative evaluation.

Hirshberg B, Livi A, Bartlett DL, et al. Forty-eight-hour fast: the diagnostic test for insulinoma. J Clin Endocrinol Metab, 2000; Vol. 85: pp. 3222–6.

Comments: This study showed that 94.5% of 127 patients with insulinoma developed fasting hypoglycemia within 48 hours of a supervised fast, underscoring the unusual need for a complete 72-hour fast to diagnose insulinoma.

Anderson MA, Carpenter S, Thompson NW, et al. Endoscopic ultrasound is highly accurate and directs management in patients with neuroendocrine tumors of the pancreas. Am J Gastroenterol, 2000; Vol. 95: pp. 2271–7.

Comments: A single center experience utilizing preoperative endoscopic ultrasound evaluation of 82 patients with pancreatic neuroendocrine tumors, showing that endoscopic ultrasound reached a sensitivity of approximately 93%.

Boukhman MP, Karam JH, Shaver J, et al. Insulinoma—experience from 1950 to 1995. West J Med, 1998; Vol. 169: pp. 98–104.

Comments: Retrospective review of 67 patients with sporadic and MEN-1 associated insulinoma treated at the University of California, San Francisco from 1950–1995, looking at presentation, diagnosis, localization studies, and medical and surgical treatment.

Service FJ, McMahon MM, O'Brien PC, et al. Functioning insulinoma—incidence, recurrence, and long-term survival of patients: a 60-year study. Mayo Clin Proc, 1991; Vol. 66: pp. 711–9.

Comments: An epidemiologic profile of insulinoma based on 224 confirmed cases seen at the Mayo Clinic from 1927 through 1986.

Demeure MJ, Klonoff DC, Karam JH, et al. Insulinomas associated with multiple endocrine neoplasia type I: the need for a different surgical approach. Surgery, 1991; Vol. 110: pp. 998–1004, discussion 1004-5.

Comments: A retrospective analysis of seven patients with insulinoma associated with MEN-1 syndrome seen at the University of California, San Francisco and a review of 53 cases reported in the English literature.

Rizza RA, Haymond MW, Verdonk CA, et al. Pathogenesis of hypoglycemia in insulinoma patients: suppression of hepatic glucose production by insulin. Diabetes, 1981; Vol. 30: pp. 377–81.

Comments: In patients with insulinoma, fasting hypoglycemia is due to suppression of glucose production rather than to acceleration of glucose utilization.

施密特综合征

Amin Sabet, MD

定义

- 施密特综合征是指自身免疫性肾上腺皮质功能不全（阿狄森氏病）与自身免疫性甲状腺功能减退和/或1型糖尿病（T1DM），是自身免疫性多个内分泌腺体综合征II型或多个腺体自身免疫综合征II型（PAS II）的一部分。
- 施密特综合征有时可以用来指PAS II。
- PASII是一种多基因疾病，其中可能包括自身免疫性甲状腺疾病（甲状腺功能低下或甲状腺功能亢进症），1型糖尿病、阿狄森氏病、原发性性腺功能低下和不太常见的甲状旁腺功能低下症或垂体功能低下。
- 也可能出现与自身免疫性疾病有关的疾病，包括特发性白癜风、腹腔疾病、脱发、恶性贫血、重症肌无力、血小板减少性紫癜、干燥综合征、类风湿关节炎。

流行病学

- 施密特综合征在一般人群中的患病率1:20 000，女性与男性的比例为3:1（Förste）。
- 发病的高峰期：30~40岁。
- 有家族聚集倾向，多个家庭成员受累。
- 可能是与某些HLA抗原（Eisenbarth）变异有关的常染色体显性遗传。
- 1型糖尿病患者中1%的患者有阿狄森氏病，2%~5%有自身免疫性甲状腺疾病（主要是甲状腺功能减退）和有腹腔病的占5%以上（Förste）。
- 1型糖尿病患者发展成自身免疫性甲状腺疾病的时间间隔为13.3 +/−11.8年。

诊断

- PASII中任何一个病症的诊断与相应的独立疾病诊断相同。
- T1DM和腹腔疾病的诊断参见别处（第6页的糖尿病的诊断与分型，第275页的乳糜泻与1型糖尿病）。
- 阿狄森氏病的诊断（自身免疫性肾上腺炎症导致的原发性肾上腺功能不全）是基于以下几点：（1）清晨（即7~9点）血清皮质醇 <3mcg/dl 或静脉推注1mcg或250mcg的促肾上腺皮质激素（ACTH），30~60分钟后血清皮质醇低于18mcg/dl；（2）血清促肾上腺皮质激素水平基础值升高；（3）其他自身免疫性疾病的存在。21−羟化酶抗体有助于诊断，推荐进行腹部CT检查可评估肾上腺皮质功能不全的其他原因（感染、出血、转移性疾病）。
- 原发性甲状腺功能减退症的诊断依据血清TSH升高和血清T4水平降低（亚临床状态下可正常），而甲状腺功能亢进症的诊断依据是TSH升高，血清T4和/或T3升高（亚临床状态下可正，抗甲状腺抗体（例如，抗甲状腺球蛋白抗体，抗微粒体的抗体，甲状腺刺激免疫球蛋白）有助于诊断。

施密特综合征

症状和体征

- 合并1型糖尿病和阿狄森氏病的患者，可能会间歇性重度低血糖和严重的疲劳，也可能出现胰岛素需求量减少，低血压，色素沉着，白癜风。
- 甲状腺功能减退症也可能出现疲劳，胰岛素需求量降低和低血糖，而甲状腺功能亢进症与胰岛素需求量增加和高血糖相关。
- 也可能会有与自身免疫性疾病相关的症状和体征（如脱发，乳糜泻）。

临床治疗

- PASII中任何一个病症的治疗与该独立病症的治疗相同。
- 原发性甲状腺功能减退症治疗：用左甲状腺素片进行生理的甲状腺激素替代治疗。典型的初始剂量是每天1.6mcg/kg（老人和心脏病患者需降低剂量），每4~6周根据血清T4和TSH调整剂量。
- 阿狄森氏病的长期治疗：糖皮质激素和盐皮质激素替代疗法，初始糖皮质激素治疗时可以用氢化可的松每天15~25mg，分2~3次给药，调整剂量以缓解糖皮质激素不足引起症状并避免糖皮质激素过多。盐皮质激素最初的方案是氟氢可的松0.1mg/d，根据需要调整剂量，避免体位性低血压并维持血钾正常。
- 阿狄森氏病的治疗期间，如有急性疾病或手术则需要根据机体状况增加糖皮质激素治疗剂量。

随访

- 抗体筛查可能有助于发现发展为自身免疫性腺体衰竭的高危患者，例如，在艾迪森患者中出现GAD65抗体可能提示发展为T1DM的风险增加，而合并T1DM的患者中21-羟化酶抗体可能提示发展为艾迪森的风险增加。然而，抗体筛查缺乏循证医学证据。

专家意见

- 建议对T1DM患者每当有症状和/或每1~2年进行甲状腺功能减退（通过测血清TSH）和腹腔疾病筛查（通过测组织转谷氨酰胺酶抗体）。
- 在没有症状的情况下，不建议常规筛查阿狄森氏病或其他与PASII有关的自身免疫性疾病。
- 注意：同时患有甲状腺功能减退症和阿狄森氏病的患者，如只是给予甲状腺素而没有糖皮质激素可诱发急性肾上腺皮质功能不全。

推荐依据

Kahaly GJ. Polyglandular autoimmune syndromes. Eur J Endocrinol, 2009; Vol. 161: pp. 11–20.
   Comments: Provides review of the pathophysiology and role of genetic testing in PAS.

Owen CJ, Cheetham TD. Diagnosis and management of polyendocrinopathy syndromes. Endocrinol Metab Clin North Am, 2009; Vol. 38: pp. 419–36, x.
   Comments: Reviews diagnosis and management of polyendocrinopathy syndromes.

Dittmar M, Kahaly GJ. Polyglandular autoimmune syndromes: immunogenetics and long-term follow-up. J Clin Endocrinol Metab, 2003; Vol. 88: pp. 2983–92.

Comments: Type 1 diabetes patients who developed autoimmune thyroid disease had an interval of 13.3 +/-11.8 years between first and second endocrinopathies.

Förster G, Krummenauer F, Kühn I, et al. Polyglandular autoimmune syndrome type II: epidemiology and forms of manifestation. Dtsch Med Wochenschr, 1999; Vol. 124: pp. 1476–81.
Comments: Reviews epidemiology of PAS II.

Eisenbarth G, Wilson P, Ward F, et al. HLA type and occurrence of disease in familial polyglandular failure. NEJM, 1978; Vol. 298: pp. 92–4.
Comments: Association of HLA antigens with PAS.

生长抑制素瘤

Amin Sabet, MD

定义
- 罕见的分泌生长激素抑制素的肿瘤,主要来源于胰腺和十二指肠。
- 与糖尿病有关,因为生长抑素升高会抑制胰岛素分泌。

流行病学
- 占胰岛细胞瘤的 1%~2%(He)。
- 确诊时,年龄的中位数为 50 岁(范围 26~84 岁),性别分布没有差异。
- 大于 50% 发生在胰腺,其中三分之二是在胰头。
- 胰腺外生长抑素瘤大部分起源于十二指肠,原发病灶极少出现在肝脏,结肠或直肠。
- 大多数为散发的,但少数与 MEN – 1 综合征相关。
- 起源于十二指肠生长抑素瘤与神经纤维瘤 1 型(NF –1)或者冯雷克林豪森病相关。
- 生长抑素瘤大多数都是恶性的,在确诊已经发生转移。
- 大多数胰腺肿瘤会导致糖尿病。
- 10% 肿瘤来源于肠道。
- 在一组病例中,36% 的生长抑素瘤患者会发生糖尿病(6 例来源于胰腺癌,5 例来源于十二指肠)(Moayedoddin)。

诊断
- 经常在腹痛、体重减轻、黄疸的患者中发现此病。也可能在一次偶然的影像学检查时发现生长抑素瘤(86% 发生在胰腺、41% 胰腺外,肿瘤大于 2 厘米),或在与本病无关的一个手术中发现。
- 如果临床上怀疑此病,但是诊断不明确的,可术前禁食,生长抑素水平 < 160pg/ml (正常范围为 10~22pg/ml)提示为生长抑素瘤。
- 影像学检查可以是结构性的(内镜超声、CT、MRI)或功能性的(奥曲肽扫描)。

症状和体征
- 最常见的症状都是非特异性的:体重减轻和腹痛。
- 可能会出现经典的三联征(生长抑素瘤综合征):糖尿病(胰岛素释放减少),胆石症(缩胆囊素释放减少,胆囊的收缩减少),腹泻与脂肪泻(抑制胰酶和碳酸氢盐分泌,引起肠道对脂类的吸收减少)。
- 经典三联征可能只发生在约 10% 的患者,在胰腺肿瘤中更为常见。
- 起源于十二指肠的生长抑素瘤很少会有经典的三联征,可能会出现梗阻性症状包括疼痛及黄疸。
- 糖尿病程度可以从葡萄糖耐受性轻度降低(比较常见)到酮症酸中毒(Jackson)。

- 有的病例会出现低血糖症状，有报道指出是由于抑制胰高血糖素和生长激素，此种情况极罕见。

临床治疗

手术治疗
- 治疗方案之一是手术切除，这是唯一可能治愈的治疗方法。
- 手术切除原发主要病灶可改善已有转移灶的患者的症状。

药物治疗
- 对于不能手术切除的患者，服用生长抑素类似物奥曲肽可降低血浆生长抑素水平、改善腹泻、高血糖和体重下降症状。
- α-干扰素治疗可以缓解50%以上的患者胰脏生长抑素瘤患者的症状，尽管肿瘤反应率很低（Schöber；Bajetta）。
- 对肝脏转移灶进行化疗栓塞可改善已发生转移的生长抑素瘤者的症状。
- 对已经发生转移的胰腺生长抑素瘤患者进行全身化疗的疗效不理想，尽管已有报道指出链佐和替莫唑胺为基础的治疗方案（Kouvaraki； Kulke）。
- 高血糖治疗与糖尿病的其他形式相同；此外，奥曲肽治疗可改善高血糖症状。

随访
- 建议手术切除后的3个月和6个月时，进行病史回顾，体格检查，影像学检查（CT/MRI），空腹生长抑素水平检测。
- 此后，建议每隔6~12个月进行一次临床、生化检查、影像学检查，为临床提供参考。
- 在44个转移性生长抑素瘤患者中，5年生存率为60%（Soga）。
- 手术治疗（如胰腺切除术）胰脏生长抑素瘤可能会发展为糖尿病，应定期监测血糖水平。

专家建议
- 与其他原因引起的继发性糖尿病相比（如肢端肥大症，Cushing的综合征），这些与胰岛素抵抗有关，而生长抑素瘤与胰岛素释放抑制有关，这可能会影响降低血糖药物的选择。
- 糖尿病通常程度较轻，发生于胰腺的生长抑素瘤更常见。
- 胰腺切除术可能会导致糖尿病的发展。

推荐依据

He X, Wang J, Wu X, et al. Pancreatic somatostatinoma manifested as severe hypoglycemia. J Gastrointestin Liver Dis, 2009; Vol. 18: pp. 221–4.
Comments: Unusual hypoglycemic presentation of somatostatinoma.

Kulke MH, Stuart K, Enzinger PC, et al. Phase II study of temozolomide and thalidomide in patients with metastatic neuroendocrine tumors. J Clin Oncol, 2006; Vol. 24: pp. 401–6.
Comments: 25% objective radiologic response rate with temozolomide/thalidomide treatment of metastatic NETs.

Moayedoddin B, Booya F, Wermers RA, et al. Spectrum of malignant somatostatin-producing neuroendocrine tumors. Endocr Pract, 2006; Vol. 12: pp. 394–400.

Comments: Diabetes occurred in 36% of patients with somatostatinoma (5 duodenal, 6 pancreatic) in this case series.

Kouvaraki MA, Ajani JA, Hoff P, et al. Fluorouracil, doxorubicin, and streptozocin in the treatment of patients with locally advanced and metastatic pancreatic endocrine carcinomas. J Clin Oncol, 2004; Vol. 22: pp. 4762–71.

Comments: 39% objective radiologic response rate with streptozocin/5-FU/doxorubicin treatment of locally advanced and metastatic pancreatic NETs.

Soga J, Yakuwa Y. Somatostatinoma/inhibitory syndrome: a statistical evaluation of 173 reported cases as compared to other pancreatic endocrinomas. J Exp Clin Cancer Res, 1999; Vol. 18: pp. 13–22.

Comments: Among 173 reported cases of somatostatinoma (83 pancreatic and 92 extrapancreatic), 5-year survival was 59.9% in patients with metastases and 100% in patients without metastases.

女性疾病

绝经期对高血糖的影响

Melissa Yates, MD, and Wanda K. Nicholson, MD, MPH, MBA

定义
- 绝经期：停经连续 12 个月（Carr）。
- 手术绝经期：先前有月经的患者，双侧卵巢都被手术移除后开始算起。

流行病学
- 糖尿病是绝经期后最常见的疾病（Wedisinghe）。
- 2 型糖尿病患者逐步增多导致绝经期后妇女中糖尿病发病率上升。65 岁以上妇女中约 20% 患有糖尿病（Shih）。
- 绝经导致的代谢改变可能与糖尿病的进展相关：向心性肥胖加重、低密度脂蛋白增高以及胰岛素抵抗加重（Shih）。
- 绝经期后胰岛素抵抗加重而胰岛素分泌相对稳定，这导致 2 型糖尿病的患病风险增加（Wedisinghe）。
- 内源性性激素包括增高的生物相容性睾丸酮、雌二醇以及降低的性激素结合球蛋白与绝经期后女性中糖尿病发病相关，这些激素变化可能与更高的肥胖率以及胰岛素抵抗有关（Kalyani）。
- 绝经期后女性代谢综合征的发生率增加了 60%（Carr）。
- 患有 1 型糖尿病的女性，其发生早闭经的概率更高，平均在 41.6 岁时发生，而未患有糖尿病的女性其绝经期平均在 51 岁（Dorman）。
- 与未患有糖尿病的绝经后女性相比，患有 1 型糖尿病的女性在绝经后髋骨骨折的相对危险系数为 12.25，2 型糖尿病者则为 1.70（Nicodemus）。

症状和体征
- 患有糖尿病的女性，其发生绝经期潮热以及阴道干燥的比率高于不患有糖尿病的女性。
- 停经前，由于内源性性激素的变化，其血糖波动也将增大（Shih）。

临床治疗
- 由于停经后心血管病（CVD）风险升高，应鼓励绝经后妇女控制 CVD 危险因素（Carr）。
- 相对于单纯的绝经的影响，体重增加对糖尿病风险的影响更大（Carr）。
- 激素替代治疗（HRT）有益于大于 60 岁的无已知心血管疾病的症状明显的糖尿病患者。对这一女性群体，建议采取最低有效剂量（Wedisinghe）。
- 由于剂量以及治疗策略的不同，外源性 HRT 对血糖的影响有好有坏（Lindheim；Cagnacci）。
- 由于女性糖尿病患者发生子宫内膜癌的风险提高，如果子宫尚完好的话，建议联合使用雌激素以及孕酮治疗（Wedisinghe）。

- 对于有症状的阴道干燥，建议日常局部应用雷波仑并考虑原位雌激素治疗如 Vagifem 或者 Estring，后两者可使全身性雌激素吸收减少。
- 对于 CVD 或者其他的危险因素，建议使用非激素治疗方法，如文拉法辛和加巴喷丁，对潮热症可使用可乐定，对骨质疏松症可使用维生素 D、钙剂以及二磷酸盐（wedisinghe）。

随访
- 鉴于患有糖尿病的绝经后女性骨质疏松症的发生风险提高，可考虑使用双光子骨密度仪进行骨密度筛查。

专家意见
- 任何绝经期后或者开始使用 HRT 后发生的阴道出血均应寻求妇产科医生的全面评估。

参考文献

Wedisinghe L, Perera M. Diabetes and the menopause. Maturitas, 2009; Vol. 63: pp. 200–3.
Comments: Review of the management of menopausal symptoms in the setting of diabetes.

Hadjidakis DI, Androulakis II, Mylonakis AM, et al. Diabetes in postmenopause: different influence on bone mass according to age and disease duration. Exp Clin Endocrinol Diabetes, 2009; Vol. 117: pp. 199–204.
Comments: Prospective, cohort study evaluating the influence of type 2 DM on bone metabolism.

Shih J, Abrahamson M. Treatment of type 2 diabetes: an update. Menopause Manage, 2009; July/August: pp. 20–26.
Comments: Review of pharmacologic management of type 2 DM in the setting of menopause.

Kalyani RR, Franco M, Dobs AS, et al. The association of endogenous sex hormones, adiposity, and insulin resistance with incident diabetes in postmenopausal women. J Clin Endocrinol Metab, 2009; Vol. 94: pp. 4127–35.
Comments: Prospective study reporting that higher bioavailable testosterone, higher estradiol and lower SHBG were associated with incident diabetes in postmenopausal women, partially explained by higher adiposity and insulin resistance.

Kernohan AF, Sattar N, Hilditch T, et al. Effects of low-dose continuous combined hormone replacement therapy on glucose homeostasis and markers of cardiovascular risk in women with type 2 diabetes. Clin Endocrinol(Oxford), 2007; Vol. 66: pp. 27–34.
Comments: Prospective, randomized, double-blind, placebo-controlled trial comparing markers for glucose homeostasis and cardiac risk in women with type 2 diabetes who took low-dose HRT.

Salpeter SR, Walsh JM, Ormiston TM, et al. Meta-analysis: effect of hormone-replacement therapy on components of the metabolic syndrome in postmenopausal women. Diabetes Obes Metab, 2006; Vol. 8: pp. 538–54.
Comments: A meta-analysis of 107 trials regarding the effect of HRT on the metabolic syndrome.

Howard BV, Hsia J, Ouyang P, et al. Postmenopausal hormone therapy is associated with atherosclerosis progression in women with abnormal glucose tolerance. Circulation, 2004; Vol. 110: pp.201–6.
Comments: Women with abnormal glucose tolerance were noted to have increased levels

of C-reactive protein and fibrinogen as well as atherosclerotic progression after 2.8 years of postmenopausal hormone therapy.

Margolis KL, Bonds DE, Rodabough RJ, et al. Effect of estrogen plus progestin on the incidence of diabetes in postmenopausal women: results from the Women's Health Initiative Hormone Trial. Diabetologia, 2004;Vol. 47: pp. 1175–87.
Comments: An evaluation of the data generated from the Women's Health Initiative in regard to the effect of HRT on incidence of diabetes and its effect on insulin resistance.

Kanaya AM, Herrington D, Vittinghoff E, et al. Glycemic effects of postmenopausal hormone therapy: the Heart and Estrogen/Progestin Replacement Study. A randomized, double-blind, placebo-controlled trial. Ann Intern Med, 2003; Vol. 138:pp.1–9.
Comments: Prospective, randomized, double-blind, placebo-controlled trial comparing combined HRT use versus placebo in women with known coronary heart disease; women were followed for an average of 4.1 years.

Carr MC. The emergence of the metabolic syndrome with menopause. J Clin Endocrinol Metab, 2003; Vol. 88:pp. 2404–11.
Comments: Review of the role that estrogen deficiency plays in development of the metabolic syndrome in postmenopausal women and how these changes may contribute to overall CVD risk.

Dorman JS, Steenkiste AR, Foley TP, et al. Menopause in type 1 diabetic women: is it premature? Diabetes, 2001;Vol. 50: pp. 1857–62.
Comments: Comparison of women with type 1 DM, their sisters, and control subjects, which determined a statistically significant younger age at menopause in women with type 1 DM resulting in a 17% decrease in reproductive years.

Nicodemus KK, Folsom AR, Iowa Women's Health Study. Type 1 and type 2 diabetes and incident hip fractures in postmenopausal women. Diabetes Care, 2001; Vol. 24: pp. 1192–7.
Comments: Prospective cohort analysis of postmenopausal women to compare the incidence of hip fracture in women with and without diabetes.

Lindheim SR, Presser SC, Ditkoff EC, et al. A possible bimodal effect of estrogen on insulin sensitivity in postmenopausal women and the attenuating effect of added progestin. Fertil Steril, 1993; Vol.60:pp.664–7.
Comments: An intervention trial examining the effect of varying doses of exogenous estrogen on insulin resistance. Moderate dose of estrogen improved insulin sensitivity but higher doses attenuated this benefit.

Cagnacci A, Soldani R, Carriero PL, et al. Effects of low doses of transdermal 17 beta-estradiol on carbohydrate metabolism in postmenopausal women. J Clin Endocrinol Metab, 1992; Vol. 74: pp. 1396–400.
Comments: Clinical trial comparing effects of oral and transdermal estrogen on glucose metabolism. Transdermal estradiol had a beneficial effect on glucose metabolism by increasing hepatic insulin clearance.

绝经期前妇女的月经周期和高血糖

Melissa Yates, MD, and Wanda K. Nicholson, MD, MPH, MBA

定义
- 月经周期指育龄女性每月的一系列生理变化,它开始于青春期的第一次月经(月经初潮),为受孕做准备。
- 与异常月经周期相关的子宫出血可以是非排卵性或是排卵性的。
- 继发性闭经:先前有月经的女性,连续6个月(或三次月经周期)没有月经。
- 月经过少:一年内月经周期少于9次,或者一个月经周期长于35天。
- 月经过频:规则的月经周期(< 21天)。
- 月经过多:规则的延长(> 7天)或者过量的子宫出血。
- 子宫出血:不规则的经常性子宫出血。
- 月经间期出血:在月经周期之间发生的子宫出血。

流行病学
- 1型糖尿病和2型糖尿病都会引起月经周期紊乱(Arrais)。
- 继发性闭经以及月经过少在1型糖尿病中的发生率为20%~30%。
- 由于月经初潮延迟以及绝经期提前,1型糖尿病患者的生育期最多会缩短17%(Arrais)。
- 患有1型糖尿病的青年人,若HbA1c > 9%,则其月经周期会延长、月经初潮会延迟,并且其月经过少的风险会提高5倍,闭经的发生率会提高12倍(Gaete)。
- 2型糖尿病与月经过少和多囊卵巢综合征相关。
- 月经过多也可见于仍分泌雌激素的1型糖尿病和2型糖尿病的无排卵患者。
- 月经周期 > 40天或者不规则到难以估计的程度的女性,其发生2型糖尿病的风险提高了两倍(Solomon)。

诊断
- 根据病史,包括:月经模式,出血时间,性行为,外伤以及感染或系统疾病的症状(例如肝病或肾病)。
- 测量血压,特别是考虑口服避孕药的影响时。
- 做盆底检查以排除其他来源的出血(如直肠),阴道或宫颈伤口以及子宫压痛。
- 考虑CBC时,进行凝血试验。
- 排除怀孕可能。
- 糖尿病患者的继发性闭经常由于促性腺激素分泌低下导致的性腺功能下降导致(低FSH,LH和雌二醇)。
- 无排卵性出血:排除高催乳素血症、甲减、甲亢、多囊卵巢综合征、库欣氏病、下丘脑功能障碍(体重减轻、饮食障碍、紧张、慢性疾病或者过度锻炼)。

- 排卵性出血：排除结构性损伤，出血性疾病（如月经过多或子宫出血）。
- 月经间期不规则出血：排除宫内节育器（IUD）、宫颈疾病或者诸如淋病等性传播疾病或者衣原体感染。
- 排卵状态的确定，最好由妇科医生确认。

症状和体征

- 血糖水平在月经周期的黄体期可能会升高，这可能与内源性性激素水平升高有关，因而需要对胰岛素用量做出相应调整（Trout）。
- 有病例报道 1 型糖尿病患者在月经期发生糖尿病酮症酸中毒（Ovalle）。
- 腹部疼痛、发热以及阴道分泌物：其他与内分泌疾病或者系统疾病相关的症状。

临床治疗

- 激素类避孕药的使用：
- 发生闭经或者月经过少时，考虑口服避孕药（OCPs），如对于没有心血管疾病的女性患者采用 Loestrin 1.5/30 以调节月经周期。
- 只含有黄体酮的激素药物如 Micronor 口服避孕药或者 Mirena 宫内节育器对代谢参数只有轻微的影响，因而可用于患有心血管疾病的女性（Visser）。
- 有少量数据表明，糖尿病患者使用宫内节育器不会导致并发症发生的增多。
- 有以下情况的患者，不建议使用激素治疗：年龄 > 35 岁、吸烟、肾病史、视网膜病变、神经病变、其他血管性疾病或者糖尿病史大于 20 年（Vicente）。铜质宫内节育器可作为一个替代品使用。
- 对于多囊卵巢综合征的患者和 / 或月经稀少的患者，应至少每三个月在月经后应用黄体酮（10mg × 10 天）以减少子宫内膜增生的风险。

随访

- 月经过频、月经过多、月经间期出血的患者需要随访，特别是需妇科医生进行检查和评估。
- 对糖尿病及月经周期紊乱的妇女均应纠正高血糖，尽管这并不能使月经恢复规律。
- 对月经紊乱的患者，除控制血糖外，应完善雌二醇、LH、FSH、催乳素、雄烯二酮、17 羟孕酮、促甲状腺激素以及 24 小时尿游离皮质醇水平检测。

专家建议

- 在育龄妇女中，将 HbA1c 降至 6.0% 可以降低胎儿畸形及妊娠自然流产的风险。

参考文献

Gaete X, Vivanco M, Eyzaguirre FC, et al. Menstrual cycle irregularities and their relationship with HbA1c and insulin dose in adolescents with type 1 diabetes mellitus. Fert Steril, 2010; Vol. 94(5): pp. 1822–6.

Comments: Prospective comparison of menstrual cycle irregularities in T1DM adoloescents and controls.

Ovalle F, Vaughan TA, Sohn JE, et al. Catamenial diabetic ketoacidosis and catamenial hyperglycemia: case report and review of the literature. Am J Med Sci, 2008; Vol. 335:

pp. 298–303.

Comments: 2 case reports of recurrent DKA at the time of the menstrual cycle.

Vicente L, Mendonça D, Dingle M, et al. Etonogestrel implant in women with diabetes mellitus. Eur J Contracept Reprod Health Care, 2008; Vol. 13: pp. 387–95.

Comments: Evaluation of the effect of the etonogestrel implant (Implanon) on carbohydrate and lipid metabo- lism in diabetic women.

Trout KK, Rickels MR, Schutta MH, et al. Menstrual cycle effects on insulin sensitivity in women with type 1 diabetes: a pilot study. Diabetes Technol Ther, 2007; Vol. 9: pp. 176–82.

Comments: Mean fasting glucose levels were higher in the luteal phase compared to the follicular phase, though the results were not significant; however, insulin adjustments may need to be made during the second half of the menstrual cycle.

Arrais RF, Dib SA. The hypothalamus-pituitary-ovary axis and type 1 diabetes mellitus: a mini review. Hum Reprod, 2006; Vol. 21: pp. 327–37.

Comments: Review of the importance of evaluation of the HPO axis in diabetic patients with adequate glyce- mic control and menstrual irregularities.

Visser J, Snel M, Van Vliet HA. Hormonal versus non-hormonal contraceptives in women with diabetes mellitus type 1 and 2. Cochrane Database Syst Rev, 2006; CD003990.

Comments: Review of 4 randomized controlled trials regarding the use of hormonal versus nonhormonal contraception in diabetic women.

Solomon, CG, Hu Fb, Dunaif, A, et al. Long or highly irregular menstrual cycles as a marker for risk of type 2 diabetes mellitus. JAMA, 2001; Vol. 286: pp. 2421–6.

Comments: Part of the Nurses Health Study II noting a significantly increased risk of T2DM in women with a history of irregular or long menstrual cycles.

la Marca A, Morgante G, De Leo V. Evaluation of hypothalamic-pituitary-adrenal axis in amenorrhoeic women with insulin-dependent diabetes. Hum Reprod, 1999; Vol. 14: pp. 298–302.

Comments: Stress induced activation of the hypothalamic-pituitary-adrenal axis may lead to hypogonoado- trophic amenorrhea.

多囊卵巢综合征

Amin Sabet, MD

定义
- 多囊卵巢综合征（PCOS）是一种异源性疾病，其主要特征包括月经失调、雄激素过多和/或多囊卵巢。

流行病学
- 是绝经前妇女中最常见的内分泌紊乱。在全世界总人口中估计患病率为6%~7%。
- 目前高达91%女性存在正常促性腺激素性排卵功能障碍（Broekmans）。
- 患PCOS的妇女中，40岁时高达35%合并糖耐量受损，10%合并2型糖尿病（Ehrmann）。
- 根据鹿特丹标准（见诊断部分），患1型糖尿病的成年妇女中，41%合并PCOS，而应用1990年NIH诊断标准，患病率为11.9%（Codner）。

诊断
- NIH标准（1990）：除外导致月经不规则和雄激素过多的其他病因，并同时存在少/无排卵导致的月经不规则和临床或生化提示高雄激素。
- 鹿特丹标准（2003）：除外导致月经不规则和雄激素过多的其他病因，并满足以下标准中的至少两条：（1）无排卵或排卵减少；（2）临床和/或生化表现为高雄激素；（3）B超提示多囊卵巢（每侧卵巢有>11个直径2~9mm的卵泡）。
- 除外PCOS的情况：妊娠，先天性肾上腺增生（CAH），分泌雄激素的肿瘤，甲状腺功能减退，高泌乳素血症，Cushing综合征。
- 实验室检查：血清HCG，泌乳素，TSH，LH，FSH，游离睾酮，DHEA-S，17羟孕酮，1mg隔夜地塞米松抑制试验（如有提示Cushing综合征的症状/体征）。
- PCOS中，LH与FSH比值常升高。雄激素包括睾酮和DHEA-S常升高。
- 卵泡期早期17羟孕酮升高常提示非典型CAH，ACTH刺激后17羟孕酮测定可确诊。
- 患分泌雄激素的肿瘤的女性的典型表现为闭经、进展性多毛、女性男性化（声音低沉、阴蒂增大），游离睾酮>150mg/dl，DHEA-S>800mcg/dl，LH降低。
- 根据NIH标准，盆腔超声不是必须检查。
- 应考虑对糖耐量异常进行筛查，包括空腹血糖和口服糖耐量试验。

症状和体征
- 月经不规则，表现为月经稀发或闭经，典型的发病时间为青春期左右（原发性闭经）或体重增加后（继发性闭经）。
- 常见无排卵性不孕。

多囊卵巢综合征

- 高雄激素血症的特点，多毛（男性型分布的肢端体毛过多），痤疮，和/或男性型脱发。
- 慢性无排卵可导致子宫内膜增生，功能性子宫出血，并可能导致子宫内膜癌。
- 此病也可见于体重正常者。

临床治疗

- 减重通常可改善高雄激素血症、月经不调和不孕。
- 多毛通常可应用雌-孕激素避孕药（OCP）（通常含 20~35mcg/d 炔雌酮和非雄激素活性的孕激素如诺孕酯、去氧孕烯或屈螺酮）。
- 安体舒通（初始剂量 50mg 每日一次或两次，可增加至 100mg 每日两次）在多毛患者中有额外获益，但在未避孕时不应使用，因为母体醛固酮应用可阻碍男胎性征正常发育。
- 二甲双胍可用于治疗 PCOS 相关的代谢紊乱（肥胖、胰岛素抵抗），可降低雄激素水平并改善月经紊乱。
- 雌孕激素（OCP）或间断孕激素治疗可保护子宫内膜，如醋酸甲羟孕酮 10mg/d，应用 7~10 天，每 1~2 个月 1 次。
- 克罗米芬是 PCOS 患者促排卵治疗的一线用药，虽然二甲双胍也可能有效。
- PCOS 患者合并高血糖的治疗和其他糖尿病患者的降糖治疗无差别。

随访

- 监测并治疗常见合并症：肥胖、胰岛素抵抗、2 型糖尿病、血脂异常（尤其甘油三酯升高和 HDL 降低）、脂肪肝和睡眠呼吸暂停。

专家建议

- 鉴于多囊卵巢的超声标准难以记录，并且正常女性也可存在多囊卵巢，我们继续应用 1990 年 NIH 标准来进行 PCOS 的诊断。
- 对于具有典型 PCOS 表现（青春期前后月经紊乱，超重/肥胖）且轻度多毛的女性可不进行血清雄激素测定，然而对于中重度或进展性多毛、任何程度的痤疮或 20 岁后月经紊乱的女性应测定血清雄激素，以鉴别是否存在雄激素分泌性肿瘤导致睾酮和 DHEA-S 过多。
- 对于超重或肥胖的 PCOS 患者，二甲双胍为一线用药，因为其有良好的改善代谢的作用，并有潜在的降低雄激素和改善月经紊乱的作用。
- 根据有限的证据（Cheung），推荐 PCOS 女性及病史中每年少于 5 个月经周期的女性进行子宫内膜活检。

推荐依据

Polycystic Ovary Syndrome Writing Committee. American Association of Clinical Endocrinologists position statement on metabolic and cardiovascular consequences of polycystic ovary syndrome. Endocr Pract, 2005; Vol. 11: pp. 126–34.

Comments: American Association of Clinical Endocrinologists' position statement regarding metabolic aspects of PCOS.

Rotterdam ESHRE/ASRM-sponsored PCOS Consensus Workshop Group. Revised 2003 consensus on diagnostic criteria and long-term health risks related to polycystic ovary syndrome (PCOS). Hum Reprod, 2004; Vol. 19: pp. 41–7.

Comments: 2003 Rotterdam consensus on PCOS diagnostic criteria.

Zawadski, JK, Dunaif, A. Diagnostic criteria for polycystic ovary syndrome: Towards a rational approach. In Dunaif A, Givens JR, Haseltine FP, Merriam GE, (Eds.), Polycystic Ovary Syndrome. Oxford, UK: Blackwell Publish- ing; 1992: pp. 59–69.

Comments: NIH diagnostic criteria for PCOS.

其他参考文献

Nestler JE. Metformin for the treatment of the polycystic ovary syndrome. NEJM, 2008; Vol. 358: pp. 47–54.

Comments: Review of metformin therapy for PCOS.

Legro RS, Barnhart HX, Schlaff WD, et al. Clomiphene, metformin, or both for infertility in the polycystic ovary syndrome. NEJM, 2007; Vol. 356: pp. 551–66.

Comments: Infertile women with PCOS treated with clomiphene had a 3-fold higher live-birth rate compared with those treated with metformin.

Broekmans FJ, Knauff EA, Valkenburg O, et al. PCOS according to the Rotterdam consensus criteria: Change in prevalence among WHO-II anovulation and association with metabolic factors. BJOG, 2006; Vol. 113: pp. 1210–7.

Comments: Using Rotterdam criteria, PCOS was present in 91% of women with euestrogenic normogonado- tropic ovulatory dysfunction.

Codner E, Soto N, Lopez P, et al. Diagnostic criteria for polycystic ovary syndrome and ovarian morphology in women with type 1 diabetes mellitus. J Clin Endocrinol Metab, 2006; Vol. 91: pp. 2250–6.

Comments: Among adult women with type 1 diabetes, 38.1% had clinical hyperandrogenism, 23.8% had bio- chemical hyperandrogenism, 19% had menstrual dysfunction, and 40.5% had PCOS based on Rotterdam crite- ria (vs 11.9% using 1990 NIH criteria).

Ehrmann DA. Polycystic ovary syndrome. NEJM, 2005; Vol. 352: pp. 1223–36.

Comments: Current review of PCOS.

Cheung AP. Ultrasound and menstrual history in predicting endometrial hyperplasia in polycystic ovary syndrome. Obstet Gynecol, 2001; Vol. 98: pp. 325–31.

Comments: Among women with PCOS, intermenstrual interval ，3 months and endometrial thickness . 7 mm were predictors of endometrial hyperplasia.

Ehrmann DA, Barnes RB, Rosenfield RL, et al. Prevalence of impaired glucose tolerance and diabetes in women with polycystic ovary syndrome. Diabetes Care, 1999; Vol. 22: pp. 141–6.

Comments: 35% and 10% prevalence of IGT and type 2 diabetes, respectively, in women with PCOS.

消化道疾病

乳糜泻与 1 型糖尿病

Octavia Pickett-Blakely, MD, MHS, and Mary Huizinga, MD, MPH

定义
- 乳糜泻是一种麦胶敏感性肠病,主要特点是由于自身免疫性肠黏膜炎症和肠绒毛结构异常而导致的小肠吸收功能不良。

流行病学
- 乳糜泻在一般美国人群中的患病率为 0.4%~1%(Collin; Green; Rewers)。
- 1 型糖尿病患者中,乳糜泻的患病率为 1%~16.4%(Rewers)。
- 乳糜泻患者中,1 型糖尿病的患病率为 5%~10%(Rewers)。
- 90% 患者中 1 型糖尿病的诊断早于乳糜泻的诊断。
- 由于疾病谱的广泛,在诊断糖尿病后,乳糜泻的出现时间尚没有明确的定义。

诊断
- 血清学试验:用于高危人群的一种无创性筛查。进食麸质食品后,检查人体内抗组织型谷氨酰胺转移酶抗体(anti-tTG),抗麦胶蛋白抗体或是抗肌内膜抗体(EM):IgA(仅有抗麦胶蛋白抗体)或是 IgG(全部)。初筛时,常同时检测抗肌内膜抗体、组织型谷氨酰胺转移酶抗体及定量 IgA。
- 诊断金标准:上消化道内窥镜检查同时行十二指肠活检,可见上皮内淋巴细胞增生、隐窝增生及绒毛增生,而无谷蛋白饮食可减轻上述现象。
- 基因检测:HIA-DR2 和 HIA-DR8 具有高度阴性预测值,常用于有乳糜泻家族史或是自身免疫性疾病史如 1 型糖尿病的无症状人群,在 1 型糖尿病患者中,并不推荐其作为常规乳糜泻筛查试验,但在其他方法不可用时可选择。

症状和体征
- 典型症状:腹泻和体重减轻。
- 其他胃肠道症状:腹胀和腹痛。
- 全身症状:乏力,生长发育缓慢。
- 生化异常:缺铁性贫血,转氨酶异常,低蛋白血症,维生素 D 缺乏导致的低钙血症。
- 骨质疏松或是骨质疏松症。
- 不孕不育。
- 神经精神症状。
- 疱疹样皮炎:发痒,红色水疱(常分布于膝、肘、臀部),伴有烧灼痛。
- 其他自身免疫性疾病(如甲状腺功能减低)。

临床治疗

- 无麸质饮食：避免食用小麦、黑麦、大麦。常见的无麸质食品包括新鲜的鱼、肉类、牛奶、奶酪、水果、蔬菜。
- 由于无麸质饮食（小麦产品）的低血糖指数，因此常鼓励糖尿病患者使用，此外无麸质食物的替代品也具有低血糖指数。
- 无麸质食物的替代品往往昂贵，且不易购买。
- 补充微量元素（如铁、维生素D、维生素B_{12}、叶酸）。
- 生育指导。

随访

- 所有乳糜泻病人应测定骨密度，筛查骨质疏松。
- 开始无麸质饮食后2~4周，患者症状及组织学检查就会有所改善。坚持这种饮食则能完全恢复。
- 患者应筛查是否存在微量元素缺乏，应由经验丰富的营养师予以评估。
- 美国糖尿病协会临床实践指南推荐在有症状或体征的1型糖尿病患者中（如缺铁性贫血、低钙血症、乏力、腹痛），提示存在乳糜泻时，应进行抗体筛查。在无症状的患者中不推荐普遍筛查（ADA）。
- 尽管没有明确的抗体复查的时间间隔，但是当患者症候群发生变化时（如体重减轻，幼儿体重不增）需重复筛查抗体（ADA）。

专家意见

- 大约有2.5%乳糜泻患者缺乏IgA，从而导致tTG、肌内膜及胶蛋白IgA抗体检查试验呈假阴性。因此在首次筛查中，需同时检查总血清IgA水平。
- 对于已严格进食无麸质食物仍有症状的患者，需评估是否有其食物是否有隐藏来源的胶蛋白，或是进行二次诊断（如乳糖吸收不良），或是否存在口炎性腹泻的并发症（如黏膜相关性T细胞淋巴瘤）。
- 对于不伴症状的1型糖尿病患者，可以使用血清学试验筛查。然而对于有持续症状的患者需使用上消化道内窥镜及小肠活检进行诊断。
- 虽然乳糜泻可增加小肠腺癌和T细胞淋巴瘤的危险性，但目前没有一个制定好的筛选准则（Disabatino）。
- 血糖控制可改善进食无麸质食物的1型糖尿病患者的乳糜泻，但是相关数据有限（Amin）。
- 网上有大量关于乳糜泻疾病的资料，如 http://www.celiac.org/ 和 http://www.gluten.net。

主要参考文献

American Diabetes association. standards of medical care in diabetes—2011. Diabetes Care, 2011; Vol. 34 suppl 1: pp. s11–61.

Comments: provides clinical practice guidelines for screening type 1 diabetes patients for CD.

其他参考文献

Sollid IM, lundin Ke. Diagnosis and treatment of celiac disease. Mucosal immunol, 2009; Vol. 2: pp. 3–7.

Comments: novel targets for treatment of CD.

Di sabatino a, Corazza GR. Celiac disease. lancet, 2009; Vol. 373: pp. 1480–93.

Comments: Review of pathogenesis of CD.

Green pH, Cellier C. Celiac disease. neJM, 2007; Vol. 357: pp. 1731–43.

Comments: excellent general review of CD.

Rewers M. epidemiology of celiac disease: what are the prevalence, incidence, and progression of celiac disease? Gastroenterology, 2005; Vol. 128: pp. s47–51.

Comments: Review of the epidemiology of CD.

Rewers M, liu e, simmons J, et al. Celiac disease associated with type 1 diabetes mellitus. endocrinol Metab Clin north am, 2004; Vol. 33: pp. 197–214, xi.

Comments: Review of the epidemiology of CD in type 1 diabetes.

Amin R, Murphy n, edge J, et al. a longitudinal study of the efects of a gluten free diet on glycemic control and weight gain in subjects with type 1 diabetes and celiac disease. Diabetes Care, 2002; Vol. 25: pp. 1117–22.

Comments: small, case-control study showing improved glycemic control in diabetics treated with a gluten-free diet.

胃轻瘫

Octavia Pickett-Blakely, MD, MHs, and Mary Huizinga, MD, MPH

定义
- 非机械性梗阻所致的胃排空延迟。
- 高血糖相关的自主神经功能紊乱及迷走神经损伤的结果。
- 除外其他导致胃排空延迟的病因(如麻醉及曾行迷走神经切断术)。

流行病学
- 糖尿病是已知的最常见的胃轻瘫的原因。
- 高达50%的糖尿病患者有胃排空延迟的客观证据,但不一定有临床表现(Kong)。
- 女性糖尿病患者中自主神经病变、视网膜病变及肾脏微血管病变是糖尿病性胃排空延迟的阳性预测因子(Jones;Koçkar)。

诊断
- 临床病史提示胃轻瘫(症状和体征)。
- 客观证据:闪烁扫描术提示固相胃排空异常,或使用上消化道内镜或X线钡餐摄影测定胃内存留物。
- 用放射性同位素标记固体和液体试餐,由闪烁扫描术测定不同时间的胃排空率(以分钟为单位)。餐后4小时胃潴留>10%为胃排空延迟(Camilleri)。
- 液相胃排空往往是正常的,因此不常用于糖尿病病人胃轻瘫的诊断(Tack)。
- 其他客观检测方法:同位素标记的呼吸试验(在美国不适用),无线胶囊内镜检查(不常用),胃肠测压术。

症状和体征
- 早饱。
- 腹痛。
- 恶心。
- 呕吐。
- 腹胀。
- 餐后饱胀。
- 体检提示血容量不足,上腹腹胀、压痛。
- 存在自主神经病变和/或其他糖尿病并发症。

临床治疗
饮食治疗
- 少食多餐,低脂、低纤维饮食。
- 如果食物摄入不能满足机体需要,需补充营养(通过口服、肠内营养或肠外营养补充)。

药物治疗

- 促胃动力药物：一线用药包括胃复安（第479页），红霉素（第476页），多潘立酮（在加拿大和欧洲可用；第473页）。
- 胃复安是美国最常用的胃动力药，但由于其神经系统副作用如导致迟发性运动障碍使该药的长期应用受到限制，而红霉素可并发QT间期延长（Haans）。
- 对症治疗：止吐药和非麻药性镇痛剂（常和prokinetics类药物联用作为二线治疗方案）。

内镜/手术治疗

- 幽门肉毒杆菌毒素注射：目前用于药物难治性胃轻瘫，其有效作用时间是不恒定的（如果有效）；尚需要大型临床随机试验来评估这种治疗方法（Haans；Desantis）。
- 胃电刺激可改善药物难治性患者的症状，但与安慰剂相比，并未从根本上改善胃排空延迟（Haans；Tack）。
- Roux-en-Y胃旁路手术可减少行减肥手术的糖尿病患者的胃轻瘫症状。

随访

- 患者应经常在门诊随访。
- 在体重明显下降和/或营养不良的患者中进行微量营养素缺乏症的筛查。
- 患者应由营养医师定期随访。
- 当患者出现胃轻瘫症状时，建议转诊胃肠病专家。另外需行上消化道内镜检查，了解是否存在其他病因。

专家意见

- 糖尿病性胃轻瘫的诊断和治疗有一定难度。
- 由于治疗的副作用限制了糖尿病性胃轻瘫患者的管理。
- 糖尿病性胃排空延迟的症状不典型或不明显，使该疾病管理更加困难。
- 由于糖尿病性胃轻瘫使患者口服摄入及吸收营养素无法预测，导致血糖控制不稳定。
- 虽然血糖控制不佳可引起胃排空延迟/胃轻瘫，并增加住院率，但是尚很少有前瞻性研究的数据显示血糖控制正常后能改善糖尿病性胃轻瘫（Uppalapati）。

参考文献

Uppalapati ss, Ramzan Z, Fisher Rs, et al. Factors contributing to hospitalization for gastroparesis exacerbations. Dig Dis sci, 2009; Vol. 54: pp. 2404–9.
  Comments: study investigating factors related to morbidity related to diabetic gastroparesis.
Tack J. Gastric motor and sensory function. Curr Opin Gastroenterol, 2009; Vol. 25: pp. 557–65.
  Comments: Review article outlining the pathophysiology of gastroparesis.
sugumar a, singh a, pasricha pJ. a systematic review of the efcacy of domperidone for the treatment of diabetic gastroparesis. Clin Gastroenterol Hepatol, 2008; Vol. 6: pp. 726–33.
  Comments: systematic review of domperidone's use in diabetic gastroparesis.

Camilleri M. Clinical practice. Diabetic gastroparesis. neJM, 2007; Vol. 356: pp. 820–9.
Comments: Review article that outlines the diagnosis and treatment of diabetic gastroparesis.

Haans JJ, Masclee aa. Review article: the diagnosis and management of gastroparesis. aliment pharmacol Ther, 2007; Vol. 26 suppl 2: pp. 37–46.
Comments: Review article outlining the diagnosis and treatment of diabetic gastroparesis.

Hasler Wl. Gastroparesis: symptoms, evaluation, and treatment. Gastroenterol Clin north am, 2007; Vol. 36: pp. 619–47, ix.
Comments: Review of the epidemiology, presentation, and treatment of diabetic gastroparesis.

Desantis eR, Huang s. botulinum toxin type a for treatment of refractory gastroparesis. am J Health syst pharm, 2007; Vol. 64: pp. 2237–40.
Comments: Review of botulinum toxin's use in gastroparesis.

Kong MF, Horowitz M. Diabetic gastroparesis. Diabet Med, 2005; Vol. 22 suppl 4: pp. 13–8.
Comments: Review of diabetic gastroparesis.

Koçkar MC, Kayahan iK, bavbek n. Diabetic gastroparesis in association with autonomic neuropathy and microvasculopathy. acta Med Okayama, 2002; Vol. 56: pp. 237–43.
Comments: study investigating the correlation between gastric emptying and parameters of autonomic neuropathy and microvasculopathy in diabetics.

Jones Kl, Russo a, stevens Je, et al. predictors of delayed gastric emptying in diabetes. Diabetes Care, 2001; Vol. 24: pp. 1264–9.
Comments: an observational study investigating the predictors of delayed gastric emptying in T1DM, T2DM, and normal controls.

非酒精性脂肪肝

Mariana Lazo, MD, ScM, PhD, and Jeanne M. Clark, MD, MPH

定义

- 非酒精性脂肪肝（NAFID）是指肝脏中脂肪浸润超过肝重的5%。活检可发现5%~10%的肝实质细胞出现脂肪变性。
- 根据定义，需排除酒精性脂肪肝。每日允许摄入的酒精量一直存在争议，一般男性酒精摄入量应小于20g/d（2 drinks），女性应小于10g/d（1 drink）被认为是安全的，而当男性酒精摄入量达到30g/d，女性达到20g/d时肝硬化风险增加。
- 原发性非酒精性脂肪肝：就是平常所指的典型性非酒精性脂肪肝，与中心性肥胖和/或2型糖尿病或胰岛素抵抗相关，而与其他病因无关。
- 继发性非酒精性脂肪肝：不伴胰岛素抵抗，与其他原因如药物使用（糖皮质激素、三苯氧胺、胺腆酮、HAART、地尔硫䓬），脂代谢异常（无β脂蛋白血症、脂代谢障碍、Weber-Christian综合征、Andersen病），全胃肠外营养及空肠回肠旁路手术相关。许多情况下，继发性非酒精性脂肪肝可能系未确诊的原发性非酒精性脂肪肝的恶化表现。
- 非酒精性脂肪性肝炎（NASH）：是非酒精性脂肪肝的一种严重形式，特征是肝活检发现炎症，肝细胞气球样变和/或肝纤维化。非酒精性脂肪肝可进展为肝硬化。

流行病学

- 在美国，非酒精性脂肪肝是最常见的慢性肝脏疾病（Clark），在世界范围内也广泛流行。
- 通过肝酶学或肝影像学检查（超声或MRI）发现，一般人群中非酒精性脂肪肝患病率为3%~30%(lazo；argo)。
- 在2型糖尿病人群中，非酒精性脂肪肝的患病率为50%~80%(lazo)。
- 与一般人群相比，2型糖尿病患者的非酒精性脂肪肝更容易进展为肝硬化(Clark；Caldwell)。
- 非西班牙裔和拉美裔人群中非酒精性脂肪肝发病风险较高。
- 更严重疾病的预测因子：年龄在40~50岁，女性，重度肥胖，高血压，糖尿病，高甘油三酯血症，ALT、AST、GGT升高，AST与ALT比值大于1。

诊断

- 患者的肝病实验室检查可能正常。
- 美国胃肠病协会（AGA）建议一个渐进的诊断方法。步骤（1）：肝脏的血清学检查，包括检测AST、ALT、碱性磷酸酶、血清胆红素、白蛋白水平及凝血酶原时间；步骤（2）：评估患者同时存在的其他可治性疾病（如丙型肝炎、自身免疫性疾病）；步骤（3）：通过患者本人或家属了解患者的饮酒情况。如果AST或ALT正常，饮酒折合乙醇含量少于20~30g/d（2~3drinks），并排除其他导致肝脏疾病的原因，则

- 进行步骤（4）：影像学检查（超声、CT扫描、MRI）。
- 目前影像学方法不能区分脂肪肝、脂肪性肝炎和肝纤维化，但是可排除胆道或是肝脏局灶性疾病。
- 对于脂肪肝的检测，超声检查要比CT扫描更敏感、便宜，且没有辐射风险。而MRI主要用于科研，如定量肝脏的脂肪含量。
- 瞬时弹性成像：基于超声技术测量组织弹性，与病毒性肝炎患者肝脏硬度数据之间存在很好的相关性，但是不能用于超重或是肥胖的非酒精性脂肪肝患者。
- 诊断的金标准是肝活检，对非酒精性脂肪肝进行分期（损伤程度）和分级（活动度）。非酒精性脂肪肝的活动评分（NAS）基于脂肪变性、炎症和肝细胞损伤的有无及程度，为0~8分。
- 纤维化评分从0~4分：0~2分为少量纤维化，3~4分为桥接纤维化和肝硬化。较高的NAS提示有更大的损害，其设计用于NASH的临床试验中。
- 肝活检的局限性：患者行动不便，潜在并发症的可能性，采样错误。
- 无创的肝纤维化标志物：纤维化评分（Fibrospect, Hepascore和Fibroscore），主要是基于血清生化检测和常规实验室检查，可以识别小的或是晚期疾病。然而大量处于灰色带的患者无法明确肝纤维化的诊断及分期。目前，FDA并未批准此种方法，在非酒精性脂肪肝中的诊断作用还不确切。
- 许多患者的胆固醇和甘油三酯水平升高。

症状和体征

- 最常见的：无症状占48%~100%，乏力占70%，右上腹疼痛高达50%。
- 肝硬化患者可出现肝掌和蜘蛛痣。
- 临床表现与代谢综合征相关。
- 儿童患者可出现肝肿大和黑棘皮病。
- 脂肪萎缩/脂肪代谢障碍。

临床治疗

非药物治疗

- 饮食和运动是治疗的基石。减轻体重5%~7%可有效改善非酒精性脂肪肝患者的肝脂肪变性及其他组织学变化，并减少疾病进展的风险(Harrison; promrat)。
- 避免体重下降过快，这可能会导致病理改变。
- 运动而不伴体重减轻：最近有证据表明这对人体是有益的。鼓励患者增加体力活动水平，即使没有实现体重下降。
- 饮食构成：特定的饮食结构对非酒精性脂肪肝患者的影响尚不清楚。美国糖尿病协会和美国心脏协会推荐均衡饮食。

药物治疗（尚未得到FDA批准）

- 噻唑烷二酮类：匹格列酮可显著改善患者肝脏组织学结果(sanya Ratziu)，同时由于在2型糖尿病治疗中的其他益处，可用于2型糖尿病伴非酒精性脂肪肝患者的治疗。

非酒精性脂肪肝

- 双胍类：二甲双胍通常只用在科研中，试验数据提示它的治疗效果喜忧参半。
- 抗氧化剂：试验数据提示维生素 E 可改善治疗效果（sanyal）。
- 细胞保护剂：胆烷酸的大型临床随机试验提示并未表现出组织学改善。

一般注意事项

- 血糖控制：理想的糖化血红蛋白水平应小于 7%。
- 酒精摄入：如果有更严重的疾病应限制摄入量。
- 服用药物时可能会加速脂肪性肝炎（如胺腆酮、他莫昔芬），需权衡用药的风险和收益。
- 避免接触肝毒性物质（如烃类溶剂）。
- 患者教育/免疫接种，预防病毒性肝炎。

随访

- 对疾病的监测尚没有确切的指南。
- 最常用的方法是：组织学检查、肝酶试验和代谢参数。
- 其他不太常用的方法：血清肝纤维化标志物，肝影像学技术。
- 当需要进行肝活检和/或实验性治疗时，建议转诊胃肠专科医生。

专家意见

- 2 型糖尿病患者中，与肝脏相关疾病的发病率和死亡率风险增高。
- 肝脏活检是对非酒精性脂肪肝患者诊断、分期、分级的金标准，但在首次评估中很少使用。
- 初次检查时，需通过实验室检查排除其他可能导致肝脏疾病的潜在原因。
- 生活方式改变仍然是疾病初期管理的基础。
- 目前，并没有获得 FDA 批准的药物治疗。尽管试验证明在 2 型糖尿病伴非酒精性脂肪肝的患者中可首选使用噻唑烷二酮类药物。

主要参考文献

american Gastroenterological association. american Gastroenterological association medical position statement: nonalcoholic fatty liver disease. Gastroenterology, 2002; Vol. 123: pp. 1702–4.available for download at http://www.aasld.org/practiceguidelines/Documents/practice%20Guidelines/position_nonfattypg.pdf.

Comments: summary of the Medical position statement.

anyal aJ, american Gastroenterological association. aGa technical review on nonalcoholic fatty liver disease. Gastroenterology, 2002; Vol. 123: pp. 1705–25.

Comments: Most comprehensive and recent ofcial review of nonalcoholic fatty liver disease.

其他参考文献

romrat K, Kleiner De, niemeier HM, et al. Randomized controlled trial testing the efects of weight loss on nonalcoholic steatohepatitis. Hepatology, 2010; Vol. 51: pp. 121–9.

Comments: small RCT of lifestyle intervention on biopsy proven nasH showing signifcant efect of 7% weight loss on liver histology: steatosis, infammation, ballooning, and nas score.

anyal aJ, et al. a randomized controlled trial of pioglitazone or vitamin e for nonalcoholic steatohepatitis (piVens) [abstract]. Hepatology, 2009; Vol. 50 (suppl): p. lb4 .

Comments: 24-month RCT of pioglitazone in biopsy proven nasH showing a signifcant efect on liver histology: steatosis, infammation, ballooning (borderline p = 0.08).

Ratziu V, Zelber-sagi s. pharmacologic therapy of non-alcoholic steatohepatitis. Clin liver Dis, 2009; Vol. 13: pp. 667–88.

Comments: excellent narrative review of treatment of naFID.

Argo CK, Caldwell sH. epidemiology and natural history of non-alcoholic steatohepatitis. Clin liver Dis, 2009; Vol. 13: pp. 511–31.

Comments: excellent narrative review of the natural History of naFID.

Ratziu V, Giral p, Jacqueminet s et al. Rosiglitazone for nonalcoholic steatohepatitis: one-year results of the randomized placebo-controlled Fatty liver improvement with Rosiglitazone Therapy (FliRT) Trial. Gastroenterology, 2008; Vol. 135: pp. 100–10.

Comments: 12-month randomized controlled trial (RCT) of rosiglitazone in nasH showing a signifcant efect on liver transaminases, insulin resistance, and steatosis.

Lazo M, Clark JM. The epidemiology of nonalcoholic fatty liver disease: a global perspective. semin liver Dis, 2008; Vol. 28: pp. 339–50.

Comments: Comprehensive narrative review of the epidemiology of naFID.

Harrison sa, Day Cp. benefts of lifestyle modifcation in naFID. Gut, 2007; Vol. 56: pp. 1760–9.

Comments: excellent review of the mechanism and experimental studies of lifestyle efects in naFID.

Harrison sa, Torgerson s, Hayashi pH. The natural history of nonalcoholic fatty liver disease: a clinical histopathological study. am J Gastroenterol, 2003; Vol. 98: pp. 2042–7.

Comments: paper that provided key data of the progression of naFID.

Marchesini G, bugianesi e, Forlani G, et al. nonalcoholic fatty liver, steatohepatitis, and the metabolic syndrome. Hepatology, 2003; Vol. 37: pp. 917–23.

Comments: This paper, along with others, has provided substantial evidence of the link between insulin resistance and naFID.

Mofrad p, Contos MJ, Haque M, et al. Clinical and histologic spectrum of nonalcoholic fatty liver disease associated with normal alT values. Hepatology, 2003; Vol. 37: pp. 1286–92.

Comments: paper that showed the limitation of liver enzymes, especially alT as surrogate marker of liver injury.

Neuschwander-Tetri ba, Caldwell sH. nonalcoholic steatohepatitis: summary of an aaslD single Topic Conference. Hepatology, 2003; Vol. 37: pp. 1202–19.

Comments: expert review of naFID. a good summary of its pathophysiology, epidemiology, and treatment, as well as current gaps in the literature.

Clark JM, brancati Fl, Diehl aM. The prevalence and etiology of elevated aminotransferase levels in the United states. am J Gastroenterol, 2003; Vol. 98: pp. 960–7.

Comments: paper that showed for the frst time the high prevalence of presumed naFID in the general population.

Clark JM, Diehl aM. nonalcoholic fatty liver disease: an underrecognized cause of cryptogenic cirrhosis. JaMa, 2003; Vol. 289: pp. 3000–4.

Comments: One of the frst studies suggesting that most cases of cryptogenic cirrhosis could be related to naFID.

Brunt eM, Janney CG, Di bisceglie aM, et al. nonalcoholic steatohepatitis: a proposal for grading and staging the histological lesions. am J Gastroenterol, 1999; Vol. 94: pp. 2467–74.

Comments: provides a widely accepted scoring system for grading and staging histologically naFID.

Matteoni Ca, younossi ZM, Gramlich T, et al. nonalcoholic fatty liver disease: a spectrum of clinical and pathological severity. Gastroenterology, 1999; Vol. 116: pp. 1413–9.

Comments: another paper that provided key data of the progression of naFID.

Caldwell sH, Oelsner DH, iezzoni JC, et al. Cryptogenic cirrhosis: clinical characterization and risk factors for underlying disease. Hepatology, 1999; Vol. 29: pp. 664–9.

Comments: One of the frst studies suggesting that most cases of cryptogenic cirrhosis could be related to naFID.

胰腺炎

Reza Alavi, MD, MHS, MBA, and Jeanne M. Clark, MD, MPH

定义
- 是指胰腺的炎症。
- 急性胰腺炎常见病因包括：胆结石，大量饮酒，高钙血症，毒品，感染和外伤。

流行病学
- 急性胰腺炎的年发生率为每十万人群中4.9~35人。与未患糖尿病的人群相比，2型糖尿病患者急性胰腺炎发生风险增加3倍（Vege）。
- 糖尿病治疗导致的药物性急性胰腺炎非常罕见。
- 极度高甘油三酯血症大于1 000mg/dl（乳糜微粒），能引发慢性胰腺炎。
- 其他病因包括囊肿性纤维化，自身免疫性疾病，胰腺结构异常（如胰腺分裂）。
- 急性胰腺炎中，50%的患者存在糖耐量异常，但仅极少数需要胰岛素治疗（Gorelick）。
- 慢性胰腺炎中，高达50%患者有糖尿病（Wakasugi），70%存在胰腺钙化（Gorelick）。
- 整体而言，急性胰腺炎住院患者死亡率约为10%（范围2%~22%）。
- 死亡率不受糖尿病状态的影响（Cavallini）。

诊断
- 血清淀粉酶在发病6~12小时内增高，通常为正常上限的3倍以上（是一种较敏感的试验）。
- 血清脂肪酶是一种更为特异的指标。
- 连续测量并不能预测预后或是改变疾病管理方式。
- 白细胞计数升高，即使在没有感染的情况下。
- 常需要检查血清电解质，特别是血钙。
- 毒理学筛查，血脂测试及血培养以找出病因。
- 胰腺CT扫描是最重要的检查方法，可发现是否存在胰腺坏死。
- 腹部平片有助于排除其他导致腹痛的原因，如肠梗阻、肠穿孔。
- 腹部超声可显示胰腺弥漫性扩大和低回声区，同时能检测胆囊结石。

症状和体征
- 上腹部疼痛。
- 恶心和呕吐。
- 发热和心动过速。
- 腹胀，上腹压痛，腹部拒按。
- 由于膈肌刺激而导致呼吸浅快。
- 在重症胰腺炎中，可出现不伴败血症的血管扩张性休克。

胰腺炎

临床治疗

- 以下重症胰腺炎需在 ICU 监测治疗：如入院时有胰腺坏死，器官功能衰竭，胸腔积液，疾病评分提示高度重症（i.e.，apaCHe-ii）。
- 在心功能允许的情况下，24~48 小时内进行液体复苏，使用等渗盐水 250~300ml/h(Tenner)。
- 纠正电解质及代谢异常。
- 供氧，保证血氧水平在 95% 以上。
- 疼痛管理：由于吗啡可增加 Oddi 括约肌的压力，故通常使用哌替啶，但并没有确切的临床证据证明吗啡可加重或引起胰腺炎或胆囊炎。
- 营养支持：如果 7 天不能进食，通常使用鼻饲，它要优于肠外营养。
- 通常不推荐常规预防性使用抗生素以防止胰腺感染（banks），即使亚胺培南或美罗培南可能对约 30% 的胰腺坏死患者有益（Villatoro）。
- 在重症胰腺炎或胆结石患者中，或是行胆囊切除术后仍有持续性胆道梗阻，可行 ERCP 手术将胆管结石取出。
- 慢性胰腺炎患者伴有顽固性疼痛时需用手术治疗。

追访

- 急性坏死性胰腺炎可导致部分 β 细胞功能丧失及胰岛素抵抗，大量患者会出现糖耐量异常（IGT）。
- 胆石性胰腺炎患者在恢复后可行胆囊切除术，轻症胰腺炎患者在恢复后 7 天内可进行该手术，重症坏死性胰腺炎在恢复后 3~4 周进行。
- 慢性胰腺炎伴 1 型或 2 型糖尿病的患者，胰腺外分泌功能常常受损。
- 胰腺外分泌功能不全时，需进食低脂饮食，并服用外源性胰腺酶。

专家意见

- 糖耐量异常发生于慢性胰腺炎，但糖尿病常发生在疾病的晚期。
- 糖尿病常与慢性钙化性疾病共同发生，特别是在钙化发生的早期。
- 伴有慢性胰腺炎的糖尿病患者常需要胰岛素治疗，但可增加低血糖的发生风险（可能是由于 α- 细胞和 β- 细胞受损）。
- 虽然初步研究显示艾塞那肽、西格列汀和西格列汀/二甲双胍增加药物性胰腺炎的风险，但是在这一点上目前没有定论（Drucker）。

参考文献

Drucker DJ, sherman si, Gorelick Fs, et al. incretin-based therapies for the treatment of type 2 diabetes: evaluation of the risks and benefts. Diabetes Care, 2010; Vol. 33: pp. 428–33.

Comments: excellent recent review of incretin-based therapies and rare adverse events including acute pancreatitis.

alani aR, Grendell JH. Drug-induced pancreatitis: incidence, management and prevention. Drug saf, 2008; Vol. 31: pp. 823–37.

Comments: Drug-induced pancreatitis.

ege ss, yadav D, Chari sT. pancreatitis. in Talley nJ, locke GR, saito ya (eds.), Gi epidemiology, 1st edition. Malden, Ma: blackwell publishing; 2007: pp. 221–225.

Comments: epidemiology of pancreatitis.

Forsmark Ce, baillie J, aGa institute Clinical practice and economics Committee, et al. aGa institute technical review on acute pancreatitis. Gastroenterology, 2007; Vol. 132: pp. 2022–44.
Comments: aGa guidelines.

Banks pa, Freeman MI, practice parameters Committee of the american College of Gastroenterology. practice guidelines in acute pancreatitis. am J Gastroenterol, 2006 Vol. 101: pp. 2379–400.
Comments: Detailed practice guidelines.

Villatoro e, bassi C, larvin M. antibiotic therapy for prophylaxis against infection of pancreatic necrosis in acute pancreatitis. Cochrane Database syst Rev, 2006; CD002941.
Comments: antibiotic therapy for severe pancreatitis.

Cavallini G, Frulloni I, bassi C, et al. prospective multicentre survey on acute pancreatitis in italy (proinf-aisp): results on 1005 patients. Dig liver Dis, 2004; Vol. 36: pp. 205–11.
Comments: italian epidemiological study of incidence, hospitalization, and mortality rates.

Tenner s. initial management of acute pancreatitis: critical issues during the frst 72 hours am J Gastroenterol, 2004; Vol. 99: pp. 2489–94.
Comments: initial management.

Malka D, Hammel p, sauvanet a, et al. Risk factors for diabetes mellitus in chronic pancreatitis. Gastroenterology, 2000; Vol. 119: pp. 1324–32.
Comments: The risk of diabetes mellitus is not infuenced by elective pancreatic surgical procedures other than distal pancreatectomy in patients with chronic pancreatitis.

Dervenis C, Johnson CD, bassi C, et al. Diagnosis, objective assessment of severity, and management of acute pancreatitis. santorini consensus conference. int J pancreatol 1999; Vol. 25: pp. 195–210.
Comments: Diagnosis using plasma concentrations of pancreatic enzymes is reliable.

Wakasugi H, Funakoshi a, iguchi H. Clinical assessment of pancreatic diabetes caused by chronic pancreatitis. J Gastroenterol, 1998; Vol. 33: pp. 254–9.
Comments: among 154 patients with chronic pancreatitis, 50% had diabetes.

Gorelick Fs. Diabetes mellitus and the exocrine pancreas. yale J biol Med, 1984; Vol. 56 pp. 271–5.
Comments: Review of epidemiology and pathophysiology of diabetes associated with pancreatitis.

血液系统疾病 / 恶性肿瘤

贫血（糖尿病）详见贫血部分，640 页

癌症和糖尿病

Hsin-Chieh Yeh, PhD, and Frederick L. Brancati, MD, MHS

定义
- 癌症或恶性肿瘤是指细胞不受控制的生长，侵入到邻近的组织内，并且通过淋巴或血液，扩散到其他的地方（转移）。
- 良性肿瘤不会侵袭或转移。

流行病学

癌症的发病
- 糖尿病与非霍奇金淋巴瘤（Chao）、乳房癌（Larsson, 2007）、大肠癌（Larsson, 2005）、子宫内膜癌（Friberg）、肝癌（El-Serag）和胰腺癌（Huxley）的发病率升高有着密切联系。
- 与前列腺癌的病发有着负性关联（Kasper）。
- 糖尿病与癌症的关联可能与以下机制相关：
  1. 胰岛素刺激细胞增殖。（Giovannucci）
  2. 高血糖促进细胞生长。（Saydah；Rinaldi）
  3. 共同的危险因素：如肥胖（Giovannucci），饮食，缺乏运动（Robert），丙型肝炎（White）和非酒精性脂肪肝（Clark）。

糖尿病和癌症死亡
- 糖尿病增加了男女患者中结肠癌和胰腺癌的死亡风险，增加了男性患者肝癌和膀胱癌的死亡风险，增加了女性患者乳腺癌的死亡风险（Coughlin）。
- 有报道指出糖尿病与男性患者中食道癌、肝癌、结直肠癌，女性患者中肝癌和宫颈癌的死亡呈正相关（Jee）。

癌症患者中的糖尿病
- 荟萃分析显示，糖尿病与多种癌症的死亡率增加相关（$HR=1.44$），子宫内膜癌（$HR=1.76$），乳腺癌（$HR=1.61$），直肠癌（$HR=1.32$）和前列腺癌（Barone；Snyder）。
- 荟萃分析显示，糖尿病与多种癌症的术后死亡率增加相关（$HR=1.5$）(Brarone)。
- 高血糖与急性淋巴细胞性白血病患者完全缓解时间短相关（Weiser）。
- 高血糖与新诊断胶质母细胞瘤患者生存期较短相关（Derr）。

糖尿病与前列腺癌
- 糖尿病与前列腺癌风险呈负相关（Kasper）。
- 去雄激素疗法引起体内成分、血脂成分的变化，降低胰岛素敏感性（Faris）。

- 去雄激素疗法显著增加了男性中患糖尿病的风险（Alibhai）。

肥胖和癌症
- 荟萃分析（Renehan）指出 BMI 与以下疾病密切相关：
  - 食道腺癌（RR 1.52），甲状腺癌（RR 1.33），结肠癌（RR 1.59）和肾癌（RR 1.24）（均为 $P<0.001$）。
  - 女性中子宫内膜癌（RR 1.59），胆囊癌（RR 1.59），食管癌（RR 1.51）和肾癌（RR 1.34）（均为 $P<0.05$）。
  - 男性中患癌症和恶性黑色素瘤，关联性较弱。
- 相比于严重的肥胖患者，胃旁路分流术后患者癌症病死率较低（Adams）。

临床治疗

糖尿病治疗和癌症风险
- 最近的研究表明二甲双胍（Currie；Bodmer）和噻唑烷二酮（Blanquicett）可能降低癌症的风险，但进一步研究正在进行。
- 长期胰岛素使用可能与癌症死亡率增加有关（Bowker），而尚未证实特定的胰岛素与患癌症率增高有绝对性的联系（Currie）。

专家意见
- 上述风险属于统计性关联，它们受一些干扰因素，不能被证明因果关系。
- 因此，在患有糖尿病的患者中，应更加谨慎地使用已有的筛查方法，例如对于结肠癌，可以有指示作用；但通常不通过强调统计数据的关联去恐吓患者。
- 同样地，治疗方面，在使用二甲双胍或胰岛素与癌症之间的相关性的临床结论需谨慎下定论。

推荐依据
Giavannucci E, Harlan DM, Archer MC, et al. Diabetes and cancer: a consensus report. CA Cancer J Clin, 2010; Vol. 60: pp. 207–21.

Comment: A consensus report from the American Diabetes Association and American Cancer Society that reviews the current state of knowledge regarding the association of diabetes and cancer, including possible biological mechanisms.

其他参考文献
Barone BB, Yeh HC, Snyder CF, et al. Postoperative mortality in cancer patients with preexisting diabetes: system- atic review and meta-analysis. Diabetes Care, 2010; Vol. 33: pp. 931–9.

Comments: The landmark systematic review reports that compared with their nondiabetic counterparts, cancer patients with preexisting diabetes are approximately 50% more likely to die after surgery.

Snyder CF, Stein KB, Barone BB, et al. Does pre-existing diabetes affect prostate cancer prognosis? A systematic review. Prostate Cancer Prostatic Dis, 2010; Vol. 13: pp. 58–64.

Comments: Reports pre-existing diabetes is associated with increased long-term, overall mortality, receiving radiation therapy, complication rates, recurrence, and treatment failure.

Faris JE, Smith MR Metabolic sequelae associated with androgen deprivation therapy for prostate cancer. Curr Opin Endocrinol Diabetes Obes, 2010; Vol. 17: pp. 240–6.

Comments: Concludes androgen deprivation therapy is associated with diabetes mellitus, and linked to cardiovascular morbidity.

Bodmer M, Meier C, Krähenbühl S, et al. Long-term metformin use is associated with decreased risk of breast cancer. Diabetes Care, 2010; Vol. 33: 1935-5548; pp. 1304–8.

Comments: Evaluates whether use of oral hypoglycemic agents is associated with an altered breast cancer risk in women.

Derr RL, Ye X, Islas MU, et al. Association between hyperglycemia and survival in patients with newly diagnosed glioblastoma. J Clin Oncol, 2009; Vol. 27: pp. 1082–6.

Comments: Reports hyperglycemia is associated with shorter survival, after controlling for glucocorticoid dose and other confounders.

Alibhai SM, Duong-Hua M, Sutradhar R, et al. Impact of androgen deprivation therapy on cardiovascular disease and diabetes. J Clin Oncol, 2009; Vol. 27: pp. 3452–8.

Comments: Continuous androgen deprivation therapy use for at least 6 months in older men is associated with an increased risk of diabetes and fragility fracture.

Currie CJ, Poole CD, Gale EA The influence of glucose-lowering therapies on cancer risk in type 2 diabetes. Diabetologia, 2009; Vol. 52: pp. 1766–77.

Comments: Examines the risk of development of solid tumors in relation to treatment with oral agents, human insulin, and insulin analogues.

Chao C, Page JH. Type 2 diabetes mellitus and risk of non-Hodgkin lymphoma: a systematic review and meta-analysis. Am J Epidemiol, 2008; Vol. 168: pp. 471–80.

Comments: Type 2 diabetes mellitus is associated with altered immune function and chronic inflammation, which are also implicated in the pathogenesis of non-Hodgkin lymphoma. This study summarizes findings from the current literature on the association between history of type 2 diabetes mellitus and risk of non-Hodgkin lymphoma.

Rinaldi S, Rohrmann S, Jenab M, et al. Glycosylated hemoglobin and risk of colorectal cancer in men and women, the European prospective investigation into cancer and nutrition. Cancer Epidemiol Biomarkers Prev, 2008; Vol. 17: pp. 3108–15.

Comments: The results of this study suggest a mild implication of hyperglycemia in colorectal cancer, which seems more important in women than in men, and more for cancer of the rectum than of the colon.

White DL, Ratziu V, El-Serag HB. Hepatitis C infection and risk of diabetes: a systematic review and meta-analysis. J Hepatol, 2008; Vol. 49: pp. 831-44.

Comments: Reports excess diabetes risk with HCV infection in comparison to non-infected controls. The excess risk observed in comparison to HBV-infected controls suggests a potential direct viral role in promoting diabetes risk.

Renehan AG, Tyson M, Egger M, et al. Body-mass index and incidence of cancer: a systematic review and meta-analysis of prospective observational studies. Lancet, 2008; Vol. 371: pp. 569–78.

Comments: This comprehensive paper reports that an increased BMI is associated with increased risk of common and less common malignancies.

Blanquicett C, Roman J, Hart CM. Thiazolidinediones as anti-cancer agents. Cancer Ther,

2008; Vol. 6: pp. 25–34.

Comments: Discusses studies employing TZDs as anti-cancer therapies for the most common types of can- cers including lung, breast, and colon, and explores the principal PPAR-gamma-dependent and -independent mechanisms by which TZDs exert their anti-tumor effects.

Larsson SC, Mantzoros CS, Wolk A. Diabetes mellitus and risk of breast cancer: a meta-analysis. Int J Cancer, 2007; Vol. 121: pp. 856–62.

Comments: This study assesses the evidence regarding the association between diabetes and risk of breast cancer. Analysis of all 20 studies showed that women with diabetes had a statistically significant increased risk of breast cancer.

Friberg E, Orsini N, Mantzoros CS, et al. Diabetes mellitus and risk of endometrial cancer: a meta-analysis. Diabetologia, 2007; Vol. 50: pp. 1365–74.

Comments: Provides a quantitative assessment of the association between diabetes and risk of endometrial cancer, including both case-control studies and cohort studies.

Adams TD, Gress RE, Smith SC, et al. Long-term mortality after gastric bypass surgery. NEJM, 2007; Vol. 357: pp. 753–61.

Comments: Concludes that long-term total mortality after gastric bypass surgery is significantly reduced, particularly deaths from diabetes, heart disease, and cancer.

El-Serag HB, Hampel H, Javadi F. The association between diabetes and hepatocellular carcinoma: a systematic review of epidemiologic evidence. Clin Gastroenterol Hepatol, 2006; Vol. 4: pp. 369–80.

Comments: A systematic review and a meta-analysis to estimate the magnitude and determinants of associa- tion between diabetes and hepatocellular carcinoma.

Kasper JS, Giovannucci E. A meta-analysis of diabetes mellitus and the risk of prostate cancer. Cancer Epidemiol Biomarkers Prev, 2006; Vol. 15: pp. 2056–62. Comments: This study suggests an inverse relationship between diabetes and prostate cancer.

Clark JM. The epidemiology of nonalcoholic fatty liver disease in adults. J Clin Gastroenterol, 2006; Vol. 40 Suppl 1: pp. S5–10.

Comments: This article reviews the prevalence of NAFLD and the factors associated with this disorder, and with the more advanced stages of NAFLD, including nonalcoholic steatohepatitis (NASH) and fibrosis.

Bowker SL, Majumdar SR, Veugelers P, et al. Increased cancer-related mortality for patients with type 2 diabetes who use sulfonylureas or insulin. Diabetes Care, 2006; Vol. 29: pp. 254–8.

Comments: Explores the association between antidiabetic therapies and cancer-related mortality in patients with type 2 diabetes, suggesting that agents that increase insulin levels might promote cancer.

Larsson SC, Orsini N, Wolk A. Diabetes mellitus and risk of colorectal cancer: a meta-analysis. J Natl Cancer Inst, 2005; Vol. 97: pp. 1679–87.

Comments: A meta-analysis of published data on the association between diabetes and the incidence and mortality of colorectal cancer. Support a relationship between diabetes and increased risk of colon and rectal cancer in both women and men.

Huxley R, Ansary-Moghaddam A, Berrington de González A, et al. Type-II diabetes and pancreatic cancer: a meta- analysis of 36 studies. Br J Cancer, 2005; Vol. 92: pp. 2076–83.

Comments: Type 2 diabetes is widely considered to be associated with pancreatic cancer, but whether this represents a causal or consequential association is unclear. This article provides a meta-analysis to examine this association.

Roberts CK, Barnard RJ. Effects of exercise and diet on chronic disease. J Appl Physiol, 2005; Vol. 98: pp. 3–30.

Comments: The purpose of this review is to 1) discuss the effects of exercise and diet in the prevention of chronic disease, 2) highlight the effects of lifestyle modification for both preventing disease progression and reversing existing disease, and 3) suggest potential mechanisms for beneficial effects.

Jee SH, Ohrr H, Sull JW, et al. Fasting serum glucose level and cancer risk in Korean men and women. JAMA, 2005; Vol. 293: pp. 194–202.

Comments: Reports elevated fasting serum glucose levels and a diagnosis of diabetes are independent risk fac- tors for several major cancers, and the risk tends to increase with an increased level of fasting serum glucose.

Weiser MA, Cabanillas ME, Konopleva M, et al. Relation between the duration of remission and hyperglycemia during induction chemotherapy for acute lymphocytic leukemia with a hyperfractionated cyclophosphamide, vincris- tine, doxorubicin, and dexamethasone/methotrexate-cytarabine regimen. Cancer, 2004; Vol. 100: pp. 1179–85.

Comments: Determines the prevalence of hyperglycemia during induction chemotherapy for acute lympho- cytic leukemia.

Saydah SH, Platz EA, Rifai N, et al. Association of markers of insulin and glucose control with subsequent colorectal cancer risk. Cancer Epidemiol Biomarkers Prev, 2003; Vol. 12: pp. 412–8.

Comments: This study supports the hypothesis that perturbations in insulin and glucose control may influence colorectal carcinogenesis.

胰腺癌

Reza Alavi, MD, MHS, MBA, and Frederick L. Brancati MD,MHS

定义
- 外分泌胰腺癌是最为常见的胰腺导管、腺泡细胞及其干细胞的腺癌。
- 内分泌（胰岛细胞）胰腺癌症通过其分泌的激素分类：胰岛素、胰高糖素、生长抑素或 VIP。

流行病学
- 美国的第四大癌症死亡原因，无论男性或女性（Jemal）。
- 45 岁之前比较罕见，但在此年龄之后，发病率急剧上升。
- 男性发病率高于女性（男女比例为 1.3：1），并且黑人高发（每 100 000 黑人男性 14.8 人患病，而总人群中，每 100 000 人中 8.8 人患病）。
- 内分泌肿瘤较罕见，而外分泌胰腺癌更为常见（例如腺癌 >95%），而内分泌肿瘤较少见。
- 与非糖尿病的患者相比，患 1 型或 2 型糖尿病的成人患者，胰腺癌的风险增加了 2 倍（Everhart）。
- 葡萄糖代谢异常也与胰腺癌的死亡率升高有关（Gapstur）。
- 约 1% 的 50 岁以上的糖尿病患者，在第一次确诊糖尿病后三年内诊断为胰腺癌（Chari）。
- 有更多的证据表明，糖尿病可导致癌症，而不是相反（例如，癌症早期由于破坏胰岛细胞导致糖尿病）(Stolzenberg)，其他的危险因素：吸烟、肥胖、饮食、缺乏体力活动、酒精和服用阿司匹林（Schernhammer）。

诊断
- 诊断和分期通常依据影像学，而不是手术探查。
- 超声内镜：敏感性为 90%，特异性为 90%，有助于分期。
- 胰腺 CT 扫描：敏感性为 90%，特异性为 95%，有助于分期。
- 超声：敏感性为 80%，特异性为 90%。
- 经内镜逆行性胰胆管造影（ERCP）：敏感性为 90%，特异性为 90%。
- 核磁共振成像扫描：敏感性为 90%，特异性为 90%。
- 细针穿刺：敏感性为 90%，特异性为 98%。
- 血清标志物（CA19-9）对于大的肿瘤有很好的敏感性和特异性，但对于诊断小的，外科手术可切除的肿瘤，作用有限。

症状和体征
- 病史：腹痛、食欲不振、黄疸、大便灰白、嗳气、体重减轻、腹胀。
- 查体结果：腹部肿块、腹水、无痛性的可触及的胆囊、左锁骨上淋巴结（Virchow's 淋巴结）。
- 出现症状时，大多数患者已无法切除病灶。
- 体形消瘦的老年人新发糖耐受异常或糖尿病，需警惕胰腺癌的可能（Chari）。

胰腺癌

- 最常见的远处转移部位包括肝脏、腹膜、肺和骨。
- 很多胰腺癌患者为高凝状态（Trousseau's 综合征）。

临床治疗
- 治疗取决于癌症的分期，以及病人是否适合外科手术（仅有 15%~20% 患者适合胰切除术）。
- 胰头肿瘤的外科治疗：标准的胰十二指肠切除术（Whipple 手术），全胰切除术，节段性胰腺切除术或保留幽门的胰十二指肠切除术。
- 胰尾肿瘤可通过远端胰腺次全切除联合脾脏切除术切除。
- 对于胰腺腺癌切除术后患者的治疗，目前并未达成共识（化疗或放疗）。
- 对于局部进展的、无法切除的非转移性疾病的治疗，目前也存在争议，治疗选择：单独放疗（RT）、化放疗和单独化疗。
- 对于进展期胰腺癌，与单独的支持治疗相比，全身化疗（吉西他滨单药治疗或 5-FU 联合治疗）可以改善疾病的相关症状和生存（Yip）。
- 胰腺切除术后是否导致糖尿病取决于手术方式（见胰腺切除术后糖尿病，95 页）。

随访
- 无论选择何种治疗，局部进展期不可切除的肿瘤患者平均生存期约 8~12 个月，已有转移的肿瘤患者为 3~6 个月。
- 绝大多数胰腺癌患者的最终的治疗重点为缓解症状。
- 可通过放置可膨胀支架来减轻黄疸。
- 可通过放置胆道支架及结肠回肠侧后吻合术治疗十二指肠梗阻。
- 可通过内镜下置入可膨胀金属支架治疗有症状的胃流出道梗阻。
- 可应用阿片类止痛药、腹腔神经丛松解术（CPN）或放射治疗缓解疼痛。
- 血栓栓塞事件的发生概率很高（包括动脉和静脉），尤其在疾病晚期。

专家意见
- 尽管糖尿病前期或糖尿病的成年人患胰腺癌的风险增高，并无确切的证据表明血糖控制影响胰腺癌的发病风险。
- 同时患有糖尿病和胰腺癌的患者，手术前后血糖控制常不稳定。
- 虽然胰腺癌可发生于新发糖尿病的老年人，在没有出现其他提示胰腺癌的症状体征时，我们不能为了可能存在的癌症，而常规地进行检查。
- 在新发糖尿病患者中诊断胰腺癌的价值需要进一步评估（例如治愈率）。
- 尽管三维重建胰腺 CT 扫描是胰腺癌诊断和分期的最好的方法，根据经验和专业知识，超声内镜检查也是很有用的。
- 应告知患者胰腺切除术可导致糖尿病，术后应仔细的随访血糖水平。

参考文献
Jemal A, Siegel R, Ward E, et al. Cancer statistics, 2009. CA Cancer J Clin, 2009; Vol. 59: pp. 225–49.
 Comments: Epidemiology of pancreatic cancer.

Yip D, Karapetis C, Strickland A, et al. Chemotherapy and radiotherapy for inoperable advanced pancreatic cancer. Cochrane Database Syst Rev, 2006; Vol. 3: CD002093.

Comments: Chemotherapy appears to prolong survival in people with advanced pancreatic cancer and can confer clinical benefits and improve quality of life.

Chari ST, Leibson CL, Rabe KG, et al. Probability of pancreatic cancer following diabetes: a population-based study. Gastroenterology, 2005; Vol. 129: pp. 504–11.

Comments: Adults with new-onset diabetes were 8 times more likely to be diagnosed with pancreatic cancer within 3 years than the general population.

Stolzenberg-Solomon RZ, Graubard BI, Chari S, et al. Insulin, glucose, insulin resistance, and pancreatic cancer in male smokers. JAMA, 2005; Vol. 294: pp. 2872–8.

Comments: Provides good evidence that the metabolic derangements related to diabetes are a cause of pancreatic cancer. The elevated risk of pancreatic cancer in people with diabetes cannot be explained solely by the cancer's effect on islet cell function during its subclinical phase.

Schernhammer ES, Kang JH, Chan AT, et al. A prospective study of aspirin use and the risk of pancreatic cancer in women. J Natl Cancer Inst, 2004; Vol. 96: pp. 22–8.

Comments: 14 tab/wk of aspirin for more than 4 years increases relative risk of pancreatic cancer by 1.8-fold.

Hochwald SN, Zee S, Conlon KC, et al. Prognostic factors in pancreatic endocrine neoplasms: an analysis of 136 cases with a proposal for low-grade and intermediate-grade groups. J Clin Oncol, 2002; Vol. 20: pp. 2633–42.

Comments: Prognosis of endocrine pancreatic cancer.

Gapstur SM, Gann PH, Lowe W, et al. Abnormal glucose metabolism and pancreatic cancer mortality. JAMA, 2000; Vol. 283: pp. 2552–8.

Comments: Abnormal glucose metabolism increases the relative risk of pancreatic cancer death by 1.5- to 2-fold

Everhart J, Wright D. Diabetes mellitus as a risk factor for pancreatic cancer. A meta-analysis. JAMA, 1995; Vol. 273: pp. 1605–9.

Comments: Diabetes increases odds of pancreatic cancer by two-fold.

感染性疾病

截肢

Lee J. Sanders, DPM

定义
- 非重大下肢截肢（lower extremity amputation, LEA）：脚趾，经跖骨，足中段截肢。
- 重大下肢截肢（LEA）：从小腿远端至胫骨结节的膝下截肢（below-knee transtibial amputation, BKA）；经过股骨的膝上截肢（above-knee amputation, AKA）。
- 切断术：对足部控制不住的脓毒败血症所行的一种开放的截肢术，通过环形切口将骨切下，以便快速去除脓毒性病灶并检查肌肉有无受到感染侵及。
- 自截：干性坏疽病变边界清楚，并可自行脱落，不需手术干预。

流行病学
- 所有 LEA 当中，约三分之二发生在糖尿病患者（主要原因）。
- 危险因素：外周动脉疾病，外周感觉神经病变，溃疡，感染，肾脏疾病，吸烟，既往截肢史。
- 约一半的 LEA 发生在 65 岁以上的患者。
- 在 2003 年，每 1 000 个美国 DM 患者中 LEA 的发生率：黑人患者为 5.0，白人患者为 3.2。
- 85% 的截肢前存在活动性足部溃疡（DFUs）。
- 糖尿病患者接受远端截肢的比例更高（脚趾、经跖骨等）；>50% 的糖尿病患者进行足部水平的截肢（40% 脚趾，13% 经跖骨）。

诊断
- 依靠对截肢危险因素的准确诊断。
- 糖尿病与股－腘动脉和胫骨（膝下）动脉粥样硬化疾病有强相关。
- 周围血管疾病（peripheral vascular disease, PVD）的诊断需要详细评估大腿、腘窝和足部脉搏是否缺失（见周围血管疾病）。
- 踝臂指数（Ankle-brachial index, ABI）：手臂收缩压除以脚踝的收缩压（正常 ABI 介于 0.91~1.30，ABI=0.4 认为存在严重缺血）(Hirsh)。
- 在 DM 患者，由于动脉壁钙化，ABI 可假性增高；10% 的患者所检动脉不能被压缩。
- 解剖研究：(1) 血管成像金标准是常规 X 线血管造影，但仅在准备进行血运重建时应用；(2) 多普勒超声（可直接查看血管状态）；(3) 磁共振血管造影（magnetic resonance angiography, MRA）（无创，风险最小）；(4) CT 血管造影（CT angiography, CTA）(Hirsh)。

- 无论使用何种成像手段，出现血管变细、血流中断、不能见到远端分支等这些征象被认为存在动脉狭窄。
- 脉搏容量记录提供了对血流的定性评估；脚趾压力大于68mmHg和经皮氧分压（transcutaneous oxygen, $TcPO_2$）大于30mmHg能够对经跖骨、足弓或膝下截肢术后能否愈合进行准确预测。
- 对于周围神经病变和足部溃疡这两个重要危险因素的诊断，见相应章节。

症状及体征

- PVD：足部脉搏消失，皮肤发红，抬高时颜色变苍白，趾背毛发缺失，有光泽、鳞屑状皮肤，脚趾增厚，间歇性跛行。
- 急性肢体缺血（Acute limb ischemia, ALI）：可能导致组织坏死的肢体灌注的突然减少；5P征：疼痛、苍白、无脉、感觉异常和麻痹。
- 严重肢体缺血（Critical limb ischemia, CLI）：前脚掌、脚趾和/或腿部的慢性缺血静息痛，缺血性溃疡，组织坏死，或由客观证实的动脉闭塞性疾病引起的。
- 中至重度需氧或厌氧菌感染伴有组织坏死。
- 评估外周动脉疾病严重程度的Rutherford分级用于评估肢体缺血及易处理程度（表3-5）（Hirsh）。

治疗

- 对ALI和CLI的治疗已在坏疽和严重肢体缺血的章节中说明。
- 在那些不能进行重建的疾病中，近40%的CLI患者在最初诊断后的6个月内需要重大截肢术（Hirsh）。
- 截肢的长短是由组织损伤和感染，组织氧灌注，患者的康复潜力，并且外科医生（皮肤温度，头发生长，组织出血，可行的肌肉和伤口无张力）的临床判断的程度来确定。
- 治疗非重大LEA目标：（1）去除没有存活的组织；（2）保留有最大机会获得治愈的足的部分；（3）提供了功能和美容上可接受的足的部分；（4）避免腿部进行重大LEA。
- 治疗重大LEA目标：（1）去除没有存活的组织；（2）保留有最大机会获得治愈的肢体残端；（3）保留最能维持长期功能的肢体残端。

随访

- 由于重大LEA术后30天报道的死亡率在4%~30%，严重疾病（心肌梗死、中风和感染）的发病率在20%~37%，因此需要密切随访。
- 由于总体预后较差，因此对所有危险因素进行强化干预是必要的；美国国家外科质量改进计划（National Surgical Quality Improvement Program, NSQIP）中接受BKA和AKA的患者3年生存期分别为57%和39%（Nehler）。
- 同时对未截肢的肢体也需要强化预防干预，最开始接受了成功的BKA术患者中的15%在2年时转而进行AKA术，这可能是由于近端肢体的动脉粥样硬化闭塞性血管疾病程度更重，膝关节屈曲挛缩以及BKA术残端伤口未愈合后病情进展所致（Nehler）。
- 最开始接受了成功的BKA术患者中还有15%接受了重大的对侧截肢术。

截肢

专家意见

- 综合性多学科参与的足部护理项目可降低 45%~85% 的截肢率。
- 这些统计数字突出了密切随访和强化预防性措施重要性。
- 重大下肢截肢术总体预后较差。

参考文献

Johannesson A, Larsson GU, Ramstrand N, et al. Incidence of lower-limb amputation in the diabetic and nondiabetic general population: a 10-year population-based cohort study of initial unilateral and contralateral amputations and reamputations. Diabetes Care, 2009; Vol. 32: pp. 275–80.

Comments: In the general population aged >45 years, the incidence of vascular lower-limb amputations at orproximal to the transmetatarsal level is 8 times higher in diabetic than in nondiabetic individuals. One in fouramputees may require contralateral amputation and/or reamputation. 74% of all amputations were transtibial.

Canavan RJ, Unwin NC, Kelly WF, et al. Diabetes-and nondiabetes-related lower extremity amputation incidencebefore and after the introduction of better organized diabetes foot care: continuous longitudinal monitoringusing a standard method. Diabetes Care, 2008; Vol. 31: pp. 459–63.

Comments: In the South Tees area of the UK, major diabetes-related LEA rates have fallen over a continuous 5-year period, while major nondiabetes LEA rates increased, after introduction of diabetes foot care program. The biggest improvement in LEA incidence was seen in the reduction of repeat major LEAs.

Ziegler-Graham K, MacKenzie EJ, Ephraim PL, et al. Estimating the prevalence of limb loss in the United States: 2005 to 2050. Arch Phys Med Rehabil, 2008; Vol. 89: pp. 422–9.

Comments: In the year 2005, 1.6 million persons were living with loss of a limb in the United States. 42% werenonwhite and 38% (608,000) had an amputation secondary to vascular disease with a comorbid diagnosis of DM.

Eskelinen E, Eskelinen A, Albäck A, et al. Major amputation incidence decreases both in non-diabetic and in diabetic patients in Helsinki. Scand J Surg, 2006; Vol. 95: pp. 185–9.

Comments: Decrease in major amputation rates among diabetic as well as nondiabetic patients attributed to increased interest in amputation prevention, with a contribution by vascular surgeons.

Jeffcoate WJ. The incidence of amputation in diabetes. Acta Chir Belg, 2005; Vol. 105: pp. 140–4.

Comments: Reported incidence of amputation varies enormously between countries, races, and communities, but gives an indication of the suffering and costs caused by disease of the foot in diabetes. Quality of care of foot disease in diabetes can, and should, be best assessed in terms of survival, function/incapacity, and well-being.

Lavery LA, Armstrong DG, Wunderlich RP, et al. Diabetic foot syndrome: evaluating the prevalence and incidence of foot pathology in Mexican Americans and non-Hispanic whites from a diabetes disease management cohort. Diabetes Care, 2003; Vol. 26: pp. 1435–8.

Comments: Incidence of amputation is higher in Mexican Americans compared to non-Hispanic whites, despite rates of ulceration, infection, vascular disease, and lower-extremity bypass.

Centers for Disease Control and Prevention (CDC). Lower extremity amputation episodes among persons with diabetes—New Mexico, 2000. MMWR, 2003; Vol. 52: pp. 66–8.

Comments: Median age of persons was 66. Incidence was twice a high for men as for women. Overall age adjusted LEA rate was 3.4 per 1000 persons with DM.

Leggetter S, Chaturvedi N, Fuller JH, et al. Ethnicity and risk of diabetes-related lower extremity amputation: a population-based, case-control study of African Caribbeans and Europeans in the United kingdom. Arch Intern Med, 2002; Vol. 162: pp. 73–8.

Comments: Amputation risk in African Caribbeans is one-third that of Europeans and is explained by low smoking, neuropathy, and peripheral vascular disease rates.

Wrobel JS, Mayfield JA, Reiber GE. Geographic variation of lower-extremity major amputation in individuals with and without diabetes in the Medicare population. Diabetes Care, 2001; Vol. 24: pp. 860–4.

Comments: Diabetes-related amputation rates exhibit high regional variation. Adjusted rate of major amputation for individuals with diabetes was 3.83 per 1000. Diabetes amputations accounted for 53% of major amputations.

Adler AI, Boyko EJ, Ahroni JH, et al. Lower-extremity amputation in diabetes. The independent effects of peripheral vascular disease, sensory neuropathy, and foot ulcers. Diabetes Care, 1999; Vol. 22: pp. 1029–35.

Comments: Prospective study to identify risk factors for LEA in individuals with diabetes. Showed that peripheral sensory neuropathy, PVD, foot ulcers, former amputation, and treatment with insulin are independent risk factors for LEA in patients with diabetes.

Centers for Disease Control and Prevention (CDC). Age-Adjusted Hospital Discharge Rates for Nontraumatic Lower Extremity Amputation per 1000 Diabetic Population, by Race, United States, 1980 to 2003. http://www.cdc.gov/diabetes/statistics/lea/diabetes_complications/fig6.htm.

Comments: From 1980 through 2003, the adjusted rate of hospital discharge for nontraumatic lower extremity amputation per 1000 persons with diabetes was higher among blacks than among whites. In 2003, the ageadjusted LEA rate per 1000 persons with diabetes was 5.0 among blacks and 3.2 among whites.

Sanders LJ. Ray and Transmetatarsal Amputations. In Fischer JE, (Ed.), Mastery of Surgery, Fifth Edition. Philadelphia: Lippincott, Williams and Wilkins; 2007: pp. 2193–2207.

Comments: This well-illustrated chapter covers minor (local) amputations of the foot, indications, criteria for wound healing, surgical techniques, complications, and functional outcomes. Attention should be directed to preserving foot function, achieving a durable, cosmetically acceptable result and whenever possible preventing major amputation of the leg.

Nehler MR, Halandres P. Major Lower Extremity Amputation. In Fischer JE, (Ed.), Mastery of Surgery, Fifth Edition. Philadelphia: Lippincott, Williams and Wilkins; 2007: pp. 2211–2220.

Comments: Nicely illustrated chapter discusses indications, preoperative planning, determining level of amputation, surgical technique, and functional outcomes for major LEA.

足部溃疡

Lee J. Sanders, DPM

定义
- 糖尿病足溃疡（Diabetic foot ulcer，DFU）：发生在糖尿病患者脚踝以下的不愈合或愈合不良的非全层或全层伤口，是糖尿病足自然病程中的关键阶段。
- 最常见的部位：脚（跖骨头和足弓）的跖面和脚趾（背侧趾间关节或远端趾尖）。
- 发病机制：DFUs经常发生于知觉丧失的脚重复受到伤害。

流行病学
- 鞋不合适是造成DFUs最常见的原因。
- DFUs危险因素：周围神经病变，周围血管病变，足部畸形（槌状趾，爪状趾，突出跖骨头，拇外翻，瓶底凸出的脚），振动觉阈值（vibratory perception threshold，VPT）高于25V，既往足部溃疡，视力障碍，糖尿病肾病（尤其是透析患者），血糖控制不佳和吸烟。
- 发病率：每年在糖尿病患者中的发病率为1.9%~2.2%。
- 患病率：根据文献报道，最低英国南亚裔1.8%，最高美国11.8%。
- DFUs罹患风险可达25%。
- DFUs最常见导致截肢的前兆，85%的截肢前存在活动性足部溃疡。
- 每次治疗溃疡相关花费平均为13 179美元（1 892~27 721美元），并随严重程度增加而递增（Stockl），主要源于住院治疗。

诊断
- 根据在神经病变的背景下是否存在缺血病变，分为神经性、缺血性或神经缺血性。在此列出几个具体的分类。
  - Wagner-Meggitt分类：基于深度，存在或不存在感染、坏疽，将足溃疡分为六个等级。除了5级之外，其他级别均可转0级糖尿病足。0级：皮肤完整；1级：浅表溃疡；2级：溃疡侵及肌腱、骨骼或关节囊；3级：侵及更深组织，并伴有脓肿、骨髓炎或沿肌腱鞘中足隔室扩展的肌腱炎；4级：单个或多个脚趾、前足的坏疽；是手术消融适应证；5级：坏疽涉及整个足部，保足治疗已不可能。需要膝下截肢（Wagner）。
  - 德克萨斯大学（University of Texas，UT）分类：UT系统评估溃疡的深度，伤口感染和缺血的征象。0级：完整的皮肤（溃疡前或已愈合的溃疡部位）；1级：表面溃疡，不累及肌腱、关节囊或骨；2级：侵及肌腱或关节囊；3级：侵及骨或关节。此级可进一步分为四期：A期：清洁伤口；B期：非缺血性感染伤口；C期：缺血性非感染伤口；D期：缺血性感染伤口（Oyibo）。
  - PEDIS：以研究为目的进行的糖尿病足溃疡分级。评估五个重要的临床特点，灌注（Perfusion），范围/大小（Extent/size），深度/组织脱落（Depth/tissue loss），感染（Infection）和感觉（Sensation）（糖尿病足国际工作组，http://www.iwgdf.org）。

症状及体征

- DFU的早期表现：轻度红斑，皮温升高，水疱形成，袜子或床单上可见浆液或血清遗留。
- 神经性溃疡：通常被结痂包围，位于脚趾尖，在趾间关节的顶部，跖骨头下方，如无感染，一般无痛感。
- 神经缺血性溃疡：通常位于足部边缘，在骨突处（第一、第五跖骨头）。溃疡周围通常有红斑光晕围绕。通常合并继发于缺血或感染的疼痛。

治疗

足部检查及危险评估

- 早期发现足部病变并积极护理可以降低截肢风险。
- 需要详细询问病史，并在光线充足的房间对足部进行仔细检查。
- 必须评估神经、血管、皮肤、骨骼肌肉等指标。
- 检查鞋子，以确定是否适合足部（长度、宽度、深度），状态（磨损状态，突出的接缝或指甲），以及是否适合患者的足部结构和功能。
- 鞋子应容纳足部畸形，保护高风险的足避免受到伤害。
- ADA危险分级（表3-10）：危险分级0~3级，由以下危险因素存在与否共同决定：伴有保护性感觉缺失（loss of protectice sensation，LOPS）的外周神经病变，外周动脉疾病（peripheral arterial disease，PAD），足畸形和既往足部溃疡或截肢史。
- 治疗和随访建议依据危险分级而定。

内科及外科治疗

- 用手术刀进行清创，去除结痂及坏死组织，可在初级保健机构进行，但最好是由糖尿病足专科人员完成。
- 伤口敷料，以控制渗出，保持湿润的环境。
- 减压力负荷（治疗足底溃疡的基石）：用全接触支具（total contact cast，TCC），苏格兰靴和可拆卸式助行器（removable cast walkers，RCWs）。一旦DFU愈合，评估是否需要定制成型鞋垫/矫形和治疗鞋类。
- 感染：糖尿病足感染需要关注局部（足）和全身性（代谢）问题，并协调跨学科足部护理团队进行感染管理。
- 避免对缺乏伤口化脓、炎症表现的非感染伤口进行抗生素治疗。
- 确定是否需要进行外科和感染性疾病专科会诊。
- 浅表溃疡合并感染：清创，针对金黄色葡萄球菌、链球菌的口服抗生素（见Johns Hopkins ABX指南，糖尿病足感染）。
- 感染的伤口可能需要：切开引流，切除感染坏死组织，局部截肢，血运重建术。
- 深部（威胁肢体）感染：紧急手术引流，清除坏死组织，静脉使用覆盖革兰阳性、革兰阴性菌及厌氧菌的广谱抗生素（见Johns Hopkins ABX指南，糖尿病足感染）。

足部溃疡

- 戒烟。

鞋类
- 鞋是最主要的可纠正的危险因素。
- 鞋子应符合脚形,具有宽敞的鞋头,可紧贴足跟,且鞋跟较低(小于5cm),内衬光滑,鞋底够厚、以防刺伤,通过系鞋带或皮带将足部固定在鞋的后方;如果可保证足够的鞋长、宽和深,运动鞋亦可。
- 为了减少摩擦,建议穿着袜子。
- 定做(定制)鞋可容纳中至重度足/踝关节畸形和部分足截肢。
- 在炎热的气候下,应穿着包住脚趾的凉鞋。

专家意见
- 最常导致 DFUs 的组合因素是周围神经病变、足部畸形和创伤。
- 最可预测溃疡的单一因素是既往溃疡史及截肢史。
- 一些发展中国家常见的赤脚习惯增加 DFUs 风险。
- 患者必须明白感觉丧失的含义,穿合适、合脚的鞋的重要性,并避免赤脚行走。

表 3-10 基于综合足部检查的危险分级

风险级别	定义	治疗建议	随访建议
0	无 LOPS,无 PAD,无畸形	患者教育,包括穿合脚鞋类的建议。	每年一次(全科医师和/或专科医师)
1	LOPS,伴或不伴畸形	考虑定制或宽松的鞋。如果足部畸形不能安全地被鞋包纳,考虑预防性手术。继续患者教育。	3~6 个月一次(全科医师或专科医师)
2	PAD,伴或不伴 LOPS	考虑定制或宽松的鞋。考虑与血管专科医师一同随访。	2~3 个月一次(专科医师)
3	有溃疡史或截肢史	同风险级别 1 如存在 PAD,考虑与血管专科医师一同随访。	1~2 个月一次(专科医师)

来源:Boulton AJ, Armstrong DG, Albert SF, et al. Comprehensive foot examination and risk assessment: a report of the task force of the foot care interest group of the American Diabetes Association, with endorsement by the American Association of Clinical Endocrinologists. Diabetes Care, 2008; Vol. 31(8): pp. 1679–85. Reprinted with permission from The American Diabetes Association.

推荐依据
Apelqvist J, Bakker K, van Houtum WH, et al. Practical guidelines on the management and prevention of the diabetic foot: based upon the International Consensus on the Diabetic Foot (2007), prepared by the International Working Group on the Diabetic Foot. Diabetes Metab Res Rev, 2008; Vol. 24 Suppl 1: pp. S181–7.

Comments: Basic principles of prevention and treatment of the diabetic foot, based upon the International Consensus on the Diabetic Foot (2007), prepared by the International Working Group on the Diabetic Foot. Five key elements of foot management: regular inspection and examination, identification of risk, education (patient, family, provider), appropriate footwear, and treatment of nonulcerative pathology.

Boulton AJ, Armstrong DG, Albert SF, et al. Comprehensive foot examination and risk assessment: a report of the task force of the foot care interest group of the American Diabetes Association, with endorsement by the American Association of Clinical Endocrinologists. Diabetes Care, 2008; Vol. 31: pp. 1679–85.

Comments: ADA Task Force Report, risk classification based on comprehensive foot examination. Can be downloaded from Diabetes Care: http://care.diabetesjournals.org/content/31/8/1679.full.pdf+html?sid=fd69ef11-8a67-4647-9f2e-5c25ed282ef0 (accessed 3/3/2011).

Lipsky BA, Berendt AR, Deery HG, et al. Diagnosis and treatment of diabetic foot infections. Clin Infect Dis, 2004; Vol. 39: pp. 885–910.

Comments: Foot infections in persons with diabetes cause severe morbidities and are the most common proximate, nontraumatic cause of amputations. This guideline provides a framework for treating all diabetic patients with a suspected foot infection.

其他参考文献

Stockl K, Vanderplas A, Tafesse E, et al. Costs of lower-extremity ulcers among patients with diabetes. Diabetes Care, 2004; Vol. 27: pp. 2129–34.

Comments: 2253 adult patients with DM who had a lower-extremity ulcer episode during 2000 and 2001 were identified by claims data. Mean age was 68.9 years, 59% of patients were male. Total ulcer-related costs averaged $13,179 per episode and increased with severity level.

Schaper NC. Diabetic foot ulcer classification system for research purposes: a progress report on criteria for including patients in research studies. Diabetes Metab Res Rev, 2004; Vol. 20 Suppl 1: pp. S90–5.

Comments: International Working Group on the Diabetic Foot (IWGDF) classification system for diabetic foot ulcers, for research purposes.

Oyibo SO, Jude EB, Tarawneh I, et al. A comparison of two diabetic foot ulcer classification systems: the Wagner and the University of Texas wound classification systems. Diabetes Care, 2001; Vol. 24: pp. 84–8.

Comments: Increasing stage, regardless of grade, associated with increased risk of amputation and prolonged healing time. UT system's inclusion of stage makes it a better predictor of outcome.

Wagner FW. The dysvascular foot: a system for diagnosis and treatment. Foot Ankle, 1981; Vol. 2: pp. 64–122.

Comments: Wagner classification of diabetic foot ulcers is based on the depth of the skin lesion and the presence or absence of infection and gangrene. It is still widely used to describe the natural history of the dysvascular foot.

Bakker K, Foster A, van Houtum W, Riley P (Eds.). Diabetes and Foot Care: Time to Act. A joint publication of the International Diabetes Federation and the International Working Group on the Diabetic Foot. 2005. ISBN 2-930229-40-3.

Comments: This publication is the fourth of the International Diabetes Federation's Time to Act series. It is written by international experts and aims to increase awareness of diabetic foot problems worldwide, to demonstrate the benefits of preventive strategies and to convince stakeholders to engage in implementing diabetic foot care services.

艾滋病毒相关糖尿病

Todd T. Brown, MD, PhD

定义
- 人类免疫缺陷病毒（Human immunodeficiency virus，HIV）是一种逆转录病毒，通过感染辅助T细胞，进而产生获得性免疫缺陷综合征（acquired immune deficiency syndrome，AIDS），导致免疫抑制和机会性感染。现代抗逆转录病毒治疗能有效控制HIV的复制，并大大改善HIV感染者的预后。
- 艾滋病毒相关糖尿病指可能没有糖尿病危险因素却发生了糖尿病的HIV感染者。

流行病学
- HIV阳性患者常发生胰岛素抵抗（Insulin resistance，IR）和糖尿病（Diabetes mellitus，DM）。
- 与HIV阴性男性相比，接受逆转录病毒治疗（highly active antiretroviral therapy，HAART）的HIV阳性男性患者糖尿病发病率升高4倍。
- 与HIV阴性相比，HIV感染者更易出现肾病、心血管疾病等并发症（Neuhaus）。
- HIV感染者发生IR/DM的危险因素：腹部脂肪堆积（即脂代谢障碍），外周脂肪萎缩，糖尿病家族史，肥胖，年龄，丙肝阳性，CD4计数降低，黑人/西班牙裔人。
- 某些蛋白酶抑制剂（protease inhibitors，PIs）可能直接影响胰岛素抵抗。在目前使用的PIs中，与IR最相关的是洛匹那韦/利托那韦。
- 司他夫定和齐多夫定也与胰岛素抵抗相关。
- HIV相关合并症其他常用影响血糖的药物：糖皮质激素，生长激素，醋酸甲地孕酮，免疫抑制剂，非典型抗精神病药。
- 患有糖尿病的HIV阳性患者发生冠心病风险增加2倍（Worm）。

诊断
- HIV感染者DM的诊断标准与无HIV相同。
- 接受HAART治疗的HIV感染者的糖化血红蛋白可能被低估约0.8%（Kim）。
- 目前临床上不使用胰岛素水平评估IR。

治疗
- 平衡膳食和规律的运动至关重要。建议ADA推荐的饮食。
- 改变生活方式确可改善HIV感染者的代谢相关指标。
- 积极控制冠心病危险因素：控制血脂，控制血压（通常使用ACEI或ARB），戒烟，避免可卡因，使用阿司匹林治疗。
- 一线治疗：二甲双胍。有些人认为吡格列酮可作为对伴有脂肪萎缩的HIV感染者一线治疗药物，因为吡格列酮可适度增加皮下脂肪。

- 二甲双胍：减轻肝脏的 IR。可减少 HIV 阳性患者的内脏脂肪含量、血压、甘油三酯（降低 10%~20%）。一些研究表明，二甲双胍可减少四肢脂肪；对伴有脂肪萎缩的患者需谨慎使用。在应用核苷类逆转录酶抑制剂（nucleoside reverse transcriptase inhibitors，NRTIs），或伴有肝脏疾病、充血性心脏衰竭时，理论上需注意乳酸酸中毒风险的增加。
- 噻唑烷二酮类（吡格列酮和罗格列酮）：通过激动过氧化物酶体增殖物激活受体（peroxisome proliferatoractivatedreceptor，PPAR）γ 而降低外周 IR。对脂肪萎缩的作用有争议。对脂肪萎缩的治疗，吡格列酮可能比罗格列酮效果更好，但没有头对头的研究。这种效果仅在未使用司他丁类或齐多夫定的患者存在。罗格列酮可能增加一些甘油三酯，但吡格列酮无类似效应。罗格列酮可能增加心血管疾病风险。对于血脂指标，罗格列酮较吡格列酮相比可能不太有利。最大的效果在数周后逐渐出现。
- 使用磺脲类、格列奈类、艾塞那肽、西格列汀或阿卡波糖作为二线治疗。
- 目前不推荐应用药物干预 IR 或糖尿病前期的做法。根据 ADA 指南，可考虑对超重、年轻的糖尿病前期患者使用二甲双胍。
- 考虑从 PI 转换为以非核苷逆转录酶抑制剂（non-nucleoside reverse transcriptase inhibitor，NNRTI）为基础的方案时，应维持控制病毒。
- 如果口服降糖药物失效，考虑小剂量（10~15U）睡前甘精胰岛素、地特胰岛素或 NPH 与口服降糖药联合。对于个体化治疗方案，胰岛素均可有效控制血糖。
- 注意：尚未发现新型的 PIs（阿扎那韦，地瑞那韦）与胰岛素抵抗相关。

随访

- 对艾滋病的常规管理中，应进行空腹血糖的监测。如血糖正常，应常规在基线、HAART 治疗开始前及 HAART 治疗后 3 个月、6 个月，以及此后每年一次，均进行空腹血糖检查。
- 如患者患有糖尿病，口服降糖药者应每天自我监测血糖 1~2 次，使用胰岛素者每天 2~4 次或更多。根据血糖控制的稳定性决定监测的密度。
- 根据控制情况，每 3~6 个月监测糖化血红蛋白。目标 < 7%，需要考虑艾滋病毒感染者检测糖化血红蛋白的准确性。
- 糖尿病前期患者应每隔 3~6 个月筛查血糖。
- 监测并发症：散瞳眼底检查；尿微量白蛋白；基线及每 6~12 个月进行足部检查，包括尼龙丝及振动觉检查（见常规预防性护理）。

专家意见

- 通过有效的 HAART 治疗，HIV 阳性患者生存期明显延长，同时，如糖尿病等与年龄相关的合并症显得越来越重要。
- 由于抗逆转录病毒药物和／或慢性感染艾滋病毒的作用，肾脏疾病和心血管疾病发生率比预期更高。
- 对多种危险因素的控制是必要的。

参考文献

Neuhaus J, Angus B, Kowalska JD, et al. Risk of all-cause mortality associated with nonfatal AIDS and serious non-AIDS events among adults infected with HIV. AIDS, 2010; Vol. 24: pp. 697–706.

Comments: A large cohort study showing the importance of non-AIDS events on mortality in HIV-infectedpersons.

Kim PS, Woods C, Georgoff P, et al. A1C underestimates glycemia in HIV infection. Diabetes Care, 2009; Vol. 32: pp. 1591–3.

Comments: Important paper demonstrating the underestimation of glycemia by A1c in HIV+ patients.

Samaras K. Prevalence and pathogenesis of diabetes mellitus in HIV-1 infection treated with combined antiretroviral therapy. J Acquir Immune Defic Syndr, 2009; Vol. 50: pp. 499–505.

Comments: Good review article regarding insulin resistance and DM in HIV+ patients.

Worm SW, Wit SD, Weber R, et al. Diabetes mellitus, preexisting coronary heart disease, and the risk of subsequent coronary heart disease events in patients infected with human immunodeficiency virus: the Data Collection on Adverse Events of Anti-HIV Drugs (D:A:D Study). Circulation, 2009; Vol. 119: pp. 805–11.

Comments: This study of 33,347 HIV-infected persons found that preexisting DM was associated with two times higher risk of heart disease.

Wohl DA, McComsey G, Tebas P, et al. Current concepts in the diagnosis and management of metabolic complications of HIV infection and its therapy. Clin Infect Dis, 2006; Vol. 43: pp. 645–53.

Comments: Recommendations regarding the management of metabolic abnormalities in HIV+ patients.

Brown TT, Cole SR, Li X, et al. Antiretroviral therapy and the prevalence and incidence of diabetes mellitus in the multicenter AIDS cohort study. Arch Intern Med, 2005; Vol. 165: pp. 1179–84.

Comments: Shows that the risk of incident DM is higher in HIV+ men on HAART compared to HIV-men.

Hadigan C, Corcoran C, Basgoz N, et al. Metformin in the treatment of HIV lipodystrophy syndrome: a randomized controlled trial. JAMA, 2000; Vol. 284: pp. 472–7.

Comments: Shows metformin may be effective in the treatment of central fat accumulation in HIV+ patients.

感染性疾病和糖尿病

Paul Auwaerter, MD

定义

- 糖尿病通常合并有较高的感染几率,但目前支持这种观点的研究结果十分有限。
- 根据 Boyko 和 Lipsky 对流行病学数据的文献综述,"很可能(probable)"指数据支持关联,"可能(possible)"指从现有的信息尚不能确定是否存在关联,"可疑(doubtful)"提示目前数据尚不支持关联。
- 风险很可能(probable)增加的感染:无症状菌尿,下肢感染,胸骨切开或全髋关节置换术后感染,B 族链球菌感染,美国印第安人结核病复发。
- 风险可能(possible)增加的感染:泌尿生殖系统感染,如细菌性膀胱炎、肾盂肾炎、念珠菌性阴道炎,呼吸道感染,包括肺炎、流感、慢性支气管炎、原发或复发肺结核,接合菌感染(如毛霉菌),恶性中耳炎,福尼耳坏疽。
- 风险可疑(doubtful)增加的感染:金黄色葡萄球菌感染,慢性鼻窦炎。

流行病学

- 基于现有数据,尚不能准确得出糖尿病(diabetes mellitus,DM)相关感染的发病率。
- 有心血管病史的糖尿病患者发生感染相关死亡率是无糖尿病患者的三倍(Bertoni)。
- 糖尿病酮症酸中毒(Diabetic ketoacidosis,DKA)和糖尿病高渗状态(hyperosmolar hyperglycemic state,HHS):感染是两者的诱发因素,其中以肺炎和尿路感染(urinary tract infections,UTIs)最为常见。
- 泌尿生殖系统(Genitourinary,GU)感染:DM 患者发生菌尿的机会升高 2~4 倍。虽然较少的数据支持糖尿病患者发生尿路感染或肾盂肾炎的风险增加,但无论男女,发生感染的几率可能是升高的。在气肿性膀胱炎的个案报告中,大部分均患有糖尿病。念珠菌性泌尿道感染,尤其是光滑念珠菌,被认为常见于糖尿病,但支持这一观点的证据不多。通常认为,糖尿病患者发生念珠菌性阴道炎较为常见,但尚无数据支持这一观点。
- 下肢(Lower extremity,LE)感染:多见,包括糖尿病足感染、蜂窝组织炎及骨髓炎。糖尿病患者截肢率较非糖尿病患者升高 15 倍。
- 手术部位感染:研究表明冠状动脉旁路移植术(coronary artery bypass graft,CABG)后胸骨伤口感染、大隐静脉移植部位感染的概率升高。糖尿病患者全髋关节置换术后发生髋部感染的概率也较高。有些研究发现较大的手术术区与发生术后感染概率增加有关(10.7% vs 1.8%),其他一些研究则发现无论是否存在糖尿病,发生术后感染的概率并无明显差别。
- 最有说服力的数据表明,美洲印第安糖尿病患者结核病发病率是增加的。
- B 族链球菌感染:多个病例报道发现,9.4%~45.8% 的 B 族链球菌感染患者存在糖尿病。

- 呼吸系统：肺炎链球菌导致社区获得性肺炎的常见原因。一些研究显示，糖尿病患者肺炎或流感的死亡率增加。
- 接合菌病：包括毛霉菌、根霉菌、小克银汉霉菌和犁头霉菌。病例报道中糖尿病患者有较高的发病率（最高达70%），DKA被认为是本病的危险因素。
- 坏死性筋膜炎/福尼耳坏疽：在病例报道中，糖尿病是本病最常见的合并症（可见于约10%的患者）。

诊断
- GU感染：无症状菌尿指在连续2个尿标本培养中出现 $>10^5$ 菌落数/ml，伴或不伴尿白细胞（white blood cells，WBCs）。膀胱炎或肾盂肾炎根据症状和尿检定义：白细胞酯酶（+），亚硝酸盐（+），尿中 >10 个白细胞/高倍视野，尿培养中 $>10^5$ 菌落数/ml。气肿性复杂UTI（膀胱炎或肾盂肾炎）中，肾或膀胱结构可见气体成分。
- DKA：白细胞计数在 $(10\sim15)\times10^9/L$ 在DKA较常见，通常并不提示感染，如果白细胞计数 $>25\times10^9/L$ 或杆状核粒细胞 $>10\%$ 则考虑存在感染，有待于循证据支持。
- 鼻脑接合菌病：患者通常有侵袭性鼻窦炎，伴焦痂形成。可进行鼻窦CT或MRI检查，并请耳鼻喉专科会诊。组织病理及培养显示菌丝以明确诊断。
- 恶性外耳炎：个案报道显示出，在糖尿病患者中有较高的发病率。病因主要是由于铜绿假单胞菌或曲霉菌属。目前影像学技术以及有效的抗生素治疗使得本病死亡率明显下降。

症状及体征
- 严重，坏死性软组织感染：坏死性筋膜炎，福尼耳坏疽可在24小时内暴发起病（如II型A组链球菌感染），或2~5天慢性起病，这通常是典型I型A组链球菌混合需氧/厌氧菌发生的感染。查体中疼痛可能缺失。如未干预，则可逐渐观察到感染部位皮肤变色、大疱、出现稀薄/污秽的渗出（非脓性分泌物）。
- 鼻脑接合菌病：鼻窦症状，可侵入骨骼和大脑，产生颅神经麻痹。
- 恶性外耳炎：耳痛、耳道红斑或焦痂。可引起面神经麻痹，进一步发展可累及第IX、X、XI及XII颅神经，伴或不伴颅骨骨髓炎。
- B族链球菌（Group B Streptococcal，GBS）感染：糖尿病患者发病风险较高，可发生皮肤/软组织感染、骨/关节感染及尿路感染，常伴发菌血症。
- GU：如果病人没有症状，无论尿液中是否存在白细胞，均提示无症状菌尿。

治疗
- 念珠菌性阴道炎：外用栓剂一线治疗（如非处方药物：克霉唑、布康唑、咪康唑、噻康唑），或外用制霉菌素10万U/天，程度较轻者短疗程（1~3天），如较严重、反复发作或患者免疫功能降低，疗程7~14天。全身治疗：氟康唑150mg单次口服（等待治疗响应3天）。硼酸600毫克凝胶胶囊阴道内给药，每日一次，共14天，对非白色念珠菌物种或难治性感

感染性疾病和糖尿病

- LE 感染：见足部溃疡和骨髓炎。应用覆盖葡萄球菌（+/−MRSA）和革兰阴性菌的抗生素（如头孢氨苄 500mg 口服、每日 4 次，阿莫西林/克拉维 875~1 000mg 口服、每日两次，或克林霉素 300mg 口服、每日三次）治疗蜂窝组织炎 14 天。
- 肺炎：在社区获得性肺炎或医院获得性肺炎的指南中糖尿病与非糖尿病患者并无治疗上的不同。糖尿病患者流感相关死亡率可能更高，因此应考虑给予早期抗病毒治疗。
- 鼻脑接合菌病：及时的手术清创是治疗的关键。抗真菌治疗使用传统的多烯类抗真菌药（两性霉素脂质体 5mg/kg IV 每 24 小时一次），但有报道，相比于单用多烯类药物，泊沙康唑及联合治疗（卡泊芬净与两性霉素 B）在抢救治疗或改善预后方面有一定作用。氟康唑，伏立康唑和棘白菌素类单药治疗无效。需要纠正潜在的酸中毒和高血糖状态。
- 恶性外耳炎：冲洗、洗耳器、耳棉芯和局部抗生素治疗（如滴耳液）。口服全身治疗通常用于联合局部治疗：环丙沙星 500mg 口服、每日两次，共 10~14 天。难治性感染或耐药菌需要通过药敏结果选用敏感药物或抗假单胞菌药物。手术治疗的作用尚不明确。
- GU 感染：无症状菌尿无需抗生素治疗。糖尿病患者出现单纯性尿路感染疗程较长（如 7~10 天），或类似于非糖尿病患者（如呋喃妥因 50~100mg 口服、每天一次，阿莫西林－克拉维酸 500/125mg 口服、每天两次，或甲氧苄氨嘧啶/磺胺甲基异噁唑双强度片一片、每天一次）。
- GBS：治疗取决于感染的位置，首选青霉素治疗。

随访

- 已经在 CABG 术后患者完成了研究，结果显示实行最佳血糖控制可降低伤口感染率。

专家意见

- 糖尿病通常被认为增加多种感染的风险。但是，绝大多数情况下，与糖尿病相关联的感染风险却并未增加。
- 高血糖状态可影响中性粒细胞的功能，使得吞噬、趋化和迁移受损，同时影响细胞内有机体的裂解。
- 其他诱发因素包括由于周围血管疾病和微循环异常引起的组织灌注不良。
- 糖尿病周围神经病变是明确的糖尿病足感染的危险因素。
- 由于自主神经病变引起的膀胱功能异常患者,发生泌尿道感染的风险较高。

推荐依据

Boyko EJ, Lipsky BA. Infection and diabetes. In Harris, MI (Ed.), Diabetes in America, 2nd edition. Washington, DC: National Institutes of Health, 1995; pp. 485–499.

Comments: Authors review available literature to establish whether there is an association with infections commonly considered to be more common in the setting of diabetes. There are some surprising findings, such as insufficient evidence to strongly link rhinocerebral mucormycosis to diabetes or DKA—although this may reflect the available data rather than a true lack of an association. Some studies that support a link date to the 1970s or earlier and relevance in the modern era may be questioned. To access online: http://

diabetes.niddk.nih.gov/dm/pubs/america/index.htm.

其他参考文献

Kitabchi AE, Umpierrez GE, Miles JM, et al. Hyperglycemic crises in adult patients with diabetes. Diabetes Care, 2009; Vol. 32: pp. 1335–43.
Comments: Although infections remain the leading cause of DKA and HHS, suggested algorithms for treatment do not incorporate any formal evaluation of infection or antibiotic therapy but leave this to the clinician to sort through.

Dooley KE, Chaisson RE. Tuberculosis and diabetes mellitus: convergence of two epidemics. Lancet Infect Dis, 2009; Vol. 9: pp. 737–46.
Comments: Authors suggest that the increasing rate of diabetes in both developing world and developing countries may be leading to increased rates of TB. Article is most helpful where highlighting issues in the comanagement of diabetes and TB infection.

Marchant MH, Viens NA, Cook C, et al. The impact of glycemic control and diabetes mellitus on perioperative outcomes after total joint arthroplasty. J Bone Joint Surg Am, 2009; Vol. 91: pp. 1621–9.
Comments: Large retrospective review examining patients with uncontrolled DM (n = 3973) and controlled DM (n = 105,485), and no DM (n = 920,555). Those with uncontrolled DM had increased odds of UTI (adjusted OR = 1.97; 95% CI = 1.61–2.42) and wound infection (adjusted OR ratio = 2.28; 95% CI = 1.36–3.81), among other conditions. Overall mortality was higher, OR 3.23, 95% CI = 1.87–5.57.

Shine TS, Uchikado M, Crawford CC, et al. Importance of perioperative blood glucose management in cardiac surgical patients. Asian Cardiovasc Thorac Ann, 2007; Vol. 15: pp. 534–8.
Comments: Although data substantiating the dangers of hyperglycemia leading to complications after cardiac surgery are robust, there is less supporting the role of tight glucose control to avoiding complications. Authors review the studies looking at intensive insulin use.

Nicolle LE, Bradley S, Colgan R, et al. Infectious Diseases Society of America guidelines for the diagnosis and treatment of asymptomatic bacteriuria in adults. Clin Infect Dis, 2005; Vol. 40: pp. 643–54.
Comments: Asymptomatic pyuria with or without the presence of WBCs is not an indication for treatment. Screening urinalysis is not recommended for diabetic women.

Bertoni AG, Saydah S, Brancati FL. Diabetes and the risk of infection-related mortality in the U.S. Diabetes Care, 2001; Vol. 24: pp. 1044–9.
Comments: Longitudinal study suggested a three-fold increased risk in mortality due to infection in patients with diabetes and cardiovascular disease (CVD), but not in those lacking CVD.

Slovis CM, Mork VG, Slovis RJ, et al. Diabetic ketoacidosis and infection: leukocyte count and differential as early predictors of serious infection. Am J Emerg Med, 1987; Vol. 5: pp. 1–5.
Comments: Given that leukocytosis is a common feature of DKA, this emergency department study of 153 patients found that only the presence of a left shift with significant bandemia (10%) correlated with the presence of actual infection (100% [19/19] and a specificity of 80% [98/122]).

骨髓炎

Paul Auwaerter, MD

定义

- 骨髓炎（Osteomyelitis, OM）：骨的感染。
- 急性 OM：出现骨髓炎表现的 2 周内，无骨坏死/死骨，通常获得途径为血行感染。
- 慢性 OM：虽无明确的定义，但应包括之前 OM 治疗的失败，症状超过 3 周，存在坏死骨/窦道或分泌物流出。
- 在糖尿病足感染（diabetic foot infection, DFI）的情况下，目前没有广泛认可针对 OM 的定义或治疗指南（见足部溃疡）。
- 可将 OM 大致分为两类：（1）在 DFI 下发生的 OM（目前最常见的）；（2）其他部位 OM。

流行病学

- 在 DFI 患者，近 20% 可能存在 OM（Berendt）。
- 由 DFI 导致的 OM 通常是因为神经病变、结痂形成和/或局部缺血引起的溃疡，进而累及了骨膜、骨所致。
- OM/DFI 的危险因素：糖尿病病程大于 10 年，周围神经病变，异常足部结构/体重不均匀地分布于跖面，周围血管疾病，吸烟，糖尿病控制不佳，皮肤/指甲疾病（如浸渍、穿刺伤、足癣、甲癣），男性。
- 急性 OM：少见，通常通过血行获得；在成人主要发生于中轴骨骼（椎间盘炎/脊椎骨髓炎）。
- 慢性 OM：多见于糖尿病患者。通常是由于连续的问题：溃疡 > 创伤 > 手术。
- 微生物：葡萄球菌最常见（金黄色葡萄球菌，包括 MRSA），链球菌（包括 A 组），肠杆菌，厌氧菌。肠球菌通常被找到，因此致病性不确定。OM 往往发生于多种微生物的感染。

诊断

- 当溃疡未能按预期愈合时应该怀疑是否存在 OM。
- 鉴别：神经骨关节病（可以共存，虽无感染，但通常行骨扫描有阳性发现）。
- 通常使用钢针探查。试验阳性增加 OM 的可能性，阴性则 OM 的可能性降低。如观察到骨质碎片，则 OM 诊断明确。
- 影像学：X 线费用较低，也易获得。如骨膜反应，软组织肿胀，骨皮质不规则，骨矿物质减少等表现相对不特异，需要其他检查辅助判断。更进一步的发现，如硬化区域周围邻近透亮或骨质破坏，则高度怀疑 OM。对于慢性 OM，X 线检查整体灵敏度较高但特异性较低。对于急性 OM，X 线改变通常在 2~3 周以后才能看到。
- MRI：评估骨和软组织的首选检查（尤其对较小的骨，对于较大的骨 CT 即可）。有时，急性夏科神经骨关节病 [见夏科关节病（糖尿病神经病性骨关节病）] 会被误读为 OM。
- 骨扫描（TC-99）：不推荐。虽然优于 X 线，但由于非感染性病因（炎症、神经骨关节病）可能产生假阳性。
- WBC 扫描：费用高，与骨扫描相比较不敏感。通常在无 MRI 检查时使用
- PET 扫描：在 OM 的价值尚不确定，相关研究较少，不能提供足够证据表明 PET 灵敏度 / 特异性情况。
- 实验室检查：血沉 > 70mm/h 或 CRP 升高；然而，如果受累的骨较少（如足趾），则血沉或 CRP 可能无变化。血沉的增快和 CRP 升高并不特异，在其他疾病活动时（如蜂窝组织炎等）可升高。血培养通常无阳性发现。
- 确诊：确诊需骨活检，可提供可能的病原学线索和慢性性质。患者应停用抗生素至少 48 小时或更长时间。从骨组织中找到一种或多种病原体即可确诊。由无受累部位进行穿刺或手术方式进行活检。由于取样问题，部分病原体（厌氧菌，不常见的放线菌或分枝杆菌）或之前抗生素治疗等可造成假阴性。由于皮肤菌群污染或伤口定植菌可造成结果假阳性。
- 目前，骨活检没有得到广泛使用。如果不能进行骨活检，需要注意的是伤口拭子结果往往不能代表实际的骨的病原体。但如果进行伤口拭子检查，大多数临床医生可用其结果来指导选用抗生素治疗，特别是对金黄色葡萄球菌（MRSA）的感染（Mackowiak）。

症状及体征
- DFI OM 最常见的部位：脚趾 > 跖骨头 > 跟骨 > 足弓（如果夏科氏神经性关节病存在的情况下）。
- 急性 OM 常伴有局部疼痛、红肿，以及全身症状、发热。
- 慢性 OM 通常无疼痛、发热或全身症状。DFI 时，如存在未愈合的溃疡或观察或探及窦道时，考虑存在 OM。

治疗
- 一般治疗：确保准确微生物学诊断（困难，需要外科医生或执行影像学引导穿刺技术的放射科医生），并清除坏死骨和无活性存在慢性感染的周围软组织。
- 在非严重、无急性感染的情况下，抗生素一般在病原学明确诊断后方可应用。如果病情严重，经验性抗生素治疗应针对革兰阳性（金黄色葡萄球菌、链球菌）、革兰阴性（若非怀疑，通常可不覆盖铜绿假单胞菌）和厌氧菌（见下文）。初始治疗可以为口服或肠胃外治疗。
- 抗生素：经验性：应覆盖链球菌、葡萄球菌和革兰氏阴性菌（gram negative bacteria, GNB），如果足部有臭味，应覆盖厌氧菌。例如：万古霉素 15mg/kg IV 每 12 小时一次（MRSA、链球菌），克林霉素 600mg IV 每 8 小时一次或 450mg 口服每 6~8 小时一次（链球菌、MSSA、一些 MRSA、厌氧菌），哌拉西林－他唑巴坦 3.375g IV 每 4~6 小时一次（MSSA、链球菌、含铜绿假单胞菌的 GNB、厌氧菌），厄他培南 1g 每 24 小时一次（MSSA、链球菌、除铜绿假单胞菌的 GNB、厌氧菌），环丙沙星 400mg IV 每 8~12 小时一次或 750mg 口服每日两次（含铜绿假单胞菌的 GNB）。
- 病原体靶向治疗：通过药物敏感性指导治疗，多种微生物感染时可能需要抗生素联合治疗。见表 3-11。
- 抑制性或巩固性治疗方案：通过药物敏感性指导治疗；一些常用的建议

骨髓炎

如下。葡萄球菌（MSSA 或 MRSA）：甲氧苄啶/磺胺甲基异噁唑双强度片 1~2 片口服、每日两次，美满霉素或强力霉素 100mg 口服、每日两次，克林霉素 300~450mg 口服、每日 3~4 次，利奈唑胺 600mg 口服、每日两次（注意贫血、血小板减少症、外周神经病变或视神经炎等长期并发症）。亦可加用利福平 600mg 口服、每日一次。链球菌，GNB，厌氧菌：阿莫西林/克拉维酸 500mg 口服、每 8 小时一次，莫西沙星 400mg、每日一次。GNB：环丙沙星 750mg 口服、每日两次，或左氧氟沙星 500~750mg、每日一次。厌氧菌：甲硝唑 500mg 口服、每日 3 次。

- 疗程：急性 OM 通常使用静脉抗生素治疗 4~6 周。慢性 OM 治疗疗程取决于病原体、清创的程度、是否有意向根治和/或预防感染复发。如果治愈为目的，使用静脉注射或口服治疗（具有良好的生物利用度的抗生素）至少 6 周，往往需要 12~24 周；有些则可根据 ESR/CRP 进行治疗，直至指标正常化（假设去除了死骨）。如不以治愈为目的，则可连续 6 周用药伴或不伴随后进一步抑制性治疗。
- 手术：对于慢性 OM 的治疗，去除坏死骨至关重要。其他的治疗包括组织、带蒂肌瓣或骨移植。是否截肢取决于是否存在足够的药物/手术治疗选择，或治疗失败。此外，截肢的水平应考虑到对结果功能性的期望和溃疡/OM 复发的可能性（例如膝上截肢或膝下截肢优于经跖骨截肢术）。
- 辅助治疗：血管重建术，向骨局部泵入抗生素，或使用抗生素浸珠，高压氧（有争议）。
- 其他对良好预后较重要的措施：良好的血糖控制，戒烟，非负重状态（如果脚涉及）。请咨询足部护理师、外科医生、或伤口护理专家。

随访

- 治疗失败的原因通常是由于清创不足、抗生素未能覆盖病原体（尤其未进行骨活检时），患者其他合并疾病（如血管功能不全、免疫抑制等），或依从性不佳。
- 目前没有很好的数据能够表明糖尿病 OM 的内科或外科治疗哪一个更优。文献报道总体成功率介于 60% ~90%（Berendt, Calhoun）。
- OM 增加病人需要截肢的可能性（如果 OM 的原因是 DFI）（见截肢）。
- 在成功治疗后，负重足动力学通常发生改变。鼓励进行足部诊疗，并随之更换鞋类。

专家意见

- 表浅溃疡或窦道培养通常是不可靠的。除非发现金黄色葡萄球菌，否则在可进行骨活检的前提下，培养结果不应指导治疗。
- 没有关于抗生素的研究显示某种药物或组合优于其他。
- 骨穿透性较好的抗生素（根据动物研究记过）：克林霉素、氟喹诺酮类、利福平。头孢唑啉和其他 β-内酰胺类药物骨穿透性较差。尚无对人的研究，因此目前不清楚这个区别对人的临床结果会产生何种影响。
- 文献中已经叙述几个关于 OM 的分期系统（Waldvogel, Cierny-Mader），但相比于初始评估或治疗，这些分期系统对外科医生更具有指导意义。
- 外科手术以及足部治疗应遵循个体化原则。使用的策略包括截肢、两阶段清创二次封闭，对出血部位进行初次清创并进行移植术（肌肉，皮肤）。

表 3-11 病原体特异性治疗

- MSSA：奈夫西林或苯唑西林 2g IV q4h，头孢唑啉 2g IV q8h，头孢曲松 2g IV q24h。
- MRSA：万古霉素 15mg/kg IV q12h（目标浓度 15~20mg/dl），达托霉素 6~8 mg/kg IV q24h。
- 葡萄球菌（MSSA，MRSA），链球菌，厌氧菌：克林霉素 600mg IV q6h 或 900mg IV q8h。
- 链球菌属：青霉素 G 2~4 MU IV q4~6h 或氨苄青霉素 2g IV q6h（对于无乳链球菌或肠球菌种，± 庆大霉素 1.0 mg/kg IV q8h）。
- GNB/厌氧菌：氨苄西林/舒巴坦 2g IV q6h，替卡西林/克拉维酸 3.1g IV q4~6h，哌拉西林/他唑巴坦 3.375g IV q4~6h，美罗培南 500~1000mg IV q8h。
- GNB：环丙沙星 400mg IV q12h（可早期过渡到口服治疗：750mg 口服 q12h）或左氧氟沙星 750mg IV（转为口服）q24h。
- GNB：头孢曲松 2g IV q24h 或头孢噻肟 2g IV q6~8h 或头孢他啶 2g IV q8h 或头孢吡肟 2g IV q12h。
- GNB，MSSA，链球菌，厌氧菌：厄他培南 1g IV q24h（方便门诊静脉治疗）。

来源：Paul Pham, PharmD, Johns Hopkins University School of Medicine

推荐依据

Berendt AR, Peters EJ, Bakker K, et al. Diabetic foot osteomyelitis: a progress report on diagnosis and a systematic review of treatment. Diabetes Metab Res Rev, 2008; Vol. 24 Suppl 1: pp. S145–61.

Comments: Systematic literature review highlights that there are insufficient data regarding medical versus surgical management or antibiotic choice to make firm recommendations.

Calhoun JH, Manring MM. Adult osteomyelitis. Infect Dis Clin North Am, 2005; Vol. 19: pp. 765–86.

Comments: Good overall review of OM including pathogenesis, diagnosis and management—both medical and surgical.

其他文献

Johnston B, Conly J. Osteomyelitis management: More art than science? Can J Infect Dis Med Microbiol, 2007; Vol. 18: pp. 115–8.

Comments: Authors present information from human and animal studies that support the rather thin evidence available for typically employed clinical recommendations.

Zuluaga AF, Galvis W, Saldarriaga JG, et al. Etiologic diagnosis of chronic osteomyelitis: a prospective study. Arch Intern Med, 2006; Vol. 166: pp. 95–100.

Comments: When carefully performed, bone culture yield was 94%. Importantly there was only a 30% correlation of bone versus non-bone cultures, although when S. aureus was present this increased to 42%. This study emphasizes that non-bone cultures are not appropriate to guide therapy.

Termaat MF, Raijmakers PG, Scholten HJ, et al. The accuracy of diagnostic imaging for the assessment of chronic osteomyelitis: a systematic review and meta-analysis. J Bone Joint Surg Am, 2005; Vol. 87: pp. 2464–71.

Comments: Useful meta-analysis that examined 23 chronic OM clinical studies compared to histological diagnosis. Sensitivity data included PET (96%), MRI (84%), Tc-99 bone scan (82%), WBC scan (61%), combined bone/wbc scans (78%). Specificity data included PET (91%), MRI (60%), Tc-99 bone scan (25%), wbc scan (84%), combined bone/wbc scans (84%). Overall, bone scans clearly suffer from lack of specificity. PET looks like the lead technology; however, it worked best on the axial skeleton and not peripheral skeleton. WBC scans might have the best diagnostic accuracy; however, sensitivity favors MRI imaging. PET imaging suffers from having relatively few, good studies to guide on its utility.

Mader JT, Shirtliff M, Calhoun JH. Staging and staging application in osteomyelitis. Clin Infect Dis, 1997; Vol. 25: pp. 1303–9.

Comments: Authors compare two commonly employed classification systems (Waldvogel, Cierny-Mader) in OM as well as others.

Mackowiak PA, Jones SR, Smith JW. Diagnostic value of sinus-tract cultures in chronic osteomyelitis. JAMA, 1978; Vol. 239: pp. 2772–5.

Comments: Often cited study showing that sinus tract cultures in chronic OM are only useful if they yield S. aureus. In this study, sinus tract cultures only yielded 44% of the pathogens retrieved from bone. However, there was ~90% correlation if S. aureus was retrieved from the sinus tract.

伤口愈合

Lee J. Sanders, DPM

定义

- 伤口愈合：真皮或表皮组织的自然再生过程。涉及激活角质化细胞、成纤维细胞、巨噬细胞血小板和血管内皮细胞等一系列级联事件。愈合包括了新的上皮细胞形成，减少伤口面积和深度，且没有渗液。
- 伤口愈合不良(Lmpaired wound healing, IWH)：缺乏有序愈合过程增加了截肢风险、死亡率和医疗费用。与 IWH 相关联病生理变化包括高血糖、糖基化终产物 (advanced glycation end products , AGE) 增加、细胞和生长因子反应降低、内皮功能障碍、局部血管生成减低等。
- 不良的愈合过程伴随血管内皮生长因子 (vascular endothelial growth factor, VEGF) 减少，损伤了血管新生和血管生成作用。骨髓衍生的内皮祖细胞 (endothelial progenitor cells, EPCs) 对新生血管形成至关重要，但糖尿病患者的 EPCs 减少。角质形成细胞和成纤维细胞的迁移和增殖也有所下降。基质金属蛋白酶 (Matrix metaloproteinases, MMPs) 在伤口愈合过程中也发挥重要作用，在伤口渗液中大量存在。
- 糖尿病足包含一系列病理状况，包括了神经病变、缺血、溃疡、感染、夏科氏足和坏疽等，其中糖尿病足溃疡 (diabetic foot ulcer, DFU) 是最具特征性。

流行病学

- 皮肤破溃后伤口愈合失败是导致截肢的最常见原因,可占81%的病例(Pecoraro)
- 诱发因素：（1）异常细胞/炎症途径；（2）外周神经病变；（3）缺血、高血糖、糖基化终末产物(AGE)及其他生理损伤原因令愈合过程复杂化，对抗感染和引起足够炎症反应的能力受损。
- 不利于伤口愈合的因素：糖尿病，衰老，肥胖，营养不良，伤口供氧降低，吸烟和肾功能受损等。

诊断

- 确定产生伤口的原因：缺血、神经病变、小的创伤、结痂、感染和/或足部畸形。
- 对是否需要住院或门诊治疗进行评估，并完善检查（伤口分泌物培养，代谢指标，血常规加白细胞分类，X光片和血管超声等）。
- 评估伤口：PEDIS– 灌注，范围/大小，深度/组织缺损，感染，感觉。
- 描述伤口解剖学位置、外观、温度、有无脓性分泌物、有无气味。
- 使用无菌探针评估伤口的深度和范围。确定皮肤边缘，窦道，脓肿，是否侵及肌腱、骨骼或关节。伤口深度对预后的判断非常重要。

症状和体征

- 由于周围感觉神经病变，未受感染的伤口症状可能非常显著。神经病变合并缺血的伤口多为中度至严重感染伤口，通常十分疼痛。

伤口愈合

- 蜂窝组织炎大于2厘米,淋巴管炎扩散,深部组织脓肿,坏疽,肌肉、肌腱关节或骨骼的受累均是中度感染的征象。
- 发热、寒战、心动过速、低血压、意识模糊、呕吐、白细胞升高、酸中毒、严重高血糖或氮质血症的存在提示全身中毒症状和/或代谢不稳定,是严重感染的特征性表现。

治疗

- 基本治疗:清洁伤口(用无菌生理盐水或伤口清洁剂),锐器伤清创,对伤口进行恰当的敷料覆盖,伤口充分减负荷设备,控制感染,控制代谢指标,缺血肢体的血运重建。
- 伤口清创:去除结痂和坏死组织。慢性伤口的维持清创的目的是促进并维持伤口在愈合状态。
- 感染控制:局部(脚)和全身性(代谢);对无感染性溃疡、无脓性分泌物或缺乏炎症表现的伤口应避免应用抗生素。伤口的细菌性污染和定植并不意味着感染。对于表浅溃疡,全身应用抗生素应针对金黄色葡萄球菌和链球菌。针对生物负载最好用清洁伤口和清创的方式处理。
- 伤口减负荷:缓解足部机械应力(压力、剪切力和重复性损伤)以治疗和预防进一步损伤,用全接触支具(total contact cast, TCC)(金标准),即时TCC(instant TCC, ITCC),可拆卸式助行器(removable cast walkers, RCWs),苏格兰靴,拐杖和轮椅。
- 敷料:根据伤口情况(干燥、渗出、感染、坏死、非全层或全层)进行选择。没有适合所有伤口的最佳敷料,而是随着愈合过程伤口的变化,敷料品种可能也随之发生改变。生理性湿润的伤口愈合环境可促进创面上皮化,并有助于防止干燥。敷料作为一个屏障,可防止伤口进一步损伤,减少感染风险,并优化伤口周围环境。常用的被动型和相互作用型敷料见表3-12所述。
- 高级治疗:局部生长因子(PDGF-BB),蛋白酶抑制剂,生物工程皮肤替代物。作为生物活性敷料,诸如低温冻存的人皮肤移植物、活性皮肤替代物可向伤口提供生长因子、细胞因子及胶原等。常用的生物活性伤口护理产品见表3-12所述。
- 负压伤口疗法(Negative pressure wound therapy, NPWT):一种开孔泡沫敷料,表面覆有粘性遮盖,并连接到真空泵产生负压。最常用的装置是封闭式负压引流(Vacuum Assisted Closure, V.A.C.)(KCI, San Antonio, TX)。尽管目前循证证据基础薄弱,但负压伤口治疗已得到广泛应用。
- 鞋类和矫形器:在伤口愈合之前,便进行评估,以确定合适的鞋子、矫形器和支撑物。
- 关键点:对高压部位进行减负荷处理,可适应足部畸形(槌状趾、拇外翻、跖骨头突出、足弓塌陷和足部分截肢)和足/踝部支撑不稳。应在伤口愈合时便提供治疗鞋类和/或支撑物,并在全重量负重前持续使用。

随访

伤口治愈的可能性随病程的延长而逐渐下降。
肾功能不全及透析是长期预后的重要预测指标。

- 4周时观察足部溃疡面积变化的百分比是在12周伤口能否愈合的重要预测指标。

专家意见

- 注：对于不同的伤口护理产品的临床疗效或优势，文献综述提供的证据水平较弱（Bergin）。对于治疗DFUs，含银敷料和外用剂价格昂贵。在标准治疗之外，细胞衍生的伤口护理产品会产生很高的费用。然而，高昂的费用可能因更快的愈合和更短的治疗周期而被抵消（Langer）。
- 由于较高的费用、较长的治疗时间以及感染和截肢的潜在风险的增加，治疗愈合较差的伤口显得非常重要。
- 慢性伤口更容易感染，更需要住院或手术治疗，并导致治疗费用的增加。
- 应不断提醒患有周围感觉神经病变的患者，他们感觉缺失可能导致反复破溃、感染、截肢的相关风险增加。
- 跨学科团队管理（包括足部治疗师或伤口护理专家）、早期发现和干预患者教育、密切监测，这些都是预防及治疗糖尿病足创伤的关键。
- 糖尿病医护人员应当对不同种类的伤口护理产品的使用有一定的了解。

表 3-12 被动型、相互作用型、生物活性伤口护理产品

类别	功能	特性	举例	适应证
被动型敷料				
藻酸纤维	吸收作用，包扎	适形和吸收作用。从褐色海藻中提取的非织制丝纤维。由藻酸钙组成，如渗出液被吸收，可通过离子交换机制（钙交换为钠），形成亲水性凝胶。可吸收高达自身20倍的重量。	Sorbsan, Kaltostat, Restore, CalciCare, Nu-derm, Algisite M, Seasorb 可作为薄片或绳使用	全层污染和感染的伤口。中度到重度渗液伤口。包扎伤口需宽松。需要辅助敷料进一步保护固定。每天换药。
泡沫材料	吸收作用，包扎	半渗透性聚氨酯泡沫。无粘性亲水性聚合物。可将渗出控制在伤口之外。	Allevyn, Lyofoam, PolyMem, Tielle, Copa	非全层和全层伤口。最小至中度渗液、感染伤口。泡沫需要盖住伤口周围皮肤，并需要额外的敷料覆盖。每3~7天更换敷料。
薄纱布	吸收作用，包扎	纺织的或无纺、无菌和非无菌。海绵状、垫状、绳状、带状和卷状。可浸渍有凡士林、抗生素和盐水。	Curity Gauze, SpongeKerlix, NuGauze Packing	非全层和全层伤口。受感染的伤口。可包扎较大的伤口。贴附于伤口组织，非选择性的清创。具有一定保湿性。需要频繁换药每天2~3次。

表 3-12 被动型、相互作用型、生物活性伤口护理产品（续）

类别	功能	特性	举例	适应证
水合胶体	吸收作用	亲水性，封闭性敷料。羧甲基纤维素，果胶或明胶。以糊剂、粉剂或薄片的形式。防渗，防水屏障。表水胶体粘合剂。	Duoderm, Restore, Tegasorb, Comfeel	非全层和全层伤口。适形。小量至中度渗出伤口。去除敷料时需小心避免撕裂皮肤。敷料与伤口渗出发生反应，在伤口内留下有气味的凝胶。每5~7天换药一次。
水凝胶	维持伤口湿润环境	以甘油或水为基础的半渗透敷料。可以薄片、粘性凝胶或颗粒的形式。薄片敷料可含有多达96%的水，保持湿润的伤口环境。自溶清创性。对伤口具有凉爽、舒缓的效果。	Aquaflo, Curafil, Hypergel, Vigilon, Intrasite gel	非全层和全层伤口。干燥或有很少渗出的伤口。坏死和感染伤口。与其他敷料配合使用。
透明薄膜	保护作用	透明的有粘性的聚氨酯薄膜。半渗透性，不吸收。自溶清创性。伤口边界需要干燥。	Op-Site, Tegaderm, Polyskin II	无渗出的非全层伤口。限制敷料下的液体排出。不建议用于感染伤口。每3~5天更换敷料。
相互作用型敷料				
元素抗生物制剂	减少生物负载	半闭合敷料含有银和碘。Cadexomer 碘在浓度达0.45%时对成纤维细胞无毒害作用。cadexomer 珠有固住细胞。银具有抑菌性能。	磺胺嘧啶银膏，含银敷料，Cadexomer 碘	可用于控制或减少伤口的生物负荷。元素抗生制剂的使用应当谨慎，仅限于2~4周。

伤口愈合

氧化再生纤维素（ORC）胶原蛋白	吸收作用，使金属蛋白酶无效	ORC 的无菌冻干基质及胶原蛋白，吸收伤口渗出物形成一种生物可降解的凝胶。与基质金属蛋白酶（MMP）化学结合，并使它们无效。在慢性伤口渗出液中升高的蛋白酶水平降低新形成的肉芽组织，从而阻碍了伤口愈合。	Promogran (Systagenix Wound Management)	非全层或全层渗出伤口。直接涂抹干整个创面。对于很少或无渗液的伤口，用生理盐水或林格氏液润湿。为了维持伤口湿润环境，可用纱布覆盖，非粘附或氢化聚合物敷料。
酶清创剂	非手术酶学清创	胶原酶和木瓜蛋白酶-尿素。减少伤口微生物负载，清除坏死组织，促进新芽组织形成。	Santyl Ointment（胶原酶），Accuzyme（木瓜蛋白酶-尿素）	非全层或全层坏死伤口。对于那些不能接受手术或需要较少损伤的清创术的患者。如果结痂出现，应用刀片在结痂上划交叉线。用生理盐水清洗伤口，将酶清创剂直接用于伤口，盖上纱布作为第二层敷料，每日一次，直至肉芽组织形成。
皮肤湿润再平衡技术（"SMRT"敷料）	湿润调节	以无纺聚酯/人造丝为衬底，加入无粘性、惰性、具有透气性的聚合物。可通过释放和吸收作用调节整个伤口的水分。湿润而无浸渍。	TheraGauze (Soluble Systems, Newport News, VA)	非全层和全层伤口。感染和未感染的伤口。干燥或伴有严重渗出的伤口。注：Fenestrate 针对中到重度渗出性伤口。需要一个覆盖敷料，透明薄膜。每周更换 2-3 次。去除敷料：如果伤口干燥，应先用生理盐水润湿。可以用于皮肤移植物和供体部位的覆盖敷料，以及局部应用预防感染或抗生素治疗。

表 3-12 被动型、相互作用型、生物活性伤口护理产品（续）

类别	功能	特性	举例	适应证
治疗糖尿病足溃疡的细胞衍生产品				
生长因子：PDGF-BB	促进伤口愈合	重组血小板衍生生长因子（PDGF）。趋化成纤维细胞并促进成纤维细胞有丝分裂。刺激细胞外基质和肉芽组织。 美国 FDA 警告： 禁用于在应用药物部位有肿瘤的患者。在一个上市后回顾性队列研究中观察到，使用 3 支以上 REGRANEX Gel 的患者中继发于治疗部位远端肿瘤的死亡率增加。 REGRANEX 凝胶应仅用于治疗获益预期大于风险的患者。	REGRANEX (becaplermin) Gel 0.01% (Ortho-McNeil)	用于治疗深入皮下组织且有血液供应充足的 DFUs。对于使用 becaplermin，清创操作是至关重要的辅助治疗措施。一天一次，每次应用恰当的剂量，并覆盖以潮湿的敷料。12 小时内更换敷料时，使用生理盐水清洁，并应用生理盐水润湿的敷料覆盖。
生物工程皮肤替代品（BSS）	促进伤口愈合	Apligraf：双层活性人皮肤替代物，具有异体真皮及分化良好的异体表皮。由在 I 型胶原蛋白基质中培养的人包皮成纤维细胞生成的新生真皮和角化细胞。可产生具有与伤口愈合相关的细胞因子和生长因子。	Apligraf (Organogenesis, Canton, MA) Dermagraft (Advanced BioHealing, La Jolla, CA)	BSS 是价格不菲，但是无溃疡时间的增加，以及感染和截肢风险的降低可抵消初始成本。 Apligraf 的适应证为治疗下肢静脉溃疡和 DFUs。

	促进伤口愈合	TheraSkin：低温冻存的人类皮肤移植物，包含表皮和真皮层。细胞得到保留。包含具有生物活性细胞外基质，可向伤口提供生长因子。提供有效的天然屏障，有助于控制感染，促进肉芽组织生成和上皮化。减少液体和蛋白质的丢失。 GammaGraft：γ 射线照射的人类皮肤移植物，表皮和真皮被保留，但没有活性细胞。在密封的铝箔和青霉素/庆大霉素溶液中封装保存。可在室温下储存2年。	TheraSkin (Soluble Systems, Newport News, VA) GammaGraft (Promethean LifeSciences, Inc., Pittsburgh, PA) GraftJacket (Wright Medical Technology, Inc., Arlington, TN)	对超过4周的保守伤口护理没有反应的糖尿病足溃疡（DFUs）和下肢静脉溃疡（VLUs）。溃疡面应无感染或潜在的骨髓炎。必须有充足的血液供应，ABI ≥ 0.65。DFUs, VLUs, 全层溃疡, 莫氏手术（Mohs surgery）部位, 植皮供皮区, 非全层伤口, 烧伤, 伤口必须清洁无感染。DFUs, 修复或替代损伤或不完整的外皮组织, 禁用于感染或非血管外科手术部位, 禁用于结缔组织疾病患者。 请参阅制造商的具体说明。
人皮肤移植物				
尸体皮肤移植物				

Dermagraft：一种低温保存的人成纤维细胞衍生的真皮替代物。由成纤维细胞、细胞外基质和可吸收支架构成。由新生包皮衍生的人类成纤维细胞制成。有助于修复真皮床，促进伤口再上皮化。

Dermagraft 的适应证为治疗6周以上通过真皮延伸的全层DFUs，同时没有肌腱、肌肉、关节囊或骨的暴露。
请参阅制造商的具体说明。

表 3-12 被动型、相互作用型、生物活性伤口护理产品（续）

类别	功能	特性	举例	适应证
		GraftJacket：脱细胞真皮组织基质。将供体皮肤中表皮和真皮细胞去除而制成。是一个支持细胞增殖和血管化的框架。在冷冻干燥的铝箔袋中密封。室温运输，冷藏储存。		

资料来源：Sanders LJ, Frykberg RG. The Charcot Foot (Pied de Charcot). In: Bowker J, Pfeifer MA, eds. Levin and O'Neal's TheDiabetic Foot. 7th ed. Philadelphia: Elsevier Inc.; 2008

推荐基于以下文献

Falanga V, Brem H, Ennis WJ, et al. Maintenance debridement in the treatment of difficult-to-heal chronic wounds. Recommendations of an expert panel. Ostomy Wound Manage, 2008; Vol. Suppl: pp. 2–13, quiz 14–5.

Comments: Consensus development conference on treatment of chronic wounds.

Bergin SM, Wraight P. Silver based wound dressings and topical agents for treating diabetic foot ulcers. Cochrane Database Syst Rev, 2006; CD005082.

Comments: Results reveal no randomized clinical trials (RCTs) or controlled clinical trials (CCTs) evaluating the effect of silver-based products on infection and healing of diabetic foot ulcers. The authors were unable to determine whether silver-based dressings and topical agents result in benefits or harms for people with diabetes-related foot ulcers.

American Diabetes Association. Consensus Development Conference on Diabetic Foot Wound Care: 7–8 April 1999, Boston, Massachusetts. Diabetes Car, 1999; Vol. 22: pp. 1354–60.

Comments: Consensus position statement on 6 questions: (1) What is the value of treating a diabetic foot wound? (2) What is the biology of wound healing? (3) How should diabetic foot wounds be assessed and classified? (4) What are the appropriate treatments for foot wounds? (5) How should new treatments be evaluated? and (6) How can recurrent foot wounds be prevented?

其他文献

Langer A, Rogowski W. Systematic review of economic evaluations of human cell-derived wound care products for the treatment of venous leg and diabetic foot ulcers. BMC Health Serv Res, 2009; Vol. 9: p. 115.

Comments: Cell-derived wound care products in addition to standard care generate very high costs. Economic analysis suggests that the initial high costs of these products may be offset by (1) restricted use to ulcers that are unresponsive to healing, (2) higher healing rates and shorter treatment periods, (3) fewer complications, and (4) fewer inpatient episodes. Further research is necessary to obtain better estimates of the clinical benefits.

Ghanassia E, Villon L, Thuan Dit Dieudonné JF, et al. Long-term outcome and disability of diabetic patients hospitalized for diabetic foot ulcers: a 6.5-year follow-up study. Diabetes Care, 2008; Vol. 31: pp. 1288–92.

Comments: 60.9% of patients had ulcer recurrence, 43.8% underwent amputation (24 minor and 15 major), and 51.7% died. The global long-term outcome of patients hospitalized for DFUs was poor. Multivariate analysis showed age and impaired renal function/albuminuria as independent predictors of wound healing failure.

Gregor S, Maegele M, Sauerland S, et al. Negative pressure wound therapy: a vacuum of evidence? Arch Surg, 2008; Vol. 143: pp. 189–96.

Comments: Institute for Research in Operative Medicine and Institute for Quality and Efficiency in Health Care systematic review of RCTs and non-RCTs comparing NPWT and conventional therapy for acute and chronic wounds. Main outcomes of interest were wound healing variables. Conclusion: Although there is some indication that NPWT may improve wound healing, the body of evidence is insufficient to clearly prove an additional clinical benefit. From 2003–2004, revenue for vacuum-assisted closure increased by 45% to $700 million.

Payne WG, Salas RE, Ko F, et al. Enzymatic debriding agents are safe in wounds with high bacterial bioburdens and stimulate healing. Eplasty, 2008; Vol. 8: p. e17.

Comments: Collagenase and papain-urea appear beneficial and safe even in wounds with high bacterial loads, and appear to significantly aid extent and rate of healing.

Brem H, Tomic-Canic M. Cellular and molecular basis of wound healing in diabetes. J Clin Invest, 2007; Vol. 117: pp. 1219–22.

Comments: Available online: http://www.jci.org/articles/view/32169/pdf.

Gallagher KA, Liu ZJ, Xiao M, et al. Diabetic impairments in NO-mediated endothelial progenitor cell mobilization and homing are reversed by hyperoxia and SDF-1 alpha. J Clin Invest, 2007; Vol. 117: pp. 1249–59.

Comments: This study aimed to determine mechanisms responsible for the diabetic defect in circulating and wound endothelial progenitor cells (EPCs). EPCs are essential in vasculogenesis and wound healing.

Bryant RA, Nix, DP. Acute and Chronic Wounds: Current Management Concepts, Third Edition. St. Louis, MO: Mosby Elsevier; 2007. ISBN-13: 978-0-323-03074-8

Comments: Comprehensive all-inclusive resource on the management of acute and chronic wounds, withemphasis on the multidisciplinary team approach to wound management.

Armstrong DG, Lavery LA, Wu S, et al. Evaluation of removable and irremovable cast walkers in the healing of diabetic foot wounds: a randomized controlled trial. Diabetes Care, 2005; Vol. 28: pp. 551–4.

Comments: Intent-to-treat analysis showed that modification of a standard RCW wrapped with a cohesive bandage or plaster bandage (iTCC), to increase patient adherence to pressure off-loading, had a higher proportion of ulcers that healed than in the RCW group (82.6 vs 51.9%). Those treated with an iTCC healed significantly sooner (41.6 + 18.7 vs 58.0 + 15.2 days, p = 0.02).

Lobmann R, Schultz G, Lehnert H. Proteases and the diabetic foot syndrome: mechanisms and therapeutic implications. Diabetes Care, 2005; Vol. 28: pp. 461–71.

Comments: Review article: the biology of normal wound healing, pathogenesis of wound healing in chronic wounds, cytokines and growth factors, MMPs in wound healing, and clinical studies with growth factors and protease inhibitors.

Lipsky BA, Berendt AR, Deery HG, et al. Diagnosis and treatment of diabetic foot infections. Clin Infect Dis, 2004; Vol. 39: pp. 885–910.

Comments: IDSA Guidelines for the evaluation, classification, and treatment of diabetic foot infections. Contains suggested empirical antibiotic regimens based on clinical severity. Can be downloaded free from http://www.journals.uchicago.edu/doi/pdf/10.1086/424846.

Sheehan P, Jones P, Caselli A, et al. Percent change in wound area of diabetic foot ulcers over a 4-week period is a robust predictor of complete healing in a 12-week prospective trial. Diabetes Care, 2003; Vol. 26: pp. 1879–82.

Comments: 276 patients randomized to either a moistened gauze dressing or a collagen/oxidized regenerated cellulose dressing (Promogran). Wound area measurements were performed at baseline and after 4 weeks. The percent change in wound area at 4 weeks in those who healed was 82%, whereas in those who failed to heal the percent change in wound area was 25%.

Armstrong DG, Nguyen HC, Lavery LA, et al. Off-loading the diabetic foot wound: a randomized clinical trial. Diabetes Care, 2001; Vol. 24: pp. 1019–22.

Comments: The proportions of healing for patients treated with TCC, RCW, and half-shoe were 89.5%, 65.0%, and 58.3%, respectively. A significantly higher proportion of patients were healed by 12 weeks in the TCC group.

Reiber GE, Vileikyte L, Boyko EJ, et al. Causal pathways for incident lower-extremity ulcers in patients with diabetes from two settings. Diabetes Care, 1999; Vol. 22: pp. 157–62.

Comments: The Rothman model of causation was applied to the diabetic foot ulcer condition. The most frequent component causes for lower-extremity ulcers were a critical triad of neuropathy, minor foot trauma, and foot deformity, present in >63% of patient's causal pathways.

Pecoraro RE, Reiber GE, Burgess EM. Pathways to diabetic limb amputation. Basis for prevention. Diabetes Care, 1990; Vol. 13: pp. 513–21.

Comments: The authors define the causal pathways responsible for 80 consecutive initial lower-extremity amputations. Most pathways were composed of multiple causes. 46% of the amputations were attributed to ischemia, 59% to infection, 61% to neuropathy, 81% to faulty wound healing, 84% to ulceration, 55% to gangrene, and 81% to initial minor trauma.

男性疾病

勃起功能障碍

Amin Sabet, MD

定义
- 不能达到或维持足够的勃起以进行令人满意的性活动。
- 糖尿病患者导致勃起功能障碍（erectile dysfunction，ED）的多种病理生理因素：内皮细胞/平滑肌功能障碍，自主神经病变，性腺功能低下症，心理/人际关系的因素，抗高血压药物副作用（如利尿剂、β受体阻滞剂）。

流行病学
- 一般人群：患病率从5.1%（40岁以前）到70.2%（70岁以后）。
- 糖尿病：20岁以上者，校正年龄后，ED发病率在糖尿病男性患者为38.6%，非糖尿病男性患者为18.4%（Selvin）。
- 与ED有关的临床情况：神经病变（周围、自主），视网膜病变，血糖控制不佳，糖尿病病史较长。
- ED是糖尿病患者发生冠心病和心脏不良事件的独立预测因素（2倍风险）（Gazzaruso）。

诊断
- 病史：性欲（与雄激素作用相关），药物使用（SSRIs、安体舒通、可乐定、噻嗪类利尿剂、β-受体阻滞剂、酮康唑、西咪替丁），使用非法药物，起病症状（起病急骤提示精神因素）。
- 查体：视野检查（垂体大腺瘤造成性腺功能低下），脉搏（股动脉、外周动脉），男性乳房发育（见于性腺功能减退），睾丸，阴茎斑块（阴茎硬结症）。
- 实验室检查：糖化血红蛋白、睾酮、泌乳素、促甲状腺激素（见男性性腺功能减退症）。
- 其他检查：邮票试验和四级勃起硬度测量带在很大程度上已被如Rigi扫描等检测设备取代，后者可对夜间勃起的刚性和膨胀程度提供更精确和可重复的信息。
- 夜间阴茎勃起试验中完全缺乏夜间/清晨勃起提示神经源性或血管疾病。

治疗
- 血糖控制不佳与ED有关，但改善血糖控制可逆转ED的证据尚不充分。
- 性腺功能减退患者ED应予雄激素治疗。
- 一线用药：PDE5抑制剂（见西地那非、伐地那非、他达拉非）。
- 二线治疗：真空勃起设备。
- 三线治疗：经尿道或海绵体内PGE1（前列地尔）。
- 四线治疗：阴茎假体植入手术。

勃起功能障碍

- PDE5 抑制剂禁用于服用硝酸酯类药物的患者；对有心肌缺血、心功能不全和使用 CYP3A4 抑制剂（减少药物清除）或 α-肾上腺素能阻滞剂（可能到导致低血压）的情况下可能有害。
- 有罕见的报道表明在使用 PDE5 抑制剂治疗时，可发生非动脉炎性前部缺血性视神经病变；但两者的因果关系尚未确立。

随访
- 泌尿科复诊，尤其是对 PDE5 抑制剂治疗效果不佳的患者。

专家意见
- PDE5 抑制剂可改善大多数 1 型和 2 型糖尿病患者的 ED（Rendell），并应首先应用，尽管对于那些非糖尿病 ED 患者并不十分有效。
- PDE5 抑制剂不应该处方给服用硝酸酯类药物的男性。
- 同时使用 PDE5 抑制剂与 α-受体阻滞剂时，需要高度注意这两个血管扩张药物合用可能会导致低血压。
- 造成 ED 的精神心理因素包括抑郁症、焦虑症、以及男女关系(包括婚姻)问题。
- 在药物治疗之外，性心理辅导作为一种辅助治疗措施是有帮助的（Melnik）。

参考文献

Gazzaruso C, Solerte SB, Pujia A, et al. Erectile dysfunction as a predictor of cardiovascular events and death in diabetic patients with angiographically proven asymptomatic coronary artery disease: a potential protective role for statins and 5-phosphodiesterase inhibitors. J Am Coll Cardiol, 2008; Vol. 51: pp. 2040–4.
Comments: ED independently predicts major adverse cardiac events (HR 2.1) in diabetics with asymptomatic CAD.

Selvin E, Burnett AL, Platz EA. Prevalence and risk factors for erectile dysfunction in the US. Am J Med, 2007; Vol. 120: pp. 151–7.
Comments: Overall prevalence of ED in men aged 20 and over is 18.4% in nondiabetic versus 38.6% (age-adjusted) in diabetic men.

Melnik T, Soares BG, Nasselo AG. Psychosocial interventions for erectile dysfunction. Cochrane Database Syst Rev, 2007; CD004825.
Comments: In men treated with sildenafil, group psychotherapy may improve ED.

Rendell MS, Rajfer J, Wicker PA, et al. Sildenafil for treatment of erectile dysfunction in men with diabetes: a randomized controlled trial. Sildenafil Diabetes Study Group. JAMA, 1999; Vol. 281: pp. 421–6.
Comments: Sildenafil improved ED in 56% of diabetic men.

Feldman HA, Goldstein I, Hatzichristou DG, et al. Impotence and its medical and psychosocial correlates: results of the Massachusetts Male Aging Study. J Urol, 1994; Vol. 151: pp. 54–61.
Comments: 52% prevalence of ED in men age 40–70 (general population).

Wein AJ, Van Arsdalen KN. Drug-induced male sexual dysfunction. Urol Clin North Am, 1988; Vol. 15: pp. 23–31.
Comments: Commonly used meds causing ED.

McCulloch DK, Campbell IW, Wu FC, et al. The prevalence of diabetic impotence. Diabetologia, 1980; Vol. 18: pp. 279–83.
Comments: Among diabetic men, ED is common and best correlates with proliferative retinopathy and symptomatic autonomic neuropathy..

男性性腺功能减退症

Amin Sabet, MD

定义
- 男性性腺功能减退是指精子生成和/或睾酮作用下降。
- 分为原发性(睾丸疾病引起)或继发性(垂体或下丘脑疾病引起)。
- 性腺功能减退可能是勃起功能障碍的一个原因,但是也应与之区分开。
- 总睾酮水平低于青年男性平均值2.5个标准差,绝对值或小于300ng/dl。
- 临床诊断标准不十分明确。

流行病学
- 在横断面研究中,男性糖尿病患者性腺功能减退症的发病率20%~64%之间,老年人中发病率更高(Dhindsa, Kalyani)。
- 糖尿病患者发生性腺功能减退症危险因素涉及多种机制,包括增加体重的性腺功能低下症,性激素结合球蛋白降低(sex hormone binding globulin, SHBG),促性腺激素释放受抑制或睾丸间质细胞分泌睾酮受抑;细胞因子介导对睾丸类固醇产生的抑制作用;芳香化酶活性增加造成雌激素相对增多。
- 尽管校正了肥胖,但低睾酮水平仍是2型糖尿病的独立危险因素,可能是由于雄激素受体基因多态性,令葡萄糖转运的改变,或降低了抗氧化作用所致(Stellato, Kalyani)。

诊断
- 诊断性腺功能减退症应用过精子数量减少和/或与年龄相匹配的参考值相比睾酮水平降低(如小于300~400mg/dl)。
- 由于睾酮存在昼夜波动,应上午8点测定睾酮,同时测定FSH、LH。
- 总睾酮水平未必准确反映肥胖患者(SHBG较低)和老年人(高SHBG)的性腺功能,如果怀疑性腺功能减退症,应进行游离或活性睾酮检测。
- 游离或活性的睾酮水平可通过总睾酮、白蛋白及SHBG水平计算(可利用 http://www.issam.ch/freetesto.htm 在线计算器)。
- 男性性腺机能减退症患者,黄体生成素(luteinizing hormone, LH)或卵泡刺激素(follicle-stimulating hormone, FSH)升高提示原发性性腺功能减退症,两者正常或偏低提示继发性性腺功能减退症。
- 原发性腺功能减退症的鉴别诊断:感染(如腮腺炎),外伤,化疗,放射线照射,隐睾,Klinefelter综合征。
- 继发性腺功能减退症的鉴别诊断:垂体功能低下,高泌乳素血症,甲状腺功能减退症,血色病,长期使用阿片类药物,肥胖。
- 全身性慢性疾病,如艾滋病、肝病/肝硬化、肾功能衰竭、糖尿病等可能有对诊断有干扰,但更可能与继发性性腺功能减退症相关(Kalyani)。
- 对于原发性腺功能减退症,进行外周血染色体核型分析以评估是否存在Klinefelter综合征(47 XXY)。

男性性腺功能减退症

- 对于继发性腺功能减退症，测定血清催乳素、甲状腺素、清晨皮质醇，铁饱和度，并行垂体 MRI 检查。

症状及体征

- 青春期后的性腺功能减退症的症状包括性功能障碍，不孕不育，男性乳房发育，精力下降，情绪低落或幸福感减退，易怒，注意力不集中，潮热，骨密度降低，乏力，疲倦，贫血，瘦体质降低并体内脂肪增加。
- 男性第二性征的减退或缺失，如体毛分布和肌肉质量，可能在性腺功能减退起病数年后发生。
- 宦官身材（下部量＞上部量，臂展较身高长 5cm 以上）提示青春期前起病。
- 查体可发现睾丸体积较小（正常 ≥ 25cc）。

治疗

- 替代治疗应当给予那些同时有低血清睾酮水平以及典型的性腺功能减退症状的患者。
- 睾酮治疗的主要治疗目标是恢复睾酮水平至正常范围，并症状改善。
- 睾酮治疗禁忌证包括存在活动性前列腺癌或乳腺癌，并可能加重红细胞增多症，阻塞性睡眠呼吸暂停，严重的下尿路症状或严重的充血性心脏衰竭。
- 经皮睾酮可作为凝胶剂、贴剂或口腔睾酮片。
- 睾酮贴剂：初始剂量是每天 5mg，但可能导致应用部位局部的不良反应。
- 1% 睾酮凝胶：初始剂量为每天 5g（50mg 睾酮），通常作为一线治疗选择，应用部位不良反应较少。
- 庚酸睾酮及环戊丙酸睾酮通过肌内注射给予。初始剂量为 150~200mg 每 2 周一次；通常是儿童患者首选的药物。通常不用于成人，这是由于这种给药方式出现非生理性的睾酮水平波动。
- 肌注睾酮治疗可改善糖尿病患者肥胖状态及血糖控制（Kapoor）。

随访

- 初始睾酮治疗后 3 个月监测症状，并定期监测。
- 初始睾酮治疗后 2~3 个月检测睾酮水平，之后每 6 个月后继续监测。如果肌注给药，应当在两次注射之间检查。
- 在治疗前，开始睾酮治疗后 3 个月，以及之后的每 6~12 个月，应进行肛门指检，并测定前列腺特异性抗原（prostate-specific antigen，PSA）和红细胞压积。
- 如果 PSA 高于 4.0ng/ml，或在任何 1 年增加超过 1.4ng/ml，或平均 PSA 增加速度超过每年 0.4ng/ml 持续两年以上，或肛门指诊有异常发现时，应就诊于泌尿外科会诊。
- 如果血细胞比容超过 54%，停止治疗，并进行缺氧和睡眠呼吸暂停的情况评估。
- 需要考虑进行血脂谱和肝功能检查。
- 对合并有骨质疏松症的性腺功能减退症患者使用睾酮治疗后 1~2 年需测量骨密度。

专家意见

- 糖尿病很可能与继发性性腺功能减退症有关。
- 睾酮治疗的益处不仅仅是改善症状,同时对糖尿病患者的血糖控制和体重控制有益。
- 常用的检测游离睾酮的方法是直接放射免疫法(direct radioimmunoassay, RIA),该方法并不十分可靠,不应被用于诊断性腺功能减退症。
- 目前所使用的最可靠有效的方法是,首先测定总睾酮水平,如果正常,则可除外性腺功能减退症;如果总睾酮水平较低,同时患者合并肥胖、糖尿病,游离睾酮可经由总睾酮、性激素结合球蛋白和白蛋白计算得出(Rosner)。
- 由于睾酮水平存在昼夜波动,即使在清晨亦是如此。因此应至少在不同时间测量两次以确认较低的睾酮水平,从而支持性腺功能减退症的诊断。
- 睾酮凝胶既避免了肌注睾酮产生的非生理性的睾酮水平波动,同时也避免了睾酮贴剂对接触皮肤区域的不良反应,是首选的治疗。但应避免所涂皮肤与妇女和儿童相接触。

推荐依据

Bhasin S, Cunningham GR, Hayes FJ, et al. Testosterone therapy in adult men with androgen deficiency syndromes: an endocrine society clinical practice guideline. J Clin Endocrinol Metab, 2006; Vol. 91: pp. 1995–2010.

Comments: Endocrine Society practice guideline on treatment of hypogonadism.

其他参考文献

Laughlin GA, Barrett-Connor E, Bergstrom J. Low serum testosterone and mortality in older men. J Clin Endocrinol Metab, 2008; Vol. 93: pp. 68–75.

Comments: Men 50 and older with testosterone levels in the lowest quartile were 40% more likely to die within 20 years than men with higher testosterone.

Selvin E, Feinleib M, Zhang L, et al. Androgens and diabetes in men: results from the Third National Health and Nutrition Examination Survey (NHANES III). Diabetes Care, 2007; Vol. 30: pp. 234–8.

Comments: Men with free and bioavailable testosterone in the lowest tertile were 4 times more likely to have diabetes than those with testosterone levels in the third tertile.

Rosner W, Auchus RJ, Azziz R, et al. Position statement: utility, limitations, and pitfalls in measuring testosterone: an Endocrine Society position statement. J Clin Endocrinol Metab, 2007; Vol. 92: pp. 405–13.

Comments: Endocrine Society position statement regarding measurement of testosterone.

Kalyani RR, Gavini S, Dobs AS. Male hypogonadism in systemic disease. Endocrinol Metab Clin North Am, 2007; Vol. 36: pp. 333–48.

Comments: Summary of manifestation and treatment of hypogonadism in various chronic systemic illnesses.

Kalyani RR, Dobs AS Androgen deficiency, diabetes, and the metabolic syndrome in men. Curr Opin Endocrinol Diabetes Obes, 2007; Vol. 14: pp. 226–34.

Comments: Describes the bidirectional association of hypogonadism and diabetes, in addition to possible mechanisms and an algorithm for evaluating suspected hypogonadism in persons with diabetes.

Kapoor D, Goodwin E, Channer KS, et al. Testosterone replacement therapy improves insulin resistance, glycaemic control, visceral adiposity and hypercholesterolaemia in hypogonadal men with type 2 diabetes. Eur J Endocrinol, 2006; Vol. 154: pp. 899–906.

Comments: Randomized-controlled crossover trial of intramuscular testosterone therapy versus placebo in hypogonadal men with diabetes for 3 months in random order. HOMA-IR, A1c, and fasting glucose all significantly improved with testosterone therapy.

Mohr BA, Guay AT, O'Donnell AB, et al. Normal, bound and nonbound testosterone levels in normally ageing men: results from the Massachusetts Male Aging Study. Clin Endocrinol (Oxford), 2005; Vol. 62: pp. 64–73.

Comments: Suggested cutoffs for abnormally low total testosterone level as less than 8.7, 7.5, 6.8, and 5.4 nm (251, 216, 196, and 156 ng/dl) for men in their 40s, 50s, 60s, and 70s, respectively.

Dhindsa S, Prabhakar S, Sethi M, et al. Frequent occurrence of hypogonadotropic hypogonadism in type 2 diabetes. J Clin Endocrinol Metab, 2004; Vol. 89: pp. 5462–8.

Comments: 33% of patient with type 2 diabetes were hypogonadal.

Stellato RK, Feldman HA, Hamdy O, et al. Testosterone, sex hormone-binding globulin, and the development of type 2 diabetes in middle-aged men: prospective results from the Massachusetts male aging study. Diabetes Care, 2000; Vol. 23: pp. 490–4.

Comments: Odds ratio for future diabetes of 1.58 for a 1 SD decrease in free testosterone.

肌肉、皮肤及骨骼疾病

骨骼疾病

Kendall F. Moseley, MD, and Todd T. Brown, MD, PhD

定义
- 骨质疏松症和骨质减少是 1 型糖尿病（type 1 diabetes mellitus，T1DM）和 2 型糖尿病（type 2 diabetes mellitus，T2DM）患者中最重要的骨骼疾病，以骨量减少和骨组织结构破坏为特征，导致骨脆性增加、易发生骨折。
- 通过双能 X 线骨密度仪（dual energy X-ray absorptiometry，DXA）测量骨密度；T 值介于 +1.0 和 −1.0 个标准差（standard deviations，SD）之间的被认为是骨密度正常，介于 −1.0 和 −2.5 个 SD 间的是骨质减少，低于 −2.5 个 SD 是骨质疏松症；Z 值用于年龄小于 50 岁的男性，以及绝经前妇女。
- 软骨病是因钙和维生素 D 代谢受损引起的骨质软化。
- Charcot 足是足或踝部骨质丢失造成的微小骨折、韧带松弛和骨破坏，并因神经病变和患者无法感知正在进行的创伤而加重的结果 [见 Charcot 关节病（糖尿病神经源性骨关节病）]。

流行病学
- 根据美国国家骨质疏松基金会（National Osteoporosis Foundation，NOF）的数据统计，50 岁以上的人超过 55% 存在骨量丢失；在美国，超过一千万人患骨质疏松症，而三千四百万人患骨量减少。
- T1DM 患者骨质疏松症和骨质疏松的患病率取决于个人是否已经达到了峰值骨量、糖尿病病程以及血糖控制的程度（Mastrandrea）。
- 与年龄匹配的对照组相比，T1DM 的中年患者中，30%~60% 存在骨量减少，10%~30% 患骨质疏松症（Wada）。
- T2DM 患者骨密度较健康对照者相比正常或偏高，尽管这个群体可能更容易发生臀部和非脊椎部位的骨折（Vestergaard）。
- T2DM 患者骨量降低和骨折的风险报道不一，取决于疾病控制，病程和终末器官损害（如神经病变、肾病、视网膜病变）（Leidig-Bruckner）。

诊断
- 请参阅具体的诊断标准部分。
- DXA 是面积密度测量的金标准（见骨密度）。
- 容积定量 CT 扫描和跟骨超声测量骨密度（bone mineral density，BMD）的替代方式。
- 筛查：没有针对糖尿病患者进行骨质疏松症或骨质疏松检查的指南建议。
- 目前 NOF 一般建议：如果没有骨质疏松症的危险因素，65 岁以上的女性及 70 岁以上的男性应进行骨密度检查（Heinemann）。
- 如果存在一个或多个骨质疏松或骨病的危险因素（如类固醇的使用、甲状旁腺功能亢进症，营养不良，产妇髋部骨折），应对50岁以上的男性及女性进行骨密度检查。
- 如果有脆性骨折史，不论年龄、性别，均应检查。
- 偶然识别出的低骨量或骨矿化较差的情况可经由常规X线进行诊断。
- 血清25-羟维生素D水平降低（小于15ng/ml）同时伴有全段甲状旁腺激素升高（intact parathyroid hormone, iPTH）提示可能存在骨软化症。
- 由于肾脏疾病或维生素D缺乏而出现的继发性甲状旁腺功能亢进患者，血清甲状旁腺激素水平的升高亦可导致骨骼疾病。

症状及体征

- 骨病的症状及体征在糖尿病与无糖尿病患者一致。
- 骨质疏松症和骨量减少通常无临床症状。
- 任何年龄段的T1DM及T2DM患者出现低创伤骨折或复发性骨折均应当提高合并骨骼疾病的警觉。
- 骨密度降低导致的脆性骨折是骨质疏松症患者疼痛和发病的主要原因。
- 突然疼痛、局部腰痛或查体中脊柱压痛提示可能存在椎体骨折。
- 跌倒后严重的髋关节疼痛、髋关节肿胀、不能行走提示可能存在髋部骨折。
- 严重的维生素D缺乏可表现为骨骼疼痛和疲劳。
- T1DM患者乳糜泻及维生素D缺乏的发病率增高，症状包括腹痛、腹胀、腹泻。
- 维生素D缺乏症/佝偻病可观察到弓形腿。

治疗

糖尿病及并发症的管理

- 优化血糖控制以减少糖基化终末产物（advanced glycation end product, AGE）在骨骼上的沉积（Schwartz）。
- 优化血糖控制和饮食，以减少营养不良的发生，特别是在T1DM早期患者。
- 糖化血红蛋白控制在小于7%的水平，虽然可以减少微血管和大血管并发症，但随之可导致和加剧骨病和摔倒的风险（Schwartz）。
- 筛查视网膜病变和神经病变，预防跌倒和减少骨折发生。
- 预防和治疗肾病，维持正常的血钙、血磷水平及维生素D羟化作用。
- 预防和减少周围血管疾病及微血管病变以优化骨骼血供并维持骨质量。
- 自主神经功能紊乱患者，若不及时治疗体位性低血压，可能会增加跌倒和骨折风险。
- 尽量减少低血糖发作，因低血糖可导致昏厥、跌倒和骨折（Schwartz）。

饮食及生活方式

- NOF推荐的饮食和生活方式适用于患有骨骼疾病的一般人群及糖尿病人群。
- 50岁以下成人每日摄入钙1 000mg和维生素D 400~800IU；50岁以上及有明确骨病的患者，每日摄入钙1200mg和维生素D 800~1 000IU。
- 如果摄入不足或吸收不良，应考虑膳食补充剂。
- 维生素D缺乏或不足者需要大剂量的维生素D。
- 每日蛋白质的摄入量应占每日卡路里摄取量的15%。

- 保持健康的体重（BMI 18.5~24.9kg/m²）。
- 进行负重运动和抗阻练习，以强化骨骼（Daly）。
- 中度有氧运动对心血管健康和维持体重有益。
- 家居安全评估和危害识别是预防跌倒的重要方面。
- 髋关节保护器对老年人具有潜在益处。

药物治疗

- 如果存在骨质疏松症和/或具有骨折高风险，通常需要在锻炼、钙剂、维生素D之外加用药物治疗（见专家意见部分）；治疗方案与没有糖尿病的骨质疏松患者相同。
- 抗骨吸收药物抑制破骨细胞介导的骨吸收发挥治疗作用，但仅限于无肾功能不全患者。
- 双磷酸盐是最常见的抗骨吸收药物（阿仑膦酸钠、利塞膦酸钠、伊班膦酸盐、唑来膦酸）。
- 剂量建议：阿仑膦酸钠70mg口服，每周一次；利塞膦酸钠35mg口服，每周一次或150mg每月一次；伊班膦酸钠150mg口服，每月一次；唑来膦酸5mg静脉注射一年一次。
- 雷洛昔芬是一种抗骨吸收和选择性雌激素受体调节剂（selective estrogen receptor modifier, SERM）：60mg口服，每日一次。
- 狄诺塞麦是一种抗RANK配体的单克隆抗体，2010年11月批准上市的新型抗骨吸收药物。
- 特立帕肽（重组PTH）是唯一批准的通过合成代谢治疗骨质疏松症用药，剂量每天20mcg，最长可使用2年。
- 对绝经后骨质疏松症的女性患者使用雌激素和/或激素替代疗法有一定争议（心血管并发症）。
- 睾酮在男性性腺机能减退症的治疗中对骨骼有益。
- 如果可能的话，应避免可能对骨代谢产生影响的药物（类固醇、抗癫痫药物、噻唑烷二酮类）（kahn）。

其他干预措施

- 物理治疗，以优化及转移受力，减少跌倒和骨折的风险。
- 行椎体成形术和内固定术缓解椎体管理和稳定脊柱。
- 需要专科处理Charcot足，包括减轻负重，全接触支具，手术干预等。
- 诊断和治疗可导致骨丢失的其他疾病（如库欣氏症、原发性甲状旁腺功能亢进、类风湿关节炎）的其他次要原因。
- 进行继发骨质疏松的检查：iPTH、24小时尿钙、睾酮、SPEP、UPEP、磷、镁、25-羟基维生素D（肾脏疾病患者考虑1,25羟维生素D）。

随访

病史和体格检查

- 骨折，骨痛。
- 跌倒史，晕厥。
- 泌尿系结石（高钙尿症）。

- 可能会恶化骨质流失的新的用药（如噻唑烷二酮、类固醇、抗癫痫、乳腺癌或前列腺癌的治疗）。
- 骨质疏松症的药物治疗的不良反应：
- 身高变化，后凸畸形的加重。
- 棘突压痛点，胫前疼痛。

实验室检查
- 糖尿病常规管理。
- 对维生素 D 缺乏的筛查目前没有明确的指南，但可考虑每年检查一次 25-羟维生素 D 水平（见维生素 D）。
- 尽管治疗干预，仍存在进行性的骨质流失，应重复进行继发骨质疏松症的原因排查。
- 对于长期药物治疗的有效性问题，可进行骨吸收标志物的测定（N-端肽或 C-端肽）。
- 特立帕肽开始治疗后 2 周测量血尿酸和血钙。

影像学
- 对新出现的腰痛、压痛点进行脊椎骨折评估，采用脊柱 X 线。
- 初始骨质疏松症治疗后应每年一次或每 2 年一次进行 DXA。
- 开始治疗时检测骨密度骨量减少的患者每年进行 DXA。
- 对那些之前骨密度正常却新发骨折时需重复 DXA。

专家意见
- 与年龄匹配的健康对照相比，虽然 2 型糖尿病患者骨密度相对较高，但发生骨折的风险增加两倍（Vestergaard）。
- 2 型糖尿病患者改善胰岛素敏感性的主要方法是减肥，尽管骨密度也会随着体质指数降低而下降。
- PPARγ 激动剂（噻唑烷二酮类）可使间充质干细胞分化为脂肪细胞，而不是成骨细胞，因此导致骨质流失和骨折的风险增加；应限于对那些被认为发生骨骼疾病风险较低的患者使用（Vestergaard）。
- 骨折风险评估工具，FRAX（http://www.shef.ac.uk/FRAX/index.htm），根据骨质流失患者的信息和风险因素，用于计算 10 年骨质疏松及髋部骨折的风险；在此模型中，1 型糖尿病被认为骨质疏松症的第二位原因。
- 对于特定患者，合并有骨质疏松症和糖尿病时，需考虑：Klinefelter 综合征，Turner 综合征，皮质醇增多症，多腺体自身免疫综合征 II 型和遗传性血色病。

参考文献
Adami S. Bone health in diabetes: considerations for clinical management. Curr Med Res Opin, 2009; Vol. 25: pp. 1057–72.
  Comments: Discussion of bone fragility in T2DM despite high BMD.
Vestergaard P. Bone metabolism in type 2 diabetes and role of thiazolidinediones. Curr Opin Endocrinol Diabetes Obes, 2009; Vol. 16: pp. 125–31.
  Comments: Discussion of PPAR gamma agonist effect on bone metabolism.
Schwartz AV, Garnero P, Hillier TA, et al. Pentosidine and increased fracture risk in older adults

with type 2 diabetes. J Clin Endocrinol Metab, 2009; Vol. 94: pp. 2380–6.

Comments: Advanced glycation end products as a cause of poor bone quality in T2DM.

Wada S, Kamiya S, Fukawa T. Bone quality changes in diabetes. Clin Calcium, 2008; Vol. 18: pp. 600–5.

Comments: Mechanisms by which diabetes affects bone remodeling and structure.

Schwartz AV, Vittinghoff E, Sellmeyer DE, et al. Diabetes-related complications, glycemic control, and falls in older adults. Diabetes Care, 2008; Vol. 31: pp. 391–6.

Comments: Reduction of diabetic complications and hypoglycemia may reduce fall risk.

Kahn SE, Zinman B, Lachin JM, et al. Rosiglitazone-associated fractures in type 2 diabetes: an Analysis from A Diabetes Outcome Progression Trial (ADOPT). Diabetes Care, 2008; Vol. 31: pp. 845–51.

Comments: Increased 5-year fracture incidence in women taking rosiglitazone compared with metformin or glyburide.

Mastrandrea LD, Wactawski-Wende J, Donahue RP, et al. Young women with type 1 diabetes have lower bone mineral density that persists over time. Diabetes Care, 2008; Vol. 31: pp. 1729–35.

Comments: Failure to achieve peak bone density in T1DM as a cause of future bone disease and fracture.

Vestergaard P. Discrepancies in bone mineral density and fracture risk in patients with type 1 and type 2 diabetes— a meta-analysis. Osteoporos Int, 2007; Vol. 18: pp. 427–44.

Comments: Meta-analysis describing higher fracture rate in T1DM and T2DM despite BMD differences in both groups.

De Liefde II, van der Klift M, de Laet CE, et al. Bone mineral density and fracture risk in type-2 diabetes mellitus: the Rotterdam Study. Osteoporos Int, 2005; Vol. 16: pp. 1713–20.

Comments: Increased nonvertebral fracture risk in T2DM (HR 1.69) compared to healthy subjects.

Daly RM, Dunstan DW, Owen N, et al. Does high-intensity resistance training maintain bone mass during moderate weight loss in older overweight adults with type 2 diabetes? Osteoporos Int, 2005; Vol. 16: pp. 1703–12.

Comments: Use of resistance exercise to minimize bone loss in attempts at weight loss in T2DM.

Malluche HH, Mawad H, Monier-Faugere MC. The importance of bone health in end-stage renal disease: out of the frying pan, into the fire? Nephrol Dial Transplant, 2004; Vol. 19 Suppl 1: pp. i9–13.

Comments: Diabetic nephropathy with resultant renal osteodystropy.

Leidig-Bruckner G, Ziegler R. Diabetes mellitus a risk for osteoporosis? Exp Clin Endocrinol Diabetes, 2001; Vol. 109 Suppl 2: pp. S493–514.

Comments: Possible pathophysiology of bone disease in T1DM versus T2DM.

Heinemann DF. Osteoporosis. An overview of the National Osteoporosis Foundation clinical practice guide. Geriatrics, 2000; Vol. 55: pp. 31–6; quiz 39.

Comments: National Osteoporosis Foundation clinical guidelines.

Barrett-Connor E, Kritz-Silverstein D. Does hyperinsulinemia preserve bone? Diabetes Care, 1996; Vol. 19: pp. 1388–92.

Comments: Fasting insulin levels positively correlated with BMD, suggesting an anabolic role.

World Health Organization Collaborating Centre for Metabolic Bone Diseases, University of Sheffield, UK. FRAX calculator. Available online http://www.shef.ac.uk/FRAX/index.htm. (accessed 3/3/2011)

Comments: Fraction risk assessment tool.

Charcot 关节病（糖尿病神经性骨关节病）

Lee J. Sanders, DPM

定义

- 糖尿病神经性骨关节病（Diabetic neuropathic osteoarthropathy，DNOAP）通常也被称为 Charcot 关节病（Charcot joint disease，CJD）。
- 是一个潜在致残的糖尿病并发症，可导致足踝畸形和残疾，进而发展为溃疡和感染，并最终导致截肢。
- 急性状态：通常在无法识别的微小创伤之后出现一个突然发生的、意外的并且往往亦是无法识别的神经性关节病；特点是局部进行性加重的炎症，伴有肿胀、红斑、皮温升高，通常与关节半脱位、脱位、骨折、骨溶解和足部畸形相关。
- 慢性状态特点：炎症、骨化旺盛、骨密度的增加、稳定性的恢复和足部畸形。

流行病学

- 是糖尿病患者足部和踝关节的神经性骨关节病的主要病因。
- 糖尿病患者中 DNOAP 的患病率为 0.08%~13%（Frykberg，Sanders）。
- DNOAP 的发病率 <1%。一项纳入 1 666 例患者的前瞻性研究发现，Charcot 关节病的发病率为 8.5/1 000 人年（Lavery）。
- 在 1 型糖尿病中：发病平均年龄为 33.5 岁，发病时平均糖尿病病程 20 年。
- 在 2 型糖尿病中：发病平均年龄为 57 岁，发病时平均糖尿病病程 15 年。
- DNOAP 与重大截肢风险和死亡率增加相关（5 年死亡率 28%）（Sohn）。
- 危险因素：周围神经病变（必备），年龄，糖尿病病程，体重，骨密度降低，局部骨量减少，既往胰肾联合移植史。
- 男性、女性发病率相等。

诊断

- 周围神经病变是诊断 DNOAP 的必备条件。
- 发病机制：多因素参与，感觉运动神经病变，自主神经病变，轻微外伤。
- 相关因素：骨密度降低，促炎症因子。
- 急性 DNOAP 的鉴别诊断：蜂窝组织炎，急性痛风性关节炎，骨髓炎和深静脉血栓形成。
- 慢性 DNOAP 的鉴别诊断：糖尿病（主要原因），酒精性神经病，麻风病，脊髓痨，脊髓空洞症，先天性痛觉不敏感。
- 实验室检查：白细胞计数正常（无感染证据），C- 反应蛋白正常，血尿酸正常，双功超声扫描阴性，骨扫描阳性（非特异性，不能区分骨髓炎或 CJD，没有感染时可出现假阳性）。
- 影像学检查：Charcot 足和骨髓炎之间无 X 线或 MRI 上的差异。
- 早期 X 线检查可以没有或有很微小的阳性发现。
- 诊断不确定时建议骨活检。

症状及体征

- 摇椅足畸形伴有足弓塌陷是 DNOAP 的标志。
- 最早的表现与早期骨关节炎一致。
- 急性 CJD 表现：急性炎症表现，伴有轻至中度疼痛、肿胀、局部红斑及皮温升高。可能会有关节积液、骨吸收、关节半脱位、脱位和不稳定。
- 三个影像学分期（Eichenholtz）：进展期、合并期及重建期，是 CJD 由急性转为慢性的过程。
- 五个解剖学分型（Sanders and Frykberg）：I 型：前掌关节；II 型：跗跖关节；III 型：跗骨间、舟楔关节；IV 型：踝和 / 或距下关节；V 型：跟骨。
- Ⅰ、Ⅱ、Ⅲ型通常与溃疡有关；Ⅳ型会导致严重的结构畸形和不稳定，截肢风险最高。
- 误诊和治疗延迟令机械应力不间断地产生患处负重，加之软组织损伤（溃疡），微骨折，骨折，脱位，半脱位，骨吸收，组织破坏和碎片化，软组织水肿，增加关节活动度及畸形。可导致截肢。
- Charcot 足病程演变：见下图 3-2。

治疗

- 治疗目标：防止进展为足 / 踝畸形，溃疡或溃疡再发。
- 生活质量的目标包括继续工作，可以独立活动，可穿鞋。
- 治疗急性 CJD 基石：立即将集中在足部的压力负荷减掉，短时间卧床休息并抬高患肢以减少肿胀，之后是支具固定，最好应用全接触支具（total contact casts，TCC）或塑件可拆式助行器（removable cast walker，RCW），避免患侧关节移动（Sanders）。
- 建议长时间不负重并在随后进行保护性负重。
- 支具和定制鞋：在肿胀、温热和红斑减轻，以及存在影像学下支持骨愈合的证据（Eichenholtz2 期、3 期）后，可过渡到部分负重的 RCW，足踝矫形器（ankle foot orthosis，AFO），Charcot 约束矫形助行器（Charcot Restraint Orthotic Walker，CROW），或髌骨肌腱轴承支架（patella-tendon-bearing brace，PTB）和定制鞋。
- 抗骨吸收药物：双膦酸盐，降钙素影响骨重建周期，但目前尚未批准用于预防或治疗 CJD。
- 手术治疗：有争议。主要适应证是保守治疗无效患者。次要适应证：足 / 踝关节不稳，畸形，慢性溃疡，进行性的关节破坏。手术并发症的发生率很高，尤其存在足部慢性溃疡患者。缺乏对术后长期效果的研究。

随访

- 令急性 CJD 缓解的外固定平均时间为 10 个月（7~15 个月）。
- 高风险人群需要专业的足部护理和终身监测，以预防、早期发现和治疗足部并发症。
- 推荐多学科团队对患者进行疾病管理。

Charcot 关节病

图 3-2 Charcot 足的病程演变

0 期 前驱期	1 期 进展期	2 期 合并期	3 期 重建期
肿胀	关节边缘碎片形成	水肿减少	进一步的修复和骨的重塑
局部温热	软骨下骨破碎	细碎屑吸收	较大碎片整合
轻度红斑	半脱位	骨折愈合	血运重建
临床不稳定	错位	较大碎片融合凝聚	硬化缩减
影像学改变缺失或很小	关节软骨侵蚀	血管的损失	稳定性恢复
	骨吸收	骨硬化	增加骨密度
	骨溶解和骨量减少		骨化丰富
	骨破碎、解体		畸形
	软组织水肿加重关节的不稳定性		

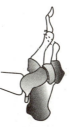

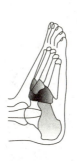

骨吸收　　　　　修复

资料来源：Sanders LJ, Frykberg RG. The Charcot Foot (Pied de Charcot). In: Bowker J, Pfeifer MA, eds. Levin and O'Neal's The Diabetic Foot. 7th ed. Philadelphia: Elsevier, Inc.; 2008.

专家意见

- 早期发现并及时治疗往往会得到更满意的预后。
- 治疗的关键是通过减轻足踝部压力负荷以预防畸形和溃疡,同时在骨和软组织愈合前避免进一步的损伤。

参考文献

Sohn MW, Lee TA, Stuck RM, et al. Mortality risk of Charcot arthropathy compared with that of diabetic foot ulcer and diabetes alone. Diabetes Care, 2009; Vol. 32: pp. 816–21.
Comments: Charcot arthropathy is associated with higher mortality risk than diabetes alone and with lower risk than foot ulcer.

Sanders LJ, Frykberg RG. The Charcot Foot (Pied de Charcot). In Bowker J, Pfeifer MA, (Eds.), Levin and O'Neal's The Diabetic Foot, Seventh Edition. Philadelphia: Elsevier Inc.; 2008: pp. 257–283.
Comments: Review of the pathogenesis, natural history, and management of the Charcot foot. Anatomic patterns of bone and joint involvement are illustrated. Emerging research is reviewed, including the putative role of antiresorptive pharmacologic agents, proinflammatory cytokines, and osteoclastogenesis and the RANKL/OPG signaling pathway.

Sanders LJ. What lessons can history teach us about the Charcot foot? Clin Podiatr Med Surg, 2008; Vol. 25: pp. 1–15, v.
Comments: Contemporary historical perspective on the Charcot foot. Contains original 19th century illustrations from primary source materials.

Frykberg RG, Belczyk R. Epidemiology of the Charcot foot. Clin Podiatr Med Surg, 2008; Vol. 25: pp. 17–28, v.
Comments: The actual incidence of CJD is likely greater than that reported. The diagnosis is delayed or missed in 25% of the cases.

Burns PR, Wukich DK. Surgical reconstruction of the Charcot rearfoot and ankle. Clin Podiatr Med Surg, 2008; Vol. 25: pp. 95–120, vii–viii.
Comments: Overview of surgical management of the Charcot foot, including basic surgical principles and techniques. Outcomes and scientific evidence-based medicine regarding Charcot ankle and hindfoot deformity is minimal.

Lavery LA, Armstrong DG, Wunderlich RP, et al. Diabetic foot syndrome: evaluating the prevalence and incidence of foot pathology in Mexican Americans and non-Hispanic whites from a diabetes disease management cohort. Diabetes Care, 2003; Vol. 26: pp. 1435–8.
Comments: A prospective study of 1666 patients from a disease management program in Texas found the incidence of Charcot arthropathy was 8.5/1000 per year.

Hoché G, Sanders LJ. On some arthropathies apparently related to a lesion of the brain or spinal cord, by Dr. J-M Charcot, January 1868. J Hist Neurosci, 1992; Vol. 1: pp. 75–87.
Comments: Translation of J-M Charcot's 1868 paper on the tabetic arthropathies. Contains 4 clinical case observations and a discussion of 2 main groups of arthropathies manifesting in the course of progressive locomotor ataxia.

Eichenholtz SN. Charcot joints. Springfield, IL: Charles C. Thomas, 1966: p. 227.
Comments: This is Sidney Eichenholtz's classic monograph on Charcot joints,

in which he describes three well-defined radiographic stages in the evolution of this condition. His classification is the most commonly accepted taxonomy of neuroarthropathy.

NIH Office of Rare Diseases and National Institute of Diabetes and Digestive and Kidney Diseases (NIDDK). Summary Report: Charcot Neuroarthropathy Workshop, September 17–18, 2008. Bethesda, MD. Report can be downloaded from the NIDDK website. http://www3.niddk.nih.gov/fund/other/neuroarthropathy/SummaryReport.pdf (accessed 3/3/2011).

Comments: NIH Office of Rare Diseases and NIDDK cosponsored workshop, Charcot Neuroarthropathy Recent Progress and Future Directions.

糖尿病患者的皮肤表现

Mary Huizinga, MD, MPH

定义
- 糖尿病患者皮肤表现较常见，并以多种形式出现（Romano）。
- 皮肤病变的发现可能有助于诊断糖尿病（例如黑棘皮病）或反映糖尿病长期并发症 [如糖尿病脂性渐进性坏死（necrobiosis lipoidica diabeticorum，NLD）]。
- 皮肤病变可能是由于糖基化终产物（advanced glycosylation end product，AGEs）的沉积、感染性病因、自身免疫性因素或与治疗糖尿病的药物（如胰岛素）相关。
- 通常情况下，皮肤表现也可反映其他共患疾病，如血脂异常。

流行病学
- 大约一半的糖尿病患者都会有一些皮肤表现（Chakrabarty，Romano）。
- 相比 T2DM，T1DM 更易出现自身免疫相关的皮肤病变表现（Romano）。
- 感染原因相关的皮肤表现多见于血糖控制不佳的糖尿病患者（Romano）。

诊断
- 诊断通常可以通过检查皮肤确定。
- 偶尔，为了确定诊断，如 NLD，需要活检、培养或影像学检查。

症状及体征
- 黑棘皮病：在皮肤皱褶处出现天鹅绒般的色素沉着，最常见部位是腋下和后颈部。是胰岛素抵抗的一个表现，通常在 2 型糖尿病和多囊卵巢综合征患者出现，无伴随症状。鉴别诊断包含伴癌综合征，胃肠道恶性肿瘤的标志或药物反应（Higgins，Ahmed）。
- 糖尿病性皮肤病（颈前色素斑）：在小腿出现成群的斑点，可消退或加重；加重的方式可为斑点数量增多，斑点面积增大，色素沉着加深和/或变暗。可见于 40% 的糖尿病患者，男性多于女性，通常合并有其他微血管并发症。可能是源于慢性创伤的愈合（Ahmed，van Hatten）。
- 糖尿病脂性渐进性坏死（necrobiosis lipoidica diabeticorum，NLD）：最初表现为紫红色片状皮损，后逐渐发展，有红色边缘和黄棕色中心区；随着时间的推移，中心区萎缩为蜡状，伴毛细血管扩张。35% 病例可发生溃疡。发病罕见，仅在 0.3% 的糖尿病患者中出现，通常发生在 30~40 岁的女性，并且可在糖尿病发病前很多年就已出现。除非发生溃烂，否则本病多无症状，仅在化妆时偶然发现（Ferringer，Cohen，Paron）。
- 糖尿病大疱病：手掌、足掌和腿部出现无痛、表面张力较大的浆液性水泡，起病较快，通常在 2~4 周内愈合。发生于病史较长糖尿病患者（Romano，Ferringer，Ahmed，van Hattem，Paron）。
- 黄色指甲、手掌、脚掌：较普遍，没有明确的病理后果。病因不明，但可能由于糖基化产物的沉积或胡萝卜素的增加有关（Paron，Ahmed，Ferringer）。

糖尿病患者的皮肤表现

- 皮肤感染：发生于20%~60%的糖尿病患者。（1）念珠菌：葡萄球菌和链球菌是常见的，多影响摩擦区域（如腹股沟、乳房下、腋窝），女性阴道炎，男性阴茎炎。常见于血糖控制不佳患者；（2）坏死性筋膜炎：皮肤和软组织的急进性感染，混合细菌感染，在那些出现脓毒症的患者发生蜂窝组织炎迹象时需考虑；（3）恶性外耳炎：侵袭性外耳道感染，最常见的是假单胞菌感染，可能会蔓延到周围结构。临床检查可发现耳廓压痛及脓性分泌物的流出。需要CT或MRI检查以确定是否存在骨受累；（4）红癣：皮肤褶皱处的常见感染（腋下、腹股沟、趾间、腹股沟），通常是棒状杆菌感染；（5）鼻脑毛霉菌病：罕见但危及生命，多发生于老年患者，由于接合菌感染，伴发热，面部蜂窝组织炎，眶周水肿，面部麻木，眼球突出和/或失明。CT/MRI用于评估受累范围（Romano，Ahmed，Chakrabarty，Carfrae）。
- 硬皮病样改变：患病率2.5%~50%。T1DM和T2DM均可出现，发病无性别或种族倾向。手部（指端硬化）和/或颈部、肩背部皮肤非对称不可凹性增厚、变硬（糖尿病硬肿症或Bushke硬肿症）。常伴发关节疾病，受累面积及硬度随病程渐进式增加（Cole，Sattar，Brik，Ahmed，Ferringer，Yosipovitch）。
- 胰岛素相关皮肤反应：（1）脂肪萎缩：受累区域皮下脂肪丢失，范围可达5~10cm。可能有免疫学基础参与，或因胰岛素促进脂肪分解作用所致。反复在同一部位注射时风险增加。胰岛素的吸收不稳定。相比牛/猪胰岛素，此类皮肤反应在使用新型胰岛素制剂时较少出现；（2）脂肪肥大：受累区域皮下脂肪明显肥大，周长1~15cm，高于皮面3~5cm。这是胰岛素治疗最常见的皮肤并发症。应用新的胰岛素制剂可消退。如脂肪萎缩一样，与反复在同一个部位注射有关，并可导致胰岛素吸收不稳定；（3）局部过敏反应：红斑、瘙痒和硬结。这些反应是一过性的，多在几周内消退（Paron，Richardson）。
- 与糖尿病相关血脂异常：（1）高甘油三酯血症：如果程度较重（>1000mg/dl），在轻度红斑的基础上，可见丘疹性黄瘤、带有白尖（甘油三酯）的斑丘疹，经常出现于四肢，随高甘油三酯血症的缓解而消退；（2）高胆固醇血症：黄色瘤（在眼睑上的黄色斑块）；肌腱黄色瘤；结节性黄色瘤（手肘、膝盖）；（3）血β脂蛋白异常：掌面黄瘤，是一种不常见的与低密度脂蛋白（VLDL）升高和乳糜微粒相关脂代谢紊乱，总胆固醇和甘油三酯>第90百分位数。

治疗

与年龄相关的

- 黑棘皮病（Acanthosis nigricans，AN）：采用减体重、运动、二甲双胍、噻唑烷二酮等减轻胰岛素抵抗的治疗方式，虽然很少有证据表明这样的方式对AN有效。乳酸软膏或视黄酸可软化病变；维甲酸会降低病变，但病变在停药后会再发（Higgins，van Hatten）。
- 糖尿病性皮肤病（颈前色素斑）：预防继发感染（Chakrabarty）。
- 糖尿病脂性渐进性坏死：没有标准的治疗。局部注射类固醇激素或使用外用药膏的结果有一定争议。严重病变可能需要植皮。
- 糖尿病大疱病：通常不进行干预便可缓解。如果存在不适，可对大疱进行抽液；外用抗生素可用于预防继发感染。

- 皮肤发黄：没有针对性治疗。

皮肤感染
- 念珠菌感染：保持患处干燥，外用抗真菌药物治疗。对浅表念珠菌病很少需要口服抗真菌药物（Hay, Guitart）。
- 蜂窝组织炎：患处抬高，维持皮肤湿润以避免开裂，经验性抗生素治疗应覆盖金黄色葡萄球菌（+/-MRSA）和革兰阴性菌。
- 坏死性筋膜炎：外科评估，迅速使用静脉抗生素治疗（Ahmed）。
- 恶性外耳炎：使用长疗程的喹诺酮类药物，可能需要清创（Ahmed, Carfrae）。
- 红癣：红霉素 250mg，每天 4 次，疗程 14 天（Holdiness）。
- 鼻脑毛霉菌病：即刻静脉注射两性霉素 B 和外科清创。
- 有关的详细信息，见感染性疾病和糖尿病。

自身免疫性
- 硬皮病样改变：治疗有不同的结果。方法包括光分离置换术、放疗、环孢素以及大剂量青霉素。尚无治疗糖尿病性硬肿症的有效方法（Van Hattem, Ferringer）。

胰岛素相关皮肤反应
- 脂肪萎缩：轮换胰岛素注射部位或给药方式。偶尔，在严重的情况下，可以考虑加用糖皮质激素。
- 脂肪肥大：轮换注射部位。偶尔，为了达到美容目的，可考虑吸脂治疗。
- 局部过敏反应：通常会自行消退，但亦可应用糖皮质激素脱敏治疗或换用胰岛素泵治疗。

共患疾病
- 血脂异常：控制血脂。

专家意见
- 糖尿病患者常见皮肤表现。
- 大多数皮肤表现与高血糖（AGEs）、自身免疫或因药物治疗或合并症导致的感染性病因有关。
- 根据皮肤病变类型不同，预后和治疗差别很大。

参考文献

Chakrabarty A, Norman RA, Phillips TJ. Cutaneous manifestations of diabetes. In Norman RA (Ed.), Diagnosis of Aging Skin Diseases. London: Springer-Verlag; 2008; Online ISBN 978-1-84628-678-0; pp. 253–263.
  Comments: Review of skin manifestations of diabetes.
Van Hattem S, Bootsma AH, Thio HB. Skin manifestations of diabetes. Cleve Clin J Med 2008; Vol. 75: pp. 772, 774, 776–7 passim.
  Comments: Review of skin manifestations of diabetes.
Carfrae MJ, Kesser BW. Malignant otitis externa. Otolaryngol Clin North Am, 2008; Vol. 41 pp. 537–49, viii–ix.
  Comments: Review of malignant otitis externa.

iggins SP, Freemark M, Prose NS. Acanthosis nigricans: a practical approach to evaluation and management. Dermatol Online J, 2008; Vol. 14: p. 2.
Comments: Review of management for acanthosis nigricans.

hmed I, Goldstein B. Diabetes mellitus. Clin Dermatol, 2006; Vol. 24: pp. 237–46.
Comments: Review of skin manifestations of diabetes.

ichardson T, Kerr D Skin-related complications of insulin therapy: epidemiology and emerging management strategies. Am J Clin Dermatol, 2003; Vol. 4: pp. 661–7.
Comments: Skin-related complications of insulin therapy.

ichardson T, Kerr D. Skin-related complications of insulin therapy: epidemiology and emerging management strategies. Am J Clin Dermatol, 2003; Vol. 4: pp. 661–7.
Comments: Review of skin-related complications of insulin therapy.

oldiness MR. Management of cutaneous erythrasma. Drugs, 2002; Vol. 62: pp. 1131–41.
Comments: Review of treatments for erythrasma.

erringer T, Miller F. Cutaneous manifestations of diabetes mellitus. Dermatol Clin, 2002; Vol. 20: pp. 483–92.
Comments: Review of skin manifestations of diabetes.

aron NG, Lambert PW. Cutaneous manifestations of diabetes mellitus. Prim Care, 2000; Vol. 27: pp. 371–83.
Comments: Review of cutaneous manifestations of diabetes.

ay RJ. The management of superficial candidiasis. J Am Acad Dermatol, 1999; Vol. 40: pp. S35–42.
Comments: Review of superficial candidiasis.

omano G, Moretti G, Di Benedetto A, et al. Skin lesions in diabetes mellitus: prevalence and clinical correlations. Diabetes Res Clin Pract, 1998; Vol. 39: pp. 101–6.
Comments: Prevalence of skin manifestations found in 60% of patients.

sipovitch G, Hodak E, Vardi P, et al. The prevalence of cutaneous manifestations in IDDM patients and their association with diabetes risk factors and microvascular complications. Diabetes Care, 1998; Vol. 21: pp. 506–9.
Comments: Cross-sectional study of 238 insulin dependent patients and 122 controls; scleroderma-like changes found in 39% of patients.

ohen O, Yaniv R, Karasik A, et al. Necrobiosis lipoidica and diabetic control revisited. Med Hypotheses, 1996; Vol. 46: pp. 348–50.
Comments: Review of necrobiosis lipoidica.

uitart J, Woodley DT. Intertrigo: a practical approach. Compr Ther, 1994; Vol. 20: pp. 402–9.
Comments: Review of superficial candidiasis.

ik R, Berant M, Vardi P. The scleroderma-like syndrome of insulin-dependent diabetes mellitus. Diabetes Metab Rev, 1991; Vol. 7: pp. 120–8.
Comments: Scleroderma-like syndromes.

attar MA, Diab S, Sugathan TN, et al. Scleroedema diabeticorum: a minor but often unrecognized complication of diabetes mellitus. Diabet Med, 1988; Vol. 5: pp. 465–8.
Comments: Cross-sectional study of 100 persons with diabetes; 14% had scleredema diabeticorum.

ole GW, Headley J, Skowsky R. Scleredema diabeticorum: a common and distinct cutaneous manifestation of diabetes mellitus. Diabetes Care, 1983; Vol. 6: pp. 189–92.
Comments: Review, case series, and prospective analysis of patients with diabetes; prevalence of scleredema in patients with diabetes was 2.5%.

坏疽和严重肢体缺血

Lee J. Sanders, DPM

定义
- 坏疽是与缺血（干性坏疽）或感染（湿性坏疽）相关的组织坏死。
- 气性坏疽是湿性坏疽的一种类型，由厌氧菌引起（梭状芽胞杆菌），特别是产气荚膜梭菌。
- 严重肢体缺血（critical limb ischemia，CLI）用于存在慢性缺血性静息痛、溃疡或由客观证实的动脉闭塞性疾病导致坏疽的患者，如果不及时治疗，在6个月内的自然病程内可导致重大截肢。
- 糖尿病足患者CLI的病理生理是复杂的，由动脉供血不足、神经病变、溃疡和感染相互作用所致，肢体灌注减少，不足以维持基础组织代谢所需血供，导致缓慢渐进的组织坏死和截肢。

流行病学
- CLI的发病率约是500~1000人每百万人年（Dormandy）。
- 慢性CLI多是由弥漫性或多节段性动脉粥样硬化动脉闭塞性发展而来。
- 跛行的CLI患者具有相同的心血管危险因素，包括吸烟、高血压、糖尿病和高脂血症。
- 糖尿病患者出现CLI的风险较大。
- 糖尿病CLI患者发生坏疽的发生率为40%，无糖尿病患者则为9%。
- 慢性CLI患者1年死亡率约20%。近50%的患者需要血运重建术保肢治疗，40%的未行血运重建术患者在初始诊断后的6个月内需要截肢（Hirsh）。
- 与仅有PAD（peripheral arterial disease，PAD）的患者相比，糖尿病合并PAD的患者可能需要截肢的风险升高10倍左右。
- 在明尼苏达州的罗彻斯特市，一项以人群为基础的糖尿病队列研究中，在无下肢动脉疾病（lower extremity arterial disease，LEAD）的糖尿病患者中新发肢体坏疽的发病率为4.5人每千人年。而同时有LEAD和糖尿病的患者，新发肢体坏疽的发生率在男性为29.6人每千人年，女性为37.1人每千人年（Melton）。
- 坏疽的危险因素包括外周动脉疾病，周围神经病变，感染，外伤和伤口愈合不良。

诊断
- 通过详细的病史（缺血性静息痛，间歇性跛行，慢性未愈合的伤口），查体（足部动脉缺失，皮肤营养不良变化，缺血性溃疡或皮肤坏死），PAD的无创性评估（ABI），实验室评估[节段性压力，脉搏量记录，术前经皮氧张力测定（transcutaneous oxygen tension，TcPO2）]，解剖学研究（多普勒超声，磁共振血管造影，血管造影）等确定诊断。
- 湿性坏疽：广泛坏死或坏疽，散发恶臭。常为多种微生物混合感染。
- 病原体：混合需氧革兰阳性球菌，包括肠球菌、肠杆菌、非发酵革兰

坏疽和严重肢体缺血

性杆菌和专性厌氧菌。
- 缺血的严重程度：Rutherford 分级 III 级（少量组织损失）和 IV 级（溃疡或坏疽）。请参阅周围血管疾病中的表 3-5。

症状及体征

- 坏疽通常会影响脚趾，在严重的情况下可累及前足。
- 在没有感染的情况下脚趾可出现"木乃伊化"和自截（干性坏疽），通常存在明确的分界线，在分界线以下皮温骤然降低，提示在分界线附近发生的灌注变化。
- 在感染存在的情况下，皮肤可能会温热，坏死组织通常潮湿和恶臭（湿性坏疽）。
- 中等程度的感染：一般情况较好，代谢状态稳定，存在以下一项或多项：蜂窝组织炎面积超过 2cm，淋巴管炎，累及浅筋膜下，深部组织脓肿，坏疽，肌肉肌腱、关节或骨受累。
- 严重感染表现：全身毒性症状或代谢不稳定（如发热，寒战，心动过速，低血压，意识模糊，呕吐，白细胞升高，酸中毒，严重高血糖状态或氮质血症）。
- 患者严重动脉供血不足表现为剧烈疼痛，常发在足或趾的远端；夜间缺血性静息痛，因跛行而导致行走能力的严重受损；足、趾背部毛发缺失；脚趾冊萎缩；抬高患肢皮肤苍白。
- 鞋的压力可令脚趾尖、足跟和曲率半径小的区域（如第一和第五跖骨头）出现动脉性溃疡。

治疗

- 强化干预危险因素：戒烟，控制血糖，积极控制血压（血管紧张素转换酶抑制剂，β-受体阻滞剂，钙通道阻滞剂），抗血小板治疗（ASA，氯吡格雷），降脂药（他汀类），以及对跛行患者的运动康复和西洛他唑治疗。
- 全身应用抗生素：在蜂窝组织炎或缺血性溃疡、坏疽合并感染时应用，同时不应该耽误其他治疗。
- 血运重建：对 CLI 理想的治疗方法是通过经皮血管成形术（percutaneous angioplasty，PTA）或支架手术处理较大的闭塞血管，消除阻塞。
- 静脉旁路移植术被认为是治疗 CLI 的金标准。
- 药物治疗：改善远端微循环低灌注压的影响。
- 高压氧（Hyperbaric oxygen，HBO）治疗：作为抗生素和积极的外科清创的辅助治疗，有一定争议，适应证可能包括坏死性筋膜炎、气性坏疽、慢性顽固性骨髓炎、感染和糖尿病足溃疡。
- 疼痛管理：所有 CLI 患者均需充分治疗缺血性疼痛，可能需要短期使用麻醉药。
- 对于 CLI 患者单一应用外用抗生素、生长因子和清创剂（酶），一般不会成功。
- 应由一个多学科小组在考虑下列问题之后提出最适当的干预决定：坏疽及感染的范围，血管病变形态，合并症，患者个体的手术风险，既往接受的治疗（旁路或血管成形术），患者预期寿命，康复潜力，以及医疗

- 团队的专业知识、特殊手术或血管内手术经验。
- 对于神经缺血性患者发生的干性坏疽，需要血管外科会诊，伤口清创，和/或截肢，或自截。
- 对于神经病变患者发生的湿性坏疽，需要静脉注射抗生素及外科清创或截肢
- 对于神经缺血性患者发生的湿性坏疽，需要静脉注射抗生素及需要手术清创和/或血运重建手术。

随访

- 患有 CLI 的糖尿病患者有非常高的发生心肌梗死、中风和血管性死亡的风险
- 未进行适当血运重建可导致外周组织灌注不良，进而可导致肢体损失。
- CLI 患者在足科和血管专科定期随诊能够提高保肢的机会。
- 有良好血供的神经病变患者发生继发感染或外伤性的脚趾坏疽的预后优于那些神经缺血性的 CLI 患者。
- CLI 是不可能被完全或永久治愈的，因外周动脉疾病仍在不断进展。
- 治疗缺血性组织损失的下肢血运重建术是否临床成功取决于患者的内在因素，而不是血运重建方法。存在坏疽的行动不便的糖尿病患者 85.2% 概率失败，而终末期肾病患者，伴随行动不便、坏疽、既往曾行血管介入的患者，失败概率高达 92.8%。

专家意见

- 鉴别缺血性疼痛（程度重，腿部抬高或行走时加重，伴随缺血征象）与神经性疼痛（与行走无关，通常相对对称出现，有神经病变的征象，无缺血征象）。患者可能同时存在两种性质的疼痛，但缺血性疼痛提示 CLI。
- 与间歇性跛行患者相比，CLI 患者预后非常差。CLI 的患者有较高的死亡率和截肢风险。

推荐依据

Hirsch AT, Haskal ZJ, Hertzer NR, et al. ACC/AHA 2005 guidelines for the management of patients with peripheral arterial disease (lower extremity, renal, mesenteric, and abdominal aortic): executive summary. A collaborative report from the American Association for Vascular Surgery/Society for Vascular Surgery, Society for Cardiovascular Angiography and Interventions, Society for Vascular Medicine and Biology, Society of Interventional Radiology, and the American College of Cardiology (ACC)/American Heart Association (AHA) Task Force on Practice Guidelines: writing Committee to Develop Guidelines for the Management of Patients With Peripheral Arterial Disease. J Am Coll Cardiol, 2006; Vol. 47: pp. 1239–312.

Comments: The ACC/AHA guidelines address the diagnosis and management atherosclerotic, aneurysmal, and thromboembolic peripheral arterial diseases (PADs

Dormandy JA, Rutherford RB. Management of peripheral arterial disease (PAD). TASC Working Group. Trans Atlantic Inter-Society Consensus (TASC). J Vasc Surg, 2000; Vol 31: pp. S1–S296.

Comments: TransAtlantic Inter-Society Consensus (TASC) document on the management of peripheral arterial disease. Comprehensive monograph on the epidemiology, natural history, risk factors, evaluation, and medical and surgical management of PVD.

其他参考文献

Taylor SM, York JW, Cull DL, et al. Clinical success using patient-oriented outcome measures after lower extremity bypass and endovascular intervention for ischemic tissue loss. J Vasc Surg, 2009; Vol. 50: pp. 534–41; discussion 541.

Comments: The purpose of this study was to retrospectively examine success after lower extremity revascularization for tissue loss using patient-oriented measures and to include patients who underwent both open surgical bypass and endovascular procedures. Type of intervention was not a significant factor in either bivariate or logistic regression analysis.

Mohler E, Giri J, American College of Cardiology, et al. Management of peripheral arterial disease patients: comparing the ACC/AHA and TASC-II guidelines. Curr Med Res Opin, 2008; Vol. 24: pp. 2509–22.

Comments: Findings and conclusions: Both documents agree on the need for aggressive management of patients with PAD. In spite of these recommendations, there is a general lack of adherence to the current guidelines—a critical concern considering the high morbidity and mortality associated with the disease.

Jather A, Bee CS, Huak CY, et al. Epidemiology of diabetic foot problems and predictive factors for limb loss. J Diabetes Complications, 2008; Vol. 22: pp. 77–82.

Comments: Detailed prospective study of 202 patients during the period January 2005–May 2006, to evaluate the epidemiology of diabetic foot problems (DFP) and predictive factors for major lower extremity amputations. Results: 192 patients had DM2, mean age 60 years, male to female ratio of 1:1. 72.8% of patients had poor endocrine control and 42.1% had sensory neuropathy. Common DPF = gangrene (31.7%), infection (28.7%), ulcer 27.7%, cellulitis (6.4%), necrotizing fasciitis (3.5%), and Charcot osteoarthropathy (2.0%). Surgery was performed in 74.8% of patients, major amputation in 27.2% (below-knee in 20.3% and above knee in 6.9%).

Saide CG, Khandelwal S. Hyperbaric oxygen: applications in infectious disease. Emerg Med Clin North Am, 2008; Vol. 26: pp. 571–95, xi.

Comments: Review article discussing the application of hyperbaric oxygen (HBO) as an adjunctive treatment of certain infectious processes.

Lipsky BA, Berendt AR, Deery HG, et al. Diagnosis and treatment of diabetic foot infections. Clin Infect Dis, 2004; Vol. 39: pp. 885–910.

Comments: Infectious Disease Society of America (IDSA) guidelines for the diagnosis and treatment of diabetic foot infections. Document can be downloaded from http://www.journals.uchicago.edu/doi/abs/10.1086/424846.

Melton LJ, Macken KM, Palumbo PJ, et al. Incidence and prevalence of clinical peripheral vascular disease in a population-based cohort of diabetic patients. Diabetes Care, 1981; Vol. 3: pp. 650–4.

Comments: Rochester, MN, population-based cohort of diabetic patients. In the cohort with diabetes and gangrene, survival was poor, with only 39% alive after 2 years.

Joslin, EP. The menace of diabetic gangrene. NEJM, 1934; Vol. 211(1): pp. 16–20.

Comments: Joslin noted that following the introduction of insulin, mortality from diabetic coma had fallen significantly from 60% to 5%. Yet, deaths from diabetic gangrene (of the foot and leg) had risen significantly. Joslin observed that gangrene increased with age and duration of diabetes. There was almost always a history of injury to the foot that could be elicited from the patient. Burns and ill-fitting shoes caused the most common injuries. Joslin firmly believed that gangrene and amputations were preventable. His remedy was a team approach to diabetes care.

肌肉骨骼疾病

Mary Huizinga, MD, MPH

定义
- 许多肌肉骨骼病（musculoskeletal disorders，MSDs）都与糖尿病相关。
- 最常受累的关节包括肩关节、手和脚关节。
- 许多与糖尿病相关的 MSDs 是系统性的。
- 无论糖尿病类型为何，对大多数 MSDs 来说，糖尿病病程是一个显著的危险因素。

流行病学
- MSD 的是常见的糖尿病。在一项研究中，有一半的糖尿病患者手部存在一个 MSD，四分之一的存在两处 MSD（Gamstedt）。
- 腕管综合征：糖尿病患者患病率 20%~75%（Gamstedt，Chaudhuri）。
- Dupuytren 挛缩：在糖尿病患者中可达 40%（Gamstedt，Noble）。
- 屈肌腱鞘炎：在糖尿病患者可达 20%，不论血糖控制情况，本病与糖尿病病程有关（Gamstedt）。
- 粘连性关节囊炎：糖尿病患者患病率 19%~29%，危险因素包括年龄增加、较长的糖尿病病程，Dupuytren 挛缩和视网膜病变（Pal，Balci）。
- 钙化性肩周炎：糖尿病患者比非糖尿病患者患病风险增加 3 倍，与年龄较长的糖尿病病程及使用胰岛素相关（Mavrikakis）。
- 关节活动受限：患病率介于 8%~58%；加重因素包括糖尿病病程、血糖控制、糖尿病视网膜病变、肾病、年龄和吸烟。
- 糖尿病肢端硬化：见糖尿病皮肤病表现。
- 僵人病：在 1 型糖尿病患者出现渐进性肌肉僵硬，是非常罕见的疾病（Helfgott）。
- 糖尿病肌肉梗死：糖尿病患者自发出现肌肉梗死的罕见并发症（Trujillo-Santos）。
- 骨关节炎：可与糖尿病相关，可能是由于肥胖（Hochberg）。
- 类风湿关节炎（Rheumatoid arthritis，RA）：RA 是慢性炎症加之长期使用糖皮质激素可能会增加 2 型糖尿病的风险，没有证据表明 T1DM 与 RA 存在联系，尽管两者均可能存在于多腺体自身免疫性疾病（Doran，Simard）。

诊断
- 腕管综合征：由于正中神经受压导致关节活动受限，Hoffmann-Tinel 征（轻敲手腕正中神经走行部位引出症状）和 Phalen 征（腕关节急性屈曲 30~60 秒引出症状）阳性，电生理检查提示正中神经功能异常（Preston）。
- Dupuytren 挛缩：由于手掌筋膜的纤维化、皮肤的三角形褶皱或屈肌腱上的结节导致的关节僵硬，同时无关节炎表现；随病程增加逐渐退化的患者可达 10%（Gudmundsson）。

肌肉骨骼疾病

- 屈肌腱鞘炎：在屈肌腱可扪及结节，拇指、中指和无名指最有可能受累，可能双侧发病（Ryzewicz）。
- 粘连性关节囊炎："冻结肩"（可逆性肩膀收缩）的进展情形，粘连形成导致活动范围的显著受限（外展和旋转）；活动受限并非由于关节炎或其他疾病引起（Sheridan）。
- 钙化性肩周炎：又称钙化性肌腱炎，是指羟基磷灰石钙结晶沉积在肩关节周围肌腱，X线下肩部肌腱钙化可以诊断（Siegal，Mavrikakis）。
- 关节活动受限：关节运动受限，特别是手部小关节，可能是由于胶原蛋白的糖基化所致，"祈祷征"（无法双手合十）和"桌面测试"（无法手掌伸平放在桌面上）阳性（Kapoor）。
- 僵人病：1型糖尿病若出现抗GAD抗体阳性则高度提示存在本病可能，查体和肌电图也有帮助（Duddy）。
- 糖尿病肌肉梗死：往往是排除诊断；肌酸激酶可能正常或升高，超声和MRI对诊断可能有帮助，肌肉活检显示肌坏死、水肿和动脉闭塞（Trujillo-Santos）。
- 骨关节炎：X线平片显示关节的恶化（Feydy）。

症状及体征

- 腕管综合征：大拇指、示指、中指及无名指的桡侧疼痛和感觉异常。
- Dupuytren挛缩：主要症状是一个或多个手指在掌指关节发生屈肌收缩。
- 屈肌腱鞘炎：在弯曲肌腱时疼痛，手上存在压痛点。
- 粘连性关节囊炎：肩膀的运动范围受限和疼痛。
- 钙化性肩周炎：仅三分之一患者出现症状（肩部疼痛）。
- 关节活动受限：无痛性关节运动受限，握力减退(也见于Dupuytren挛缩)。
- 僵人病：主要影响脊柱和下肢，并与自身免疫性疾病（如T1DM）相关。
- 糖尿病肌肉梗死：通常会影响下肢，很少影响上肢。三分之一的病例对称出现，50%的病例在同一部位复发；疼痛，肿胀，压痛，并可能出现轻度发热。
- 骨关节炎：关节痛，最常见的部位是膝盖。

治疗

一般治疗

- 关节活动受限：优化控制血糖，停止吸烟，被动伸展物理治疗。虽然极少证据支持，但青霉胺、醛糖还原酶抑制剂、糖皮质激素注射已在临床应用（Kapoor）。
- 僵人病：最有效的治疗方法是苯二氮䓬和运动（Duddy）。
- 糖尿病肌肉梗死：最好的治疗尚不清楚，但方案包括：(1)休息和镇痛药；(2)抗血小板药物和/或消炎药；(3)手术切除（Trujillo-Santos）。
- 骨关节炎：物理疗法，NSAID，糖皮质激素注射，手术置换关节（Crosby）。

手关节

- 腕管综合征：排除甲状腺功能低下，治疗方法包括夹板固定手腕，NSAID类药物，糖皮质激素注射和手术（Preston）。

- Dupuytren挛缩：初期，被动伸展和羊毛脂按摩；进展期，糖皮质激素注射，手术松解筋膜（Trojian）。
- 屈肌腱鞘炎：糖皮质激素注射或手术，偶尔需要二次手术（Ryzewicz）。

肩关节
- 粘连性关节囊炎：物理治疗，糖皮质激素注射，关节内扩张，外科手术（Sheridan）
- 钙化性肩周炎：关节吸引术，糖皮质激素注射或手术切除（Siegal）。

脚
- Charcot关节（或足）：见Charcot关节病（糖尿病性骨关节病）。

随访
- 许多治疗需要转至专科医生，如风湿科、皮肤科、整形外科或物理治疗师

专家意见
- MSDs常见于糖尿病患者。
- 良好的血糖控制，规律的体力活动，戒烟可减少一些MSDs的风险。
- 对于糖尿病患者主诉关节疼痛或活动受限时应考虑存在糖尿病相关的MSDs。
- 治疗团队应当包含专科医师，以制定适当的管理计划。

参考文献

Siegal DS, Wu JS, Newman JS, et al. Calcific tendinitis: a pictorial review. Can Assoc Radiol J, 2009; Vol. 60: pp. 263–72.
Comments: A review of calcific tendinitis with examples of radiographic findings.

Duddy ME, Baker MR. Stiff person syndrome. Front Neurol Neurosci, 2009; Vol. 26: pp. 147–65.
Comments: Review of stiff-person syndrome.

Feydy A, Pluot E, Guerini H, et al. Role of imaging in spine, hand, and wrist osteoarthritis. Rheum Dis Clin North Am, 2009; Vol. 35: pp. 605–49.
Comments: Review of imaging in osteoarthritis.

Crosby J. Osteoarthritis: managing without surgery. J Fam Pract, 2009; Vol. 58: pp. 354–61.
Comments: Review of nonsurgical treatment of osteoarthritis.

Doran M. Rheumatoid arthritis and diabetes mellitus: evidence for an association? Rheumatol, 2007; Vol. 34: pp. 460–2.
Comments: Discussion of the links between diabetes and rheumatoid arthritis.

Simard JF, Mittleman MA. Prevalent rheumatoid arthritis and diabetes among NHANES participants aged 60 and older. J Rheumatol, 2007; Vol. 34: pp. 469–73.
Comments: NHANES III examination of the association between diabetes and rheumatoid arthritis. No significant association was found.

Trojian TH, Chu SM. Dupuytren's disease: diagnosis and treatment. Am Fam Physician, 2007; Vol. 76: pp. 86–9.
Comments: Review of Dupuytren's contracture.

Ryzewicz M, Wolf JM. Trigger digits: principles, management, and complications. J Hand

Surg Am, 2006; Vol. 31: pp. 135–46.
Comments: Description of stenosing flexor tenosynovitis.

Sheridan MA, Hannafin JA. Upper extremity: emphasis on frozen shoulder. Orthop Clin North Am, 2006; Vol. 37: pp. 531–9.
Comments: Description of adhesive capsulitis and frozen shoulder.

Lindsay JR, Kennedy L, Atkinson AB, et al. Reduced prevalence of limited joint mobility in type 1 diabetes in a UK clinic population over a 20-year period. Diabetes Care, 2005; Vol. 28: pp. 658–61.
Comments: Decreased prevalence of limited joint mobility from 1981–2002 (from 43%–23%). Authors hypothesized this was due to better glycemic control.

Trujillo-Santos AJ. Diabetic muscle infarction: an underdiagnosed complication of long-standing diabetes. Diabetes Care, 2003; Vol. 26: pp. 211–5.
Comments: Systematic review of case reports of diabetic muscle infarction. 166 episodes were found in the literature.

Smith LL, Burnet SP, McNeil JD. Musculoskeletal manifestations of diabetes mellitus. Br J Sports Med, 2003; Vol. 37: pp. 30–5.
Comments: Review of various arthropathies seen in diabetes, including adhesive capsulitis.

Cagliero E, Apruzzese W, Perlmutter GS, et al. Musculoskeletal disorders of the hand and shoulder in patients with diabetes mellitus. Am J Med, 2002; Vol. 112: pp. 487–90.
Comments: 200 diabetes and 100 nondiabetes patients enrolled and examined for hand and shoulder disorders. MSDs of hand and shoulder found in 39% of persons with diabetes and 9% of controls.

Frost D, Beischer W. Limited joint mobility in type 1 diabetic patients: associations with microangiopathy and subclinical macroangiopathy are different in men and women. Diabetes Care, 2001; Vol. 24: pp. 95–9.
Comments: Limited joint movement is associated with microvascular disease in men.

Gudmundsson KG, Arngrimsson R, Jónsson T. Eighteen year follow-up study of the clinical manifestations and progression of Dupuytren's disease. Scand J Rheumatol, 2001; Vol. 30: pp. 31–4.
Comments: Cohort to study progression of Dupuytren's contracture; not limited to persons with diabetes.

Helfgott SM. Stiff-man syndrome: from the bedside to the bench. Arthritis Rheum, 1999; Vol. 42: pp. 1312–20.
Comments: Review of the stiff-person syndrome and its association with diabetes.

Balci N, Balci MK, Tüzüner S. Shoulder adhesive capsulitis and shoulder range of motion in type II diabetes mellitus: association with diabetic complications. J Diabetes Complications, 1999; Vol. 13: pp. 135–40.
Comments: Shoulder adhesive capsulitis was found in 29%; associated with other MSDs, increasing age, duration of diabetes, retinopathy.

Preston DC, Shapiro BE. Median neuropathy. In Electromyography and Neuromuscular Disorders: Clinical-Electrophysiologic Correlations. Boston: Butterworth-Heinemann; 1998.
Comments: Description of carpal tunnel syndrome.

Arkkila PE, Kantola IM, Viikari JS. Limited joint mobility in type 1 diabetic patients: correlation to other diabetic complications. J Intern Med, 1994; Vol. 236: pp. 215–23.
Comments: Limited joint mobility found in 58% of persons with diabetes and

14% of controls. Limited joint mobility was associated with duration of diabetes, retinopathy, and nephropathy.

Gamstedt A, Holm-Glad J, Ohlson CG, et al. Hand abnormalities are strongly associated with the duration of diabetes mellitus. J Intern Med, 1993; Vol. 234: pp. 189–93.

Comments: Cross-sectional study of 100 persons with diabetes; one hand abnormality found in 50%, more than one abnormalities found in 26%. Associated with duration of diabetes but not glycemic control.

Eadington DW, Patrick AW, Frier BM. Association between connective tissue changes and smoking habit in type 2 diabetes and in non-diabetic humans. Diabetes Res Clin Pract, 1991; Vol. 11: pp. 121–5.

Comments: Cigarette smoking was associated with limited joint mobility and Dypuytren's contracture in persons with and without diabetes.

Hochberg MC. Epidemiology of osteoarthritis: current concepts and new insights. J Rheumatol Suppl, 1991; Vol. 27: pp. 4–6.

Comments: Review of several studies for prevalence of osteoarthritis.

Mavrikakis ME, Drimis S, Kontoyannis DA, et al. Calcific shoulder periarthritis (tendinitis) in adult onset diabetes mellitus: a controlled study. Ann Rheum Dis, 1989; Vol. 48: pp. 211–4.

Comments: Examination of calcific shoulder periarthritis (tendinitis)—32% of patients with diabetes had shoulder calcification compared to 10% of the control group.

Chaudhuri KR, Davidson AR, Morris IM. Limited joint mobility and carpal tunnel syndrome in insulin-dependent diabetes. Br J Rheumatol, 1989; Vol. 28: pp. 191–4.

Comments: Carpal tunnel is present in 75% of persons with diabetes who have limited joint mobility.

Kapoor A, Sibbitt WL. Contractures in diabetes mellitus: the syndrome of limited joint mobility. Semin Arthritis Rheum, 1989; Vol. 18: pp. 168–80.

Comments: Description of limited joint mobility.

Pal B, Anderson J, Dick WC, et al. Limitation of joint mobility and shoulder capsulitis in insulin- and non-insulindependent diabetes mellitus. Br J Rheumatol, 1986; Vol. 25: pp. 147–51.

Comments: Limitation of shoulder mobility found in 49% of patients with T1DM, 52% of patients with T2DM, and 20% of controls. Those with joint limitations had longer duration of diabetes and increased prevalence of retinopathy. Shoulder capsulitits was found in 19% of persons with diabetes and 5% of controls.

Noble J, Heathcote JG, Cohen H. Diabetes mellitus in the aetiology of Dupuytren's disease. J Bone Joint Surg Br, 1984; Vol. 66: pp. 322–5.

Comments: 42% of persons with diabetes had signs of Dupuytren's contracture.

神经系统疾病

周围神经病变

Michael Polydefkis, MD, MHS, and Donna Westervelt, CRNP, MS, CDE

定义
- 糖尿病周围神经病变（diabetic peripheral neuropathy, DPN）是糖尿病最常见的神经病变。
- DPN 是一个长度依赖性、以感觉神经为主的周围神经病变，症状始于最长的外周神经末端（如足部）。
- 糖尿病患者神经病变可能不仅由糖尿病所致（Gorson）。

流行病学
- DPN 的患病率从近 25%（调查问卷）到 70%（自主神经功能检查，神经传导测试和定量感觉测试）（Laughlin）。
- DPN 的危险因素包括血糖控制不佳，糖尿病病程，以及心血管危险因素如高血压、胆固醇升高、吸烟和高甘油三酯血症。身高和体重指数也增加了发病风险。
- DPN 可发生在糖尿病早期，可以是一个已经存在症状，并能与糖耐量减低（impaired glucose tolerance, IGT）相关。
- DPN 是截肢的危险因素。

诊断
- DPN 的诊断基于患者病史、体格检查和诊断试验（England）。
- 神经病变通常始于脚趾和脚，并向近端发展。
- 床边感觉检测包括单丝、振动阈值、本体感觉和针刺试验。这些检测评估不同类型的感官神经。上述检查均可检测出脚趾感觉缺失，虽然出现受损的顺序因患者而异。
- 单丝感觉的丧失（保护性感觉丧失）是糖尿病足溃疡和截肢的一个危险因素。
- 糖尿病周围神经病变相关的电生理变化可通过神经传导检查评估大的有髓感觉神经纤维。传导速度的降低表示大感觉神经纤维脱髓鞘，振幅降低表示轴突损失。DPN 患者此项检查结果可能正常，因为所测纤维仅包括 20% 的感觉神经纤维。
- 打孔皮肤活检（Punch skin biopsy）是一种相对无创的检测方式，需要使用 3mm 的皮肤钻孔器。组织学处理后，可观察到神经纤维。这个检查可评估小无髓感觉神经纤维，较神经传导速度（nerve conduction velocity, NCV）相比对 DPN 诊断的敏感性更高（Griffin）。
- IGT 相关 DPN 患者通常皮肤活检异常，并逐渐累及大的有髓纤维。
- 其他诊断试验包括定量感觉测试和自主功能测试。

周围神经病变

症状及体征
- DPN 的症状是感觉性的,以从足部向头部进展的方式,对称出现。可表现为明显的神经性疼痛,或很少、没有症状。
- 尽管有些患者存在明显的神经性疼痛,但也有的主要症状为感觉缺失(麻木感)。
- DPN 的疼痛常被描述为电击感样烧灼痛。
- 症状亦可表现为针刺样刺痛感,令患者痛苦和恼怒。症状通常在长时间站立或行走时加重,夜间尤甚,痛觉异常可干扰睡眠。
- 当症状到达下肢膝关节水平时,手指的症状通常开始出现。同样,症状到达前胸和腹部时,在上肢可延伸至肘部水平。虽然不典型,但是也有手部有症状而脚部无症状的患者。
- 有些糖尿病患者虽然多年糖尿病控制不佳,也可能很少或根本没有发展为 DPN,而也有的在非常早期的糖尿病阶段即出现 DPN 症状和体征。
- DPN 可见于葡萄糖耐量受损状态(即 IGT)。

治疗

预防
- 对 DPN 最好的预防措施是改善血糖控制。这将使得病情进展速度放慢,并可稳定已存在的周围神经病变。
- 但血糖控制不太可能令 DPN 逆转;周围神经功能在损伤后通常不会获得改善,尽管许多患者在血糖控制改善后感觉疼痛程度有所减轻。

神经再生治疗
- 尽管醛糖还原酶抑制剂(aldose reductase inhibitors,ARI)对 DPN 有一定作用,但目前尚无 FDA 批准的用于稳定、逆转或治疗 DPN 药物。这类药物中有一些在部分国家已由于肝或肾毒性被撤回,另外一种药物在日本仍在使用。目前在美国和欧洲有一个正在进行 ARI 的大型试验(Oates)。

对症治疗
- 两个 FDA 批准的药物可用于治疗 DPN 相关的神经性疼痛——度洛西汀和普瑞巴林。其他如三环类抗抑郁药和阿片类药物也有一定疗效。见神经性疼痛的治疗。

随访
- 对 DPN 患者的随访需要常规及详细的检查,以及反复的咨询和教育。
- 请注意其他可引起对糖尿病患者神经病变的原因,通常这些原因可导致神经系统疾病的快速进展。如果病情变化快速,需考虑维生素缺乏,毒物因素,或自身免疫性神经病。
- 二甲双胍可能会影响维生素 B_{12} 的吸收,应检查维生素 B_{12} 水平以排除维生素 B_{12} 缺乏是神经病变的原因(Bell)。

专家意见
- 诊断试验包括实验室检查筛查, NCV 测试和 / 或打孔皮肤活检,以明确 DPN 诊断并排除其他原因。其他类似 DPN 的疾病包括腰神经根病变,局灶神经压迫和足部疾患（足底筋膜炎或关节病）。
- 如果症状发生明显变化，应当重新评估：乏力的进展，神经性疼痛的变化或以非长度依赖方式发展的病情变化。
- 关注血糖的同时也应当关注心血管疾病危险因素，因为高血压和胆固醇升高也对 DPN 有影响（Tesfaye）。
- 一些研究提示了他汀类药物和外周神经病变之间的关联，但基于他汀类药物对心血管的益处，目前还没有足够的证据来证明 DM 患者停止使用他汀类药物。
- 手术减压是用于治疗 DPN 的一种方法。手术减压的适应证是证实存在局部因压迫引起的局部脱髓鞘病变，但目前尚不清楚外科减压可否改善糖尿病周围神经病变本身的症状。

参考文献

Bell DS. Metformin-induced vitamin B12 deficiency presenting as a peripheral neuropathy. South Med J, 2010; Vol. 103: pp. 265–7.
  Comments: A recent report that metformin may interfere with B12 absorption.

Laughlin RS, Dyck PJ, Melton LJ, et al. Incidence and prevalence of CIDP and the association of diabetes mellitus. Neurology, 2009; Vol. 73: pp. 39–45.
  Comments: Review of chronic inflammatory demyelinating polyneuropathy (CIDP) in diabetes.

England JD, Gronseth GS, Franklin G, et al. Practice parameter: evaluation of distal symmetric polyneuropathy: role of laboratory and genetic testing (an evidence-based review). Report of the American Academy of Neurology, American Association of Neuromuscular and Electrodiagnostic Medicine, and American Academy of Physical Medicine and Rehabilitation. Neurology, 2009; Vol. 72: pp. 185–92.
  Comments: A recent`practice parameter on diagnosis of peripheral neuropathy.

Oates PJ. Aldose reductase, still a compelling target for diabetic neuropathy. Curr Drug Targets, 2008; Vol. 9: pp. 14–36.
  Comments: A pertinent review of ARI trials and their potential for success.

Gorson KC, Ropper AH. Additional causes for distal sensory polyneuropathy in diabetic patients. J Neurol Neurosurg Psychiatry, 2006; Vol. 77: pp. 354–8.
  Comments: A first-rate review of other causes of neuropathy in diabetes.

Tesfaye S, Chaturvedi N, Eaton SE, et al. Vascular risk factors and diabetic neuropathy. NEJM, 2005; Vol. 352: pp. 341–50.
  Comments: An excellent longitudinal study that demonstrates cardiovascular risk factors associated with DPN.

Griffin JW, McArthur JC, Polydefkis M. Assessment of cutaneous innervation by skin biopsies. Curr Opin Neurol, 2001; Vol. 14: pp. 655–9.
  Comments: Reviews the role of different nerve fibers in peripheral neuropathy and for skin biopsy in diagnosis.

Brownlee M. Biochemistry and molecular cell biology of diabetic complications. Nature, 2001; Vol. 414: pp. 813–20.
  Comments: A detailed review of the postulated pathogenesis of DPN with a focus on oxidative stress.

肌萎缩

Michael Polydefkis, MD, MHS

定义
- 未诊断时可有多种叫法,包括"糖尿病近端肌萎缩","糖尿病腰骶神经丛病变","糖尿病患者腰骶部神经根病变","多发性缺血性单神经病变","股神经–坐骨神经病变","股神经病变","糖尿病恶病质",简称"Bruns–Garland 综合征"。
- 经典病变,以剧烈疼痛发作数周后的急性或亚急性、进行性、不对称性下肢肌肉无力(如背部、臀部或大腿)为特点的单相疾病,并有不同程度的恢复。
- 患者通常也有糖尿病周围神经病变(diabetic peripheral neuropathy,DPN)。
- 通过受累的空间范围、时间进程以及明显运动神经受累特点与糖尿病多神经病变相鉴别。
- 诊断糖尿病性肌萎缩(diabetic amyotrophy,DA)很重要,原因是因为治疗上不同于 DPN。

流行病学
- 没有很好的流行病学描述,但总体患病率约为 1%,T2DM 患者多于 T1DM 患者。
- 本病典型见于中年、老年患者,但在青少年也有报道。
- 越来越多的证据表明,潜在的致病机制可能是免疫介导的小血管炎导致的神经缺血性损伤(Chan)。
- 常与血糖控制不佳有关。

诊断
- 诊断基于临床表现,与 DPN 的不同点和电生理检查。
- 本病特点是下肢近端无力,可能是不对称的。
- 电生理检查:肌电图可见脊柱旁和腿部肌肉的多灶失神经支配,神经传导测试提示感觉和运动动作电位减低。
- 神经活检:对于诊断来说通常不需要神经活检。病理表现为显著的缺血性损伤和小血管炎,这促使医师在疾病诊断的早期治疗使用免疫调节疗法,虽然并没有证据表明免疫调节治疗对患者有益(Chan)。
- 腰椎穿刺:脑脊液蛋白通常升高。
- MRI 检查:腰椎及腰骶丛成像有助于排除浸润性疾病导致的亚急性患者。
- 与 DA 类似的疾病包括 ALS,多发性单神经病变,肢带型肌营养不良症,急性神经根病,以及其他神经丛病,如癌性浸润或放射性神经丛炎。

症状及体征
- 疼痛严重,甚至具有较高忍耐力的患者可能也需要紧急救治,需要包括阿片类药物在内的多种止痛药物干预。

肌萎缩

- 乏力通常比较显著，约50%的患者将依赖轮椅。
- 与DPN的远端感觉异常相比，本病多见于小腿近端肌肉（股四头肌、臀部屈肌、伸肌）的无力。
- 膝反射通常消失。
- 症状可数月内逐渐发展，一个研究报道中发现平均时间为6.2个月（Bastron）。
- 然而，持续时间是可变的，可从数月至数年。
- 一般为单侧，但也可以对称出现，甚至可涉及胸椎神经。
- 患者通常出现近50磅的大幅体重下降。
- 糖尿病的一个罕见并发症。

治疗

- 早期诊断对治疗非常关键，如类固醇激素或静脉注射免疫球蛋白（intravenous immunoglobulin，IVIg）。
- 免疫治疗方案包括IVIg或静脉注射甲基强的松龙（methylprednisolone，MP）。MP会升高血糖或增加对胰岛素的需求（见类固醇糖尿病）和IVIg有导致急性肾功能衰竭的风险。患者的肾小球滤过率（glomerular filtration rate，GRF）<50ml/min，应给予充分水化并密切监测。
- 未进行药物治疗时恢复较慢，由于患病率较低，目前缺乏关于治疗的确切证据。
- 主要以支持治疗为主，包括止痛和物理治疗，很少需要住院治疗。
- 对坐轮椅或卧床的有DVT风险的患者进行治疗。
- 患者可能需要亚急性康复和门诊物理治疗。

随访

- 大多数患者功能在12~24个月内能够获得恢复良好。偶有复发可能。
- 很少有证据表明血糖控制可影响预后，尽管通常建议这样做。

专家意见

- 最重要的识别和诊断DA，并与DPN作以区分。
- 虽然DA比DPN更令人担心，但通常预后较好。
- 虽然DA患者通常自发改善，大多数神经病学者在DA患者诊断后给予早期静脉注射免疫球蛋白或甲基强的松龙治疗。

参考文献

Chan YC, Lo YL, Chan ES. Immunotherapy for diabetic amyotrophy. Cochrane Database Syst Rev, 2009; CD006521.

Comments: This systemic review of the literature found only one clinical trial for DA and concluded "there is presently no evidence from RCT to support any recommendation on the use of any immunotherapy treatment in diabetic amyotrophy."

Dyck PJB, Brien P, Bosch EP, et al. The multi-centre double-blind controlled trial of IV methylprednisolone in diabetic lumbosacral radiculoplexusneuropathy. Neurology, 2006; Vol. 66 (5, Suppl 2): p. A191.

Comments: This abstract reports a trend toward a beneficial effect of IV methylprednisolone in DA.

Dyck PJ, Windebank AJ. Diabetic and nondiabetic lumbosacral radiculoplexus neuropathies: new insights into pathophysiology and treatment. Muscle Nerve, 2002; Vol. 25: pp. 477–91.

Comments: Describes the pathology of DA from fascicular nerve biopsies.

Barohn RJ, Sahenk Z, Warmolts JR, et al. The Bruns-Garland syndrome (diabetic amyotrophy). Revisited 100 years later. Arch Neurol, 1991; Vol. 48: pp. 1130–5.

Comments: An excellent historical review of DA as well as a case series that demonstrates the heterogeneity of DA presentations.

Bastron JA, Thomas JE. Diabetic polyradiculopathy: clinical and electromyographic findings in 105 patients. Mayo Clin Proc, 1981; Vol. 56: pp. 725–32.

Comments: Includes 105 patients with diabetic amyotrophy: age of onset 36–83 years; symptoms progressed over mean of 6.2 months; 9.5% of patients had painless muscle weakness.

Casey EB, Harrison MJ. Diabetic amyotrophy: a follow-up study. Br Med J, 1972; Vol. 1: pp. 656–9.

Comments: Early case reports of DA describing age of onset and other clinical features.

自主神经病变

Michael Polydefkis, MD, MHS, and Kathleen Burks, MSN, CRNP

定义
- 糖尿病自主神经病变（Diabetic autonomic neuropathy，DAN）是糖尿病的一个常见的却被低估的并发症，对生存和生活质量具有显著的负面影响。
- 糖尿病患者自主神经的受累是以长度依赖方式呈现。迷走神经是最长的自主神经，通常首先受累。迷走神经提供了75%的副交感神经张力，具有广泛的影响。
- 之后也可出现交感神经功能丧失。

流行病学
- DAN的患病率估计取决于研究人群以及所使用的方法。在一般情况下，患病率与执行检测的手段高级程度呈正相关。
- 一个以人群为基础的研究中，基于症状诊断的内脏自主神经病变大约患病率5.5%（Dyck）。
- 与此相反，另一种以社区为基础的研究显示，由心率变异率（heart rate variability，HRV）检查异常诊断的DAN患病率为16.7%（Ziegler）。
- 在22个欧洲糖尿病中心1 171糖尿病患者中，通过6项心脏自主神经功能检查中超过2项结果异常诊断为心血管自主神经病变，T1DM患病率为25.3%，T1DM患病率为34.3%（Ziegler）。
- DAN患者发生心血管（cardiovascular，CV）事件和死亡的风险增加。DAN患者具有发生心肌梗死（myocardial infarction，MI）相反的昼夜变化，较少发生在早上，多在傍晚出现。
- 影响心血管系统DAN患者（C-DAN）较无C-DAN者5年死亡率增加5倍（Valensi）。

诊断
- DAN的诊断依据受影响器官系统。
- 糖尿病患者最突出的自主神经症状和体征可累及瞳孔、汗腺、泌尿生殖系统、胃肠道、肾上腺髓质和心血管系统。
- C-DAN导致心率控制异常，和中央及外周血管张力异常。C-DAN最早症状可表现为静息心率增加，这是由于迷走神经张力首先受损所致，伴有心率变异率增加，心脏射血分数降低，心脏收缩功能障碍，舒张期充盈降低。随着症状进展，可由于交感和副交感神经功能均丧失而出现固定心率。
- 体位性低血压（站立时收缩压降低30mmHg以上）很常见，归因于内脏血管舒缩纤维失去交感神经支配以及外周阻力的降低。
- C-DAN诊断可能需要在心脏临床实验室中进行倾斜试验、心率变异率测定，肌电图检查。
- 排汗功能障碍：四肢无汗，有时伴有躯干代偿性多汗；随着病变进展，可出现弥漫无汗。
- 可见味觉出汗,即进食后面部、头部、颈部、肩部和胸部出汗异常。
- 排汗功能障碍的诊断:通过轴突反射汗水定量试验(通过响应乙酰胆碱产生汗水)或温度调节出汗测定(通过湿度敏感粉评估出汗的地区的方法,受试者躺在受控制的桑拿室里,汗水产生后与皮肤上的湿度敏感粉接触出现颜色变化)。
- 糖尿病胃肠自主神经症状(Gastrointestinal diabetic autonomic symptoms, GI-DAN):常见,通常表现为上消化道或下消化道自主神经病变。
- 胃肠道症状是迷走神经(负责食管和胃蠕动)和肠固有神经元的反映。通常通过如食管造影、胃排空试验等胃肠道运动检查很难对两者进行区分。本病病理提示胃黏膜神经失去支配。
- 胃排空延迟可导致胃石,也妨碍小肠对营养的吸收,并导致糖尿病血糖控制不稳。
- 糖尿病腹泻的典型表现是通常量多、水泻,持续数小时或数天,并经常出现腹泻便秘交替(见胃轻瘫)。
- 勃起功能障碍(Erectile Dysfunction,ED):多因素所致,包括神经病变,血管病变,代谢控制,营养,内分泌紊乱,心理因素和药物。阴茎的副交感神经功能障碍导致阴茎海绵体松弛和血流量减少(见勃起功能障碍)。
- 神经源性膀胱:通过残余尿量大于150ml,并存在尿路感染(urinary infections, UTIs)的危险因素而诊断。一年内两个以上的尿路感染提示可能为神经源性膀胱。膀胱失去交感神经、副交感神经和躯体神经支配,糖尿病患者中最早的与膀胱感觉受损的功能障碍表现为排尿反射阈值升高(见糖尿病膀胱疾病)。

症状及体征

- DAN的自主神经病变临床症状一般不会发生,除非糖尿病病史较长。但可在诊断T2DM后1年内以及诊断T1DM的5年内发生亚临床自主神经功能紊乱。
- DAN症状是基于所累及的器官系统。
- C-DAN:典型的症状包括头晕、乏力、疲劳和视力模糊。较严重的C-DAN症状包括体位性低血压,运动不耐受,无症状性心肌缺血,术中心血管状态不稳定。C-DAN也增加了由心肌梗死所致的死亡风险。
- 排汗功能障碍:症状通常不易被发现,包括不耐热和躯干多汗。足部缺乏汗水被认为可能导致溃疡形成。
- GI-DAN:分为上、下消化道症状。上消化道症状,包括烧心,吞咽困难(固体),早饱,厌食,恶心,呕吐,上腹不适,腹胀;而下消化道受累可引起腹泻与便秘交替。
- ED:见勃起功能障碍。
- 神经源性膀胱:症状多变,包括排尿延迟,尿流变细,尿流滴沥。最终,不能完全排空膀胱,膀胱过度膨胀和尿潴留,并使患者易出现UTIs。

治疗

- C-DAN：强化血糖和多因素的治疗可减慢 C-DAN（Gaede）进展，有证据表明，医药级 α-硫辛酸（美国市场没有）亦减慢发展。停止用药，可产生/加重体位性低血压。可使用盐皮质激素（如 9α-氟氢可的松，0.1mg/d 起始后逐渐增加，可能需要每天 0.5mg）和外周交感神经活动相关药物（如米多君，剂量为 2.5mg 至 10mg，每天 3 次）治疗体位性低血压。不幸的是，直至液体潴留和水肿出现时症状一般才获改善。
- 排汗功能障碍：抗胆碱能药如苯海索、丙胺太林或东莨菪碱，虽然药效可能因出现其他抗胆碱能作用而受限，如口干、尿潴留和便秘。抗摧涎素（Glycopyrolate）对部分味觉出汗患者有效。作为一种局部治疗，皮内注射 A 型肉毒毒素亦有效。
- GI-DAN：每天少量多餐（4~6 次），同时减少食物中的脂肪成分亦有帮助。治疗胃轻瘫可使用促动力药物，包括甲氧氯普胺、多潘立酮、红霉素、左舒必利。糖尿病性腹泻的严重和间歇性使治疗和评估变得困难，最好在胃肠门诊进行。
- ED：停止违禁药物，并联合心理辅导、药物或手术治疗。药物治疗包括鸟嘌呤磷酸 5 型磷酸二酯酶抑制剂，该药可增加阴茎海绵体的血液与性刺激。其他疗法包括向海绵体内注射血管活性物质如罂粟碱、酚妥拉明和前列腺素 E_1；经尿道使用的血管活性剂，以及机械装置，如真空勃起装置或收缩环。如果上述治疗失败或病人不耐受，可考虑阴茎假体植入。
- 神经性膀胱：指导患者触诊膀胱，如果患者无法在膀胱充满时触发排尿，则可每 4 小时采用 Crede 氏动作促进排尿。拟副交感神经药，如氨甲酰甲胆碱（每天 10~30mg，每天 3 次），有时有部分疗效。可用多沙唑嗪等 α_1 受体阻滞剂松弛括约肌。可能还需要间歇性导尿。

随访

- 对 DAN 患者进行定期随访以评估症状和药物效果。
- ADA 共识表明，应在 T2DM 诊断时及 T1DM 诊断 5 年后筛查 DAN。筛选通常包括自主神经功能紊乱的症状、体征，其中对 Valsalva 动作、直立或呼吸动作引起的心率变异情况最为重要。
- 每年进行重复筛查，如果筛查阳性，则应当进行适当的诊断检查及对症治疗。

专家意见

- 会出现导致残疾或影响生活质量的自主神经症状。
- 每年进行系统的自主神经症状评估是诊断的关键。
- 治疗最好由专科医院进行。

参考文献

Pop-Busui R, Low PA, Waberski BH, et al. Effects of prior intensive insulin therapy on cardiac autonomic nervous system function in type 1 diabetes mellitus: the Diabetes Control and Complications Trial/Epidemiology of Diabetes Interventions and Complications study (DCCT/EDIC). Circulation, 2009; Vol. 119: pp. 2886–93.

Comments: After 13–14 years follow-up from DCCT close-out, prevalence of cardiac autonomic neuropathy significantly lower in former intensive glycemia group (28.9%) versus former conventional glycemia group (35.2%, p=0.02).

Vinik AI, Ziegler D. Diabetic cardiovascular autonomic neuropathy. Circulation, 2007; Vol. 115: pp. 387–97.

Comments: An excellent recent review of the cardiac manifestations of DAN.

Boulton AJ, Vinik AI, Arezzo JC, et al. Diabetic neuropathies: a statement by the American Diabetes Association. Diabetes Care, 2005; Vol. 28: pp. 956–62.

Comments: ADA position statement for DPN.

Vinik AI, Maser RE, Mitchell BD, et al. Diabetic autonomic neuropathy. Diabetes Care, 2003; Vol. 26: pp. 1553–79.

Comments: An older, but still relevant general review of autonomic neuropathy in diabetes.

Valensi P, Sachs RN, Harfouche B, et al. Predictive value of cardiac autonomic neuropathy in diabetic patients with or without silent myocardial ischemia. Diabetes Care, 2001; Vol. 24: pp. 339–43.

Comments: Small study that assesses the predictive value of cardiac autonomic neuropathy on major cardiac events.

Gaede P, Vedel P, Parving HH, et al. Intensified multifactorial intervention in patients with type 2 diabetes mellitus and microalbuminuria: the Steno type 2 randomised study. Lancet, 1999; Vol. 353: pp. 617–22.

Comments: An important study that demonstrated that intensive multifactorial intervention reduced C-DAN by 68%.

Dyck PJ, Kratz KM, Karnes JL, et al. The prevalence by staged severity of various types of diabetic neuropathy, retinopathy, and nephropathy in a population-based cohort: the Rochester Diabetic Neuropathy Study. Neurology, 1993; Vol. 43: pp. 817–24.

Comments: A widely cited natural history study of diabetic neuropathy.

Ziegler D, Gries FA, Spüler M, et al. The epidemiology of diabetic neuropathy. Diabetic Cardiovascular Autonomic Neuropathy Multicenter Study Group. J Diabetes Complications, 1992; Vol. 6: pp. 49–57.

Comments: Reviews epidemiology of diabetic neuropathy.

Pfeifer MA, Weinberg CR, Cook DL, et al. Autonomic neural dysfunction in recently diagnosed diabetic subjects. Diabetes Care, 1984; Vol. 7: pp. 447–53.

Comments: Reviews the evidence that subclinical autonomic neuropathy can develop early in diabetes.

卒中

Martinson K. Arnan, MD, and Rebecca Gottesman, MD, PhD

定义
- 是任何原因引起的血液流向大脑的中断，随着时间增加可致细胞死亡并表现出局灶性神经症状。
- 出血性卒中：由血液从血管漏入脑组织引起。
- 缺血性卒中：由血管闭塞引起。
- 缺血性卒中可按机制或卒中的病因进一步细分，包括大血管动脉粥样硬化、栓塞和小血管病变。
- 卒中的其他原因包括血液高凝状态、夹层、镰状细胞贫血以及一些不确定的原因（Adams）。

流行病学
- 在美国，卒中是导致死亡的第三大原因（美国心脏协会）。
- 在美国，卒中是致残的首要原因。
- 在美国，每年超过 700 000 人确诊卒中，其中超过 160 000 人最终死亡（美国心脏协会）。
- 糖尿病是大血管动脉粥样硬化及小血管病变的诱发因素，这两者均可导致中风。
- 易患卒中的糖尿病患者一般同时合并有其他心血管危险因素，如高血压、肥胖、高脂血症。
- 糖尿病是卒中的一个独立的危险因素（美国预防服务工作组）。与非糖尿病患者相比，糖尿病患者发生卒中的风险增加 2~5 倍（Manson, Stamler）。
- 约 15%~33% 的缺血性卒中患者有糖尿病（Karapanayiotides; Megherbi; Woo）。
- 虽然糖尿病通常与小血管、腔隙型卒中相关（Karapanayiotides），但糖尿病也与其他类型的卒中风险增加相关，包括心源性和其他非腔隙型卒中（Abbott）。
- 相比非糖尿病患者，有糖尿病患者发生出血性卒中的风险较低（Jorgensen）。
- 不同于非糖尿病人群，糖尿病患者使用阿司匹林并不伴有出血性卒中风险的增加（ETDRS 调查）。
- 糖尿病史与卒中较差的预后相关（Lindsberg）。
- 因急性卒中入院的患者近 1/3 存在高血糖（Williams, Scott）。
- 高血糖与缺血性卒中较差的预后有关（Bruno, 1999; Bruno, 2002; Alvarez-Sabin）。高血糖可能是卒中的一个严重程度的标志（Candelise）。

诊断
- 卒中的诊断基于患者的病史、体格检查（包括美国国立卫生研究院卒中评分）和确诊诊断。
- 脑影像学检查：确诊位置、类型、大小和卒中的时间。通常情况下，在初始评估时进行非显影剂的头颅CT。大多数患者进行头部MRI检查，因其具有识别卒中的更高的灵敏度/特异性。
- 血管成像：通过CT血管造影，磁共振血管造影或超声检查，以确定是否存在血管阻塞。
- 灌注显像：通过CT或MRI获得，以期检出可挽救的处于危险的脑组织。
- 超声心动图：排除心脏来源的栓子。通常经胸超声心动图是首选检查。
- 血液学检查：识别与卒中类似或增加卒中可能性的临床情况。常规检查包括血糖、电解质、心电图、心肌标志物、血小板计数及凝血功能。
- 如果允许，通常可进行感染相关检查。
- 对易患卒中的患者进行其他检查[如血脂，血压，连续监测除外阵发性房颤（Christensen）]。

症状及体征
- 取决于受累脑的部分。
- 在所有卒中患者，症状基本总是突发的。
- 常见的症状包括：（1）面部、手臂和/或腿部麻木和/或无力；（2）说话困难或理解困难；（3）头晕，步态不稳，不协调；（4）视力障碍（Lloyd-Jones），包括复视，单侧视力减退或视野缺损。
- 出血性卒中往往伴有头痛、恶心、呕吐，否则，卒中很少引起疼痛。
- 在感染或血糖异常（包括低血糖或高血糖）的情况下出现既往神经功能缺损的再现可被误认为是卒中。
- 很少见的情况下，低血糖症可引起局灶性神经症状和体征，出现卒中样症状（Wallis），甚至在没有卒中史的情况下。

治疗

预防
- 血糖控制：类似于其他形式的大血管疾病，英国前瞻性糖尿病研究长期随访和糖尿病控制与并发症研究（EDIC）建议，血糖控制对减少卒中风险非常重要。
- 高血压：较高的血压与缺血性卒中风险直接相关（Rodgers）。血压降低后卒中减少30%~40%（Lawes）。在糖尿病患者，相比血压控制不佳患者，血压良好控制的患者卒中风险降低44%（UKPDS 38）。
- 高血脂：低密度脂蛋白的目标是70mg/dl（Grundy）。在心脏保护研究，他汀类药物的使用可降低糖尿病患者28%的卒中风险，这种风险的降低独立于基线LDL、糖尿病类型或病程、先前存在的血管疾病或充分的血糖控制（Collins）。
- 戒烟。
- 改变生活方式：多个大规模的前瞻性研究表明，超重与脑卒中风险呈正相关（Rexrode；Kurth；Song）。
- Look AHEAD研究是一项正在进行中的对糖尿病患者进行强化生活方式干预的随机试验，研究结果包括卒中在内的心血管终点，目前的中期分析已经显示出心血管危险因素的显著减少（Look AHEAD研究组）。
- 虽然卒中的风险计算器通常不在临床实践中应用，但对于需要在改变生活方式之前完全了解卒中风险的患者可能有帮助。可用的风险计算器已在 UKPDS 60 中包括。

急性卒中治疗

- 进行安全的溶栓治疗取决于症状出现的持续时间，即症状发作的确切时间。如果患者从睡眠中醒来时出现症状，那么症状出现的时间点应推定为最后一次患者被视为正常的时候。
- 症状出现后的 4.5 小时内静脉注射组织型纤溶酶原激活剂（tissue plasminogen activator，tPA）可显著降低缺血性卒中的破坏性影响（Hacke）。
- 前循环卒中患者不适合静脉应用 tPA，但在 6 小时时间窗内的患者可考虑进行动脉内 tPA 注射（Chalela，Choi）。对于后循环卒中患者，动脉注射 tPA 的时间窗可延长至 24 小时（Ogawa）。这两种治疗方法均需要血管介入和血管神经科医师参与。
- 取栓设备是一种通过去除阻塞在动脉的栓子而达到血流重建的方法，现在正在积极研究中（Yu，Schumacher）。在脑栓塞机械取栓（Mechanical Embolus Removal in Cerebral Embolism，MERCI）试验中应用的 MERCI 装置用于取栓治疗，虽然该设备的使用对于改善脑卒中预后的仍然不清楚（Smith）。
- 大多数急性缺血性卒中患者住院期间不需要抗凝治疗。存在心尖部血栓或心脏机械瓣膜患者在入院后可能需要抗凝治疗。
- 推荐 24~48 小时内给予急性缺血性卒中患者 325mg 阿司匹林（Coull）。阿司匹林虽不会控制急性卒中的后果，但可帮助预防卒中复发。
- 对于急性缺血性脑卒中，积极的血压管理与较差的预后相关（Castillo）。仅在收缩压高于 220mmHg 或舒张压高于 120mmHg 时予以干预。一个可接受的范围是在第一天内将血压降低 15%~25%（Grossman）。但是，如果收缩压高于 185mmHg 或舒张压高于 110mmHg 时，存在应用 tPA 的禁忌（美国国家神经疾病和卒中研究所 rt-PA 卒中研究组）。
- 在卒中治疗期间，血糖应保持在正常范围内。
- 在卒中的第一个 24 小时内持续存在的高血糖是卒中加重的独立预测因素（Baird）。因为高血糖增加了脑部的代谢需要，因此可能恶化脑水肿，血糖控制在卒中的早期阶段非常重要。
- CT 血管成像或增强 CT 中需要应用造影剂，因此为了减少乳酸性酸中毒的风险，二甲双胍需短暂停用。

随访

- 详尽询问病史，以排除卒中的并发症，如癫痫发作、疼痛综合征、挛缩或抑郁症。
- 详细的查体有助于确定康复概率，多数患者会在发生卒中事件后 1~1.5 年内会恢复部分功能。
- 优化血糖控制。
- 对干预的危险因素进行常规实验室检查（如脂质谱）。
- 抗血小板药物治疗，如阿司匹林，除非患者有心源性病因，在这种情况下，华法林是首选的。
- 询问目前行为/生活方式的改变情况，如戒烟、体育锻炼、减轻体重，保持低盐饮食。
- 物理治疗，职业治疗和语言治疗方面密切随访。
- 有卒中病史患者再发生卒中的风险增加。具有卒中史的患者需要教育以了解卒中可能的症状，并且如果他们遇到任何类似症状应当立即寻求医疗帮助。

专家意见
- 糖尿病患者卒中比一般人群更常见，并且预后较差。
- 糖尿病患者发生缺血性卒中较出血性卒中更常见，可能部分与合并如高脂血症和高血压等有关。
- 糖尿病患者使用阿司匹林是安全的，与出血性卒中的风险无关。
- 心血管危险因素的改善及血糖控制可以减少卒中的风险
- 生活方式的干预也可以减少卒中的风险。
- 早期识别卒中症状和抵达医院并确定患者是否可进行溶栓，这会影响卒中的预后。
- 糖尿病患者是否合并肾病影响着采用血管或灌注成像方法进行检查的决定，因造影剂肾病和/或肾源性系统性纤维化的风险在这部分患者是增加的。
- 颈部（但不是头部）CT 血管造影或 CT 灌注需要碘对比剂，而 MR 灌注或磁共振血管造影需要钆。
- 对于卒中的康复成功，包括物理治疗、职业治疗、言语治疗等多学科方法都很重要。

推荐依据
Sacco RL, Adams R, Albers G, et al. Guidelines for prevention of stroke in patients with ischemic stroke or transient ischemic attack. Stroke, 2006; Vol. 37: pp. 577–617.

Comments: Describes recommendations for prevention of stroke, including a section on risk factor control in persons with diabetes.

其他参考文献
Look AHEAD Research Group, Wing RR. Long-term effects of a lifestyle intervention on weight and cardiovascular risk factors in individuals with type 2 diabetes mellitus: four-year results of the Look AHEAD trial. Arch Intern Med, 2010; Vol. 170: pp. 1566–75.

Comments: Effect of lifestyle interventions in diabetics on cardiovascular risk factors.

Lloyd-Jones D, Adams R, Carnethon M, et al. Heart disease and stroke statistics—2009 update: a report from the American Heart Association Statistics Committee and Stroke Statistics Subcommittee. Circulation, 2009; Vol. 119: pp. e21–181.

Comments: Stroke statistics and symptoms.

Hacke W, Kaste M, Bluhmki E, et al. Thrombolysis with alteplase 3 to 4.5 hours after acute ischemic stroke. NEJM, 2008; Vol. 359: pp. 1317–29.

Comments: Alteplase use in acute stroke is safe in the 3- to 4.5-hour window.

Ogawa A, Mori E, Minematsu K, et al. Randomized trial of intraarterial infusion of urokinase within 6 hours of middle cerebral artery stroke: the middle cerebral artery embolism local fibrinolytic intervention trial (MELT) Japan. Stroke, 2007; Vol. 38: pp. 2633–9.

Comments: Clot lysis interventions in the posterior circulation may be done in an extended time window.

Choi JH, Bateman BT, Mangla S, et al. Endovascular recanalization therapy in acute ischemic stroke. Stroke, 2006; Vol. 37: pp. 419–24.

Comments: Time window for intra-arterial tPA.

Ohira T, Shahar E, Chambless LE, et al. Risk factors for ischemic stroke subtypes: the Atherosclerosis Risk in Communities study. Stroke, 2006; Vol. 37: pp. 2493–8.

Comments: Stroke in diabetic patients.

Christensen H, Fogh Christensen A, Boysen G. Abnormalities on ECG and telemetry predict stroke outcome at 3 months. J Neurol Sci, 2005; Vol. 234: pp. 99–103.

Comments: Stroke predictors.

Smith WS, Sung G, Starkman S, et al. Safety and efficacy of mechanical embolectomy in acute ischemic stroke: results of the MERCI trial. Stroke, 2005; Vol, 36: pp. 1432–8.

Comments: Safety and efficacy data for MERCI clot removal.

Karapanayiotides T, Piechowski-Jozwiak B, van Melle G, et al. Stroke patterns, etiology, and prognosis in patients with diabetes mellitus. Neurology, 2004: Vol. 62: pp. 1558–62.

Comments: Stroke in diabetic patients.

Lindsberg PJ, Roine RO. Hyperglycemia in acute stroke. Stroke, 2004: Vol. 35: pp. 363–4.

Comments: Stroke prognosis in diabetic patients.

Castillo J, Leira R, García MM, et al. Blood pressure decrease during the acute phase of ischemic stroke is associated with brain injury and poor stroke outcome. Stroke, 2004; Vol. 35: pp. 520–6.

Comments: Blood pressure management in acute stroke management.

Alvarez-Sabín J, Molina CA, Ribó M, et al. Impact of admission hyperglycemia on stroke outcome after thrombolysis: risk stratification in relation to time to reperfusion. Stroke, 2004; Vol. 35: pp. 2493–8.

Comments: Post-tPA stroke prognosis in the setting of hyperglycemia on admission.

Lawes CM, Bennett DA, Feigin VL, et al. Blood pressure and stroke: an overview of published reviews. Stroke, 2004; Vol. 35: pp. 776–5.

Comments: Effect of reduction of blood pressure management on strokes.

Grundy SM, Cleeman JI, Merz CN, et al. Implications of recent clinical trials for the National Cholesterol Education Program Adult Treatment Panel III guidelines. Circulation, 2004; Vol. 110: pp. 227–39.

Comments: Management of hyperlipidemia.

Song YM, Sung J, Davey Smith G, et al. Body mass index and ischemic and hemorrhagic stroke: a prospective study in Korean men. Stroke, 2004; Vol. 35: pp. 831–6.

Comments: Weight as a risk factor stroke in Korean men.

American Heart Association. Heart Disease and Stroke Statistics—2004 Update. Dallas, TX: American Heart Association; 2003.

Comments: Stroke statistics;

Megherbi SE, Milan C, Minier D, et al. Association between diabetes and stroke subtype on survival and functional outcome 3 months after stroke: data from the European BIOMED Stroke Project. Stroke, 2003; Vol. 34: pp. 688–94.

Comments: Diabetes and stroke subtypes.

Yu W, Binder D, Foster-Barber A, et al. Endovascular embolectomy of acute basilar artery occlusion. Neurology, 2003; Vol. 61: pp. 1421–3.

Comments: Mechanical clot removal of posterior circulation strokes.

Schumacher HC, Meyers PM, Yavagal DR, et al. Endovascular mechanical thrombectomy of an occluded superior division branch of the left MCA for acute cardioembolic stroke. Cardiovasc Intervent Radiol, 2003; Vol. 26: pp. 305–8.

Comments: Mechanical clot removal in MCA strokes.

Baird TA, Parsons MW, Phanh T, et al. Persistent poststroke hyperglycemia is independently associated with infarct expansion and worse clinical outcome. Stroke 2003; Vol. 34: pp. 2208–14.

Comments: Hyperglycemia and infarct expansion.

Collins R, Armitage J, Parish S, et al. MRC/BHF Heart Protection Study of cholesterol-lowering with simvastatin in 5963 people with diabetes: a randomised placebo-controlled trial. Lancet, 2003; Vol. 361: pp. 2005–16.

Comments: Benefit of statin use.

Williams LS, Rotich J, Qi R, et al. Effects of admission hyperglycemia on mortality and costs in acute ischemic stroke. Neurology, 2002; Vol. 59: pp. 67–71.

Comments: Hyperglycemia in acute stroke patients.

Bruno A, Levine SR, Frankel MR, et al. Admission glucose level and clinical outcomes in the NINDS rt-PA Stroke Trial. Neurology, 2002; Vol. 59: pp. 669–74.

Comments: Relevance of admission serum glucose levels in stroke management.

Coull BM, Williams LS, Goldstein LB, et al. Anticoagulants and antiplatelet agents in acute ischemic stroke: report of the Joint Stroke Guideline Development Committee of the American Academy of Neurology and the American Stroke Association (a division of the American Heart Association). Stroke, 2002; Vol. 33: pp. 1934–42.

Comments: Aspirin use in acute strokes.

Kurth T, Gaziano JM, Berger K, et al. Body mass index and the risk of stroke in men. Arch Intern Med, 2002; Vol. 162: pp. 2557–62.

Comments: Weight as a risk factor for stroke in men.

Chalela JA, Katzan I, Liebeskind DS, et al. Safety of intra-arterial thrombolysis in the postoperative period. Stroke, 2001; Vol. 32: pp. 1365–9.

Comments: Safety of IA tPA.

Woo D, Gebel J, Miller R, et al. Incidence rates of first-ever ischemic stroke subtypes among blacks: a populationbased study. Stroke, 1999; Vol. 30: pp. 2517–22.

Comments: Strokes in black diabetic patients.

Scott JF, Robinson GM, French JM, et al. Prevalence of admission hyperglycaemia across clinical subtypes of acute stroke. Lancet, 1999; Vol. 353: pp. 376–7.

Comments: Hyperglycemia in different stroke subtypes.

Bruno A, Biller J, Adams HP, et al. Acute blood glucose level and outcome from ischemic stroke. Trial of ORG 10172 in Acute Stroke Treatment (TOAST) Investigators. Neurology 1999; Vol. 52: pp. 280–4.

Comments: Prognosis in acute strokes in the setting of hyperglycemia.

Grossman E, Ironi AN, Messerli FH. Comparative tolerability profile of hypertensive crisis treatments. Drug Saf, 1998; Vol. 19: pp. 99–122.

Comments: Treatment options for blood pressure management.

UK Prospective Diabetes Study Group. Tight blood pressure control and risk of macrovascular and microvascular complications in type 2 diabetes: UKPDS 38. BMJ, 1998; Vol. 317: pp. 703–13.

Comments: Blood pressure management in diabetes.

Rexrode KM, Hennekens CH, Willett WC, et al. A prospective study of body mass index, weight change, and risk of stroke in women. JAMA, 1997; Vol. 277: pp. 1539–45.
Comments: Weight as a risk factor for stroke in women.

US Preventive Services Task Force. Guide to Clinical Preventive Services. 2nd ed. Baltimore, MD: Williams & Wilkins; 1996.
Comments: Primary prevention of stroke.

Rodgers A, MacMahon S, Gamble G, et al. Blood pressure and risk of stroke in patients with cerebrovascular disease. The United Kingdom Transient Ischaemic Attack Collaborative Group. BMJ, 1996; Vol. 313: pp. 147.
Comments: Blood pressure as a risk factor for stroke.

The National Institute of Neurological Disorders and Stroke rt-PA Stroke Study Group. Tissue plasminogen activator for acute ischemic stroke. NEJM, 1995; Vol. 333: pp. 1581–7.
Comments: Checklist for administering tPA safely.

Jørgensen II, Nakayama H, Raaschou HO, et al. Stroke in patients with diabetes. The Copenhagen Stroke Study. Stroke, 1994; Vol. 25: pp. 1977–84.
Comments: Types of strokes in diabetic patients.

Adams HP, Bendixen BH, Kappelle LJ, et al. Classification of subtype of acute ischemic stroke. Definitions for use in a multicenter clinical trial. TOAST. Trial of Org 10172 in Acute Stroke Treatment. Stroke, 1993; Vol. 24: pp. 35–41.
Comments: Classifies subtypes of stroke.

Stamler J, Vaccaro O, Neaton JD, et al. Diabetes, other risk factors, and 12-yr cardiovascular mortality for men screened in the Multiple Risk Factor Intervention Trial. Diabetes Care, 1993; Vol. 16: pp. 434–44.
Comments: Cardiovascular risk factors in men.

ETDRS Investigators. Aspirin effects on mortality and morbidity in patients with diabetes mellitus. Early Treatment Diabetic Retinopathy Study report 14. JAMA, 1992; Vol. 268: pp. 1292–300.
Comments: Aspirin is safe to use in diabetes.

Manson JE, Colditz GA, Stampfer MJ, et al. A prospective study of maturity-onset diabetes mellitus and risk of coronary heart disease and stroke in women. Arch Intern Med, 1991; Vol. 151: pp. 1141–7.
Comments: Cardiovascular risk factors in women.

Abbott RD, Donahue RP, MacMahon SW, et al. Diabetes and the risk of stroke. The Honolulu Heart Program. JAMA, 1987; Vol. 257: pp. 949–52.
Comments: Stroke in diabetic patients.

Candelise L, Landi G, Orazio EN, et al. Prognostic significance of hyperglycemia in acute stroke. Arch Neurol, 1985; Vol. 42: pp. 661–3.
Comments: Acute stroke prognosis in the setting of hyperglycemia.

Wallis WE, Donaldson I, Scott RS, et al. Hypoglycemia masquerading as cerebrovascular disease (hypoglycemic hemiplegia). Ann Neurol, 1985; Vol. 18: pp. 510–2.
Comments: Focal neurological symptoms in hypoglycemia.

眼科疾病

视网膜病变

Sachin D. Kalyani,MD

定义
- 糖尿病视网膜血管病变分类：增殖型、非增殖型。
- 糖尿病非增殖型视网膜病变（NPDR）：糖尿病视网膜病变的早期改变，由视网膜小血管损伤引起。
- 糖尿病增殖型视网膜病变（PDR）：糖尿病视网膜病变的晚期改变，伴有视网膜表面新生血管形成。

流行病学
- 在美国20至74岁人群中，糖尿病视网膜病变是导致失明的最主要原因。
- 每年有5 000新发失明患者继发于糖尿病视网膜病变。
- 在1型糖尿病及2型糖尿病人群中，糖尿病的患病时间和血糖升高的严重程度与糖尿病视网膜病变发生率的升高直接相关。
- Wisconsin糖尿病视网膜病变流行病学研究显示，20年以上的糖尿病病史，将导致99%的1型糖尿病患者和>60%的2型糖尿病患者发生不同程度的糖尿病视网膜病变。
- 在45岁以上人群中，糖尿病视网膜病变的发生率在非西班牙裔黑人和墨西哥裔美国人中分别是27%和33%，高于非西班牙裔白人的18%。

诊断
- 轻度糖尿病非增殖型视网膜病变：仅仅有微血管瘤。
- 中度糖尿病非增殖型视网膜病变：除了微血管瘤，还存在以下一种或几种病变，微出血、硬性渗出或棉絮斑，但是不足以诊断重度糖尿病非增殖型视网膜病变。
- 重度糖尿病非增殖型视网膜病变：采用糖尿病非增殖型视网膜病变的4∶2∶1规则进行诊断，符合以下3条中任一条即可诊断，符合2条以上诊断为非常严重的糖尿病非增殖型视网膜病变：(1)4个象限内出现弥漫性视网膜内出血和微血管瘤；(2)2个象限内出现静脉串珠样改变；(3)1个象限内出现视网膜血管畸形（IRMA）。
- 糖尿病增殖型视网膜病变：虹膜或视网膜上新生血管形成，血管壁脆，易出血。
- 糖尿病非增殖型视网膜病变的严重程度分级，对于将在更严重的视网膜病变中是否会用到激光光凝治疗具有提示意义。
- 有些患者可以终生不出现糖尿病增殖型或非增殖型视网膜病变。
- 散瞳后眼底检查是糖尿病视网膜病变诊断的最好方法。
- 在缺少眼科医生的地区，眼底照相检查也可以作为诊断糖尿病视网膜病变的手段。

视网膜病变

症状和体征

糖尿病非增殖型视网膜病变：微血管瘤，点状视网膜内出血，硬性渗出，视网膜水肿，静脉出血，视网膜内微血管异常（IRMA），棉絮斑（神经纤维层梗塞），毛细血管无灌注区域。

糖尿病增殖型视网膜病变：除了糖尿病非增殖型视网膜病变体征外，视盘新生血管形成（NVD），视网膜新生血管形成（NVE），视网膜前出血，玻璃体出血，玻璃体表面维管组织形成，牵拉视网膜脱离。

虽然具有临床意义的黄斑水肿更多地被当做是视网膜病变进展的标志，但其实它在视网膜病变的任意阶段都可以出现。

常常没有症状，但也可以导致视物模糊、视力下降、视力波动（也可以由于高血糖或低血糖所致的折射误差引起）、飞蚊症、夜视障碍、阴影和视野缺损。

临床治疗

药物治疗

主要目标是通过良好的血糖控制，预防糖尿病视网膜病变发生。

糖尿病控制和并发症试验（DCCT）：在1型糖尿病患者中，强化血糖控制，76%患者可以减少视网膜病变发生风险，54%患者可以减缓病程进展。

英国前瞻性糖尿病研究（UKPDS）：在2型糖尿病患者中，强化血糖控制，25%患者可以减少微血管并发症发生风险，其中，减少视网膜光凝治疗占了其中大部分比例。

还是UKPDS研究：强化血压控制，可以减少37%微血管并发症发生率，减少34%视网膜病变进展，减少47%渐进性的视力丧失。

高血压、颈动脉闭塞性疾病、进展性糖尿病肾病以及贫血对糖尿病视网膜病变有不利影响。

FIELDS研究：2型糖尿病患者使用非诺贝特治疗，可以减少糖尿病视网膜病变激光治疗风险，效果不依赖于血脂的改变。

ACCORD研究眼病研究小组：最近报道，在心血管疾病高危风险的2型糖尿病人群中，与标准血糖控制人群（7%~7.9%）相比，强化血糖控制人群（<6%）患视网膜病变的风险下降，与单独使用辛伐他汀的人群相比，联合使用非诺贝特、辛伐他汀的人群视网膜病变的发生风险下降40%。强化血压控制组未见到明显差别。

糖尿病视网膜病变早期治疗研究（ETDRS）：阿司匹林没有益处也没有坏处。

尽管抗血管内皮生长因子已经应用在严重的糖尿病非增殖型视网膜病变与糖尿病增殖型视网膜病变中，但当前证据不支持其常规应用。

当常规治疗失败后，在永久失明的眼睛，向玻璃体内注射类固醇激素可以作为治疗方法。

妊娠与视网膜病变的短暂、可逆的加重有关系。

激光治疗

治疗严重糖尿病非增殖型视网膜病变和糖尿病增殖型视网膜病变的最佳治疗方法是全视网膜的热激光光凝治疗，以此来减缓疾病进展。

糖尿病视网膜病变研究（DRS）：全视网膜光凝治疗（PRP）5年后比较，

手术治疗

- 玻璃体出血和牵拉性视网膜脱离（都是糖尿病增殖型视网膜病变的并发症）可以通过外科玻璃体切除术治疗。
- 玻璃体切除术的目的是解除玻璃体视网膜的牵拉，促进视网膜重新附着。
- 糖尿病视网膜病变玻璃体切除手术研究（DRVS）：对于1型糖尿病严重玻璃体出血的患者，早期进行视网膜切除手术是有益的；但是，此观点在2型糖尿病人群中没有得到证实。
- 最近共识：如果还没有进行过 PRP 手术，在糖尿病视网膜病变严重玻璃体出血患者中，早期手术治疗时推荐的。
- 在视网膜脱离牵拉累及黄斑时，建议进行玻璃体切除手术。
- 进行完整眼科病史收集和眼科检查的推荐（包括散瞳眼底镜检查）。
- 1型糖尿病：发生糖尿病后第五年检查一次，如无视网膜病变发生，以后每年检查一次。
- 2型糖尿病：诊断时检查一次，如无视网膜病变发生，以后每年检查一次。
- 妊娠期糖尿病：孕前检查，妊娠期每三个月一次，产后每3~6个月一次。
- 表3-13 显示了发现视网膜病变后的随诊检查推荐。

表 3-13. 糖尿病视网膜病变基础上的检查时间表

视网膜病变	建议的随访时间
正常或少见的微动脉瘤	每年一次
轻度糖尿病非增殖型视网膜病变	每9个月1次
中度糖尿病非增殖型视网膜病变	每6个月1次
重度糖尿病非增殖型视网膜病变	每4个月1次
有临床意义的黄斑水肿	每2~4个月1次
糖尿病增殖型视网膜病变	每2~3个月1次

来源：Regillo C. Basic and clinical science course, section 12: retina and vitreous American Academy of Ophthalmology, 2004–2005.
由 Minnesota 非盈利机构美国眼科协会允许转载.

专家意见

- 重要推荐：有意义的糖尿病视网膜病变（DR）可以完全没有症状。
- 视力丧失可以有或没有视网膜病变。
- 成功治疗糖尿病视网膜病变（DR）的关键是早期诊断、正确治疗，来防远期眼科并发症的进展。
- 白内障手术可能加重糖尿病视网膜病变或加重视网膜病变的进展。
- 糖尿病视网膜病变，包括黄斑水肿在内，应该在白内障手术前治疗（提是白内障的严重程度没有影响到视网膜的观察）。

推荐依据

Fong DS, Aiello L, Gardner TW, et al. for the American Diabetes Association. Retinopathy in diabetes. Diabetes Care, 2004; Vol. 27: pp. s84–87.

其他参考文献

ACCORD Study Group, ACCORD Eye Study Group, Chew EY, et al. Effects of medical therapies on retinopathy progression in type 2 diabetes. NEJM, 2010; Vol. 363: 233–44.

Comments: The ACCORD Eye Study Group recently reported that in 2856 participants with type 2 diabetes at high risk for cardiovascular disease, participants who had intensive versus standard glycemic treatment (< 6% vs 7%–7.9%) had 33% lower rate of retinopathy progression (7.3% vs 10.4%, p = 0.003). Those who had fenofibrate and simvastatin versus simvastatin alone also had 40% lower rates of retinopathy progression (6.5% vs 10.2%, p = 0.0006). However, no significant beneficial effect was seen with intensive blood pressure control (< 120 mmHg) versus standard control (< 40 mmHg).

Keech AC, Mitchell P, Summanen PA, et al. Effect of fenofibrate on the need for laser treatment for diabetic retinopathy (FIELD study): a randomised controlled trial. Lancet, 2007; Vol. 370: pp. 1687–97.

Comments: Study showed that treatment with fenofibrate in individuals with type 2 diabetes mellitus reduces the need for laser treatment for diabetic retinopathy.

Mohamed Q, Gillies MC, Wong TY. Management of diabetic retinopathy: a systematic review. JAMA, 2007; Vol. 298: pp. 902–16.

Comments: Objective was to review the best evidence for primary and secondary intervention in the management of diabetic retinopathy, including diabetic macular edema.

American Academy of Ophthalmology. Basic and Clinical Science Course, Section 12: Retina and Vitreous; 2004: pp. 99–112.

Comments: Good summary in diabetic retinopathy chapter, including epidemiology, diagnosis, and treatment of the disease.

Kaiser PK, Friedman NJ, Pineda II R. The Massachusetts Eye and Ear Infirmary Illustrated Manual of Ophthalmology. Philadelphia: Elsevier Science, 2004; Vol. 2: pp. 317–22.

Comments: Good summary in diabetic retinopathy chapter, including epidemiology, diagnosis, and treatment of the disease.

Eliott D, Lee MS, Abrams GW. Proliferative diabetic retinopathy: principles and techniques of surgical treatment. In Ryan, SJ, (Ed). Retina. 3rd edition. St. Louis: Mosby, 2001; Vol. 3: pp. 2436–76.

Comments: Chapter with excellent summary on diabetic retinopathy.

Harris MI, Klein R, Cowie CC, et al. Is the risk of diabetic retinopathy greater in non-Hispanic blacks and Mexican Americans than in non-Hispanic whites with type 2 diabetes? A US population study. Diabetes Care, 1998; Vol. 21: pp. 1230–5.

Comments: This study compared the risk for diabetic retinopathy in non-Hispanic white, non-Hispanic black, and Mexican-American adults with type 2 diabetes in the US population.

UK Prospective Diabetes Study (UKPDS) Group. Intensive blood-glucose control with sulphonylureas or insulin compared with conventional treatment and risk of complications in patients with type 2 diabetes (UKPDS 33). Lancet, 1998; Vol. 352: pp. 837–53.

Comments: Results showed that intensive blood-glucose control by either sulphonylureas or insulin substantially decreases the risk of microvascular complications, but not macrovascular disease, in patients with type 2 diabetes.

1 UK Prospective Diabetes Study Group. Tight blood pressure control and risk of macrovascular and microvascular complications in type 2 diabetes: UKPDS 38. BMJ, 1998; Vol. 317: pp. 703–13.

Comments: Study concluded that tight blood pressure control in patients with hypertension and type 2 diabetes achieves a clinically important reduction in the risk of deaths related to diabetes, complications related to diabetes, progression of diabetic retinopathy, and deterioration in visual acuity.

American Academy of Ophthalmology, Preferred Practice Patterns Committee. Retina Panel, Diabetic Retinopathy. San Francisco; 1998.

Comments: The American Academy of Ophthalmology's recommendations for follow-up of patients with diabetes and diabetic retinopathy.

Chew EY, Mills JL, Metzger BE, et al. Metabolic control and progression of retinopathy. The Diabetes in Early Pregnancy Study. National Institute of Child Health and Human Development Diabetes in Early Pregnancy Study. Diabetes Care, 1995; Vol. 18: pp. 631–7.

Comments: This study evaluated the role of metabolic control in the progression of diabetic retinopathy during pregnancy.

Diabetes Control and Complications Trial Research Group. Progression of retinopathy with intensive versus conventional treatment in the Diabetes Control and Complications Trial. Ophthalmology, 1995; Vol. 102: pp. 647–61.

Comments: More detailed analysis regarding the effect of intensive diabetes management on retinopathy in insulin-dependent diabetes mellitus.

The Diabetes Control and Complications Trial Research Group. The effect of intensive treatment of diabetes on the development and progression of long-term complications in insulin-dependent diabetes mellitus. NEJM, 1993; Vol. 329: pp. 977–86.

Comments: Results showed that intensive therapy effectively delays the onset and slows the progression of diabetic retinopathy, nephropathy, and neuropathy in patients with IDDM.

Early Treatment Diabetic Retinopathy Study Research Group. Early photocoagulation for diabetic retinopathy. ETDRS report no. 9. Ophthalmology, 1991; Vol. 98: pp. 766–85.

Comments: This study evaluated when and with what type of laser photocoagulation should be initiated in patients with diabetic retinopathy.

The Diabetic Retinopathy Vitrectomy Study Research Group. Early vitrectomy for severe proliferative diabetic retinopathy in eyes with useful vision. Results of a randomized trial-Diabetic Retinopathy Vitrectomy Study Report 3. Ophthalmology, 1988; Vol. 95: pp. 1307–20.

Comments: The study showed that early vitrectomy for type 1 diabetics with advanced PDR was beneficial.

Klein R, Klein BE, Moss SE, et al. The Wisconsin epidemiologic study of diabetic retinopathy. II. Prevalence and risk of diabetic retinopathy when age at diagnosis is less than 30 years. Arch Ophthalmol, 1984; Vol. 102: pp. 520–6.

Comments: Younger-onset persons with diabetes were examined using standard protocols to determine the prevalence and severity of diabetic retinopathy and associated risk factors.

The Diabetic Retinopathy Study Research Group. Photocoagulation treatment of proliferative diabetic retinopathy. Clinical application of Diabetic Retinopathy Study (DRS) findings, DRS Report No. 8. Ophthalmology, 1981; Vol. 88: pp. 583–600.

Comments: Photocoagulation reduces the risk of severe visual loss by 50% or more in eyes with severe PDR.

黄斑水肿

Sachin D. Kalyani, MD

定义

黄斑大概是长在视网膜中心的一个小的、高敏感性的区域,刚好在视神经颞侧。

黄斑水肿的发生是由于黄斑血管水、蛋白质渗出引起黄斑肿胀、变厚。

局灶性黄斑水肿是由于容易引起液体渗出的中心血管异常导致,主要是微血管瘤。

弥漫性黄斑水肿是由于视网膜微血管扩张引起。

具有临床意义的黄斑水肿(CSME)的定义早期是由治疗糖尿病视网膜病变研究小组(ETDRS)提出,具体定义见诊断部分。

流行病学

占 3/4 视力丧失与糖尿病相关(Sutter)。

青年发病(< 30 岁)或老年发病(> 30 岁)的糖尿病患者 CSME 发病率分别是 5.9% 和 7.5%(Hirai)。

黄斑水肿的发病率升高与以下因素相关,男性、严重的糖尿病视网膜病变、高糖化血红蛋白、蛋白尿、高收缩压与高舒张压以及长期吸烟史(Klein)。

可以发生在糖尿病视网膜病变的任意阶段,最常发生在糖尿病视网膜病变进展时。

在老年发病的糖尿病患者中,CSME 与生存率下降有关(Hirai)。

诊断

ETDRS 定义有临床意义的黄斑水肿如下:(1) 视网膜水肿局限在黄斑中心 500 μm 以内(包含);(2) 如果与毗邻的视网膜增厚相关,硬性渗出在中心 500 μm 以内(包含);(3) 如果局限在黄斑中心视盘内,增厚区域大于视盘区域(ETDRS)。

诊断最好由眼科医生采用后极接触透镜式的裂隙灯双目立体检眼镜进行。

采用直接眼底镜进行眼底检查可以发现黄斑内和黄斑周围的硬性渗出、微血管瘤,但是不能为诊断提供立体图。

症状体征

视力模糊在中央视野中心或一侧。

视力丧失可以经过数月时间缓慢进展。

视力灵敏度在一些 CSME 病例中可以达到 20/20。

病人可能以不能清楚聚焦为主诉。

症状可以是单眼或双眼。

临床治疗

激光治疗是一线治疗:局灶(适于局灶病变)和网格(适用于弥漫病变)。

ETDRS 已证实,与对照组未经治疗的 CSME 相比,经过氩激光光凝治疗后眼睛可以得到获益。治疗后可以减少50%患者缓慢进展的视力丧失，同时可以增加视力恢复的机会，以及使视野缺损局限在小面积内(ETDRS)。
- 眼睛患有视网膜水肿，但却没有达到 CSME 标准的，治疗组与对照组无显著性差异。
- 局灶激光治疗黄斑水肿的时机，要在高风险的糖尿病增殖型视网膜病变接受全视网膜激光治疗之前，同时也要在白内障手术之前，因为手术会增加黄斑水肿加重的风险。
- 局灶激光治疗的副反应有：旁中心盲点，暂时的水肿加重，视力下降，脉络膜新生血管形成，激光光凝疤痕膨胀，意外的孔状烧伤(Kim)。
- ETDRS 已证实，激光治疗后的患者视网膜下纤维化少于对照组未接受治疗的患者。
- 在一些难治的 CSME 患者中，类固醇激素的玻璃体内治疗已经被证实有效，使用激素的副反应包括增加白内障再次手术机会的2~3倍，眼压增加了4~8倍。
- 睫状体扁平部玻璃体切除和玻璃体后脱离在治疗糖尿病黄斑水肿中同样有效 (Kaiser)。
- 药物治疗包括局部NSAIDS治疗和类固醇激素滴眼液，但是激光治疗更有效。
- 控制高血压、高血脂、高血糖等危险因素在预防黄斑水肿加重中同样重要 (Ciulla)。

随访
- 全面眼底检查需要每2~4个月进行一次，直到诊断有临床意义的黄斑水肿

专家意见
- 视觉灵敏度并不是诊断和/或治疗有临床意义的黄斑水肿的标准，但是在后续的临床过程中有用。
- 诊断需要专科医生采用立体镜检查。

参考文献

Klein R, Knudtson MD, Lee KE, et al. The Wisconsin Epidemiologic Study of Diabetic Retinopathy XXIII: the twenty-five-year incidence of macular edema in persons with type diabetes. Ophthalmology, 2009; Vol. 116: pp. 497–503.
Comments: This study examined the 25-year cumulative incidence of macular edema (ME) and its relation to various risk factors.

Hirai FE, Knudtson MD, Klein BE, et al. Clinically significant macular edema and survival type 1 and type 2 diabetes. Am J Ophthalmol, 2008; Vol. 145: pp. 700–6.
Comments: Investigation of the association of CSME and long-term survival type 1 and type 2 diabetics.

Sutter FK, Gillies MC, Helbig H. In Holze FG, Spaide RF (Eds.), Diabetic Macular Edema in Medical Retina. Springer; 2007; pp. 131–146.
Comments: Review of current treatments for macular edema.

Ciulla TA, Amador AG, Zinman B. Diabetic retinopathy and diabetic macular edema pathophysiology, screening, and novel therapies. Diabetes Care, 2003; Vol. 26: pp 2653–64.
Comments: Review of pathophysiology and treatments for diabetic retinopathy and

macular edema.

Martidis A, Duker JS, Greenberg PB, et al. Intravitreal triamcinolone for refractory diabetic macular edema. Ophthalmology, 2002; Vol. 109: pp. 920–7.

Comments: The purpose of this study was to determine if an intravitreal injection of triamcinolone acetonide is safe and effective in treating diabetic macular edema unresponsive to prior laser photocoagulation.

Kaiser PK, Riemann CD, Sears JE, et al. Macular traction detachment and diabetic macular edema associated with posterior hyaloidal traction. Am J Ophthalmol, 2001; Vol. 131: pp. 44–9.

Comments: Reviewed the clinical, photographic, fluorescein angiographic, and optical coherence tomographic findings in patients with diabetic macular traction and edema (DMTE) associated with posterior hyaloidal traction (PHT).

Kim JW, Ai E. Diabetic retinopathy. In Regillo, CD, Brown, GC, Flynn Jr, HW, (Eds.), Vitreoretinal Diseases: The Essentials. New York: Georg Thieme; 1999: p. 147 (Table 3).

Comments: This table examines the side effects and complications of focal laser photocoagulation.

Early Treatment Diabetic Retinopathy Study Research Group. Focal photocoagulation treatment of diabetic macular edema. Relationship of treatment effect to fluorescein angiographic and other retinal characteristics at baseline: ETDRS Report no. 19. Arch Ophthalmol, 1995; Vol. 113: pp. 1144–55.

Comments: This study's objective was to determine whether the efficacy of photocoagulation treatment of diabetic macular edema may be influenced by degree of capillary closure, severity or source of fluorescein leakage, extent of retinal edema, presence of cystoid changes, or severity of hard exudates.

Early Treatment Diabetic Retinopathy Study Research Group. Photocoagulation for diabetic macular edema. ETDRS Report no. 1. Arch Ophthalmol, 1985; Vol. 103: pp. 1796–806.

Comments: Examined if laser photocoagulation helped reduce the risk of vision loss secondary to CSME.

白内障

Sachin D. Kalyani, MD

定义
- 眼中一个布满云雾状或不透明的天然晶状体。
- 当晶体内血糖升高时（如高血糖状态），山梨醇通路激活大于糖酵解，山梨醇在晶体内累积、保留。
- 伴随着山梨醇，果糖在高糖环境中同样在晶体内积累。
- 这两种糖分增加晶体内渗透压，使水分内流。
- 结果导致晶体纤维肿胀，正常的细胞结构遭到破坏，最后晶体混浊(Andley)。

流行病学
- 糖尿病患者随着年龄的增长晶体改变风险增加，与非糖尿病病人的年龄相关白内障相比无差异。
- 与非糖尿病患者相比，糖尿病患者的晶体改变发生更年轻(Flynn)。
- 与同年龄人群相比，糖尿病患者的皮层和被膜下混浊发生更早。
- 1型糖尿病患者有20%患白内障，与年龄、视网膜激光治疗史、高血脂酮状态和高血压相关(Esteves)。
- 到2050年，40岁及40岁以上人群中患白内障的人数大概会增长235%。

诊断
- 如果视力影响患者的日常活动(ADLs)(如开车、读书、看电视)，需要病史进行评价。
- 综合眼科检查来评估白内障，包括视觉灵敏度、裂隙灯检查和散瞳眼底镜。
- 检查中，眼底镜检查可以看到云雾状的晶体，视网膜检查困难、模糊。

症状体征
- 云雾状或视物模糊。
- 闪光（车头灯或日光可能使视力下降），光周光晕。
- 夜视力下降
- 色觉减弱。
- 单眼复视，或单眼中多个图像。
- 白内障通常双眼受累，但是，可能在检查时发现一只眼进展更快。

临床治疗
- 早期白内障可以通过更换眼镜、增加照明亮度、使用防眩光太阳镜或者使用放大镜改善。
- 如果这些措施不能奏效，手术是唯一有效的治疗手段，通常白内障摘除术与超声乳化白内障吸出术和晶体置换术同时进行。
- 白内障手术只有在视力下降影响日常生活活动(ADLs)时才建议进行。
- 其他白内障手术适应证：当白内障影响其他眼部疾病的检查和治疗时，如糖尿病视网膜病变或者年龄相关黄斑变性。

白内障

- 糖尿病视网膜病变在白内障手术术后可能会进展(Jaffe)。
- 因此,对于患有临床有意义的黄斑水肿(CSME)、严重的糖尿病非增殖型视网膜病变(NPDR)或者糖尿病增殖型视网膜病变(PDR)而言,激光光凝术要在白内障手术之前进行。

随访

- 对于所有患有糖尿病视网膜病变的白内障术后患者重新评估。
- 接受超声乳化白内障吸出术的糖尿病患者,在术后 12 个月内糖尿病视网膜病变进展速度加倍(Hong)。
- 但是研究结果表明,白内障囊内摘除术和白内障囊外摘除术后进展减缓。(Jaffe)

专家意见

- 在白内障摘除术前适当的时候进行糖尿病视网膜病变治疗。
- 白内障通常双眼受累,但是可以有一只眼进展更快。
- 白内障摘除术后最好的纠正视觉敏感度的方法是,限制其在糖尿病视网膜病变治疗后进行。

参考文献

National Eye Institute: Cataracts. http://www.nei.nih.gov/health/cataract/cataract_facts.as p, 2009. Accessed November 1, 2009.

Comments: The National Eye Institute's website on cataracts.

Hong T, Mitchell P, de Loryn T, et al. Development and progression of diabetic retinopathy 12 months after phacoemulsification cataract surgery. Ophthalmology, 2009; Vol. 116: pp. 1510–4.

Comments: This study evaluated whether phacoemulsification cataract surgery exacerbates the development and progression of diabetic retinopathy.

Esteves JF, Dal Pizzol MM, Sccoco CA, et al. Cataract and type 1 diabetes mellitus. Diabetes Res Clin Pract, 2008; Vol. 82: pp. 324–8.

Comments: Evaluated the prevalence and possible risk factors of cataract formation in type 1 diabetics.

Saaddine JB, Honeycutt AA, Narayan KM, et al. Projection of diabetic retinopathy and other major eye diseases among people with diabetes mellitus: United States, 2005–2050. Arch Ophthalmol, 2008; Vol. 126: pp. 1740–7.

Comments: Estimates the number of people with cataracts among Americans 40 years or older with diabetes for the years 2005–2050.

Flynn HW, Jr., Smiddy WE. Diabetes and ocular disease: past, present, and future therapies. Ophthalmology Monograph 14, American Academy of Ophthalmology: 2000; Vol. 226: pp. 49–53.

Comments: Focuses on the epidemiology of cataracts in patients with diabetes.

Andley UP, Liang JJN, Lou MF. Biochemical mechanisms of age-related cataract. Albert DM, Jakobiec FA, (Eds.), Principles and Practice of Ophthalmology, 2nd edition. Philadelphia: WB Saunders Publishers; 2000: pp. 1428–1449.

Comments: Describes pathophysiology of cataract formation.

Jaffe GJ, Burton TC, Kuhn E, et al. Progression of nonproliferative diabetic retinopathy and visual outcome after extracapsular cataract extraction and intraocular lens implantation. Am J Ophthalmol, 1992; Vol. 114: pp. 448–56.

Comments: Looked at the progression of diabetic retinopathy after cataract surgery.

耳科疾病

听力障碍

Nisa M. Maruthur, MD, MHS

定义
- 以下两点符合任意一点即可诊断，(1) 感音神经性听力障碍，表现为声音频率相关的听觉障碍和音高相关的听觉障碍；(2) 传导性听力损失。
- 糖尿病患者感音神经性听力障碍的患病率增加，可能与糖尿病微血管病变有关。

流行病学
- 糖尿病患者中，发生感音神经性听力障碍的可能性大约是没有糖尿病患者群的 2 倍 (Bainbridge)。
- 糖尿病患者中，低频和高频听力障碍更常见。
- 糖尿病患者中，轻度或重度高频听力障碍经年龄调整的患病率是 54.1%（没有糖尿病是 32%）。
- 糖尿病患者中，轻度或重度低频听力障碍经年龄调整的患病率是 21.3%。
- 如果存在微血管病变，年龄、噪声、耳毒性药物和吸烟将会增加听力障碍患病风险。

诊断
- 病史：是否存在主观听力障碍，发生时间，职业史，外伤，药物，家族病史，家庭成员的回答。
- 自我报告：由纯音测听测定听力阈值。回答"是的"的阳性似然比 (LR) 为 2.5(95%CI:1.7~3.6)。回答"不"的阴性似然比为 0.13 (95%CI:0.09~0.19)。家庭成员的回答可能会有一些价值。
- 低声音声感知：测试医生站在患者身后，用手指塞住不测试的耳朵，考官低语 3 个数字和字母的组合，也可以重复一次。如果可以重复 3/6 的字母或数字，即是正常；无法感知低语声音的阳性似然率为 6.1(95%CI:4.5~8.4)。正常感知的阴性似然率为 0.03(95%CI:0~0.24)。
- 韦伯测试：额头正中放置振动音叉，如果其中一侧更响亮（偏侧性），即为阳性。结果提示声音大的一侧传导性听力障碍或声音小的一侧感音神经性听力障碍。因为测试取决于偏侧性，如果双边、对称听力丧失，则无意义。异常结果：阳性似然率为 1.6(95%CI:1.0~2.3)。
- Rinne 测试：为传导性听力损失评估，将振动的音叉放在乳突（骨传导 (BC)）直到声音是没有听到，然后搬到 1 英寸于外部道 [空气传导 (AC)]，看看声音仍然存在。正常：AC < BC。异常测试：阳性似然率 2.7~62。正常测试阴性似然率 0.01~0.85。
- 评估其他医疗听力障碍的原因，如梅毒等（即。螺旋体免疫荧光法测试）。
- 耳镜检查评估外部耳道和鼓膜。
- MRI 或 CT 成像评估听神经瘤或其他异常。

听力障碍

- 通过听觉病矫治专家进行听力学检查。

症状体征

- 低或高频率和/或不同的声音强度的进行性听力障碍。
- 由自我报告,低语的声音感知、韦伯测试或 Rinne 测试证实的听力障碍。
- 可能伴随眩晕和耳鸣。

临床治疗

- 治疗外耳道和中耳疾病(如耵聍栓塞和中耳炎)。
- 避免/停止耳毒性药物(如氨基糖苷类,循环利尿剂,水杨酸盐和非甾体类抗炎药,万古霉素和红霉素)。
- 与听力学家和/或耳鼻喉科专家协商,采用助听器和其他听力辅助设备。

随访

- 通过定期询问主观听力障碍筛查。
- 建议使用助听器。
- 如果怀疑听力障碍,推荐进行正规的听力学检查。

专家意见

- 在定期的糖尿病随访期间,每6个月询问主观听力障碍。
- 通过询问家庭成员,可能有助于确定听力障碍的存在和程度。
- 虽然目前没有令人信服的数据,但如果糖尿病相关听力障碍确实是由于微血管疾病引起,那么进行血压和血糖控制应该在预防和治疗并发症中起重要作用。
- 对官方的听力障碍测试进行比较表明,推荐的听力测试是基于病人主观报告听力丧失和/或异常的低声声音感知测试,而韦伯测试和 Rinne 测试的价值有限(Bagai)。
- 严重、先天性或母系遗传耳聋是线粒体糖尿病的可能性大(见线粒体糖尿病,159页)。

参考文献

Roberts HA. Sensorineural hearing loss: evaluation and management in adults; etiology of SNHL (pharmacologic toxicity). In Cummings CW, Haughey BH, Thomas JR, (Eds.), Cummings Otolaryngology: Head and Neck Surgery, 4th edition. Philadelphia: Elsevier Mosby; 2005.
Comments: Preeminent reference for otolaryngology.

US Preventive Services Task Force. Screening for Hearing Impairment in Older Adults, Topic Page. US PreventiveServices Task Force. Agency for Healthcare Research and Quality (AHRQ), Rockville, MD. http://www.ahrq.gov/clinic/uspstf/uspshear.htm, Accessed August 9, 2009.
Comments: Screening guidelines for hearing impairment in the US from US Preventive Services Task Force.

Bainbridge KE, Hoffman HJ, Cowie CC. Diabetes and hearing impairment in the United States: audiometric evidence from the National Health and Nutrition Examination Survey, 1999 to 2004. Ann Intern Med, 2008; Vol. 149: pp. 1–10.

Comments: Nationally representative analysis of the relationship between diabetes and hearing impairment in the US.

Bagai A, Thavendiranathan P, Detsky AS. Does this patient have hearing impairment JAMA, 2006; Vol. 295: pp. 416–28.

Comments: Systematic review of bedside clinical maneuvers to evaluate hearing impairment.

Korsch B. Commentary: screening for psychosocial problems. Pediatrics, 1976; Vol. 58 pp. 471–2.

Comments: Results from a cohort study of aging in Wisconsin showing a modest association between type 2 diabetes and hearing loss but no association between glycemic control and hearing loss.

精神疾病

糖尿病相关抑郁

Sherita Hill Golden, MD, MHS

定义
- 抑郁症是一种精神疾病,从根据《精神障碍的诊断与统计手册》(DSM-IV) 中的标准进行诊断,表现为在大多数活动中抑郁情绪和/或缺少快乐(快感缺乏),伴随表 3-14 中所描述的症状和体征。
- 必须出现症状至少 2 周。

流行病学
- 抑郁症是一种有重大意义的糖尿病相关疾病,在世界范围内,大约有 4300 万糖尿病病人患有抑郁症。
- 糖尿病患者患有抑郁症的风险是非糖尿病患者的两倍 (Anderson)。
- 根据一个糖尿病的 meta 分析,重度抑郁症 (MDD) 的总患病率是 11.4%,而高抑郁症的患病率升高,大约在 31%(Anderson)。
- 高抑郁症状患者患 2 型糖尿病的风险大约增加 30%~60%,2 型糖尿病患者发展为高抑郁症的风险增加大约 12%~50% (Mezuk;Golden)。
- 糖尿病患者中的抑郁症与血糖控制较差以及糖尿病微血管和大血管并发症相关 (Lustman;deGroot)。

诊断
- 抑郁症最准确地诊断标准是基于 DSM-IV 的格式化临床访谈。两个常用的临床访谈是抑郁状态问卷 (DIS) 和障碍定式临床检查 (SCID)。
- 抑郁症诊断标准基于 DSM-IV 标准,如表 3-14 所示。
- 抑郁症状也可以通过自我或访谈式问卷调查评估。患者健康问卷抑郁量表 -9(PHQ-9) 是最常用在初级保健中用来筛查 MDD 和明显的抑郁症状 (Kroenke)。五个症状大于 10 分(包括平常活动中的抑郁情绪或缺乏快乐)持续超过半天可以诊断中都抑郁症。
- 另一个临床中筛查重度抑郁症的有效工具是 PHQ-2,是缩减版的 PHQ-9(Kroenke)。

症状和体征
- 见表 3-14 中列出的症状。

表 3-14. 基于 DSM-IV 准则的抑郁症的诊断标准

	重度抑郁症	轻度抑郁障碍	精神抑郁
需要存在一个抑郁情绪症状			X
需要存在至少一个症状抑郁情绪或快感缺乏	X	X	
许多额外的症状	至少有 5 个： 抑郁情绪 明显对大部分或全部活动兴趣或乐趣减少（快感缺乏） 明显的体重减轻或体重增加（>5% 体重 / 月），或者食欲减少或增加 失眠或嗜睡 精神运动激越或迟缓 疲劳或缺乏精神 自觉毫无价值或不恰当的负罪感 思考或集中能力下降，犹豫不决 反复出现死亡或自杀的想法	至少两个但小于 5 个重度抑郁症的症状	两个或两个以上的： 食欲不振或暴饮暴食 失眠或嗜睡 精神不振或疲劳 缺乏自信 注意力不集中或犹豫不决 感到绝望
症状持续时间	每天发作持续至少 2 周	每天发作持续至少 2 周	一半以上时间发作持续 2 年以上症状持续存在超过 2 个月

来源：由 Sherita Hill Golden 提供．

临床治疗

抑郁症的心理疗法

- 心理疗法治疗糖尿病相关抑郁症的研究包括抑郁症的认知行为治疗（CBT）和解决问题治疗。这两种心理治疗都可以改善糖尿病患者的抑郁症状 (Petrak)。
- 认知行为治疗的一项研究中，治疗 3 个月后认知行为治疗组的糖化血红蛋白较低 (9.5%)，对照组的糖化血红蛋白是 10.9%；但解决问题治疗并没有导致显著改善血糖控制 (Petrak)。

抑郁症的药物治疗

- 目前已经证明药物疗法可以改善糖尿病患者的抑郁症状,其中包括选择性5-羟色胺再摄取抑制剂(SSRIs),氟西汀、舍曲林、帕罗西汀(Kroenke)。
- 药物治疗需要4~6周起效,4~6周之后如果症状没有改善,剂量应该逐渐增加直到症状改善。推荐的初始剂量调整和最大剂量如表3-15所示。

随访

- 如果首次药物治疗抑郁症状没有改善(使用PHQ-9再评估),抗抑郁药物剂量可以根据表3-15推荐进行调整。

专家意见

- 对于一个经过强化治疗后血糖仍控制不佳的患者,临床医生应该怀疑抑郁症的可能性,并使用PHQ-2或PHQ-9筛查抑郁症。
- 高抑郁症状与不健康的生活习惯有关,如增加卡路里的摄入量和缺乏身体活动,从而导致超重、肥胖加重,导致血糖控制差。
- 行为治疗抑郁症还应该激励患者参与身体活动和调整健康的生活方式。
- 与心理健康提供者(即心理学家或精神病学家)协作工作来治疗糖尿病的这种伴随疾病。

表3-15. 糖尿病抑郁症治疗中选择性5-羟色胺再摄取抑制剂的剂量选择和调整

	初始剂量	剂量调整	最大剂量
氟西汀	20mg/d	如果需要,每个月剂量增加10~20mg	80mg/d(如果每天总剂量>80mg,可以在早餐和午餐前分开服用)
舍曲林	25mg 或 50mg/d	剂量调整至少间隔一个星期	200mg/d
帕罗西汀	20mg/d(老年人10mg/d)	按照每周剂量增加10mg	50mg/d(老年人40mg/d)

来源:由 Sherita Hill Golden 提供

推荐依据

Petrak F, Herpertz S. Treatment of depression in diabetes: an update. Curr Opin Psychiatry, 2009; Vol. 22: pp. 211-7.

Comments: Provides an excellent overview of psychotherapies and pharmacologic treatments for depression. In summary, most depression treatments improve depressive symptoms but do not significantly improve glycemic control in diabetes.

Kroenke K, Spitzer RL, Williams JB. The Patient Health Questionnaire-2: validity of a two-item depression screener. Med Care, 2003; Vol. 41: pp. 1284-92.

Comments: Describes the validity of using the PHQ-2 screening questionnaire to identify individuals at increased risk for having a depressive disorder.

Kroenke K, Spitzer RL, Williams JB. The PHQ-9: validity of a brief depression severity measure. J Gen Intern Med, 2001; Vol. 16: pp. 606–13.
Comments: Describes the validity of using the PHQ-9 questionnaire to identify individuals with depressive disorders.

其他参考文献

Mezuk B, Eaton WW, Albrecht S, et al. Depression and type 2 diabetes over the lifespan: a meta-analysis. Diabetes Care, 2008; Vol. 31: pp. 2383–90.
Comments: This is the first meta-analysis demonstrating that depression is associated with an increased risk of type 2 diabetes and that type 2 diabetes is associated with an increased risk of depression.

Golden SH, Lazo M, Carnethon M, et al. Examining a bidirectional association between depressive symptoms and diabetes. JAMA, 2008; Vol. 299: pp. 2751–9.
Comments: Population-based study in a multiethnic cohort showing that there is a bidirectional relationship between elevated depressive symptoms and type 2 diabetes.

Anderson RJ, Freedland KE, Clouse RE, et al. The prevalence of comorbid depression in adults with diabetes: a meta-analysis. Diabetes Care, 2001; Vol. 24: pp. 1069–78.
Comments: This is the most comprehensive study describing the prevalence of major depressive disorder and elevated depressive symptoms in diabetes.

De Groot M, Anderson R, Freedland KE, et al. Association of depression and diabetes complications: a metaanalysis. Psychosom Med, 2001; Vol. 63: pp. 619–30.
Comments: This meta-analysis demonstrates that depression is associated with increased microvascular and macrovascular diabetes complications.

Lustman PJ, Anderson RJ, Freedland KE, et al. Depression and poor glycemic control: a meta-analytic review of the literature. Diabetes Care, 2000; Vol. 23: pp. 934–42.
Comments: This meta-analysis demonstrates that depression is associated with poor glycemic control.

Maheux P, Ducros F, Bourque J, et al. Fluoxetine improves insulin sensitivity in obese patients with non-insulin-dependent diabetes mellitus independently of weight loss. In J Obes Relat Metab Disord, 1997; Vol. 21: pp. 97–102.
Comments: This study suggests that fluoxetine improves insulin sensitivity in diabetes patients independent of weight loss.

糖尿病的饮食紊乱

Mariana Lazo, MD, ScM, PhD, and Mary Huizinga, MD, MPH

定义

- 这组精神疾病包括神经性厌食症、神经性暴食症和未另有规定的其他进食障碍（如暴食症、夜间进食综合征），可能会危及生命的健康影响。
- 厌食症的特点是绝食和过度减肥，以及对体重增加的强烈恐惧。
- 暴食症的特点是周期性的暴食（吃大量食物 – 比大多数人一顿饭吃的多 – 短时间多次进餐），其次是清除（通过呕吐、滥用泻药或过度运动摆脱食物和热量）。
- 在 1 型糖尿病患者，最常见的清除表现是故意遗漏和限制胰岛素。
- 暴食症（没有清除）会导致体重增加和可能糖尿病管理恶化。

流行病学

- 1 型糖尿病的饮食失调非常普遍。据报道，遗漏或限制胰岛素注射在青春期前的女孩中占 2%，在十来岁孩子中占 11%~15%，在青少年和成年早期中占 30%~39%(Nielsen; Jones; Colton)。
- 公开的 1 型糖尿病进食障碍综合征的患病率在从 0~11% 不等，阈下进食障碍的患病率范围是 7%~35%(Colton)。
- 厌食症合并 1 型糖尿病患者的死亡率升高 [10 年期死亡率 =34.6/(1 000 人年)]，高于任一单种疾病的死亡率 [1 型糖尿病：10 年死亡率 =2.2/(1 000 人年)；厌食症：10 年期死亡率 =7.3/(1 000 人年)]（尼尔森）。
- 1 型糖尿病合并饮食失调的糖尿病并发症（主要是视网膜病变、酮症酸中毒、神经病变）发生率更高 (Rydall; Peveler)。
- 2 型糖尿病患者更有可能有暴食症，由于频繁反复超重或肥胖与控制体重交替（饮食限制）(Herpertz)。
- 2 型糖尿病饮食失调的患病率估测范围 6.5%~9%。
- 危险因素：女性，进食障碍的家族史，节食的历史，对自己身体不满，高 BMI，抑郁和焦虑障碍，人格障碍（强迫性、完美主义者、戏剧的特征、冲动），年轻（虽然也观察到后来发作）。

诊断

- 患者常常并不诉饮食失调，饮食失调是隐匿的。
- 故意遗漏胰岛素注射是一种常见的行为，并且患者最初可能否认。
- 饮食失调最常见的体征和症状请参考 3-16。
- 厌食：正式诊断基于 DSM-IV 标准，包括：(1) 拒绝维持体重达到或超过基于身高、体型、年龄和活动水平所定的最低限度正常体重（不到 85% 的预期）；(2) 尽管剧烈的减肥，仍强烈害怕体重增加或变"胖"或感觉"胖"或超重；(3) 月经失调；(4) 极端关注体重和体形。
- 暴食症：DSM-IV 标准包括：(1) 在离散时间反复发作的暴饮暴食，比大多数人会吃更多的食物，发作期间强烈的失去控制的感觉；- (2) 反复不恰当的补救行为，防止体重增加，如呕吐、滥用泻药、利尿剂、灌肠剂或其他药物、禁食或过度运动；(3)暴食和不恰当的补救手段的发生平均3个月内至少每周两次；(4)极端关注体重和体形。
- 临床征兆：整体心理社会功能恶化、抑郁症状、身体形象差/自尊心低、低体重、家庭成员表现出担忧、难治的代谢紊乱、闭经以及青春期、性成熟和长身高的延迟。

表 3-16. 饮食失调最常见的体征和症状

饮食失调	症状	体征
神经性食欲缺乏	虚弱、疲乏、疲劳、心悸、头晕、四肢冷并且不耐受、冷漠、注意力下降、腹胀、便秘、脱发、性欲减退	低体重、脱水、低体温、恶病质、心动过缓、直立性高血压、脉弱不规则、焦虑、易怒或情绪低落、低体温、腹部肠鸣音、良性腮腺增生、汗毛、皮肤异常、月经不调、不孕、性抑制进展
暴食症	无力、心悸、冷漠、注意力不集中、反流、烧心、腹痛和腹胀、体重波动、牙齿脱落、咽痛、不孕	心律失常、焦急、易怒或情绪低落、唾液腺增生、胃炎、呕吐物混血、食管炎、胃食管反流和侵蚀、胰腺炎、手背疤痕(Russell 征)、瘀斑、呕吐后结膜出血、牙釉质腐蚀产生龋齿(特别是门齿的舌侧)、咽部红斑、腭部划痕、多言症、闭经

来源：由 Mariana Lazo and Mary Huizinga 提供.

精神疾病
- 糖尿病相关特殊迹象：高血糖、尿糖、不明原因的糖化血红蛋白水平升高、反复糖尿病酮症酸中毒(DKA)。
- 其他行为/态度与饮食失调：过度的体力活动和限制饮食。
- 拓展工具(问卷调查)用于饮食失调的正式评估。通常由训练有素的面试官执行、评分，但在糖尿病中没有经验(Criego)。
- 临床医生接诊糖尿病患者应该使用开放式筛选问题，来了解病人的当前对体重的满意度、胰岛素的使用模式和整体饮食行为：(1)你昨天吃了什么？(2)你吃的是不是比你想吃的多或是否使用非处方泻药、利尿剂、减肥药？(3)你们胰岛素用量小于治疗剂量吗？(4)你认为你瘦吗？

临床治疗
一般考虑
- 这些诊断是非常严重的，尤其是与糖尿病共存时；它们的重要性不应该被忽略或忽视。
- 血糖控制不佳的糖尿病患者，建议住院治疗，直到医疗安全。一般来说，1型糖尿病伴饮食失调的患者更难以治疗。

- 推荐采用住院患者的综合医护管理团队进行护理,包括:内分泌学家、心理学家、精神病学家、普通内科医生、专业营养师和糖尿病教育家。
- 护理水平的选择:需要综合考虑患者的生理和心理条件、行为和社会环境,而不是仅仅依靠诸如体重这样一个或多个物理参数。
- 基本的实验室分析:葡萄糖、糖化血红蛋白、血清电解质、血尿素氮、血清肌酐(解释必须纳入体重的评估)、促甲状腺激素测试、包括分类的完整血细胞计数、红细胞沉降率、肝功能、尿检。
- 专业测试:心电图,骨量减少和骨质疏松症的评估(闭经>6个月),女性患者查血清雌二醇,男性患者查血清睾酮。
- 饮食失调询证医学治疗指南适用于一般人群治疗(美国精神病协会),但是在糖尿病患者中的效果和有效性并没有被清楚地显示。只有很少小型研究在进行这项人群研究。

糖尿病管理
- 设置小增量的目标,调整适当的胰岛素剂量,改善总体血糖控制,规范饮食模式。
- 糖化血红蛋白目标水平遵守在安全指导方针;阻止过分追求完美目标糖化血红蛋白和(空腹、餐后)血糖(Goebel–Fabbri, 2009)。
- 预计血糖改善可能发生胰岛素水肿和液体潴留,同时可能会增加复发的风险。
- 坚持血糖自我检测和胰岛素管理(1型糖尿病)。调整药物治疗,改变体重预防低血糖。

营养康复
- 热量摄入水平开始通常控制在每天30~40kcal/kg(约1000~1600 kcal/d)。一些病人在体重增加阶段,摄入量可以逐步增加到每天70~100kcal/kg;许多男性患者需要大量的热量增加体重。
- 为使热量达标通常需要三餐加三顿小食。
- 持续呕吐的患者推荐定期监测血清钾水平。低钾血症应口服或静脉注射补钾和补液治疗。
- 硫胺素也可能降低患者的呕吐。
- 如果有严重营养不良,患者应密切监测再进食综合征。再进食综合征需要仔细监测电解质(特别是低磷酸盐血症)、神经和心肺系统。
- 推荐补充钙、维生素D、维生素B_{12}治疗。
- 避免关注食品标签,因为这可能是导致食品限制。
- 长期目标是有一个与胰岛素(或糖尿病药物)治疗保持一致饮食的模式。

心理治疗
- 家庭干预措施来促进家庭支持糖尿病管理。
- 开发灵活的食品和膳食计划。
- 个人或团体疗法提高自尊,接受自己的身体。
- 如果严重的精神病症状,可能需要正式的评估和治疗。

药物治疗
- 选择性血清素再吸收抑制剂广泛用于治疗神经性厌食和持续性抑郁、焦虑或强迫性症状和暴食症的患者,来改善他们的体重。
- 氟西汀是这方面最好的研究,是FDA唯一批准的暴食症药物(推荐剂量调整到60mg/d,并需要定期评估)。

随访
- 监测病人的体重变化(每周,每月),血压、脉搏和其他心血管参数,葡萄糖和其他代谢参数。
- 监控病人的态度和行为,检测早期复发的迹象。

专家意见
- 1型或2型糖尿病比一般人群的饮食失调发生率更高,他们可能担心强化糖尿病治疗导致体重增加。
- 过分关注食品、部分控制和膳食计划可能会使态度/行为变的消极,加重饮食失调。
- 需要注意,进食障碍患者常常竭尽全力合理化、否认或隐藏他们。
- 与单纯糖尿病相比,糖尿病合并饮食失调的死亡率和糖尿病并发症的发生率均增高,这可能由于反复发作低血糖症风险的增加以及总体糖尿病控制不佳。
- 建议早期和常规筛查。饮食失调可能出现严重的并发症才被发现。临床医生应该警惕精神疾病的警报迹象。饮食失调所造成体重下降可能被误认为饮食控制的结果。
- 遗漏或限制胰岛素可以掩盖暴饮暴食。"代谢清除"是指人们不采用胰岛素,这样他们会吃却不会增加体重,是一种危险的做法。
- 许多患者,尤其是年轻的患者,同时存在多种饮食失调症状,不能严格分为厌食症和暴食症。
- 需要多学科协作的护理模式。

推荐依据
American Psychiatric Association. Treatment of patients with eating disorders, Third Edition. American Psychiatric Association. Am J Psychiatry, 2006; Vol. 163: pp. 4–54.
Comments: This is the most recent official medical guideline by the American Psychiatric Association for the treatment of eating disorders in the general population.

其他参考文献
Colton P, Rodin G, Bergenstal R, Parkin C. Eating disorders and diabetes: introduction and overview. Diabetes Spectrum, 2009; Vol. 22: pp. 138–42.
Comments: Narrative review of the topic. First invited article of a section in one of the leading journals of diabetes education.
Goebel-Fabbri AE. Disturbed eating behaviors and eating disorders in type 1 diabetes: clinical significance and treatment recommendations. Curr Diab Rep, 2009; Vol. 9: pp. 133–9.
Comments: Comprehensive review of the literature on type 1 diabetes and eating disorders.
Goebel-Fabbri AE, Fikkan J, Franko DL, et al. Insulin restriction and associated morbidity

and mortality in women with type 1 diabetes. Diabetes Care, 2008; Vol. 31: pp. 415–9.
Comments: Paper that provided evidence of the role of insulin restriction as predictor of mortality.

American Psychiatric Association. Treatment of patients with eating disorders, Third Edition. American Psychiatric Association. Am J Psychiatry, 2006; Vol. 163: pp. 4–54.
Comments: This is the most recent official medical guideline by the American Psychiatric Association for the treatment of eating disorders in the general population.

Peveler RC, Bryden KS, Neil HA, et al. The relationship of disordered eating habits and attitudes to clinical outcomes in young adult females with type 1 diabetes. Diabetes Care, 2005; Vol. 28: pp. 84–8.
Comments: Provides data on complications associated with eating disorders and diabetes.

Nielsen S. Eating disorders in females with type 1 diabetes: an update of a meta-analysis. Eur Eat Dis Rev, 2002; Vol. 10: pp. 241–54.
Comments: Summary of the evidence of the epidemiology of eating disorders in patients with type 1 diabetes, including data on long-term mortality.

Jones JM, Lawson ML, Daneman D, et al. Eating disorders in adolescent females with and without type 1 diabetes: cross sectional study. BMJ, 2000; Vol. 320: pp. 1563–6.
Comments: This study provides a snapshot of the epidemiology of eating disorders in people with diabetes and nondiabetes among teenage girls.

Herpertz S, Albus C, Lichtblau K, et al. Relationship of weight and eating disorders in type 2 diabetic patients: a multicenter study. Int J Eat Disord, 2000; Vol. 28: pp. 68–77.
Comments: One of the few studies on the association between eating disorders and type 2 diabetes.

Rydall AC, Rodin GM, Olmsted MP, et al. Disordered eating behavior and microvascular complications in young women with insulin-dependent diabetes mellitus. NEJM, 1997; Vol. 336: pp. 1849–54.
Comments: This paper was one of the first to provide evidence of higher rates of microvascular complications among people with diabetes and eating disorders.

肺疾病

囊性纤维化相关糖尿病

Sherita Hill Golden, MD, MHS

定义

- 囊性纤维化(CF)：一种常染色体隐性疾病，符合以下两条即可诊断，(1) 至少在一个器官系统临床症状符合囊性纤维化；(2) 囊性纤维化横跨膜电导调节体(CFTR)功能障碍的证据，其中包括两次高氯化汗水>60mmol/L，检测到两个CFTR致病突变(最常见的突变是δF508)，或鼻电位差异常。
- 临床表现：呼吸道疾病、鼻窦疾病、外分泌胰腺功能不全、胎粪性肠梗阻和远端回肠阻塞、胆道疾病、不孕症、肌肉骨骼疾病(骨矿物质含量减少、肥厚性骨关节病)、肾结石、肾钙质沉着症和复发性静脉血栓形成。
- 囊性纤维化相关糖尿病(CFRD)：与1型或2型糖尿病不同，有β细胞功能障碍的证据，但有关胰岛素抵抗的结果相互矛盾。由于留存基础胰岛素分泌，患者不容易患酮症。

流行病学

- 患病率随着年龄增长而稳步上升，在儿童中2%，在青少年中19%，在成年人中40%~50% (Moran)。
- 估计发病率为每年每100人中2.7例(Moran)。
- 整体囊性纤维化患者人群中，估测葡萄糖耐量减低(IGT)患病率为15%~30%(Moran)。
- CFRD风险因素：delta F508基因突变为纯合性，高龄，女性，胰腺功能不全，严重的肺病，肺病急性加重，营养状况受损，口服/植入避孕药物使用，痰中混杂铜绿假单胞菌或拟杆菌，肝脏疾病，过敏性支气管肺曲霉病(ABPA)(Marshall)。

诊断

- CFRD的诊断标准同糖尿病。
- 1型糖尿病可以独立于囊性纤维化出现，一个10岁以前的孩子出现酮症应怀疑此病。

症状体征

- 囊性纤维化患者多尿、烦渴。
- 尽管给予适当的营养干预，仍未能增长或维持体重。
- 生长速度缓慢。
- 青春期延迟。
- 不明原因的慢性肺功能下降。

囊性纤维化相关糖尿病

临床治疗

药物治疗
- 餐后高血糖是 CFRD 常见的情况,需要启动餐前胰岛素(营养胰岛素)治疗,胰岛素剂量的确定基于碳水化合物摄入量(如 1 单位 / 10 克碳水化合物),建议使用速效胰岛素(天冬胰岛素或赖脯胰岛素)之一,目标是餐后两个小时血糖 < 180mg/dl。
- 如果患者没有空腹高血糖,首次治疗没有必要使用基础胰岛素。
- 空腹高血糖患者启动基础胰岛素,提供患者每日 40%~50% 的总胰岛素剂量。每天一次基础胰岛素类似物(甘精胰岛素或地特胰岛素)或在早晨和睡前使用 NPH。目标是空腹血糖 80~120mg/dl。
- 口服药物治疗不是 CFRD 的有效治疗手段。

医学营养治疗
- 由于囊性纤维化患者代谢需求的增加,总能量摄入量推荐日食量增加到 120%~150% 来恢复增长,达到基于身高的目标体重的 100%,实现身高体重指数至少达到 $21kg/m^2$。
- 为弥补吸收不良,能量摄入的 40% 由脂肪提供。
- 摄入碳水化合物量要提高,精制碳水化合物可以随意进食(含糖饮料、零食除外)。
- 蛋白质摄入不能减少,即使有肾病基础。
- 由于吸收不良和营养不良,纤维摄入量要减少。
- 盐摄入量增加。

随访
- 查糖化血红蛋白来监测平均血糖控制。
- 为对 CRFD 患者进行最佳保健,需要每 3 个月访问一个糖尿病专家,糖尿病护理教育者和 / 或营养学家。
- 没有空腹高血糖的 CRFD:开始医学营养治疗,锻炼和并发症筛查;密切监测空腹高血糖;如有急性疾病发生,监测血糖频率增加。
- 胰岛素治疗的适应证:体重下降,增长缓慢,青春期延迟,不明原因的肺活量恶化。
- 餐后高血糖的患者应该考虑餐前胰岛素(营养胰岛素)治疗(两个小时血糖 > 180mg/dl)。

专家建议
- 与 1 型糖尿病患者不同,CRFD 患者有残余的 β 细胞功能,通常不出现空腹高血糖。
- 通常,在最初诊断时是餐后血糖升高,在初始胰岛素治疗是餐前胰岛素(营养胰岛素),而不是基础胰岛素。
- 囊性纤维化患者的营养需求大大增加,因此医学营养治疗与大多数糖尿病患者不同。

推荐依据

Brennan AL, Gyi KM, Wood DM, et al. Relationship between glycosylated haemoglobin and mean plasma glucose concentration in cystic fibrosis. J Cyst Fibros, 2006; Vol. 5: pp. 27–31.

Comments: This study determined whether hemoglobin A1c was an accurate measure of glycemic control in patients with CFRD. The study showed that hemoglobin A1c correlated with mean plasma glucose in patients with CFRD just as it does in patients with type 1 diabetes.

Moran A, Hardin D, Rodman D, et al. Diagnosis, screening and management of cystic fibrosis related diabetes mellitus: a consensus conference report. Diabetes Res Clin Pract, 1999; Vol. 45: pp. 61–73.

Comments: This comprehensive consensus statement provides current guidelines regarding the diagnosis, screening, and treatment of CFRD.

其他参考文献

Moran A, Dunitz J, Nathan B, et al. Cystic fibrosis-related diabetes: current trends in prevalence, incidence, and mortality. Diabetes Care, 2009; Vol. 32: pp. 1626–31.

Comments: This provides the most up-to-date statistics on the epidemiology (prevalence, incidence, and mortality) of CFRD.

Marshall BC, Butler SM, Stoddard M, et al. Epidemiology of cystic fibrosis-related diabetes. J Pediatr, 2005; Vol. 146: pp. 681–7.

Comments: This article provides an excellent summary of the epidemiology of CFRD from the Epidemiology Study of Cystic Fibrosis. This is one of the largest populations of cystic fibrosis patients and at baseline includes 8247 adolescents and adults with the disease in the United States.

Yung B, Noormohamed FH, Kemp M, et al. Cystic fibrosis-related diabetes: the role of peripheral insulin resistance and beta-cell dysfunction. Diabet Med, 2002; Vol. 19: pp. 221–6.

Comments: This study demonstrates beta-cell dysfunction in CFRD with similar levels of insulin resistance among CF patients with and without diabetes.

睡眠呼吸暂停

Naresh Punjabi, MD, PhD

定义
- 睡眠呼吸暂停综合征是一种 2 型糖尿病患者中常见的医学疾病，持续气道正压 (CPAP) 治疗可以改善血糖控制。

流行病学
- 一般成年人中，25% 的男性和 9% 的女性患有阻塞性睡眠呼吸暂停 (OSA)(Young)。
- 多达 80% 的 2 型糖尿病患者有阻塞性睡眠呼吸暂停综合征，其中 20% 病情严重 (Foster)。
- 2 型糖尿病患者潮式呼吸患病率增加 (Resnick)。
- 存在自主神经病变的患者睡眠呼吸暂停综合征患病率较高 (Bottini)。
- 阻塞性睡眠呼吸暂停综合征可能与心血管疾病相关。
- CPAP 治疗阻塞性睡眠呼吸暂停综合征可以改善血糖控制和血压控制 (Babu)。

诊断
- 过夜睡眠研究（多导睡眠图）是进行诊断的金标准。
- 呼吸暂停事件：睡眠中的气流完全停止。
- 低通气事件：睡眠中气流下降，导致血氧饱和度下降或从睡眠中觉醒。
- 阻塞性事件：用力呼吸后出现气流减少或消失。
- 核心事件：气流减少或消失，同时没有呼吸动作。
- 低通气指数 (AHI)：睡眠中每小时窒息和低通气次数之和。
- 睡眠呼吸暂停：AHI > 5 次/小时。
- 阻塞性睡眠呼吸暂停综合征：睡眠中大于 50% 的异常呼吸事件由阻塞引起。
- 中枢性睡眠呼吸暂停综合征：睡眠中大于 50% 的异常呼吸事件由中枢引起。
- 睡眠监测技术（如血氧定量法、气流）是在家中诊断的设备。

症状体征
- 经配偶（床上伴侣）或家庭成员证实的，睡眠期间的大声打鼾和呼吸暂停 (Steier)。
- 夜间发作的窒息和喘气。
- 睡眠障碍（焦躁不安、辗转反侧）和因夜尿觉醒。
- 晨起头痛，日间困倦和疲劳，阳痿。
- 专注、注意力和记忆障碍。
- 性格变化（攻击性、易怒、焦虑或抑郁）。
- 颈围超过 40 厘米。
- 颌后缩，上齿突出（向前挤压的上门齿超过了下门齿）。

- 小口咽，扁桃体肿大，巨大舌，悬雍垂水肿或红斑。
- 超重或肥胖（BMI > 28 kg/m²），腹围增大，高血压，下肢水肿

临床治疗
- CPAP 是中度到重度阻塞性睡眠呼吸暂停综合征一线治疗。
- 减肥至关重要，可以治愈。适度减肥（10%）可以缓解轻度睡眠呼吸紊乱（Peppard）。
- 轻度的或 CPAP 不耐受的病人可以选择口腔矫正器（如下颌拉伸设备）。
- 上呼吸道手术治疗对于 CPAP 治疗不能耐受的病人是一种选择。尚未有共识把手术治疗作为阻塞性睡眠呼吸暂停综合征的最佳治疗手段。
- 补充氧气对睡眠相关严重低氧血症是必要的。
- 避免酒精、镇静剂和麻醉剂等可导致在睡眠期间上呼吸道塌陷的药物。
- 优化夜间睡眠习惯，避免睡眠不足，可缓解缺氧和高碳酸血症下的通气反应。
- 经过充分 CPAP 治疗阻塞性睡眠呼吸暂停综合征后残余的嗜睡症状，可以使用兴奋剂疗法（如莫达非尼）治疗。

随访
- 确诊后，需要进行夜间 CPAP 滴定研究来确定治疗压力。
- 最初 1~3 个月之间评估临床改善程度和 CPAP 耐受性。
- 每年常规随访评估 CPAP 耐受性。
- 如果 CPAP 治疗后仍有睡意，体重增加或减少 10%~15% 以上，患者经上呼吸道手术治疗或口腔矫正器治疗，需进行重复睡眠测试。

专家意见
- 卫生专业人员诊治 2 型糖尿病或阻塞性睡眠呼吸暂停综合征的高危人群时，应进行临床检查，来确定患者是否罹患另一种疾病。
- 应该对 2 型糖尿病患者的打鼾、睡眠中窒息和白天嗜睡情况进行评估。
- 推荐 2 型糖尿病应用一个低阈参考范围作为阻塞性睡眠呼吸暂停综合征的诊断标准，因为相关治疗对白天嗜睡、生活质量、血糖控制和高血压有确定的疗效。
- 治疗阻塞性睡眠呼吸暂停综合征应该首先关注减肥。
- CPAP 是当前治疗中度到重度阻塞性睡眠呼吸暂停综合征的最好方案。

参考文献
Foster GD, Sanders MH, Millman R, et al. Obstructive sleep apnea among obese patients with type 2 diabetes. Diabetes Care, 2009; Vol. 32: pp. 1017–9.
   Comments: Demonstration of high prevalence of untreated sleep apnea in patients with type 2 diabetes.
Bazzano LA, Khan Z, Reynolds K, et al. Effect of nocturnal nasal continuous positive airway pressure on blood pressure in obstructive sleep apnea. Hypertension, 2007; Vol. 50: pp. 417–23.
   Comments: This study demonstrated significant reductions in mean systolic and diastolic blood pressure of ~2 mmHg in those OSA patients treated with versus without CPAP.
Babu AR, Herdegen J, Fogelfeld L, et al. Type 2 diabetes, glycemic control, and continuous

positive airway pressure in obstructive sleep apnea. Arch Intern Med, 2005; Vol. 165: pp. 447–52.

Comments: Treatment of obstructive sleep apnea with CPAP reduces hemoglobin A1c levels in patients with type 2 diabetes.

Stierer T, Punjabi NM. Demographics and diagnosis of obstructive sleep apnea. Anesthesiol Clin North Am, 2005; Vol. 23: pp. 405–20, v.

Comments: General review of the demographic factors associated with obstructive sleep apnea and the methods for diagnosis.

Resnick HE, Redline S, Shahar E, et al. Diabetes and sleep disturbances: findings from the Sleep Heart Health Study. Diabetes Care, 2003; Vol. 26: pp. 702–9.

Comments: Largest community-based study demonstrating the higher prevalence of periodic breathing (Cheyne-Stokes respiration) in those with type 2 diabetes.

Bottini P, Dottorini ML, Cristina Cordoni M, et al. Sleep-disordered breathing in nonobese diabetic subjects with autonomic neuropathy. Eur Respir J, 2003; Vol. 22: pp. 654–60.

Comments: Autonomic neuropathy in patients with type 2 diabetes associated with a higher prevalence of obstructive sleep apnea.

Shamsuzzaman AS, Gersh BJ, Somers VK. Obstructive sleep apnea: implications for cardiac and vascular disease. JAMA, 2003; Vol. 290: pp. 1906–14.

Comments: This systematic review describes the association of OSA with cardiovascular diseases.

Peppard PE, Young T, Palta M, et al. Prospective study of the association between sleep-disordered breathing and hypertension. N Engl J Med, 2000; Vol. 342: pp. 1378–4.

Comments: Describes the dose-response association of sleep-disordered breathing with presence of hypertension four years later.

Peppard PE, Young T, Palta M, et al. Longitudinal study of moderate weight change and sleep-disordered breathing. JAMA, 2000; Vol. 284: pp. 3015–21.

Comments: Observation longitudinal study describing the association between weight increase and decrease and the propensity for sleep apnea.

Young T, Palta M, Dempsey J, et al. The occurrence of sleep-disordered breathing among middle-aged adults. NEJM, 1993; Vol. 328: pp. 1230–5.

Comments: Population-based study on prevalence of obstructive sleep apnea in adult men and women. Approximately 9% of women and 25% of men have obstructive sleep apnea.

肾和泌尿系统疾病

肾病

Donna I. Myers, MD

定义
- 糖尿病肾病(DN)是一种更常见的糖尿病的长期的、微血管的并发症。
- 特点最初由微量蛋白尿(30~300 毫克白蛋白/克肌酐),然后是大量蛋白尿("严重"或"临床"蛋白尿)(> 300 毫克白蛋白/克肌酐),再然后的是尿素氮和肌酐升高,最后终末期肾病(ESRD)。
- 肾脏病理变化为典型结节性肾小球硬化症,同时组织学变化可能包括许多其他特性。

流行病学
- 发生在任何类型的糖尿病,流行率类似,均为 25%。
- 微量蛋白尿预测肾病进展的价值在 1 型糖尿病中是最强的。
- 1 型糖尿病患者在 10 年之后几乎都进展到微量蛋白尿,糖尿病患者患病 16 年之后都高度预测会发生微量蛋白尿(30% 会进展)。
- 2 型糖尿病患者微量蛋白尿的预测价值较弱;2 型糖尿病患者有 25% 将在 10 年之内出现微量蛋白尿,但只有 20%~40% 将进展为大量蛋白尿。
- 尽管随着治疗的进步,改善血压(BP)控制、阻断肾素血管紧张素醛固酮系统(RAAS)治疗可以改善糖尿病肾病的结局,但糖尿病患病率的增长仍增加了糖尿病和 ESRD 患者的数量。
- 在 1 型糖尿病中,如果父母有高血压(HTN),患慢性肾脏疾病(CKD)的风险会增加。
- 大多数患有大量蛋白尿的 1 型糖尿病患者有糖尿病视网膜病变的迹象,但只有 50% 的 2 型糖尿病、有明显的蛋白尿患者同时患有糖尿病视网膜病变。

诊断
- 慢性肾脏疾病(CKD)根据蛋白尿和肾小球滤过率(GFR)[ml/(min·1.73m^2)] 分类如下:1 期:持续蛋白尿 > 3 个月,GFR > 90;2 期:GFR=60~89;3 期:GFR:30~59;4 期:GFR:15~29;5 期:GFR<15。
- 25%~50% 的糖尿病患者在早期出现肾小球高滤过状态(GFR > 120)。这种情况的出现提示糖尿病肾病患病风险提升三倍。
- 微量蛋白尿或大量蛋白尿的诊断可以基于不同一天的随机尿样中的白蛋白和肌酐水平。随机尿样可以提供相对较好数据,更接近日常白蛋白排泄情况;24 小时尿液收集并不经常用于诊断,并且也不太实用(见蛋白尿,661 页)。
- 大量蛋白尿预示着肾小球滤过率(GFR)下降,发展为终末期肾病(ESRD)自然病程为 3~5 年。

肾病

- 糖尿病肾病的早期几乎均伴有高血压或静息BP > 140/90mmHg；如果不伴有高血压，则诊断糖尿病肾病需谨慎。
- 如果出现以下情况，应怀疑并非糖尿病肾脏疾病：糖尿病病程<5年；突发大量蛋白尿；肾小球滤过率降低，但不伴蛋白尿；急性肾功能衰竭；尿沉渣阳性；无糖尿病视网膜病变（特别是1型糖尿病）。

症状和体征

- 糖尿病肾病以及慢性肾脏病1~2期通常没有任何症状，可能只伴有高血压。
- 肾病综合征（> 3g蛋白尿/天）可以导致肾钠潴留、泡沫尿、弥漫性水肿所致体重增加与难治性高血压和心脏衰竭，以及扰乱睡眠的夜尿增多。
- 影像学通常提示肾脏大小正常或增大，甚至糖尿病肾病的晚期慢性肾脏病同样如此。
- 尿沉渣符合肾病表现（仅伴有脂肪尿），显微血尿可能出现。
- 慢性肾脏病3期可能出现贫血、进展的代谢性酸中毒、高磷血症、继发性甲状旁腺功能亢进和血钾过高。
- 尿毒症晚期的症状包括厌食、体重减轻（经常颜面部水肿）、清晨恶心、缺乏精神和嗜睡，同时可能出现金属异味。
- 慢性肾脏病进展缓慢，症状为无痛性，病人可能没有意识到他们。
- 因为常伴随冠心病等并发症，糖尿病肾病的终末期肾病早期（GFR 10~15）即需要进行透析（见透析开始和管理，416页），而其他原因的终末期肾病进行透析需要肾小球滤过率更低（<10）。
- 评估糖尿病视网膜病变等并发症（如肥胖、阻塞性睡眠呼吸暂停）。

临床治疗

血糖控制

- 糖尿病早期严格控制血糖，降低高滤过状态发生率。
- 在糖尿病肾病的早期阶段（慢性肾脏病1~3期）优化血糖控制，可以稳定甚至逆转肾脏疾病；建议糖化血红蛋白6%~7%。
- 教育患者，使其了解糖尿病控制不佳与潜在并发症糖尿病肾病之间的关系。
- 慢性肾脏病4~5期，最初有胰岛素抵抗和血糖控制不佳，胰岛素需要量增加；之后出现肾脏降解胰岛素减少，在ESRD可能出现低血糖进而需要降低胰岛素剂量。
- 接近终末期肾病时，密切监控低血糖并进行调整；病人可能完全脱离胰岛素。
- 肾小球滤过率<90或血肌酐> 1.5mg/dl时，二甲双胍禁忌使用，因为会增加乳酸酸中毒的风险。

高血压管理

- 见糖尿病肾病。
- 在家中及每次就诊时监控血压(BP)。
- 降压目标BP<130/80mmHg。
- 饮食钠限制在100mmol/d(2.3 g)，限制酒精摄入，减肥（如果需要），锻炼。

- 单侧或双侧肾动脉狭窄(RAS)通常与糖尿病肾病共存；在慢性肾脏病1~2期，通过钆增强MRA诊断双肾动脉狭窄；而慢性肾脏病3~5期，最好采用肾动脉多普勒血流或非增强MRA。
- 大多数患高血压的糖尿病患者需要多种降压药物来达到降压目标，噻嗪类利尿剂或袢利尿剂是很多病人的一线治疗。
- 血管紧张素转换酶抑制剂(ACE-I)或血管紧张素受体拮抗剂(ARB)等RAAS阻断剂可以控制血压、降低蛋白尿和改善左心室收缩功能障碍，联合使用ACE-I和ARB可能恶化肾功能，如果必须使用，需要密切检测肾功能。ACE-I和ARB对于以下人群禁用：试图怀孕的育龄妇女、容易脱水的患者、难治性高钾血症患者或开始治疗后血清肌酐上升0.6mg/dl。
- β受体阻滞剂是有益的，特别是有充血性心力衰竭病史的患者，但应该在有哮喘病史患者中小心使用。
- 二氢吡啶(DHP)和非二氢吡啶类钙通道阻滞剂(CCBs)是有益，非二氢吡啶类对保护肾脏更有意义，但可能抑制心肌功能。CCBs可能导致下肢水肿和便秘。
- 尽可能简化治疗方案，尽可能提高依从性。

微量/大量蛋白尿
- 建议使用随机尿尿白蛋白肌酐比筛查微量蛋白尿。
- RAAS阻断剂应该在1型糖尿病伴微量白蛋白尿时即开始使用，不论有或没有高血压(见以前的高血压管理部分)。
- 使用RAAS阻断剂过程中，密切监测避免低血压和脱水。检查血钾和肌酐的基线值，并在开始治疗或剂量增加后的7~10天复查。
- 如果微量蛋白尿进展，可以在血压允许的情况下调整RAAS阻断剂的剂量。
- 大量蛋白尿的管理类似于微蛋白尿管理，然而膳食钠限制在这个阶段通常是必要的，<100mmol/d(<2.3g)。
- 如果糖尿病患者没有蛋白尿，RAAS阻断剂的使用是有争议的，它可以改善心血管功能但促进肾功能恶化。
- 在慢性肾脏病4~5期适度减少每日蛋白质摄入量，补充蛋白质0.8g/kg体重。
- 在慢性肾脏病的所有阶段避免减肥饮食。
- 慢性肾脏病的高蛋白质摄入会引起肾小球高滤过、氮质血症增加、代谢性酸中毒和疲劳。

水肿管理
- 膳食建议：减少精加工食品和盐。
- 水钠潴留的初始治疗是钠摄入的控制，<2g/d。
- 利尿剂只有在饮食控制不能缓解水肿时应用。
- 在早期慢性肾病(1~2期)使用噻嗪类利尿剂，在慢性肾脏病3~5期，袢利尿剂(呋喃苯胺酸)是首选，需要每日两次的治疗方案。
- 为保证舒适性，避免在晚上使用利尿剂。
- 为减轻双下肢水肿，在服用利尿剂后，坐位时应抬高下肢(臀部高度)。

- 建议起床前和白天使用弹力袜，可以加强利尿剂效果，减少皮肤破裂和感染的风险。
- 所有使用利尿剂的患者应密切监测血清电解质、肌酐和血尿素氮。
- 轻度肾前性氮质血症可容许，但严重的肾前肾功能衰竭应该避免。
- 国家肾脏基金会网站是患者教育资源(http://www.kidney.org)。

肾脏病学会推荐
- 尽早转诊患者到肾内专科会降低发病率、促进更及时的透析治疗、帮助尽早准备肾移植、降低总体成本，提高生存。
- 拖后转诊意味着在6个月内开始透析。
- 透析的开始和管理见416页。

随访
- 1型糖尿病患病5年之后每年检查尿微量白蛋白，2型糖尿病在发病时即开始，阳性结果需要再次确认。
- 每次就诊均需检查血压，为得到正确的结果，需在仰卧位、坐着、站位分别测量。
- 在糖尿病肾病、慢性肾脏病1~2期，至少每6个月监测肾功能。
- 在糖尿病肾病、慢性肾脏病3~5期，每三个月监测以下指标，血清电解质（钠、钾、氯、二氧化碳）、骨代谢情况（钙、磷、完整的甲状旁腺素）、营养状况（血白蛋白、尿素氮）、贫血指标（血红蛋白、红细胞压积、铁检验）以及肾小球滤过率估测值（血清肌酐）和随机尿尿微量白蛋白。
- 在早期糖尿病肾病（慢性肾脏病1~2期），尤其是在1型糖尿病，采用严格的血糖、血压控制和RAAS阻滞剂的使用进行治疗，目标是逆转疾病。
- 中期糖尿病肾病（慢性肾脏病3~4期）的目标是延缓疾病的进展，细致观察治疗干预结果，避免肾损伤药物。
- 晚期糖尿病肾病（慢性肾脏病5期）的目的是避免慢性肾疾病急性加重（如对比研究）、平稳过渡到及时的透析或移植治疗。

专家建议
- 慢性肾脏病3期应当转诊到肾科医生：评估导致慢性肾脏病的其他原因，进行关于终末期肾病的管理措施教育，安排转诊血管手术规划和预先做好肾移植的计划。
- 应该在糖尿病的所有阶段找出潜在的可逆的并存疾病，如阻塞性睡眠呼吸暂停、吸烟、病态肥胖、高血脂、双肾动脉狭窄、膀胱出口梗阻所致的肾盂积水和/或感染、肾损伤药物的持续暴露（如非甾体类抗炎药）。
- 预计妊娠的患者应该停用RAAS阻断剂。孕期糖尿病肾病可能恶化，有时不可逆转。

推荐依据
KDOQI. KDOQI Clinical Practice Guidelines and Clinical Practice Recommendations for Diabetes and Chronic Kidney Disease. Am J Kidney Dis, 2007; Vol. 49: pp. S12–154.
Comments: The Kidney Disease Outcomes Quality Initiative (K/DOQI) has published this comprehensive reference text for the clinician involved in managing

diabetic patients with chronic kidney disease. Reviews national (US) guidelines for management and the rationale for these therapies.

Chobanian AV, Bakris GL, Black HR, et al. The seventh report of the Joint National Committee on Prevention, Detection, Evaluation, and Treatment of High Blood Pressure: the JNC 7 report. JAMA, 2003; Vol. 289: pp. 2560–72.

Comments: A landmark report outlining stricter guidelines for blood pressure control.

其他参考文献

Magee GM, Bilous RW, Cardwell CR, et al. Is hyperfiltration associated with the future risk of developing diabetic nephropathy? A meta-analysis. Diabetologia, 2009; Vol. 52: pp. 691–7.

Comments: A meta-analysis of 10 cohort studies in type 1 diabetes mellitus to determine the predictive value of early glomerular hyperfiltration for future diabetic nephropathy.

Onuigbo MA. Reno-prevention vs. reno-protection: a critical re-appraisal of the evidence-base from the large RAAS blockade trials after ONTARGET—a call for more circumspection. QJM, 2009; Vol. 102: pp. 155–67.

Comments: An important review article outlining the need for close monitoring to avoid acute kidney injury when using RAAS blockade in advanced CKD.

Locatelli F, Del Vecchio L, Cavalli A. Inhibition of the renin-angiotensin system in chronic kidney disease: a critical look to single and dual blockade. Nephron Clin Pract, 2009; Vol. 113: pp. c286–c293.

Comments: A comprehensive review article of the benefits and risks of RAAS blockade in CKD patients.

Mann JF, Schmieder RE, Dyal L, et al. Effect of telmisartan on renal outcomes: a randomized trial. Ann Intern Med, 2009; Vol. 151: pp. 1–10, W1–2.

Comments: Summarizes the renal outcomes of the TRANSCEND trial that randomized patients with diabetes or cardiovascular disease to telmisartan versus placebo and found a positive effect of ARB therapy on cardiac outcomes but a negative impact on renal outcomes.

Parfrey PS. Angiotensin-receptor blockers in the prevention or treatment of microalbuminuria. Ann Intern Med, 2009; Vol. 151: pp. 63–5.

Comments: An editorial that reviews the adverse or neutral effects of ARB therapy on renal outcome in diabetic patients without baseline renal disease.

Waden J, Forsblom C, Thorn LM, et al. A1C variability predicts incident cardiovascular events, microalbuminuria, and overt diabetic nephropathy in patients with type 1 diabetes. Diabetes, 2009; Vol. 58: pp. 2649–55.

Comments: A Finnish study of 2107 patients with type 1 diabetes showed that increasing A1c levels were associated with microalbuminuria, progressive CKD and CVD events, confirming and expanding the original findings of the Diabetes Control and Complications Trial (DCCT).

Diabetes Control and Complications Trial/Epidemiology of Diabetes Interventions and Complications (DCCT/ EDIC) Research Group, Nathan DM, Zinman B, et al. Modern-day clinical course of type 1 diabetes mellitus after 30 years' duration: the diabetes control and complications trial/epidemiology of diabetes interventions and complications and Pittsburgh epidemiology of diabetes complications experience (1983–2005). Arch Intern Med, 2009; Vol. 169: pp. 1307–16.

Comments: An update on the importance of the DCCT and other longitudinal trials that changed the course of type 1 diabetes over the last 25 yrs by intensive diabetic management, resulting in a 50% reduction in microvascular complications.

Kalaitzidis R, Bakris GL. Effects of angiotensin II receptor blockers on diabetic nephropathy. J Hypertens, 2009; Vol. 27 Suppl 5: pp. S15–21.

Comments: A comprehensive review of the importance of targeting proteinuria as a risk factor for both renal and cardiovascular disease.

Mauer M, Zinman B, Gardiner R, et al. Renal and retinal effects of enalapril and losartan in type 1 diabetes. NEJM, 2009; Vol. 361: pp. 40–51.

Comments: A small but meticulous study of the effects of RAAS blockade on renal and retinal outcomes in normotensive subjects with type 1 diabetes. There were no renal benefits by biopsy, but they did receive retinal benefits. Surprisingly, ARB therapy was associated with a higher incidence of developing microalbuminuria than placebo or ACE-I therapy.

Fioretto P, Caramori ML, Mauer M. The kidney in diabetes: dynamic pathways of injury and repair. The Camillo Golgi Lecture 2007. Diabetologia, 2008; Vol. 51: pp. 1347–55.

Comments: An elegant review of general interest regarding current and future directions for the treatment of diabetic nephropathy.

Wolf G, Müller N, Mandecka A, et al. Association of diabetic retinopathy and renal function in patients with types 1 and 2 diabetes mellitus. Clin Nephrol, 2007; Vol. 68: pp. 81–6.

Comments: Underscores the variability of diabetic retinopathy and renal disease in types 1 and 2 diabetes mellitus.

Atkins RC, Briganti EM, Lewis JB, et al. Proteinuria reduction and progression to renal failure in patients with type 2 diabetes mellitus and overt nephropathy. Am J Kidney Dis, 2005; Vol. 45: pp. 281–7.

Comments: A comparison trial (The Irbesartan Diabetic Nephropathy Trial, IDNT) of an ARB (irbesartan) and a calcium channel blocker (amlodipine) for proteinuria reduction in type 2 diabetes.

Morales E, Valero MA, Leon M, et al. Beneficial effects of weight loss in overweight patients with chronic proteinuric nephropathies. Am J Kidney Dis, 2003; Vol. 41: pp. 319–27.

Comments: A study that looks at the association of obesity with proteinuria, and protection by weight loss.

Adler AI, Stratton IM, Neil HA, et al. Association of systolic blood pressure with macrovascular and microvascular complications of type 2 diabetes (UKPDS 36): prospective observational study. BMJ, 2000; Vol. 321: pp. 412–9.

Comments: A multicentered observational study (UK Prospective Diabetes Study Group 36) of hypertension and vascular complications of type 2 diabetes.

糖尿病中的肾脏疾病

Donna I. Myers, MD

定义
- 糖尿病中的肾脏疾病可能是由于糖尿病导致,也可能由于其他病因引起与糖尿病共存。
- 对于糖尿病患者,没有其他原因的持续性蛋白尿是糖尿病肾病的第一个迹象。

流行病学
- 糖尿病是世界上终末期肾病(ESRD)最常见的原因(Harvey)。
- 只有25%的1型和2型糖尿病患者会出现典型的糖尿病肾病、高血压肾病;然而,肾小球硬化、动脉粥样硬化性肾动脉狭窄、非糖尿病患者肾小球疾病、急性和慢性肾盂肾炎、肾乳头坏死和IV型肾小管酸中毒(RTA)在糖尿病患者中都更普遍(Mazzucco)。
- 1型和2型糖尿病中,由于糖尿病肾病的蛋白尿大多在经过10年糖尿病病史后缓慢起病(Mazzucco; Harvey)。

诊断
- 肾脏疾病分期只需要一个随机尿的尿白蛋白肌酐比率、一个血清肌酐水平和使用修改后MDRD公式计算的肾小球滤过率(见国家肾脏基金会肾小球滤过率计算器,http://www.kidney.org/professionals/kdoqi/gfr_calculator.cfm)。
- 慢性肾脏疾病(CKD)根据尿白蛋白和肾小球滤过率(GFR)[ml/(min·1.73m^2)]进行分期:1期:蛋白尿,肾小球滤过率 > 90;2期:蛋白尿,肾小球滤过率60~89;3期:肾小球滤过率30~59;4期:肾小球滤过率15~29;5期:肾小球滤过率<15。
- 进一步评估包括一个完整的尿检验、血清电解质和肾超声;肾活检在某些情况下可能是必要的(见肾功能,656页)。
- 任何糖尿病伴高钾血症的患者,在没有急进性肾小球肾炎、补钾或使用保钾利尿剂证据时,都应怀疑IV型肾小管酸中毒(低肾素低醛固酮血症可能性;轻度代谢性酸中毒通常表现阴离子间隙正常(见醛固酮减少症,617页)。
- 如果有以下情况,需怀疑肾动脉狭窄:恶性高血压、严重的周围性血管疾病、腹部和大腿的杂音、肾脏大小不对称(差异1.5厘米)和/或使用血管紧张素转换酶抑制剂(ACE-I)或血管紧张素受体阻滞剂(ARB)后血清肌酐上升 > 0.6mg/dl。

症状和体征
- 肾脏疾病的实验室征象包括蛋白尿、肾小球滤过率下降、血尿素氮升高、血钾升高和IV型肾小管酸中毒。
- 早期肾脏疾病的阳性体征包括高血压和水肿。
- 肾脏疾病的早期症状包括厌食、口中"金属"味道、清晨恶心、泡沫尿(> 3g蛋白尿)、夜尿症、疲劳和过度睡眠。

糖尿病中的肾脏疾病

- 中间症状包括注意力不集中、肌肉组织的减少、不安腿和嗜睡。
- 晚期症状包括尿毒症的恶臭、扑翼样震颤、周围神经病变、精神状态改变和癫痫发作。

临床治疗

治疗的目标

- 目前对患有慢性肾病的糖尿病患者没有统一的血糖控制指南,但控制好血糖可以延缓进展。
- 在慢性肾病 1~4 期时,遵循一般治疗原则,维持糖化血红蛋白在 6% ~7% 之间。
- 糖化血红蛋白检验受以下因素干扰:尿毒症、酸中毒、红细胞寿命缩短,它们可能不合逻辑的影响慢性肾脏病 5 期和终末期肾病患者的 HbA1c 水平。
- 遵循 JNC7 指南的血压控制标准(<130/80mmHg),注意由于药物和糖尿病自主神经病变引起的心态改变。
- 对所有肾病患者使用肾素血管紧张素系统(RAAS)阻断剂治疗。
- 限制膳食钠 2.0g/d(100mmol),包括"隐藏"的膳食钠(即罐头食品)。
- 不可控的高钾血症和血清肌酐上升 > 0.6mg/dl 限制治疗。
- 肥胖患者应该节食并锻炼来改善高血压、阻塞性睡眠呼吸暂停、二级焦和由于肾毛细血管细胞膜高滤过状态引起的节段性肾小球硬化症。
- 高脂血症管理可以降低动脉粥样硬化的风险,动脉粥样硬化经常伴随糖尿病肾脏疾病。
- 戒烟可以减少蛋白尿。

肾小球滤过率(GFR)下降后的药物调整

- 糖尿病伴随进展性肾脏疾病的病人,由于胰岛素敏感性下降可能出现血糖控制差,胰岛素治疗需要的剂量越来越高。
- 邻近终末期肾病的患者,由于胰岛素从肾脏清除减少,胰岛素的需求可能下降。
- 避免二甲双胍在慢性肾脏病 3 期、4 期和 5 期病人中使用(增加乳酸酸中毒的风险)。肌酐 > 1.5mg/dl 为禁忌。
- 所有糖尿病药物因为肾小球滤过率下降的剂量调整(见表 3 - 17)。
- Ⅳ型肾小管酸中毒应该限制和避免饮食中的补充 K^+;一些病人可能有必要中止 ACE-I 或 ARB 治疗。

表 3-17. 高血糖治疗药物根据肾功能的剂量调整 *

种类	药物	慢性肾脏病 3~5 期	透析
第一代磺脲类药物	乙酰苯磺酰环己脲	避免	避免
	氯磺丙脲	GFR50~70ml/min 调整剂量；GFR<50ml/min 避免使用	避免
	甲磺吖庚脲	避免	避免
	甲苯磺丁脲	避免	避免
第二代磺酰脲类药物	格列吡嗪	选择口服的药物	选择口服的药物
	格列本脲	避免	避免
	格列美脲	减小剂量使用	避免
α 糖苷酶抑制剂	阿卡波糖	如果肌酐 >2mg/dl, 避免使用	避免
	米格列醇	如果肌酐 >2mg/dl, 避免使用	避免
双胍类药物	二甲双胍	如果肌酐 >1.5mg/dl(男) 1.4mg/dl(女), 避免使用	避免
氯茴苯酸类药物	瑞格列奈	谨慎使用	谨慎使用
	那格列奈	减小剂量使用	避免
噻唑烷二酮类药物	吡格列酮	谨慎使用	谨慎使用
	罗格列酮	谨慎使用	谨慎使用
肠促胰岛素类似物	艾塞那肽	GFR<30 ml/min 避免使用	避免
胰淀素类似物	普兰林肽	谨慎使用	未研究
DPP-4 抑制剂	西格列汀	如果 GFR>50ml/min, 需要剂量调整	需要剂量调整

* 改编自国家肾脏基金会 KDOQI 临床实践指南、糖尿病和慢性肾脏病和临床实践的建议。

高血压管理
- 生活方式：锻炼、限制饮酒、减肥、限制钠盐 2g/d(100mmol)。
- 检查仰卧位和站立血压。
- 如果需要利尿剂，在慢性肾脏病 1~3 期使用噻嗪类利尿剂，慢性肾脏病 4~5 期使用祥利尿剂(呋喃苯胺酸)，可能需要每天两次；慢性肾脏病 期、4 期、5 期应当谨慎使用保钾利尿剂。
- ACE-I 和 ARBs 类 RAAS 阻断剂可以减少尿蛋白、保护肾脏、控制血压；也可以改善充血性心力衰竭或左心室功能障碍。

糖尿病中的肾脏疾病

联合 ACE 和 ARB 治疗可能会进一步降低蛋白尿,但也整体恶化肾功能,需要密切监测。

开始使用或增加 ACE-I 药物剂量后,应 7 天内监测高钾血症和急性肾损伤情况。

容量不足的病人使用利尿剂和 ACE-I 或 ARB 联合治疗可能导致急性肾功能衰竭。

与选择性 $β_1$ 受体阻滞剂对比,非选择性 β 受体阻滞剂可以改善胰岛素敏感性、降低蛋白尿。

非二氢吡啶类药物可以更有效地降低蛋白尿,但可能导致抑制心肌功能。

避免肾损伤药物

避免慢性肾病患者使用非甾体抗炎药,伴随糖尿病将进一步增加乳头状坏死的风险。

影像学对比剂是剂量依赖性的肾毒性药物;风险因素包括糖尿病、蛋白尿、无效的肾灌注(充血性心力衰竭、肝硬化)和慢性肾脏病 3~5 期。

如果对比剂至关重要,使用低渗透压的非离子对比剂,并在对比剂负荷当天及前一天做好预防措施。

预防措施:N-乙酰半胱氨酸 1 200 毫克每天两次口服 2 天(见乙酰半胱氨酸 587 页),盐水水化,停止 ACE-I/ARB 或利尿剂。

减少对比剂负荷量是最重要的。

增强 MRI 中所用的钆,只有在慢性肾脏病早期可以谨慎使用,在慢性肾脏病 4~5 期禁忌使用,因为会导致肾发生系统性纤维化的风险。

肾小球滤过率 <30ml/min,双磷酸盐禁忌使用(慢性肾脏病 4~5 期)。

含磷酸盐药物进行肠道准备可能会导致严重的高磷血症和不可逆的急性肾损伤,应当避免慢性肾脏病病人使用。

随访

慢性肾脏病的年度筛查 2 型糖尿病从确诊时开始,1 型糖尿病从诊断 5 年后开始,使用随机尿的尿白蛋白肌酐比值、血清肌酐、估测肾小球滤过率筛查。

涉及糖尿病伴随慢性肾脏病 1~2 期,同时肾脏病变诊断不明确的患者。

在可行的情况下,慢性肾脏病 3 期转诊至肾脏科。

慢性肾脏病 4~5 期或者前终末期肾病的病人应该立即肾脏科就诊。

专家意见

通知病人治疗管理的目标。

使用 RAAS 阻断剂和利尿剂治疗是一把双刃剑:风险是这些药物可以引起脱水,导致急性肾损伤。

没有糖尿病性视网膜病变共存,糖尿病肾病是罕见的,应考虑肾脏疾病的其他病因。

许多糖尿病药物,包括胰岛素和口服药物,都需要根据肾脏疾病的进展进行剂量调整。

推荐依据

Bakris GL, Sowers JR, American Society of Hypertension (ASH) Writing Group. ASH position paper: treatment of hypertension in patients with diabetes—an update. J Clin Hypertens (Greenwich), 2008; Vol. 10: pp. 707–13, discussion 714-5.

Comments: A consensus report from the American Society of Hypertension (ASH) on managing HTN in patients with diabetes.

The Kidney Disease Outcomes Quality Initiative (K/DOQI). K/DOQI clinical practice guidelines and clinical practice recommendations for diabetes and chronic kidney disease. Am J Kidney Dis, 2007; Vol. 49(2 Suppl 2): S12– 154.

Comments: The Kidney Disease Outcomes Quality Initiative (K/DOQI) has published this comprehensive reference text for the clinician involved in managing diabetic patients with chronic kidney disease; reviews national (US) guidelines for management and the rationale for these therapies.

Chobanian AV, Bakris GL, Black HR, et al. The seventh report of the Joint National Committee on Prevention, Detection, Evaluation, and Treatment of High Blood Pressure: the JNC 7 report. JAMA, 2003; Vol. 289: pp. 2560–72.

Comments: A landmark report updating stricter guidelines for blood pressure control. 13372_SEC_3_COMP_25_Printer.indd 371 5/24/11 1:27 PM

Bakris GL, Williams M, Dworkin L, et al. Preserving renal function in adults with hypertension and diabetes: a consensus approach. National Kidney Foundation Hypertension and Diabetes Executive Committees Working Group. Am J Kidney Dis 2000; Vol. 36: pp. 646–61.

Comments: National guidelines on hypertension management in patients with diabetes and CKD.

其他参考文献

Appel LJ, American Society of Hypertension Writing Group, Giles TD, et al. ASH Position Paper: dietary approaches to lower blood pressure. J Clin Hypertens (Greenwich) 2009; Vol. 11: pp. 358–68.

Comments: An ASH position paper on dietary management of HTN.

Wetzels JF. Renal outcomes in the ONTARGET study. Lancet, 2008; Vol. 372: p. 202 author reply 2020–1.

Comments: A trial with some evidence that the combination of ACE-I and ARB therapy may impact negatively on renal outcome in diabetes.

Bakris GL, Fonseca V, Katholi RE, et al. Differential effects of beta-blockers on albuminuria in patients with type 2 diabetes. Hypertension, 2005; Vol. 46: pp. 1309–15.

Comments: A comparison of selective versus nonselective beta-blockers diabetes.

Grossman E, Messerli FH. Are calcium antagonists beneficial in diabetic patients with hypertension? Am J Med, 2004; Vol. 116: pp. 44–9.

Comments: A meta-analysis of 14 studies using calcium antagonists hypertensive patients with diabetes and outcomes of cardiovascular protection

Harvey, John N. Trends in the prevalence of diabetic nephropathy in type 1 and type 2 diabetes. Curr Opin Nephrol Hypertens, 2003; Vol. 12(3): pp. 317–322.

Comments: A concise epidemiologic review article of the increasing prevalence diabetic nephropathy worldwide.

Ansari A, Thomas S, Goldsmith D. Assessing glycemic control in patients with diabetes and end-stage renal failure. Am J Kidney Dis, 2003; Vol. 41: pp. 523–31.

Comments: A focused review of monitoring glycemic control in end-stage renal disease patients.

azzucco, G., Bertani T, Fortunato, M, et al. Different patterns of renal damage in type 2 diabetes mellitus: a multicentric study on 393 biopsies. Am J Kidney Dis, 2002; Vol. 39(4): pp. 713–720.

Comments: An original article that underscores the prevalence of nondiabetic nephropathy in patients with diabetes.

nslie-Smith AM, Boyle DI, Evans JM, et al. Contraindications to metformin therapy in patients with type 2 diabetes— a population-based study of adherence to prescribing guidelines. Diabet Med, 2001; Vol. 18: pp. 483–8.

Comments: An article that reveals widespread prescribing of metformin against pharmaceutical precautions and yet a very low incidence of lactic acidosis.

eFronzo RA. Pharmacologic therapy for type 2 diabetes mellitus. Ann Intern Med, 1999, Vol. 131: pp. 281–303.

Comments: An article that includes precautions for using metformin in diabetic patients with CKD.

透析开始和管理

Donna I. Myers, M[...]

定义
- 终末期肾病(ESRD)的治疗方案包括维持血液透析(HD)、腹膜透析(PD[...]和肾移植(Tpl)。

流行病学
- 约 40%~50% 的透析人群是由于糖尿病肾病(DN)继发终末期肾[...](ESRD),糖尿病成为 ESRD 最常见的病因。
- 糖尿病患者的透析生存率比没有糖尿病的患者更低。
- 在大多数研究中,血液透析和腹膜透析的生存率是相似的。糖尿病肾[...]患者腹膜透析的 5 年生存率是 24% 左右,血液透析约为 27%,总体[...]析人群的 5 年生存率是 33%。
- 50% 的无症状的糖尿病和晚期慢性肾脏病(CKD)患者患有以前未知[...]冠心病。
- 肾脏替代治疗的死因大多数是心血管疾病加重和感染。

诊断
- 见肾病(404 页)和糖尿病肾病(410 页)。

症状和体征
- 尿毒症是指由于含氮废物积累引起的多器官体征和症状的总和。
- 症状和体征构成开始透析的"硬性"(绝对)适应证,包括尿毒症或消[...]道出血、难治性水肿与反复发作的充血性心力衰竭、尿毒症浆膜炎(心[...]炎、胸膜炎或腹膜炎)、无法控制的代谢性酸中毒和/或高钾血症以及[...]有明显其他病因的精神状态改变。
- 开始透析的"软性"(相对)适应证,包括厌食、恶心、金属味、体重下降[...]液体潴留、注意力不集中以及未能迅速进展的慢性肾脏病 5 期[患者[...]小球滤过率 <15 ml/(min·1.73m^2)]。

临床治疗

总体管理和病人的准备
- 在慢性肾脏病 1~3 期时尽早安排患者就诊于肾脏专科可能会逆转或延[...]糖尿病肾病发展。如果肾小球滤过率(GFR)下降不可逆转,应该在慢[...]肾脏病 3 期时开始患者教育。
- 糖尿病病人合并肾脏疾病和尿毒症症状时,应该在肾小球滤过[...] <15ml/(min·1.73m^2) 时开始透析,而不是 <10ml/(min·1.73m^2)。
- 治疗方式(HD、PD、Tpl)的选择由病人的合并症情况和患者的偏好决定[...]
- 腹膜透析是糖尿病病人的一种选择。限制因素:视力低下、缺乏家庭条件[...]操作能力不足、未控制的糖尿病(1 型)、多次腹部手术后和病态肥胖。
- 血液透析也是一种选择。限制因素:创造一个永久性血管通路困难、[...]析期间血流动力学不稳定和机动性问题。

透析开始和管理

如果病人是肾脏移植的候选人，并且有合格的有或无血缘关系的供者，肾脏移植是首选治疗（见肾移植 423 页）。肾移植的五年生存率高于透析人群，达 69%。

安排后期肾脏学 (6 个月内开始透析) 发生在 25%~50% 的患者和 25% 与贫穷相关的结果。

病人准备：终末期肾病前告知患者治疗方案。最佳方案是透析护士、肾脏移植代表、肾营养师和社会工作者均在场。

选择血液透析或腹膜透析之前，需参考血管外科医生意见，评估自体动静脉瘘(AVF)、瘘管/移植物(AVF/G) 或 Tenckhoff 腹膜透析导管的可行性。

对于血液透析来说，自体瘘（使用患者自己的静脉和动脉）远远比移植物合适，这本身就是一个合适的导管。AVF 的成熟时间至少 3~6 个月、瘘管/移植物需要 4~6 周。导管可以立即使用。

见并发症

广泛的周围性血管疾病使盗血综合征的风险增加（由于血流高速通过动静脉瘘或瘘管/移植物造成远端缺血）；腹膜透析可能是一个更好的选择。

临时或长期血液透析导管可能会导致中心静脉狭窄、血栓形成和威胁生命的感染，以上并发症应该尽可能避免。

伴有病态肥胖或多个腹部手术的患者，腹部腹膜透析不可行，但可以考虑胸骨前腹膜透析。腹膜透析导管的准备时间是 3~4 周。

感染的可能性使血液透析和腹膜透析复杂化。

腹膜透析的导管相关性并发症：细菌性腹膜炎在治疗中每 30 个月发生一次。体征和症状：腹痛、透析液浑浊，通常没有菌血症。治疗通常是门诊开具腹腔内抗生素。

血液透析并发症：没有其他明确来源的感染，开始为未被发现的间歇性菌血症，进而发展到明显的脓毒症症状（寒颤、发热、恶心、呕吐）。常见的是细菌性心内膜炎（葡萄球菌），伴或不伴细菌栓子。导管的感染几率是自体动静脉瘘的 10~20 倍。

如果有合适的捐赠者，糖尿病伴慢性肾脏病 4~5 期优先考虑肾脏移植。需要透析前 6 个月内开始评价。如果患者可以耐受手术，可以开始透析后即进行肾脏移植。

末期肾病的液体和电解质并发症

终末期肾病的高血压通常是容量相关的。容量负荷过重的其他并发症：充血性心力衰竭和血液透析过程中血流动力学不稳定。

通过饮食咨询（限制钠）和血糖控制来避免烦渴和过度饮水，以此减少两次透析之间水负荷。

透析相关低血压在血液透析中的发生率高达 30%。在老年患者、自主功能障碍（糖尿病）、水负荷过重或心脏储备差的人群中更常见的。

血液透析中反复发作的透析相关低血压的治疗方法包括膳食咨询、使用低温透析液、钠调整（改变透析液钠浓度）以及透析前甲氧胺福林治疗。改为腹膜透析此问题可解决。

血液透析的并发症包括肌肉痉挛疼痛、增加中风和心肌缺血的风险，慢性水负荷过重和心脏功能恶化形成恶性循环。

- 许多新透析患者没有少尿(尿液输出 > 500ml/d)。保护剩余的肾小球滤过率(GFR)对提高腹膜透析患者的生存率很重要，对于血液透析患者也是有利的；因此对于腹膜透析和血液透析患者避免非紧急静脉对比剂和非甾体类抗炎药使用，延长其有尿时间。
- 常规血液透析超滤每周进行3次，每次3~4小时。理想的每小时液体排出量(超滤率)<500ml，以避免血流动力学不稳定。两次透析之间的入液量经常超过这一目标，此时超滤率需要 > 1L/h。每天家庭血液透析(不是随时的)和每日腹膜透析可以使用更低的、耐受性好的超滤率。
- 对于腹膜透析，高血糖限制通过渗透梯度排出液体，而且透析液可能反被吸收。
- 慢性高钾血症是少尿的血液透析患者需要面对的一个问题，饮食限钾是必要的。
- 腹膜透析患者经常出现低血钾，需要进行个体化饮食补钾或药物补钾治疗(与之前的限钾患者容易混淆)。
- 所有的终末期肾病患者都要监测钙、磷、甲状旁腺素(PTH)。K/DOQI指南：血清钙 8.4~9.5mg/dl，磷 3.5~5.5mg/dl，磷酸钙产物 <55，全甲状旁腺素 150~300pg/ml。
- 对于高磷血症，可以在吃饭时服用不含铝的磷酸盐结合剂(司维拉姆、磷酸钙和碳酸镧)。
- 血清磷酸盐 <5.5mg/dl，但 iPTH 仍高于目标，则需要添加维生素 D 类药物(骨化三醇、帕立骨化醇、度骨化醇)。如果仍然 iPTH > 300pg/ml 或钙 > 8.4mg/dl，使用钙受体调节剂(西那卡塞)治疗；这些药物效过好，但由于胃肠道(GI)的不良反应耐受性差。

心血管疾病(CVD)
- 血液透析和腹膜透析合并心血管疾病的死亡率为 40%~50%。
- 甚至在年轻的透析病人中可以见到冠状动脉钙化。慢性肾脏病患者中中层钙化比内膜钙化更常见。
- 透析患者发生加速动脉粥样硬化的原因尚不清楚，贫血、左心室肥大、高血压、慢性容量超负荷和电解质失衡都是假设。
- 终末期肾病患者可以通过治疗高磷血症、甲状旁腺功能亢进、维生素缺乏和慢性炎症预防血管钙化。
- 下肢周围性血管疾病在血液透析患者中的发生率是 25%。危险因素：吸烟、糖尿病、年龄、男性、高血压。
- 一些透析诊所对他们的糖尿病患者每月安排一次足部检查，以减少感染和残肢的风险。

营养和贫血
- 尽管指南推荐，但除非透析患者正在准备移植或者 BMI > 40kg/m², 不应强调减肥。规律锻炼是有益的。
- 蛋白质-能量营养不良与终末期肾病的失望率相关。维持即使血清白蛋白在正常范围，血清白蛋白水平和透析生存率之间仍存在线性关系。透析前停止"肾病饮食"，透析时开始"肾病饮食"，因为"肾病饮食"限制了蛋白质。

透析开始和管理

腹膜透析患者容易发生低白蛋白血症,这是由于蛋白质经透析液浪费。腹膜透析患者应该接受1.2g/(kg·d)的蛋白质摄入。如果出现持续的低白蛋白血症,尤其是术后或化疗期间,可能需要临时或永久改为血液透析。

进行血液透析或腹膜透析的终末期肾病患者进行促红细胞生成素类药物(ESAs)治疗。不良反应有炎症、慢性移植排斥、艾滋病毒、不明原因感染和严重的甲状旁腺功能亢进。

大多数透析患者需要补充铁剂,血液透析或每月失血的腹膜透析进行静脉补铁治疗。所有的透析病人都要补充叶酸、维生素B和维生素C。

慢性肾脏病的贫血管理指南建议血红蛋白目标为11~12g/dl。

血糖管理:可以在透析时检查血糖,而无需测指尖血糖,可以及时调整胰岛素。

标准透析液的葡萄糖浓度为200mg/dl。

大量的透析间液体摄入需要增加每小时超滤率(血液透析),或者增加透析强度(腹膜透析),结果导致发病率和死亡率增加。建议患者限制膳食钠的摄入,避免无法控制的高血糖,从而减少液体摄入。

即使在透析人群中,糖化血红蛋白也是用于监测长期血糖水平的指标。糖化血红蛋白结果的假性升高,可能由于高氮酸中毒和缺铁导致非免疫学检测方法出现误差。

糖化血红蛋白的控制目标为:1型糖尿病6%~7%,2型糖尿病7%~8%。如果糖化血红蛋白水平降低,并且除外营养不良因素,提示预后较好。

终末期肾病患者避免使用二甲双胍(乳酸酸中毒的风险)和罗格列酮(心血管死亡率)。磺酰脲类药物如格列吡嗪需要谨慎使用,避免使用格列本脲、氯磺丙脲(长效)。慢性肾脏病患者不推荐使用α糖苷酶抑制剂(见糖尿病中的肾脏疾病,410页)。

虽然建议腹膜透析患者使用腹腔内胰岛素,但剂量难以确定,同时添加了一个潜在的污染源。糖尿病患者进行腹膜透析可以考虑无糖透析液的解决方案(艾考糊精),尽管它不是现成的。

如果血糖高,腹膜透析不能达到合适的超滤;如果长期血糖控制不佳,血液透析可能是一个更好的选择。

对于少尿或无尿而又出现严重高血糖及酮症酸中毒的患者可以采用低剂量静脉注射胰岛素治疗。补液是不必要的,并且存在潜在的危险。

对于伴发高血糖的终末期肾病患者来说,高钾血症是一种潜在威胁生命的并发症。胰岛素治疗中逆转细胞内外的钾转换。对未确定血糖情况的意识障碍者,避免常规补充浓缩糖治疗。如果慢性肾脏病(甚至终末期肾病前期)患者的意识障碍是由于高血糖引起,进行浓缩糖补充治疗而非胰岛素治疗可能加重高钾血症,导致心律失常。

随访

认真确定主治医师,建议组成终末期肾病医疗团队。

每三个月监测透析病人的糖化血红蛋白水平,告知患者和主要照顾者。

早期研究提示的血液透析加速糖尿病性视网膜病变进展尚未被证实。眼科常规检查还是必要的。

鉴于慢性肾脏病患者中心血管疾病的高发生率,建议进行心脏病咨询。

- 常规进行足部检查，如果确定病变尽早安排血管手术。在透析中每月进行足检查，直到需要进行保肢治疗。

专家意见

- 相比血液透析或者腹膜透析，肾脏移植在所有终末期肾病患者中的获益均更高，尽管这可能混有部分选择偏倚。
- 关于进行血液透析和腹膜透析的终末期肾病患者的相对生存率，目前尚未达成共识。其高低决定于患者的个人喜好、伴随症状、服务可用性和社会支持网络。
- 所有透析患者都需警惕营养不良-慢性炎症复合体综合征。它与总体预后差有关。
- 糖尿病透析患者的生存率已有所改善，但仍然很低，再次强调糖尿病肾病早期阶段的预防治疗。

推荐依据

Slinin Y, Foley RN, Collins AJ. Calcium, phosphorus, parathyroid hormone, and cardiovascular disease in hemodialysis patients: the USRDS waves 1, 3, and 4 study. Am Soc Nephrol, 2005; Vol. 16: pp. 1788–93.

Comments: Using the USRDS database, this article links disorders of calcium homeostasis with cardiovascular events in HD patients.

K/DOQI Workgroup. K/DOQI clinical practice guidelines for cardiovascular disease dialysis patients. Am J Kidney Dis, 2005; Vol. 45: pp. S1–153.

Comments: Practice guidelines for evaluation and management of cardiovascular disease in ESRD patients.

National Kidney Foundation. K/DOQI clinical practice guidelines for bone metabolism and disease in chronic kidney disease. Am J Kidney Dis, 2003; Vol. 42: pp. S1–201.

Comments: K/DOQI guidelines for mineral bone metabolism in ESRD.

其他参考文献

Kalantar-Zadeh K, Regidor DL, Kovesdy CP, et al. Fluid retention is associated with cardiovascular mortality in patients undergoing long-term hemodialysis. Circulation 2009; Vol. 119: pp. 671–9.

Comments: This article stresses the importance of reducing interdialytic fluid gain in intermittent HD patients.

Kalantar-Zadeh K, Lee GH, Miller JE, et al. Predictors of hyporesponsiveness erythropoiesis-stimulating agents in hemodialysis patients. Am J Kidney Dis, 2009; Vol. 53: pp. 823–34.

Comments: In maintenance HD patients, erythropoietin-stimulating agent (ESA) hyporesponsiveness was associated with high turnover bone disease, hyperparathyroidism and low iron stores.

Kovesdy CP, Kalantar-Zadeh K. Review article: biomarkers of clinical outcomes advanced chronic kidney disease. Nephrology (Carlton), 2009; Vol. 14: pp. 408–15.

Comments: Markers of protein-energy wasting, especially albumin, remain the strongest predictors of survival in advanced CKD.

Kovesdy CP, Kalantar-Zadeh K. Why is protein-energy wasting associated with mortality chronic kidney disease? Semin Nephrol, 2009; Vol. 29: pp. 3–14.

Comments: A discussion of the possible mechanisms why protein-energy wasting is such a strong marker for mortality on dialysis.

Ramirez SP, Albert JM, Blayney MJ, et al. Rosiglitazone is associated with mortality in chronic hemodialysis patients. J Am Soc Nephrol, 2009; Vol. 20: pp. 1094–101.

Comments: Association of rosiglitazone with worse outcome in 2393 HD patients.

US Renal Data System (RSRDS). Morbidity and mortality. USRDS 2008 Annual Data Report, 2008; Vol. 2, Chapter 6: pp. 269–280. Available online at http://www.usrds.org/ (accessed 3/4/2011).

Comments: A comprehensive review of mortality trends in ESRD patients in the US from the exhaustive USRDS 2008 database.

Cosio FG, Hickson LJ, Griffin MD, et al. Patient survival and cardiovascular risk after kidney transplantation: the challenge of diabetes. Am J Transplant, 2008; Vol. 8: pp. 593–9.

Comments: Compared to nondiabetic patients receiving kidney transplantation, diabetic patients had more pretransplant cardiovascular disease and worse posttransplant survival.

Ishimura E, Okuno S, Taniwaki H, et al. Different risk factors for vascular calcification in end-stage renal disease between diabetics and nondiabetics: the respective importance of glycemic and phosphate control. Kidney Blood Press Res, 2008; Vol. 31: pp. 10–5.

Comments: Review article of vascular calcification in pre-ESRD and ESRD diabetic patients emphasizing the role of glycemic and phosphate control.

Dinavahi R, Akalin E. Preemptive kidney transplantation in patients with diabetes mellitus. Endocrinol Metab Clin North Am, 2007; Vol. 36: pp. 1039–49, x.

Comments: A review article summarizing the data in favor of preemptive renal transplantation in diabetic patients with ESRD prior to starting dialysis.

Westra WM, Kopple JD, Krediet RT, et al. Dietary protein requirements and dialysate protein losses in chronic peritoneal dialysis patients. Perit Dial Int, 2007; Vol. 27: pp. 192–5.

Comments: PD patients using the automated cycler machine at night may have higher 24-hour protein losses than patients performing manual exchanges.

Kalantar-Zadeh K, Kopple JD, Regidor DL, et al. A1C and survival in maintenance hemodialysis patients. Diabetes Care, 2007; Vol. 30: pp. 1049–55.

Comments: In another large study on survival of diabetic patients on dialysis followed for 3 years, unadjusted higher A1c levels were paradoxically associated with lower death rates. However, after adjusting for anemia, malnutrition, and inflammation, glycemic control correlated with improved survival.

Berns JS, Szczech LA. What is the nephrologist's role as a primary care provider? We all have different answers. Clin J Am Soc Nephrol, 2007; Vol. 2: pp. 601–3.

Comments: Reviews the complex issues involved in caring for dialysis patients and coordinating care with other physicians.

Rajagopalan S, Dellegrottaglie S, Furniss AL, et al. Peripheral arterial disease in patients with end-stage renal disease: observations from the Dialysis Outcomes and Practice Patterns Study (DOPPS). Circulation, 2006; Vol. 114: pp. 1914–22.

Comments: Data from the Dialysis Outcomes and Practice Patterns Study (DOPPS) on >29,000 HD patients reviews associations between PVD and underlying clinical variables.

Williams ME, Lacson E, Teng M, et al. Hemodialyzed type I and type II diabetic patients in the US: characteristics, glycemic control, and survival. Kidney Int, 2006; Vol. 70: pp. 1503–9.

Comments: In a large population of HD patients with diabetes, survival did not vary with HbA1c at 12 months.

Vonesh EF, Snyder JJ, Foley RN, et al. The differential impact of risk factors on mortality in hemodialysis and peritoneal dialysis. Kidney Int, 2004; Vol. 66: pp. 2389–401.

Comments: The relative risk of hemodialysis versus peritoneal dialysis varies by time on dialysis and comorbidities.

Kalantar-Zadeh K, Rodriguez RA, Humphreys MH. Association between serum ferritin and measures of inflammation, nutrition and iron in haemodialysis patients. Nephrol Dial Transplant, 2004; Vol. 19: pp. 141–9.

Comments: Overview of the malnutrition-inflammation syndrome in ESRD patients.

肾移植

Bassam G. Abu Jawdeh, MD, and Nada Alachkar, MD

定义

- 将肾脏从供者转移给另外一个人的移植手术。(allograft 同种异体移植)。
- 肾移植发生在同卵双胞胎之间为同系异体移植。
- 胰腺和肾脏联合移植手术(SPK)已经成功在继发于1型糖尿病的终末期肾病患者身上进行。其他移植手术还包括肾脏移植之前或之后的胰腺或胰岛细胞移植。
- 大多数接受肾脏移植(以及所有胰腺移植)的患者是同种异体移植受者,需要终生免疫抑制治疗,来防止对移植物的免疫反应。
- 本篇肾移植章节中所提到的糖尿病,包括移植前诊断的糖尿病和移植后糖尿病(PTDM)。

流行病学

- 每年新确诊的慢性肾脏病有45%患糖尿病。
- 2007年,新登记的肾移植患者中40%患有糖尿病。
- 对于大多数糖尿病患者,这是终末期肾脏疾病需要进行肾脏和/或胰腺移植的原因。
- 另外,每年5%~25%的非糖尿病肾移植受者将发展为移植后糖尿病(PTDM)。
- 移植后3个月、12个月和36个月的移植后糖尿病的发病率分别是9%、16%和24%。
- 移植后糖尿病是移植失败和生存率降低的强大的、独立的预测信号。
- 移植后糖尿病的不可控危险因素包括年龄、家族史、女性、西班牙裔和非裔美国人。
- 移植后糖尿病的可控危险因素包括肥胖(BMI > $30kg/m^2$)、丙型肝炎和使用他克莫司。

诊断

- 肾移植仍然是终末期肾脏病患者肾脏替代治疗首选的方案,特别是对那些不存在影响手术或免疫抑制剂治疗的并发症的人群。
- 只有肾小球滤过率<20ml/(min·$1.73m^2$)的患者才能被允许进入器官共享联合网络(UNOS)注册申请尸体肾脏移植,例外是当肾脏和其他器官同时需要移植时。
- 通常,以下疾病的患者不被考虑成为肾移植候选人:严重阻塞性或限制性肺疾病、慢性肠道吸收不良和腹泻、非法使用毒品或损害社会救助系统。
- 肥胖是肾移植的相对禁忌证,与同种异体移植预后差以及伤口愈合不佳相关。大多数程序排除BMI>$40kg/m^2$患者的移植。
- 在肾移植之前需要评估现症感染、恶性肿瘤和心血管疾病风险的情况。
- 移植候选人应该筛选乙型肝炎病毒(HBV)、丙型肝炎病毒(HCV)、巨细胞病毒(CMV)、爱泼斯坦巴尔病毒(EBV)、水痘带状疱疹病毒(VZV)、人类免疫缺陷病毒(HIV)、梅毒(RPR)的血清学指标，同时行 PPD 检查排除肺结核。
- 潜在的候选人也应该进行每年适龄的癌症筛查，包括结肠镜检查、乳房 X 线检查，女性的子宫颈涂片检查和男性的 PSA 检查。
- 关于心血管疾病危险度分层，无症状移植候选人需要心脏压力测试，如果症状常常需要进行心导管检查。如发生不稳定心绞痛或心肌梗死，必须在移植之前进行血运重建治疗。
- 整个评估过程是由肾脏移植科医师指导下的移植协调员进行。
- 最终决定批准移植候选人是多学科委员会。

症状和体征
- 慢性肾脏疾病相关的体征和症状(见肾病,404 页,糖尿病中的肾脏疾病,410 页)。

临床治疗

免疫抑制
- 移植受者要终生维持免疫抑制治疗。
- 常见的方案包括小剂量糖皮质激素、抗增殖剂包括麦考酚酯(骁悉)、麦考酚酸(霉酚酸)或更少用的硫唑嘌呤(依木兰)，以及钙调神经磷酸酶抑制剂，常用的他克莫司(普乐可复)或不常用的环孢霉素(新山地明,Gengraf)。
- 西罗莫司(雷帕鸣)是一种 m-TOR 抑制剂，不常用。
- 节制激素免疫抑制方案与亚临床的活检证实的免疫反映发病率升高有关，最终导致同种异体移植病人的纤维化和瘢痕增加，所以这些方法并不常用。
- 另外，移植受者要分别预防性使用缬更昔洛韦、复方新诺明和克霉唑等抗生素治疗，来预防巨细胞病毒、卡氏肺孢子虫肺炎(PCP)和真菌(念珠菌)感染。
- 预防治疗在移植后一天开始，持续 3~6 个月。

移植后糖尿病(PTDM)
- 使用糖皮质激素会导致类固醇性糖尿病(见 171 页)。
- 钙调神经磷酸酶抑制剂(通常用于移植后免疫抑制治疗)，尤其是他克莫司，可导致胰岛素抵抗，可能与 β 细胞损伤有关。
- 他克莫司治疗与没有他克莫司治疗的患者相比，患移植后糖尿病风险升高了 53%，呈剂量依赖性。
- 西罗莫司(m-TO 抑制剂)联合钙调神经磷酸酶抑制剂治疗后，移植后糖尿病的风险也增加了。西罗莫司可能改变 β 细胞功能、降低胰岛素敏感性。
- 经肾脏代谢清除的口服降糖药(即磺酰脲类药物)应避免用于同种异体移植后肾脏功能紊乱的患者。
- 同种异体移植后肾脏功能紊乱的患者使用胰岛素剂量需要降低计量，因为胰岛素清除率下降。
- 胰腺移植后，患者的空腹血糖和糖化血红蛋白通常可以达到正常水平。肾脏移植后胰腺移植(PAK)和胰腺肾脏联合移植(SPK)后，糖尿病微血管和大血管并发症的进展均可以得到抑制。

其他移植后并发症

- 手术后免疫抑制治疗中可能发生机会性感染和恶性肿瘤。
- 明显的感染可以是原发感染或既往感染再复发，如黏膜单纯疱疹病毒的再活化。
- 感染容易在移植后第一年发生，包括巨细胞病毒、单纯疱疹病毒、卡式肺囊虫肺炎。
- EBV 感染与移植后淋巴组织增生性疾病有关。
- BK 病毒感染与同种异体移植肾脏病变有关。
- 非黑色素皮肤癌是肾移植受者中最常见恶性肿瘤，发生率是一般人群的 50 倍。
- 与非糖尿患者相比，糖尿病患者在肾移植之前和之后患心血管疾病的风险都更高。

随访

- 移植受者应由具有移植经验的肾移植科医生或普通肾科医生随访。
- 因为移植后记性排斥反应和机会性感染的风险高，患者在前 3~6 个月应密切随访，之后可减少随访频率。
- 肾功能测、完整的血细胞计数、验尿、钙调神经磷酸酶抑制剂谷浓度的是移植后常规实验室检测。
- 另外，病人应该定期检查全段甲状旁腺激素，25-OH-Vitamin D（维生素 D）。如果同种异体移植物功能正常，全段甲状旁腺激素通常在移植不久降到正常范围内，然而，有些患者需要 1 年。
- 每月、每季度检查血清 BK 病毒的 PCR，第一年之后每年检查一次。
- 如果病人有流感样症状或巨细胞病毒感染的症状，应行巨细胞病毒 PCR 检测血清。
- 移植肾肾功能恶化可能由尿路梗阻和血流动力学介导（肾前性）的氮质血症导致。
- 移植肾活检可以鉴别急性同种异体排斥反应、基本肾病复发和其他病因。

专家意见

- 肾移植仍然是终末期肾病患者最好的肾脏替代治疗方式。
- 肾移植潜在候选人应该称为肾脏科。
- 胰肾联合移植对于 1 型糖尿病的终末期肾病是一个很好的选择。
- 相对于终末期肾患者群的增长，可移植器官相对短缺，肾移植后应密切管理，按时服药、定期化验、定期随诊。
- 对有可疑感染或恶性肿瘤症状或体征的移植患者，需要保持。如果需要，及时咨询移植传染病专家。
- 照顾移植患者是一个复杂的长期的过程，需要多学科小组协作。

参考文献

Razonable RR. Strategies for managing cytomegalovirus in transplant recipients. Expert Opin Pharmacother, 2010; Vol. 11: pp. 1983–97.
  Comments: Reviews strategies for managing cytomegalovirus in transplant recipients.

Sharif A, Baboolal K. Risk factors for new-onset diabetes after kidney transplantation. Nat Rev Nephrol, 2010; Vol. 6: pp. 415–23.
Comments: A recent review of risk factors associated with post-transplant diabetes mellitus.

Sis B, Mengel M, Haas M, et al. Banff '09 meeting report: antibody mediated graft deterioration and implementation of Banff working groups. Am J Transplant, 2010; Vol. 10: pp. 464–71.
Comments: The most recent Banff classification of renal allograft pathology.

Desai NM, Schnitzler M, Jendrisak MD, et al. Maintenance steroid therapy for kidney recipients—not ready for relegation. Am J Transplant, 2009; Vol. 9: pp. 1263–4.
Comments: Discusses corticosteroid withdrawal from maintenance immunosuppressive therapy; argues that it is still early to adopt this strategy.

Cimbaluk D, Pitelka L, Kluskens L, et al. Update on human polyomavirus BK nephropathy. Diagn Cytopathol, 2009; Vol. 37: pp. 773–9.
Comments: A comprehensive review on BK virus nephropathy.

Morath C, Schmied B, Mehrabi A, et al. Simultaneous pancreas-kidney transplantation in type 1 diabetes. Clin Transplant, 2009; Vol. 23 Suppl 21: pp. 115–20.
Comments: A review of simultaneous pancreas-kidney transplantation in diabetes mellitus type 1.

Evaluation of kidney transplant candidates. In: Hricik DE, ed. Kidney Transplantation, 2nd ed. Lincolnshire, IL: Remedica Publishing; 2007: .
Comments: Discusses the approach for evaluation of potential transplant recipients.

Ekberg H, Tedesco-Silva H, Demirbas A, et al. Reduced exposure to calcineurin inhibitors in renal transplantation. NEJM, 2007; Vol. 357: pp. 2562–75.
Comments: Shows that the use of a regimen that includes mycophenolate, corticosteroids, and low-dose tacrolimus is advantageous for renal function, allograft survival, and acute rejection rates.

Ciancio G, Burke GW, Gaynor JJ, et al. A randomized long-term trial of tacrolimus/sirolimus versus tacrolimums/mycophenolate versus cyclosporine/sirolimus in renal transplantation: three-year analysis. Transplantation, 2006; Vol. 81: pp. 845–52.
Comments: Shows better graft function and fewer endocrine side-effects in mycophenolate/tacrolimus regimen when compared to sirolimus/tacrolimus regimen.

Larsen JL, Bennett RG, Burkman T, et al. Tacrolimus and sirolimus cause insulin resistance in normal Sprague dawley rats. Transplantation, 2006; Vol. 82: pp. 466–70.
Comments: Shows that tacrolimus and sirolimus have a synergistic effect on islet cell apoptosis in Sprague Dawley rats.

Vajdic CM, McDonald SP, McCredie MR, et al. Cancer incidence before and after kidney transplantation. JAMA, 2006; Vol. 296: pp. 2823–31.
Comments: Highlights the role of the interaction between the immune system and common viral infections in the etiology of cancer.

Moloney FJ, Comber H, O'Lorcain P, et al. A population-based study of skin cancer incidence and prevalence in renal transplant recipients. Br J Dermatol, 2006; Vol. 154: pp. 498–504.
Comments: Demonstrates a biphasic increase in skin cancer incidence following kidney transplantation; this was determined by the age at transplantation.

Ojo AO. Cardiovascular complications after renal transplantation and their prevention Transplantation, 2006; Vol. 82: pp. 603–11.

Comments: Discusses risk factors that confer greater risk of CVD morbidity and mortality in the posttransplant period.

Numakura K, Satoh S, Tsuchiya N, et al. Clinical and genetic risk factors for posttransplant diabetes mellitus in adult renal transplant recipients treated with tacrolimus. Transplantation, 2005; Vol. 80: pp. 1419–24.

Comments: Suggests that certain genetic polymorphisms may predict patients' risk for developing post-transplant diabetes mellitus.

Webster AC, Woodroffe RC, Taylor RS, et al. Tacrolimus versus ciclosporin as primary immunosuppression for kidney transplant recipients: meta-analysis and meta-regression of randomised trial data. BMJ, 2005; Vol. 331: p. 810.

Comments: A meta-analysis showing a higher risk for developing post-transplant diabetes mellitus with tacrolimus compared to cyclosporine.

Teutonico A, Schena PF, Di Paolo S. Glucose metabolism in renal transplant recipients: effect of calcineurin inhibitor withdrawal and conversion to sirolimus. J Am Soc Nephrol, 2005; Vol. 16: pp. 3128–35.

Comments: Shows that sirolimus is associated with worsening insulin resistance.

Cosio FG, Kudva Y, van der Velde M, et al. New onset hyperglycemia and diabetes are associated with increased cardiovascular risk after kidney transplantation. Kidney Int, 2005; Vol. 67: pp. 2415–21.

Comments: Demonstrates a significant relationship between post-transplant hyperglycemia and cardiovascular events.

Markell M. New-onset diabetes mellitus in transplant patients: pathogenesis, complications, and management. Am J Kidney Dis, 2004; Vol. 43: pp. 953–65.

Comments: A review that discusses the pathogenesis, complications, and management of post-transplant diabetesmellitus.

Kasiske BL, Snyder JJ, Gilbertson DT, et al. Cancer after kidney transplantation in the United States. Am J Transplant, 2004; Vol. 4: pp. 905–13.

Comments: Shows that the rates for most malignancies are higher after transplantation; concludes that cancerprevention should be a main focus in kidney transplant recipients.

Kasiske BL, Snyder JJ, Gilbertson D, et al. Diabetes mellitus after kidney transplantation in the United States. Am J Transplant, 2003; Vol. 3: pp. 178–85.

Comments: Analyzes data from the United Renal Data System and identifies risk factors associated with posttransplant diabetes mellitus.

Montori VM, Basu A, Erwin PJ, et al. Posttransplantation diabetes: a systematic review of the literature. Diabetes Care, 2002; Vol. 25: pp. 583–92.

Comments: Shows that immunosuppressive regimens including high-dose calcineurin inhibitors increase risk for post-transplant diabetes mellitus.

Harden PN, Fryer AA, Reece S, et al. Annual incidence and predicted risk of nonmelanoma skin cancer in renaltransplant recipients. Transplant Proc, 2001; Vol. 33: pp. 1302–4.

Comments: Identifies risk factors for developing non-melanoma skin cancer post-transplantation.

Sung RS, Althoen M, Howell TA, et al. Peripheral vascular occlusive disease in renal transplant recipients: risk factors and impact on kidney allograft survival. Transplantation, 2000; Vol. 70: pp. 1049–54.

Comments: Shows that peripheral vascular disease after transplantation is associated with reduced survival; it appears that transplantation does not accelerate or retard its progression.

Fishman JA, Rubin RH. Infection in organ-transplant recipients. NEJM, 1998; Vol. 338: pp. 1741–51.

Comments: A comprehensive review on infections in organ-transplant recipients.

National Institutes of Health, National Institute of Diabetes and Digestive and Kidney Diseases. US Renal Data System. USRDS 2008 Annual Data Report: Atlas of Chronic Kidney Disease and End-Stage Renal Disease in the United States. Bethesda, MD. Available at: http://www.usrds.org/2008/view/ckd_00_intro.asp (accessed 3/4/2011).

Comments: The national data registry that collects and analyzes information on the end-stage renal disease population in the US.

U.S. Department of Health and Human Services, Health Resources and Services Administration, Healthcare Systems Bureau, Division of Transplantation, 2008 Annual Report of the U.S. Organ Procurement and Transplantation Network and the Scientific Registry of Transplant Recipients: Transplant Data 1998–2007. Rockville, MD. Available at: http://optn.transplant.hrsa.gov/ar2008/ (accessed 3/4/2011).

Comments: Organ Procurement and Transplantation Network and the Scientific Registry of Transplant Recipients.

糖尿病的膀胱疾病

Nisa M. Maruthur, MD, MHS

定义
- 糖尿病(DM)的膀胱功能障碍包括从下尿路症状(LUTS)(如膀胱失禁)到糖尿病膀胱病变的一系列症候群。
- 逼尿肌、神经和泌尿道上皮细胞功能障碍是糖尿病膀胱功能障碍的基础。
- 急迫性尿失禁:当感觉要小便时不知觉的排尿。由神经源性逼尿肌过度活跃所致(也就是指痉挛性膀胱)。
- 压力性尿失禁:在身体活动时无意识的排尿,如咳嗽、喷嚏、大笑或运动。通常由于骨盆底肌肉无力。
- 糖尿病性膀胱:膀胱感觉和收缩障碍导致尿潴留,是糖尿病中最严重的膀胱疾病。通常由于自主神经病变(也称为神经性膀胱)。

流行病学
- 超过50%的糖尿病患者有膀胱功能障碍(如尿失禁),糖尿病性膀胱罕见(Brown)。
- 美国糖尿病女性,35%的人至少每周发生一次尿失禁,26%至少每周一次急迫性尿失禁,30%的人至少每周一次压力失禁;相应的,那些血浆葡萄糖正常的各种尿失禁发生率(NHANES)是17%、8%和14%(Brown、Vittinghoff)。
- 良性前列腺增生是一种常见的疾病,可能与下尿路症状及男性糖尿病人膀胱功能障碍有关。
- 在糖尿病预防计划中,强化生活方式干预,减轻体重和增加活动量,可以减少二甲双胍和安慰剂治疗的高危女性的每周尿失禁患病率(Brown, Wing, 2006)。

诊断
- 符合膀胱功能障碍的症状和体征通常即可诊断。
- 尿动力学测试可以由泌尿科医生进行:膀胱内测量法、括约肌肌电图、尿疗、尿道压力。

症状和体征
- 下尿路症状:尿频,尿急、夜尿症和尿失禁。
- 糖尿病膀胱:尿意减少,膀胱排空不完全,排尿频率减少。
- 尿动力学结果随不同的膀胱功能障碍阶段发生变化,但可以显示膀胱容量的增加,随着时间的推移逼尿肌收缩力减低,残余尿增加。
- 经过排尿反射减少,证实糖尿病膀胱可以导致膀胱迟缓。
- 其他自主神经病变(如体位性低血压)也可能被发现。
- 膀胱功能障碍可能会导致尿路感染。

临床治疗
- 压力性尿失禁:膀胱和女性盆腔肌肉训练。
- 急迫性尿失禁:抗胆碱能药物(如奥昔布宁,604页)。

- 定期排尿，固定时间间隔。
- 血糖控制很重要，因为神经病变可能导致膀胱功能障碍。然而 DCCT/EDIC 男性进行强化血糖控制的下尿路症状患病率并无减少 (Van Den Eeden)。
- 糖尿病膀胱：胆碱能受体激动剂（如氨甲酰甲胆碱，601 页）。
- 异常严重的病例间断导尿治疗。
- 泌尿科咨询。

专家意见
- 定期评估可能的膀胱功能障碍的症状。
- 突发膀胱症状的改变应该通过尿检和 / 或尿培养评估感染。

参考文献

Danforth KN, Townsend MK, Curhan GC, et al. Type 2 diabetes mellitus and risk of stress, urge and mixed urinary incontinence. J Urol, 2009; Vol. 181: pp. 193–7.
Comments: Study showing that DM is associated with incident urinary incontinence (urge incontinence in particular) in the Nurses' Health Study.

Brown JS. Diabetic cystopathy—what does it mean? J Urol, 2009; Vol. 181: pp. 13–4.
Comments: Editorial on meaning of diabetic cystopathy.

Van Den Eeden SK, Sarma AV, Rutledge BN, et al. Effect of intensive glycemic control and diabetes complications on lower urinary tract symptoms in men with type 1 diabetes: Diabetes Control and Complications Trial/Epidemiology of Diabetes Interventions and Complications (DCCT/EDIC) study. Diabetes Care, 2009; Vol. 32: pp. 664–70.
Comments: Potentially underpowered analysis of UroEDIC cohort showing no effect of intensive glucose control on LUTS.

Brown JS, Vittinghoff E, Lin F, et al. Prevalence and risk factors for urinary incontinence in women with type 2 diabetes and impaired fasting glucose: findings from the National Health and Nutrition Examination Survey (NHANES) 2001–2002. Diabetes Care, 2006; Vol. 29: pp. 1307–12.
Comments: Nationally representative study (NHANES) evaluating prevalence of urinary incontinence in women with DM, impaired glucose tolerance, and normal fasting glucose.

Brown JS, Wing R, Barrett-Connor E, et al. Lifestyle intervention is associated with lower prevalence of urinary incontinence: the Diabetes Prevention Program. Diabetes Care, 2006; Vol. 29: pp. 385–90.
Comments: Analysis of Diabetes Prevention Program data showing decreased prevalence of weekly urinary incontinence in the lifestyle intervention relative to the metformin and placebo groups.

Brown JS, Wessells H, Chancellor MB, et al. Urologic complications of diabetes. Diabetes Care, 2005; Vol. 28: pp. 177–85.
Comments: Unstructured review of urologic complications of DM.

Sasaki K, Yoshimura N, Chancellor MB. Implications of diabetes mellitus in urology. Urol Clin North Am, 2003; Vol. 30: pp. 1–12.
Comments: Review of urologic complications in DM.

Wein, AJ. Lower urinary tract dysfunction in neurologic injury and disease. In Wein, AJ (Ed.), Campbell-Walsh Urology, 9th edition, Philadelphia: Saunders Elsevier; 2007: chapter 59.
Comments: Chapter from Campbell's urology reviewing bladder dysfunction in DM.

第四部分

药物

心血管疾病	433
补充和替代医学	440
脂代谢紊乱	445
勃起功能障碍	469
胃轻瘫	473
降糖治疗	482
升高血糖	523
高血压	545
肾病	587
神经病变	590
肥胖	595
泌尿系统	601

心血管疾病

抗凝药物使用

Sheldon H. Gottlieb, MD, and Paul A. Pham, PharmD

适应证

FDA（美国食品药品监督管理局）
阿司匹林
- 二级预防：短暂性脑缺血发作（transient ischemic attack，TIA）和缺血性脑卒中（ischemic stroke）的治疗；预防反复发作的心肌梗死（myocardial infarction，MI）；降低心肌梗死及不稳定型心绞痛和慢性稳定型心绞痛突发猝死的风险；用于血管成形术、冠状动脉搭桥术和颈动脉内膜切除术后。

氯吡格雷
- 二级预防：急性冠状动脉综合征（不稳定型心绞痛，非 ST 段抬高型心肌梗死）的患者，包括那些准备进行冠状动脉血管重建术的患者；ST 段抬高型心肌梗死的患者；心梗后、脑卒中后和确诊为外周血管疾病的患者。

华法林
- 二级适应证：预防和治疗心房纤颤、机械心瓣引起的血栓栓塞，降低心梗后脑卒中或心梗复发的风险，预防和治疗高危患者发生静脉血栓或血栓栓塞。

非 FDA 批准的用法
阿司匹林
- 糖尿病患者发生心血管事件的一级预防（见"日常预防保健"，72 页）。

氯吡格雷
- 一级预防：尚未建立。

华法林
- 一级预防：尚未建立。

机制
- 阿司匹林：不可逆地结合（乙酰化）环氧合酶（cyclooxygenase，COX），并抑制其功能，从而预防血小板聚集血栓烷 A2 形成复合物。
- 氯吡格雷：氯吡格雷的活性代谢产物可与血小板 ADP 受体的 P2Y12 亚型不可逆地结合，从而抑制血小板聚集。
- 华法林：抑制对维生素 K 有依赖性的凝结因子，从而抑制血液凝结。

成人通常使用的药物剂量
- 阿司匹林：每天 75~325mg。

- 氯吡格雷：每天 75mg。老年人无剂量调整。
- 华法林：剂量有很强的个体化差异，与遗传因素（CYP2C9 和 VKORC1 基因型）、是否服用维生素 K 以及同时服用的其他药物有很大关系。通常每日剂量在 2~7.5mg 之间。对于老年人、CYP2C9 和 VKORC1 基因型的患者推荐使用较小剂量。根据目标的 INR 范围调整剂量。

剂型
- 见表 4-1。

特殊人群的用药剂量

肾病的患者
- 阿司匹林：严重肾衰的病人禁用（GFR<10ml/min）。
- 氯吡格雷：数据有限，使用需慎重。
- 华法林：进行性肾衰竭需使用较小剂量。透析患者应用时需非常谨慎；其效益可能较小并且可能增加血管硬化（Bennett）。

肝病的患者
- 阿司匹林：严重肝功能不全的患者禁用。
- 氯吡格雷：无剂量调整。
- 华法林：慎重使用；剂量有很强的个体化特点；中至重度肝功能不全的患者具有很高的发生出血并发症的危险。

孕妇
- 阿司匹林：C 类。妊娠早期和中期的孕妇只有当明显需要时方可使用。妊娠晚期禁用，因为此时阿司匹林对胎儿循环系统有潜在影响（可能导致动脉导管闭锁），且可增加孕妇的出血倾向。
- 氯吡格雷：B 类。对动物妊娠期的研究尚未证明对胎儿的危险，但缺乏人群方面的数据。
- 华法林：X 类。孕妇和可能将要怀孕的女性禁用。华法林可通过胎盘屏障。具有很高的致胎儿死亡和畸形的危险。

哺乳期女性
- 阿司匹林：在母乳中有分泌，所以哺乳期应该谨慎使用。
- 氯吡格雷：避免使用，尚不知在人类母乳中是否有分泌。
- 华法林：在母体血液循环中有很高的蛋白结合能力；在母乳中分泌很少，因此哺乳期使用相对安全。

药物不良反应

一般
- 所有抗凝药都可能增加出血风险。

常见
- 阿司匹林：胃肠道不耐受（呈剂量依赖性）。

偶见

- 阿司匹林：耳鸣（大剂量且/或长期使用）；食管、胃、消化道溃疡；肾毒性（如急性间质性肾炎或肾前性急性肾小管坏死），尿酸增加（呈剂量依赖性）；反跳性头痛（长期使用阿司匹林）；大剂量使用引起酸碱平衡紊乱（如代谢性酸中毒或呼吸性碱中毒）。

罕见

- 阿司匹林：严重过敏，皮疹；血细胞减少症（如白细胞减少症、血小板减少症、粒细胞缺乏症、再生障碍性贫血）；过敏反应；雷氏综合征（水痘病毒感染后）；肝炎。
- 氯吡格雷：中性粒细胞减少症；血栓性血小板减少性紫癜（TTP）；过敏反应；严重过敏；肝炎。
- 华法林：继发于胆固醇微血栓形成的紫趾综合征（用药后3~10周间起病），表现为脚趾变紫、疼痛、敏感。如果不停用华法林，可能会导致坏疽、组织坏死、皮疹、气管支气管钙化。

药物相互作用

- 阿司匹林：非甾体类抗炎药干扰阿司匹林与血小板的结合。大多数副作用和剂量有关。
- 氯吡格雷：氯吡格雷在肝中被细胞色素 P450 2C19（CYP2C19）转变为活性代谢产物，所以 CYP2C19 的抑制剂（如奥美拉唑、埃索美拉唑、甲氰咪胍、氟康唑、酮康唑、伏立康唑、依曲韦林、非氨酯、氟西汀、氟伏沙明）可能降低氯吡格雷的效果，避免这些药和氯吡格雷同服。
- 华法林：和华法林有潜在的相互作用的药物包括：破坏止血或凝血因子合成的药物，对维生素K有竞争性的拮抗作用的药物；和华法林有药代动力学方面的相互作用的药物包括：具有肝酶诱导作用的药物（如利福平）或肝酶抑制作用的药物（如氟康唑），能够降低血浆结合力的药物；或因存在其他共存的疾病而影响华法林的药代动力学，这些共存疾病包括但不仅限于血液病、癌症、胶原血管病、心衰、腹泻、发热、肝功能异常、甲亢、营养缺乏（包括维生素K缺乏）、脂肪痢。

  - 能使华法林的抗凝作用增加的药物包括：磺胺甲基异噁唑、红霉素、氟康唑、异烟肼、甲硝哒唑、胺碘酮、氯贝丁酯、丙胺苯丙酮、心得安、磺吡酮、苯基丁氮酮、吡罗昔康、酒精、甲氰咪胍、奥美拉唑。

  - 具有降低华法林抗凝作用效果的药物：灰黄霉素、利福平、乙氧萘青霉素、巴比妥酸盐、卡马西平、甲氨二氮卓、消胆胺、硫糖铝。

  - 和华法林相互作用的药物很多，其他的与其相互作用的药物详见网站：http://www.drugs.com/drug-interactions.warfarin.html.

- 应对患者进行关于华法林可能的药物相互作用的教育（见表4-2）。

专家意见

- 尚无明确证据显示，阿司匹林作为糖尿病患者发生心血管疾病的一级预防用药，可使糖尿病患者获益；但阿司匹林可能对有很高的心血管疾病发生风险的糖尿病患者获益最大（比如 >10%）。然而，FDA 只批准阿司匹林作为二级预防用药（而非一级预防用药）。
- 最近的指南认识到阿司匹林治疗可增加潜在的出血风险，所以限制了阿司匹林作为心血管疾病的一级预防用药，即使患者可能获益于服用阿司匹林来预防心血管疾病。
- 每位患者服用阿司匹林都需个体化。
- 氯吡格雷和华法林更推荐于血栓栓塞性疾病或不适合使用阿司匹林的患者。

药代动力学

表 4-1 抗凝药的药代动力学和剂型

药物	吸收	代谢	清除	剂型	价格
阿司匹林	快速持续时间：4~6小时	在酯酶的作用下水解成有活性的水杨酸。水杨酸在肝中结合代谢。	经尿；原药的$T_{1/2}$为15~20分钟；水杨酸的$T_{1/2}$有剂量依赖性：小剂量（300~600mg）为3小时，中等剂量（1~2g）为5~6小时，较大剂量（>2~4g）为10小时。	一般剂型包括：可嚼服81mg；常规的包有肠溶衣的为81、325、500mg；控释剂为800mg；包有肠溶衣的为975mg	不同厂商价格有差异。可嚼服81mg剂型（36片）为11.99美元，325mg剂型（100片）为11.99美元，控释片800mg剂型（100片）为125.53美元，包有肠溶衣的975mg剂型（90片）为11.25美元。
氯吡格雷	吸收良好	完全在肝中通过CYP450介导而氧化为活化的硫醇代谢物。	经尿、便；$T_{1/2}$约为6小时	唯一厂家生产，75mg和300mg片剂。	75mg（30片）为165.99美元。

表 4-1 抗凝药的药代动力学和剂型（续）

药物	吸收	代谢	清除	剂型	价格
华法林	吸收快速且完全。起效时间：24~72小时。完全起治疗所用的时间：5~7天。持续时间：2~5天。	S-华法林（更强效的异构体）在肝中经CYP2C9代谢。少量通过CYP2C8、2C18、2C19、1A2、3A4代谢（R-华法林）	经尿；$T_{1/2}$=20~60小时，平均约40小时，个体差异较大（基于CYP2C9和VKORC1基因型的差异）。	一般可获得的片剂：1、2、2.5、3、4、5、7.5和10mg。	1mg（30片）为13.99美元，2mg（30片）为14.88美元，2.5mg（30片）为14.99美元，3mg（30片）为15.99美元，4mg（30片）为14.99美元，5mg（30片）为13.99美元，7.5mg（30片）为23.21美元，10mg（30片）为24.24美元。

表 4-2. 对服用香豆素类药的患者进行的解释

1. 为什么需要这样的治疗。
2. 药物是如何作用的。
3. 为什么需要监测。
4. 为什么每天固定时间服药很重要。
5. 酒精如何影响到抗凝效果，并如何增加出血的风险。
6. 食物的改变如何影响疗效。
7. 药物相互作用可能是如何影响到治疗的。
8. 为什么应该将改变用药告诉诊所的工作人员。
9. 应该采取什么样的措施来预防出血。
10. 如何识别出血的症状和体征。

*Green D. Avoiding "sticker" shock. Blood, 2009; Vol. 114: pp. 930 - 1. Reproduced with permission of The American Society of Hematology (ASH).

参考文献

Würtz M, Grove EL, Kristensen SD, et al. The antiplatelet effect of aspirin is reduced by proton pump inhibitors in patients with coronary artery disease. Heart, 2010; Vol. 96: pp. 368–71.

Comments: Proton pump inhibitors (PPI) may reduce aspirin effect on platelet aggregation. This topic remains controversial; PPI use should be monitored and dose adjusted to effect.

Pignone M, Alberts MJ, Colwell JA, et al. Aspirin for primary prevention of cardiovascular events in people with diabetes: a position statement of the American Diabetes Association, a scientific statement of the American Heart Association, and an expert consensus document of the American College of Cardiology Foundation. Diabetes Care, 2010; Vol. 33: pp. 1395–402.

Comments: This position statement by the ADA, AHA, and ACC outlines recommendations for use of low dose ASA (75–162 mg/day) in the primary prevention of cardiovascular disease in diabetes.

De Berardis G, Sacco M, Strippoli GF, et al. Aspirin for primary prevention of cardiovascular events in people with diabetes: meta-analysis of randomised controlled trials. BMJ 2009; Vol. 339: p. b4531.

Comments: This meta-analysis of 6 trials found that though ASA reduced risk of cardiovascular outcomes by 6–17%, no significant difference was found compared to placebo. Increased risk of bleeding and GI symptoms was noted in a few studies but not significant. ASA significantly reduced MI risk in men but not women.

Antithrombotic Trialists' (ATT) Collaboration, Baigent C, Blackwell L, et al. Aspirin in the primary and secondary prevention of vascular disease: collaborative meta-analysis of individual participant data from randomised trials. Lancet, 2009; Vol. 373: pp. 1849–60.

Comments: The use of aspirin in primary prevention remains controversial; the authors recommend that guidelines be "relaxed" until more information is available. See Expert Opinion section.

Haynes R, Bowman L, Armitage J. Aspirin for primary prevention of vascular disease in people with diabetes. BMJ, 2009; Vol. 339: p. b4596.

Comments: A review of the uncertainty surrounding the use of aspirin for prevention of CV events, and a call to encourage patients to enroll in clinical trials to help determine who should receive aspirin.

Price HC, Holman RR. Primary prevention of cardiovascular events in diabetes: is there a role for aspirin? Nat Clin Pract Cardiovasc Med, 2009; Vol. 6: pp. 168–9.

Comments: This article summarizes the evidence for use of aspirin in primary prevention of CVD.

Connolly SJ, Ezekowitz MD, Yusuf S, et al. Dabigatran versus warfarin in patients with atrial fibrillation. NEJM, 2009; Vol. 361: pp. 1139–51.

Comments: This was a non-inferiority trial of dabigatran, an oral direct thrombin inhibitor, versus warfarin, in patients with atrial fibrillation. Outcomes were similar. Dabigatran scheduled to be reviewed by the FDA in the summer of 2010.

Singer DE, Chang Y, Fang MC, et al. The net clinical benefit of warfarin anticoagulation in atrial fibrillation. Ann Intern Med, 2009; Vol. 151: pp. 297–305.

Comments: Study documents risks and benefits of warfarin use in patients with atrial fibrillation, based on CHADS(2) score. Older high-risk patients benefit the most, despite risk of hemorrhage.

Green D. Avoiding "sticker" shock. Blood, 2009; Vol. 114: pp. 930–1.

Comments: Practical review of laboratory monitoring of anticoagulation with useful patient information.

Singla A, Antonino MJ, Bliden KP, et al. The relation between platelet reactivity and glycemic control in diabetic patients with cardiovascular disease on maintenance aspirin and clopidogrel therapy. Am Heart J, 2009; Vol. 158: pp. 784.e1–6.

Comments: In patients with type 2 diabetes treated with dual antiplatelet agents, poor glycemic control is associated with greater platelet reactivity; these patients may require adjustment of antiplatelet regimen.

Bennett WM. Should dialysis patients ever receive warfarin and for what reasons? Clin J Am Soc Nephrol, 2006; Vol. 1: pp. 1357–1359.

Comments: This article reviews the use of warfarin in dialysis patients.

Vane JR, Botting RM. The mechanism of action of aspirin. Thromb Res, 2003; Vol. 110: pp. 255–8.

Comments: VComments: Vane won the Nobel Prize for his studies of aspirin effects.

Savi P, Nurden P, Nurden AT, et al. Clopidogrel: a review of its mechanism of action. Platelets, 1998; Vol. 9: pp. 251–5.

Comments: In-depth review of important drug.

US Food and Drug Administration (FDA). Aspirin: Questions and Answers. Available online at http://www.fda.gov/ Drugs/ResourcesForYou/Consumers/QuestionsAnswers/ucm071879.htm (accessed 7/15/2010).

补充和替代医学

草药

Todd T. Brown, MD, PhD, and Paul A. Pham, PharmD

定义
- 草药是指利用植物或植物的一部分达到医治目的。
- 也称为植物医学或植物药学。
- 在不同文化中很多不同的草药被用来治疗糖尿病。
- 但很少被系统地评估其有效性和安全性。
- 这一章将讨论一些经科学评估的草药。

流行病学
- 在美国,超过 1/3 的糖尿病患者使用草药或传统治疗方案(Egede)。

临床治疗
人参
- 最被广泛使用的草药之一。
- 两种主要类型:亚洲人参(Panax ginseng)和美洲人参(也称花旗参,Panax quinquefolius)。
- 人参皂苷被认为是有效成分(仅同一种类的人参含皂苷可达 20~30 种,不同人参含有的人参皂苷种类有所不同);非人参皂苷成分可能也有一定的生理作用(Attele,1999)。
- 机制:临床前期数据显示人参皂苷可改善胰岛素抵抗(Attele,2002)。
- 效果:临床数据有限。人参根被使用得最普遍(Vuksan),剂量 1~3g/d。人参的其他部分也被尝试使用过(包括其果实和叶子等)。
- 不良反应:高血压、恶心、头痛、失眠、精神紧张。
- 草药 – 药物相互作用:与华法林同时使用可降低华法林的治疗作用(Yuan)。

肉桂(学名:Cinnamon cassia)
- 机制:可能增强胰岛素信号传导,增加糖原合成酶活性(Qin)。
- 效果:人群的临床试验使用剂量是 1~6g/d。短期使用对降低空腹血糖有一定效果(5%~24%),但结果尚不一致(Kirkham)。
- 安全性:尚没有不良反应报道。
- 草药 – 药物相互作用:尚不知。

苦瓜(学名:Momordica charantia)
- 在很多不同文化中苦瓜被作为传统的治疗糖尿病药物,包括印度草药医学(阿育吠陀医学)。
- 机制:可能通过活化 AMP 激酶改善胰岛素抵抗(Miura;Cheng)。

- 临床效果：在很多案例中显示有一定益处，但两个随机对照研究显示没有效果（Leung）。显示其有效果的研究使用苦瓜汁或新鲜苦瓜，而不是苦瓜干。最近的综述发现没有足够证据推荐苦瓜来治疗2型糖尿病（Ooi）。
- 不良反应：有一些报道显示有胃肠道不适，葡萄糖-6-磷酸酶缺乏症患者食用苦瓜籽可引发蚕豆病。
- 草药–药物相互作用：尚未知。

葫芦巴（或称"苦豆"，Trigonella foenum-graecum）

- 在亚洲和地中海文化中葫芦巴是传统植物。印度草药医学使用葫芦巴的叶子和种子作为药物。
- 机制：葫芦巴含有的4-羟基异亮氨酸可能促进胰岛素释放（Sauvarie）。此外，葫芦巴富含纤维。
- 效果：有限，短期数据显示结果不一致。剂量：10~100g葫芦巴粉用餐时口服（Basch）。
- 不良反应：短暂的腹泻、胃肠气胀、眩晕（Basch）。
- 草药–药物相互作用：尚未知。

匙羹藤（学名：Gymnema sylvestre）

- 在印度草药医学中匙羹藤叶子被用来治疗糖尿病、高胆固醇血症和肥胖。在印度语中还有一名字叫"gurmar"（意为"灭糖者"）。
- 机制：不清楚。一些证据显示它对胰岛素分泌有效果（Liu）。
- 效果：在一些小型的质量有限的临床试验中显示有一些益处（将糖化血红蛋白降低约0.6%）。使用剂量：匙羹藤液提取物200~400mg，每天两次（Leach）。
- 不良反应：尚无报道。
- 草药–药物相互作用：尚未知。

专家意见

在很多文化中草药来源的成分被用来治疗糖尿病。

虽然一些研究显示部分草药成分有一定益处，但是目前没有足够证据推荐任何一种草药来治疗糖尿病。

虽然已使用的草药剂量一般都能被人体耐受，但有些草药成分有明显的药物相互作用（比如人参和华法林同用），这些尚需进一步研究。

参考文献

Ooi CP, Yassin Z, Hamid TA. Momordica charantia for type 2 diabetes mellitus. Cochrane Database Syst Rev, 2010; Vol. 2: CD007845.

Comments: Cochrane review of 3 randomized trials found insufficient evidence to recommend Momordica charantia for treatment of type 2 diabetes.

Arkham S, Akilen R, Sharma S, et al. The potential of cinnamon to reduce blood glucose levels in patients with type 2 diabetes and insulin resistance. Diabetes Obes Metab, 2009; Vol. 11: pp. 1100–13.

Comments: Good review of human cinnamon/diabetes studies.

Leung L, Birtwhistle R, Kotecha J, et al. Anti-diabetic and hypoglycaemic effects of Momordica charantia (bitter melon): a mini review. Br J Nutr, 2009; Vol. 102: pp. 1703–8.

Comments: Good review of human bitter melon/diabetes studies.

Liu B, Asare-Anane H, Al-Romaiyan A, et al. Characterisation of the insulinotropic activity of an aqueous extract of Gymnema sylvestre in mouse beta-cells and human islets of Langerhans. Cell Physiol Biochem, 2009; Vol. 23: pp. 125–32.
Comments: New study investigating the mechanisms underlying fenugreek.

Cheng HL, Huang HK, Chang CI, et al. A cell-based screening identifies compounds from the stem of Momordica charantia that overcome insulin resistance and activate AMP activated protein kinase. J Agric Food Chem, 2008; Vol. 56: pp. 6835–43.
Comments: This paper provides some evidence that Momoridica charantia may improve insulin resistance.

Vuksan V, Sievenpiper JL. Herbal remedies in the management of diabetes: lessons learned from the study of ginseng. Nutr Metab Cardiovasc Dis, 2005; Vol. 15: pp. 149–60.
Comments: Good review of clinical effect by research team who have completed many of the human studies.

Yuan CS, Wei G, Dey L, et al. Brief communication: American ginseng reduces warfarin effect in healthy patients: a randomized, controlled trial. Ann Intern Med, 2004; Vol. 141: pp. 23–7.
Comments: Identifies important interaction between ginseng and warfarin.

Qin B, Nagasaki M, Ren M, et al. Cinnamon extract (traditional herb) potentiates in vivo insulin regulated glucose utilization via enhancing insulin signaling in rats. Diabetes Res Clin Pract, 2003; Vol. 62: pp. 139–48.
Comments: Shows potential mechanism of cinnamon.

Basch E, Ulbricht C, Kuo G, et al. Therapeutic applications of fenugreek. Altern Med Rev, 2003; Vol. 8: pp. 20–7.
Comments: Good review of clinical studies on fenugreek.

Egede LE, Ye X, Zheng D, et al. The prevalence and pattern of complementary and alternative medicine use in individuals with diabetes. Diabetes Care, 2002; Vol. 25: pp. 324–9.
Comments: Survey of CAM usage among patients with diabetes.

Attele AS, Zhou YP, Xie JT, et al. Antidiabetic effects of Panax ginseng berry extract and the identification of an effective component. Diabetes, 2002; Vol. 51: pp. 1851–8.
Comments: Shows effect of ginseng on insulin resistance.

Miura T, Itoh C, Iwamoto N, et al. Hypoglycemic activity of the fruit of the Momordica charantia in type 2 diabetic mice. J Nutr Sci Vitaminol (Tokyo), 2001; Vol. 47: pp. 340–4.
Comments: Further evidence that Momoridica charantia may improve insulin resistance.

Attele AS, Wu JA, Yuan CS. Ginseng pharmacology: multiple constituents and multiple actions. Biochem Pharmacol, 1999; Vol. 58: pp. 1685–93.
Comments: Good review of ginseng pharmacology.

Sauvaire Y, Petit P, Broca C, et al. 4-Hydroxyisoleucine: a novel amino acid potentiator of insulin secretion. Diabetes, 1998; Vol. 47: pp. 206–10.
Comments: Identifies a potential active compound and mechanism for fenugreek.

非草药方面

Todd T. Brown, MD, PhD, and Paul A. Pham, PharmD

定义

- 非草药方面的治疗是指不是利用植物为基础的治疗糖尿病的补充或替代医学方法。
- 很少被系统地评估效果或安全性。
- 本章讨论那些已经有对照评估的非草药方法。

临床治疗

铬

- 在碳水化合物和脂肪代谢中有重要作用的必要成分。铬缺乏导致可逆性的胰岛素抵抗和糖尿病。
- 最常见的剂型是吡啶甲酸铬和啤酒酵母。
- 近期的一项荟萃分析显示:以200~1 000g的剂量,服用6~26周,可将糖化血红蛋白水平平均降低0.6%(95%CI:-0.9~0.2),且能将空腹血糖平均降低1mmol/L(95%CI:-1.4~0.5)。但是超过半数的相关研究质量都很差(Pittler)。
- 随机对照研究显示铬可能对控制体重有一些作用(6~14周减轻1.1kg体重)(Pittler),并且可能减轻服用磺脲类药物所致的体重增加(Martin)。
- 在综述所提的文章中未报道铬有明显不良反应。
- 和其他药物的相互作用尚不知。
- 虽然有一些初步的临床试验看起来显示铬的作用尚可,但能否利用铬来治疗糖尿病尚需大型的设计质量高的临床研究。

钒

- 钒可能通过抑制酪氨酸磷酸酶从而影响胰岛素受体(Verma)。
- 在小型的无对照的研究中,硫酸氧钒或偏钒酸钠以50~300mg/d的剂量给药3~6周,可降低空腹血糖13~40mg/dl,并降低糖化血红蛋白0.4%~0.8%(Smith)。一项近期的研究(Jacques-Camerena)显示钒对胰岛素敏感性无影响,但可增加甘油三酯水平。
- 常见不良反应包括胃肠道不适、胀气、恶心等。
- 不推荐使用钒来治疗糖尿病。

钙和维生素D

- 观察研究证明2型糖尿病和维生素D缺乏相关。
- 可能的机制:维生素D参与beta细胞功能和胰岛素作用,并减少炎症反应。钙可能也影响胰岛素作用和分泌。
- 临床试验未证明钙或维生素D对治疗高血糖有明确益处。对一随机临床试验的事后分析显示:糖耐量受损的患者每天口服700IU维生素D3和钙500mg超过三年,可减少血糖的升高和胰岛素抵抗(Pittas)。

- 尚需进一步研究来证实维生素 D 和钙对糖尿病的益处，并决定最佳剂量。因为糖尿病患者骨质疏松和骨折很常见，为了骨骼健康，推荐糖尿病患者每日钙的剂量为 1 000~1 200mg，每日维生素 D 的剂量为 800~1000IU。
- 见维生素 D（613 页）。

专家意见
- 铬对改善糖尿病患者的糖代谢可能有一些益处。但需要经过大型的长期的研究来证实铬是否可被推荐为常规药物。

参考文献

Jacques-Camarena O, Gonz.lez-Ortiz M, Martz-Abundis E, et al. Effect of vanadium on insulin sensitivity in patients with impaired glucose tolerance. Ann Nutr Metab, 2008; Vol. 53: pp. 195–8.
Comments: Well-designed negative study on effect of vanadium on insulin sensitivity.

Smith DM, Pickering RM, Lewith GT. A systematic review of vanadium oral supplements for glycaemic control in type 2 diabetes mellitus. QJM, 2008; Vol. 101: pp. 351–8.
Comments: Good review of existing evidence of safety and efficacy of vanadium on diabetes and insulin resistance.

Smith DM, Pickering RM, Lewith GT. A systematic review of vanadium oral supplements for glycaemic control in type 2 diabetes mellitus. QJM, 2008; Vol. 101: pp. 351–8.
Comments: Review of vanadium effect on glycemia.

Pittas AG, Lau J, Hu FB, et al. The role of vitamin D and calcium in type 2 diabetes. A systematic review and metaanalysis. J Clin Endocrinol Metab, 2007; Vol. 92: pp. 2017–29.
Comments: Well-designed meta-analysis summarizing the data on the effect of calcium and vitamin D on glucose outcomes.

Martin J, Wang ZQ, Zhang XH, et al. Chromium picolinate supplementation attenuates body weight gain and increases insulin sensitivity in subjects with type 2 diabetes. Diabetes Care, 2006; Vol. 29: pp. 1826–32.
Comments: Well-designed randomized trial of chromium's effect on insulin sensitivity.

Pittler MH, Stevinson C, Ernst E. Chromium picolinate for reducing body weight: meta-analysis of randomized trials. Int J Obes Relat Metab Disord, 2003; Vol. 27: pp. 522–9.
Comments: Good meta-analysis of chromium's effect on glucose and weight.

Verma S, Cam MC, McNeill JH. Nutritional factors that can favorably influence the glucose/insulin system: vanadium. J Am Coll Nutr, 1998; Vol. 17: pp. 11–8.
Comments: Review about potential mechanisms of vanadium on glucose metabolism.

脂代谢紊乱

胆汁酸螯合剂

Simeon Margolis, MD, PhD, and Paul A. Pham, PharmD

适应证

FDA

高胆固醇血症：预防心血管疾病或其并发症。

控制欠佳的 2 型糖尿病：降低 HbA1c（考来维仑）。

缓解局部胆道梗阻相关的瘙痒感（考来烯胺）。

机制

在肠内和胆汁酸结合，继而随大便排泄。为代偿胆汁酸的减少，肝将更多的胆固醇转化为胆汁酸。

肝中胆固醇的减少使 LDL 受体合成增加，从而增加血中 LDL 的清除，并降低血清中总胆固醇和 LDL 胆固醇。

常成人使用的剂量

考来烯胺粉剂：可给予 1~2 袋或 1~2 勺，qd 或 bid。维持剂量：每天 2~4 袋或勺（8~16g 无水考来烯胺酯），分两次与餐同服。

考来替泊片剂：每天 2~16g（2~16 片），1 次或分次口服；起始剂量：2g,qd 或 bid；每 1~2 个月递增 2g 至维持剂量。或考来替泊颗粒：5~30g（1~6 袋或勺，1 次或分次口服），治疗起始阶段予 2g, qd 或 bid。

考来维仑盐酸盐：6 片（3.75g）qd 或 3 片（1.875g）bid，与餐或水同服。食用前，充分搅拌或用华林牌搅拌器将粉剂混匀。

剂型

商品名	通用名	剂型	价格
消胆胺（多家制药公司生产）	考来烯胺	4g（口服粉剂）	2.12 美元
降脂树脂 2 号（Pfizer 和其他一些制药公司）	考来替泊	5g（口服颗粒） 7.5g（口服颗粒，添加矫味剂） 1g（口服片剂）	2.7 美元 3.17 美元 0.84 美元
WelChol（SANKYO 制药公司）	考来维仑盐酸盐	625mg（口服片剂）	1.36 美元

特殊人群的用药剂量

肾病患者
- 尚无数据。参照常用剂量。

肝病患者
- 商务数据。参照常用剂量。

孕妇
- B 类。

哺乳期女性
- 在母乳中未发现有存在；但胆汁酸螯合剂会干扰脂溶性维生素的吸收，所以哺乳期妇女需谨慎使用。

药物不良反应

一般
- 除了引起便秘，一般人对胆汁酸螯合剂耐受性很好。

常见
- 便秘。

偶见
- 嗳气，胃胀。

罕见
- 胃痛。
- 恶心和呕吐。

药物相互作用
- 能够干扰多种口服药物的吸收。
- 为减少药物相互作用，其他药物需在服用考来烯胺前至少 1 小时或服后至少 4~6 小时，或在服用考来维仑前 4 小时。
- 和以下的药物相互作用，可导致药物治疗作用的消失：噻嗪类利尿剂、呋塞米、格列吡嗪、普萘洛尔、口服的青霉素、口服的万古霉素、四素、脂溶性维生素（如维生素 A、D、E、K），铁补充剂、左旋甲状腺素、雷洛昔芬、地高辛、甲氨蝶呤、熊去氧胆酸、丙咪嗪、丙戊酸、一些甾体类抗炎药、吉非贝齐、以及非诺贝特。
- 华法林：和华法林同服可能升高或降低 INR。
- 依泽替米贝：作用可能会下降。依泽替米贝的服用应该在服用胆汁酸合剂前至少 2 小时或服用后至少 4 小时。

药代动力学
- 吸收：胆汁酸螯合剂不被吸收。它们在肠内起作用。
- 代谢：不被消化酶水解。
- 排泄：和胆汁酸形成复合物随大便排出，<1% 经肾。

胆汁酸螯合剂

专家意见

胆汁酸螯合剂可降低 LDL 胆固醇 15% 至 25%（和口服剂量有关），并可增加 HDL 胆固醇达 2%。

可升高甘油三酯水平（Crouse），因此，高甘油三酯血症的患者不可服用。

粉剂和颗粒剂需和液体完全混匀后服用，因此不很方便。考来替泊片剂较大，吞咽可能困难。

考来维仑最常用，服用较方便，且不良反应较小（Davidson）。

为避免干扰其他药物的吸收，其他药物的服用需在服用考来烯胺和考来替泊前 1 小时或后 4~6 小时，或在服用考来维仑前 4 小时。

胆汁酸螯合剂尤其可干扰脂溶性维生素的吸收。

2 型糖尿病患者口服考来维仑，可轻度降低 HbA1c（Fonseca；Bays）。

有胆管或肠道梗阻、胃轻瘫或有其他胃肠动力疾病的患者不可服用胆汁酸螯合剂。

有吞咽困难或其他吞咽问题的患者慎用考来维仑和考来替泊片剂。

参考文献

Fonseca VA, Rosenstock J, Wang AC, et al. Colesevelam HCl improves glycemic control and reduces LDL choles- terol in patients with inadequately controlled type 2 diabetes on sulfonylurea-based therapy. Diabetes Care, 2008; 31: 1479–84.

Comments: Colesevelam improved glycemic control and reduced LDL cholesterol levels in patients with type 2 diabetes receiving sulfonylurea-based therapy.

Bays HE, Goldberg RB. The "forgotten" bile acid sequestrants: is now a good time to remember? Am J Ther, 2007; 14: 567–80.

Comments: Bile acid sequestrants should be considered for the treatment of patients with type 2 diabetes to lower LDL cholesterol and improve diabetic control.

Davidson MH, Dillon MA, Gordon B, et al. Colesevelam hydrochloride (cholestagel): a new, potent bile acid seques- trant associated with a low incidence of gastrointestinal side effects. Arch Intern Med, 1999; 159: 1893–900.

Comments: Colesevelam has fewer gastrointestinal side effects than the other bile acid sequestrants.

Crouse JR. Hypertriglyceridemia: a contraindication to the use of bile acid binding resins. Am J Med, 1987; 83: 243–8.

Comments: Bile acid sequestrants can raise triglyceride levels and should not be used in patients with elevated triglycerides.

[No authors listed]. The Lipid Research Clinics Coronary Primary Prevention Trial results. II. The relationship of reduction in incidence of coronary heart disease to cholesterol lowering. JAMA, 1984; 251: 365–74.

Comments: The Lipid Research Clinics clearly demonstrated for the first time that lowering cholesterol levels significantly reduced the number of coronary events in men with elevated cholesterol levels.

依泽替米贝（依折麦布）

Simeon Margolis, MD, PhD, and Paul A. Pham, Pharm

适应证
FDA
- 降低总胆固醇和 LDL 胆固醇，从而预防心血管疾病或事件。

机制
- 依泽替米贝选择性抑制胆固醇和相关植物固醇在小肠内吸收。

通常成人使用的剂量
- 每天 10mg，与或不与食物同服皆可。
- 可以用作单药治疗，但通常和他汀类药物一起服用。

剂型

商品名	通用名	剂型	价格
Zetia（Merck 制药公司）	依泽替米贝（依折麦布）	10mg（口服片剂）	4.03 美元

特殊人群使用剂量
肝病患者
- 中重度肝损害患者不推荐使用。

孕妇
- C 类。

哺乳期女性
- 不推荐使用，除非其潜在的获益高于对胎儿可能的危险。

药物不良反应
一般
- 一般没有明显的药物不良反应，除非依泽替米贝和他汀类药物一起服用
- 和安慰剂相比，依泽替米贝一般都能被耐受。

罕见
- 关节痛。
- 头晕。

药物相互作用
- 环孢菌素：环保菌素和依泽替米贝同服，血药浓度可增加。环保菌素血浓度/时间曲线下面积增加 15%。若二者同服需监测环保菌素血药浓度
- 非诺贝特：非诺贝特和吉非贝齐可分别增加依泽替米贝浓度约 50%、70% 共同给药的数据有限；若共同给药需严密监测增加胆石症的潜在危险。

依泽替米贝

考来烯胺和其他胆汁酸螯合剂：依泽替米贝血药浓度（浓度/时间曲线下面积）下降55%。依泽替米贝的服用需在胆汁酸螯合剂服用前至少2小时或后4小时。

香豆素类抗凝药：有案例报道显示，与依泽替米贝共同给药，可增加国际标准化比值（INR）。若两者共同给药，严密监测INR。

当和他汀类药物结合使用，药物副作用和相对适应证与单服他汀相同。

药代动力学

吸收：虽然大部分依泽替米贝很快被吸收并被葡萄糖醛酸化，但已知该药仅在肠内发挥作用。

代谢和排泄：在小肠和肝中通过葡萄糖醛酸化作用代谢。约80%发现随大便排泄，10%以葡萄糖醛酸化物的形式经尿排泄。

最高血药浓度，最低血药浓度和药物浓度/时间曲线下面积：依泽替米贝药物原形的最高血药浓度为3.4~5.5ng/ml（服药后4~12小时）。葡萄糖醛酸化物的最高血药浓度为45~71ng/ml（服药后1~2小时）。

半衰期：20~30小时。

专家意见

依泽替米贝加他汀可进一步降低15%的LDL醛固酮，但不影响2型糖尿病患者颈动脉内膜/中膜的厚度（Fleg）。

因为依泽替米贝一般无明显药物不良反应，所以，使用最高剂量的他汀药仍不能有效控制LDL胆固醇至目标值的患者，可加用依泽替米贝（Brown）。

依泽替米贝不抑制甘油三酯、脂溶性维生素、乙炔雌二醇或黄体酮的吸收（van Heek）。

依泽替米贝抑制植物固醇（如谷固醇和油菜甾醇）的吸收，所以可用于治疗谷固醇血症。

参考文献

Fleg JL, Mete M, Howard BV, et al. Effect of statins alone versus statins plus ezetimibe on carotid atherosclerosis in type 2 diabetes: the SANDS (Stop Atherosclerosis in Native Diabetics Study) trial. J Am Coll Cardiol, 2008; Vol. 52: pp. 2198–205.

Comments: Reducing LDL-C to aggressive targets resulted in similar regression of carotid artery intima-media thickness in patients with type 2 diabetes who attained equivalent LDL-C reductions from a statin alone or statin plus ezetimibe.

Kastelein JJ, Akdim F, Stroes ES, et al. ENHANCE Investigators. Simvastatin with or without ezetimibe in familial hypercholesterolemia. NEJM, 2008; Vol. 358: pp. 1431–43.

Comments: In patients with familial hypercholesterolemia, combined therapy with Vytorin (ezetimibe and simvastatin) did not result in a significant difference in changes in carotid intima-media thickness, as com- pared with simvastatin alone, despite greater decreases in levels of LDL cholesterol and C-reactive protein in those treated with Vytorin.

Brown BG, Taylor AJ. Does ENHANCE diminish confidence in lowering LDL or in ezetimibe? NEJM, 2008; Vol. 358: pp. 1504–7.

Comments: In response to the disappointing findings of ENHANCE: continue use ezetimibe in patients who fail to meet their LDL cholesterol targets despite maximal use of other cholesterol-lowering drugs, and await the outcomes further studies.

Pearson T, Ballantyne C, Sisk C, et al. Comparison of effects of ezetimibe/simvastatin versus simvastatin versus atorva] statin in reducing C-reactive protein and low-density lipoprotein cholesterol levels. Am J Cardiol, 2007; Vol. 99: pp. 1706–1713.

Comments: Ezetimibe plus simvastatin (Vytorin) was significantly more effective than simvastatin alone in lowering LDL cholesterol, 53% versus 38%, and lowering C-reactive protein levels.

Clarenbach JJ, Reber M, Lütjohann D, et al. The lipid-lowering effect of ezetimibe in pure vegetarians. J Lipid Res, 2006; Vol. 47: pp. 2820–4.

Comments: Ezetimibe 10 mg lowered LDL cholesterol by 17% in vegetarians who had a very low cholesterol intake.

Patrick JE, Kosoglou T, Stauber KL, et al. Disposition of the selective cholesterol absorption inhibitor ezetimibe in healthy male subjects. Drug Metab Dispos, 2002; Vol. 30: pp. 430–7.

Comments: Although known actions of ezetimibe are limited to the intestine, most of the administered drug is rapidly absorbed. It is possible that absorbed ezetimibe may exert additional benefits.

van Heek M, Farley C, Compton DS, et al. Ezetimibe selectively inhibits intestinal cholesterol absorption in rodents in the presence and absence of exocrine pancreatic function. Br J Pharmacol, 2001; Vol. 134: pp. 409–17.

Comments: Ezetimibe selectively inhibited the absorption of cholesterol, with no effect on the absorption of triglycerides, fat-soluble vitamins, ethinylestradiol, progesteron.

Bays HE, Moore PB, Drehobl MA, et al. Effectiveness and tolerability of ezetimibe in patients with primary hyper- cholesterolemia: pooled analysis of two phase II studies. Clin Ther, 2001; Vol. 23: pp. 1209–30.

Comments: Ezetimibe 10 mg lowered LDL cholesterol by 15% or more and raised HDL cholesterol slightly.

纤维酸衍生物

Simeon Margolis, MD, PhD, and Paul A. Pham, PharmD

适应证

FDA

- 高甘油三酯血症：预防心血管疾病和事件（Buse）。
- 混合型脂代谢紊乱：预防心血管疾病和事件（Buse）。

非 FDA 批准的使用

- 预防继发于严重高甘油三酯血症所致的急性胰腺炎。

机制

- 激活 PPAR alpha，从而降低 apo AIII 的合成。Apo AIII 是脂蛋白脂酶活性的抑制剂（van Dijk），脂蛋白脂酶可降解循环血中的甘油三酯（Hertz）。
- PPAR alpha 的激活还可以促进 apo AV 的合成，从而降低血中甘油三酯水平（Prieur）。

通常成人使用的剂量

- 非诺贝特（Tricor）：每日 48~145mg。
- 非诺贝特（Fenoglide）：每日 20~120mg。
- 非诺贝特，微粒化的剂型（Antara, Lofibra）：Antara 每日 43~130mg；Lofibra 每日 67~200mg；Trilipix 每日 45~135mg。与食物同服。
- 吉非贝齐（Lopid）：120mg，bid。
- 甘油三酯水平高于 500mg/dl 的患者从最大剂量起始。
- 在服用 4~6 周时，根据患者对其反应（血甘油三酯水平的变化）进行剂量调整。

剂型

商品名	通用名	剂型	价格
Tricor（Fournier 制药公司[专利]）	非诺贝特	48mg（口服的纳米晶片剂）	1.50 美元
Lofibra（Gate 制药公司）	非诺贝特（微粒化的剂型）	67mg（口服的微粒化的片剂） 134mg（口服的微粒化的片剂） 200mg（口服的微粒化的片剂）	1.04 美元 2.00 美元 3.12 美元
Fenoglide（Sciele 制药公司）	非诺贝特	40mg（口服的片剂） 120mg（口服的片剂）	1.6 美元 4.8 美元
Antara（Oscient 制药公司）	非诺贝特（微粒化的剂型）	43mg（口服的微粒化的片剂） 130mg（口服的微粒化的片剂）	1.57 美元 4.70 美元

商品名	通用名	剂型	价格
Lopid（Pfizer 和一些专利生产商）	吉非贝齐	60mg（口服的片剂）	1.25 美元
Trilipix（Abbott 实验室）	非诺贝特缓释剂	45mg（口服的缓释胶囊） 135mg（口服的缓释胶囊）	1.62 美元 4.92 美元

特殊人群的使用剂量
肾病患者
- 严重肾疾病（GFR<30ml/min）或透析患者禁忌服用。
- 中度肾疾病（GFR 为 30~60ml/min），减少使用剂量。

肝病
- 活动性肝病和原发性胆汁性肝硬化禁忌使用。

孕妇
- C 类。

哺乳期女性
- 禁忌。

药物不良反应
一般
- 和他汀一起使用时，最大的顾虑是引起严重肌炎和横纹肌溶解。

常见
- 无常见不良反应。

偶见
- 肝功能异常。
- 腹痛。
- 胃部不适。
- 肌炎。
- 头痛、头晕。

罕见
- 当和他汀一起使用时，出现严重肌炎、横纹肌溶解、肾衰竭。
- 胆结石。
- 骨髓移植。

药物相互作用
- 他汀：该类药物与他汀类药物同服可增加横纹肌溶解的危险。监测横纹肌溶解的症状和体征。吉非贝齐增加瑞舒伐他汀血药浓度/时间曲线下面积（AUC）90%（所以使用非诺贝特和瑞舒伐他汀一起）。
- 华法林：可能增加 INR。若两药一起给，需严密监测 INR。

纤维酸衍生物

- 胆汁酸螯合剂：可减少非诺贝特吸收。非诺贝特的口服应在服用胆汁酸螯合剂前 1 小时或后 4~6 小时。
- 格列苯脲：有案例报道示，吉非贝齐和格列苯脲一起给药增加低血糖反应。一起给药时需严密监测血糖。
- 瑞格列奈：吉非贝齐可使瑞格列奈血清浓度增加 8.1 倍；因此，一起给药是禁忌的。非诺贝特和瑞格列奈无明显相互作用。
- 吡格列酮和罗格列酮：和纤维酸衍生物一起给药可能增加低血糖反应。吉非贝齐增加吡格列酮和罗格列酮的血药浓度/时间曲线下面积（AUC）分别达 226%、130%。
- 熊去氧胆汁酸：效果可能会降低。

药代动力学

- 吸收：吉非贝齐 97% 可被吸收，非诺贝特 60%~90% 可被吸收。
- 代谢和排泄：吉非贝齐：经肝代谢，以原型 70% 经肾排出，6% 经大便排出。非诺贝特：广泛的被葡萄糖醛酸化，也在肾中转化为非诺贝酸，继而 60%~90% 经肾排出，10%~25% 经便排出。
- 半衰期：吉非贝齐为 1.3 小时，非诺贝特为 20 小时。

专家意见

- 贝特类降低甘油三酯 25%~50%，并增加 HDL 胆固醇约 8%，但对甘油三酯 >500mg/dl 的患者可能增加 LDL 胆固醇。
- 贝特类和他汀一起给药可能发生严重肌溶解。
- 他汀和吉非贝齐一起给药发生肌炎的危险高于和非诺贝特一起给药。
- 当甘油三酯水平在 200~500mg/dl 且 LDL 升高，可开始他汀治疗。如果甘油三酯仍然 >200mg/dl，考虑加用非诺贝特。目标是非 HDL 胆固醇水平 <100mg/dl（非 HDL 胆固醇 = 总胆固醇 –HDL 胆固醇）。
- 若患者 LDL 胆固醇正常且甘油三酯在 200~500mg/dl，或甘油三酯 >500mg/dl，可使用贝特类单药治疗。
- 一项对 2 型糖尿病人群的大型临床试验显示非诺贝特未减少冠心病发病率和病死率（Keech）。
- 非诺贝特可降低糖尿病视网膜病变需要激光治疗的概率（Keech）。
- 降低体重和控制血糖应该持续在贝特类治疗前和治疗过程中，从而降低甘油三酯水平。
- 近期的临床研究（ACCORD）：给 5 518 位口服他汀药且有心血管事件高危险的糖尿病患者加服非诺贝特，以观察非诺贝特的效果。非诺贝特组和安慰剂组的 LDL 胆固醇均较低（约 80mg/dl），非诺贝特和辛伐他汀一起给药并不比辛伐他汀单药治疗获益更多（Ginsberg）。

参考文献

ACCORD Study Group, Ginsberg HN, Elam MB, et al. Effects of combination lipid therapy in type 2 diabetes mellitus. NEJM, 2010; Vol. 362: pp. 1563–74.

Comments: The ACCORD Study tested the effect of intensive glucose control, intensive blood pressure control, and addition of fenofibrate. In this report, patients starting with triglyceride .200 mg/dl and low HDL had benefit from fenofibrate—not surprising, since the fibrates are generally used to tread hypertriglyceridemia. However, no overall benefit observed with addition of fenofibrate to statin therapy on the risk of cardiovascular outcomes.

Buse JB, Ginsberg HN, Bakris GL, et al. Primary prevention of cardiovascular diseases in people with diabetes mellitus: a scientific statement from the American Heart Association and the American Diabetes Association. Circulation, 2007; Vol. 115: pp. 114–26.

Comments: Recommendations from AHA and ADA for the primary prevention of cardiovascular heart disease in patients with diabetes.

Keech AC, Mitchell P, Summanen PA, et al. Effect of fenofibrate on the need for laser treatment for diabetic retinopathy (FIELD study): a randomised controlled trial. Lancet 2007; Vol. 370: pp. 1687–97.

Comments: Treatment with fenofibrate in individuals with type 2 diabetes mellitus reduced the need for laser treatment for diabetic retinopathy.

Sarwar N, Danesh J, Eiriksdottir G, et al. Triglycerides and the risk of coronary heart disease: 10,158 incident cases among 262,525 participants in 29 Western prospective studies. Circulation, 2007; Vol. 115: pp. 450–8.

Comments: Prospective studies in Western populations consistently indicate moderate and highly significant associations between triglyceride values and coronary heart disease risk.

Keech A, Simes RJ, Barter P, et al. Effects of long-term fenofibrate therapy on cardiovascular events in 9795 people with type 2 diabetes mellitus (the FIELD study) randomised controlled trial. Lancet, 2005; Vol. 366: pp. 1849–61.

Comments: Fenofibrate did not significantly reduce the risk of the primary outcome of coronary events. It did reduce total cardiovascular events.

Grundy SM, Vega GL, Yuan Z, et al. Effectiveness and tolerability of simvastatin plus fenofibrate for combined hyperlipidemia (the SAFARI trial). Am J Cardiol, 2005; Vol. 95 pp. 462–8.

Comments: The combination of a statin and fenofibrate is beneficial in the treatment of combined hyper- lipidemia.

van Dijk KW, Rensen PC, Voshol PJ, et al. The role and mode of action of apolipoproteins CII and AV: synergistic actors in triglyceride metabolism? Curr Opin Lipidol, 2004; Vol. 15: pp 239–46.

Comments: Apo CIII raises triglyceride levels by inhibiting lipoprotein lipase activity Apo AV lowers plasma triglyceride levels.

Prieur X, Coste H, Rodriguez JC. The human apolipoprotein AV gene is regulated by peroxisome proliferator- activated receptor-alpha and contains a novel farnesoic X-activated receptor response element. J Biol Chem, 2003; Vol. 278: pp. 25468–80.

Comments: Apo AV formation is stimulated by activation of PPAR alpha.

Expert Panel on Detection, Evaluation, and Treatment of High Blood Cholesterol in Adults Executive Summary of The Third Report of The National Cholesterol Education Program (NCEP) Expert Panel on Detection, Evalu- ation, And Treatment of High Blood Cholesterol In Adults (Adult Treatment Panel III). JAMA, 2001; Vol. 285: pp. 2486–97.

Comments: General guidelines for management of blood lipid abnormalities—risk factors, normal and abnor- mal cholesterol levels, when to initiate treatments, targets for treatment.

►Hertz R, Bishara-Shieban J, Bar-Tana J. Mode of action of peroxisome proliferators as hypolipidemic drugs. Suppression of apolipoprotein C-III. J Biol Chem, 1995; Vol. 270: p. 134705.

Comments: Fibrates exert their effects by activating PPAR alpha, which inhibits the formation of apo CIII.

烟酸类

Simeon Margolis, MD, PhD, and Paul A. Pham, PharmD

适应证
FDA
- 高脂血症（尤其 HDL 胆固醇较低的患者）。
- 预防动脉粥样硬化和心肌梗死。
- 烟酸缺乏和糙皮病。

机制
- 烟酸类药物可结合脂肪细胞和免疫细胞上的一种 G 蛋白偶联受体(Tunaru)。
- 受体的激活可降低 cAMP 水平，从而降低激素敏感性脂酶的活性，该脂酶在脂肪组织中将甘油三酯转化为脂肪酸（Tunaru）。
- 烟酸类药物可降低血浆中游离脂肪酸的产生。游离脂肪酸在肝中被利用来合成甘油三酯（Tunaru），甘油三酯由极低密度脂蛋白（VLDL）携带运输，VLDL 在血中转化为低密度脂蛋白（LDL）。
- 烟酸类药物和免疫细胞上的受体结合也可致皮肤红疹伴瘙痒(药物副作用)。

通常成人服用的剂量
- Niaspan ER（烟酸缓释剂）或 Slo-Niacin（烟酸控释剂）：睡前 500~2 000mg。逐渐加量的流程：睡前 500mg（第 1~4 周）；睡前加至 1g（第 5~8 周）。可每四周增加 500mg（最大剂量为 2g 每日）。
- Niacor(烟酸速释剂)：500~1 000mg，每天 2~3 次。逐渐加量的流程：起始剂量 100mg tid，在 5~8 周时间内逐渐增加至平均 1g tid 的剂量(最大剂量为每天 6g)。
- Niacin SR：睡前 500mg 逐渐加至维持剂量 1~2g tid。
- 和食物同服以减少胃肠不适；若出现皮肤红疹，可考虑口服阿司匹林(Guyton)。

剂型

商品名	通用名	剂型	价格
Niaspan ER（Abbott 实验室）	烟酸缓释剂	500mg（缓释片）	$2.49
		750mg（缓释片）	$3.55
		1 000mg（缓释片）	$4.40
Slo-niacin（可作为非处方药）（Upsher-Smith 制药公司）	烟酸控释剂	250mg（口服的控释片）	$0.09
		500mg（口服的控释片）	$0.13
		750mg（口服的控释片）	$0.18
Niacor（Upsher-Smith）	晶状制剂或烟酸速释剂	500mg（口服的片剂）	$0.28

烟酸类

商品名	通用名	剂型	价格
Niacin（可作为非处方药）（多家专利厂商）	晶状制剂或烟酸速释剂	50mg、100mg、125mg、250mg、500mg、1 000mg（口服的片剂）	$0.01~0.06
Niacin SR（多家专利厂商）	烟酸持续释放剂型	250mg（口服的片剂）500mg（口服的片剂）	$0.04 $0.05

特殊人群的用药剂量
肾病患者
- 明显肾脏疾病（GFR<50）的患者需慎用。

肝病患者
- 肝病活跃期或无法解释的肝酶升高禁用烟酸类药物。
- 既往有肝病史或大量饮酒的人群慎用。

孕妇
- C 类。

哺乳期女性
- 禁用。哺乳期需停止使用烟酸类药物，若使用，则需停止哺乳。

药物不良反应
常见
- 皮肤红疹（常在治疗起始阶段出现，继续使用一段时间后可消失）。在口服烟酸 30 分钟前口服阿司匹林可帮助防止皮肤起红疹（Guyton）。
- 肝酶异常。
- 增加尿酸水平。
- 瘙痒（出现时，可考虑使用抗组胺药）。

偶见
- 加重消化性溃疡。
- 恶心、呕吐，腹痛。
- 痛风发作。
- 升高碱性磷酸酶，降低磷的含量（平均降低 13%）。
- 升高血糖水平（Elam）。

罕见
- 肝毒性（使用烟酸持续释放剂型，其发生率可能更高）。
- 黑棘皮症。
- 当和他汀一起给药时可出现横纹肌溶解。
- 血小板减少症。

- 皮疹。

药物相互作用
- 他汀类药物:辛伐他汀和洛伐他汀与烟酸一起给药,可能增加肌病的危险。但是,在一项前瞻性研究中 1g/d 的烟酸和 40mg/d 的洛伐他汀一起给药未增加肌病的发生率(Bays)。当患者口服辛伐他汀 10mg/d 或洛伐他汀 20mg/d 作为维持剂量时,可考虑一起给药。
- 口服的降糖药:烟酸可能降低口服降糖药的效果。二者一起给药时,监测降糖药的治疗效果。
- 考来烯胺:可能减少烟酸的吸收。将二者给药时间错开 4~6 小时。
- 酒精或热饮:可能增加皮肤红疹和瘙痒的出现。进食酒精或热饮时,需避免使用烟酸药物(Guyton)。

药代动力学
- 吸收:60%~76% 可被吸收。
- 代谢和排泄:主要在肝中代谢,代谢产物 90% 经尿排出。
- 半衰期:20~45 分钟。

专家意见
- 烟酸类药物是升高 HDL 胆固醇最有效的药。
- 烟酸类药物可升高 HDL20%~35%,降低总胆固醇和 LDL 胆固醇 15%~25%,并能降低甘油三酯 30%~50%(Pan)。一些报道显示烟酸类药物也能降低脂蛋白(a)。
- 烟酸类有非处方制剂,但必须在医师的指导下服用,因为其存在不良反应。
- Slo-Niacin 的肝毒性高于其他烟酸类制剂(Myers)。
- 烟酸类药物对 2 型糖尿病患者有益之处在于它能降低 LDL 胆固醇和甘油三酯,并增加 HDL 胆固醇,但这类药物可能使一些患者的血糖控制欠佳(Elam)。
- 在服用烟酸类药物前 30 分钟口服阿司匹林或其他非甾体类抗炎药(NSAID)可减少皮肤红疹的发生。
- 烟酸类药物和热饮或食物一起同服可能使皮肤红疹更加严重。长期使用烟酸类药物,皮肤红疹的反应会减少(Guyton)。
- 虽然很多专家均推荐增加 HDL 胆固醇水平,但尚无明确证据说明升高 HDL 胆固醇对心血管有益处(Briel)。

参考文献
Briel M, Ferreira-Gonzalez I, You JJ, et al. Association between change in high density lipoprotein cholesterol and cardiovascular disease morbidity and mortality: systematic review and meta-regression analysis. BMJ, 2009; Vol. 338: p. b92.

Comments: Conclusions of the authors: "Available data suggest that simply increasing the amount of circu- lating HDL cholesterol does not reduce the risk of coronary heart disease events, coronary heart disease deaths, or total deaths. The results support reduction in LDL cholesterol as the primary goal for lipid modifying interventions."

Guyton JR, Bays HE. Safety considerations with niacin therapy. Am J Cardiol, 2007; Vol. 99: pp. 22C–31C.
Comments: This article describes ways to overcome the side effects of niacin, including the use of aspirin to prevent or reduce flushing. The authors argue that niacin is underused because of excessive concern about side effects. No-flush niacin does not cause flushing, but it has no effects on blood lipids or lipoproteins.

Tunaru S, Kero J, Schaub A, et al. PUMA-G and HM74 are receptors for nicotinic acid and mediate its anti-lipolytic effect. Nat Med, 2003; Vol. 9: pp. 352–5.
Comments: Activation of a niacin receptor in adipose tissue is responsible for the lipid-lowering effect of the drug.

Meyers CD, Carr MC, Park S, et al. Varying cost and free nicotinic acid content in over-the-counter niacin prepara- tions for dyslipidemia. Ann Intern Med, 2003; Vol. 139: pp. 996–1002.
Comments: This review identified the following formulations of over-the-counter niacins: 10 immediate release, 9 slow (sustained)-release, and 10 "no-flush" formulations.

Bays HE, Dujovne CA, McGovern ME, et al. Comparison of once-daily, niacin extended-release/lovastatin with standard doses of atorvastatin and simvastatin (the ADvicor Versus Other Cholesterol-Modulating Agents Trial Evaluation [ADVOCATE]). Am J Cardiol, 2003; Vol. 91: pp. 667–72.
Comments: No drug-induced myopathy was seen in a trial using Niaspan and lovastatin.

Pan J, Lin M, Kesala RL, et al. Niacin treatment of the atherogenic lipid profile and Lp(a) in diabetes. Diabetes Obes Metab, 2002; Vol. 4: pp. 255–61.
Comments: In this small study of patients with type 2 diabetes, HDL cholesterol rose by 31% while the follow- ing decreased: LDL cholesterol (20%), triglycerides (52%), and lipoprotein a (40%). The percentage of small dense LDL also fell.

Elam MB, Hunninghake DB, Davis KB, et al. Effect of niacin on lipid and lipoprotein levels and glycemic control in patients with diabetes and peripheral arterial disease: the ADMIT study: A randomized trial. Arterial Disease Multiple Intervention Trial. JAMA, 2000; Vol. 284: pp. 1263–70.
Comments: Niacin can be safely used in people with diabetes, but the drug may result in worsening of glycemic control in some patients.

Capuzzi DM, Guyton JR, Morgan JM, et al. Efficacy and safety of an extended-release niacin (Niaspan): a long- term study. Am J Cardiol, 1998; Vol. 82: pp. 74U–81U; discussion 85U–86U.
Comments: Niaspan is equally effective and associated with fewer side effects than other forms of niacin.

McKenney JM, Proctor JD, Harris S, et al. A comparison of the efficacy and toxic effects of sustained vs immediate- release niacin in hypercholesterolemic patients. JAMA, 1994; Vol. 271: pp. 672–7.
Comments: Slow-release niacin is associated with an increased risk of severe hepatotoxicity compared with other forms of niacin.

Brown G, Albers JJ, Fisher LD, et al. Regression of coronary artery disease as a result of intensive lipid-lowering therapy in men with high levels of apolipoprotein B. NEJM, 1990; Vol. 323: pp. 1289–98.
Comments: Treatment with colestipol plus large doses of niacin was associated with reduced frequency of coro- nary artery disease progression and increased frequency of regression compared with conventional treatment.

OMEGA-3 脂肪酸（鱼油）

Simeon Margolis, MD, PhD, and Paul A. Pham, PharmD

适应证
FDA
- 成人服用可降低极高甘油三酯水平（>500mg/dl）（饮食之外的辅助食品）。

非 FDA 批准的使用
- 对已患心血管疾病的患者，可预防心血管事件和猝死（二级预防）（GISSI；Rupp；Oikawa）。
- 预防心律不齐（Rupp）。

机制
- 机制不明，但 omega-3 脂肪酸可抑制肝中甘油三酯形成，并降低极低密度脂蛋白（VLDL）的释放，从而降低血甘油三酯水平（Chan；Harris）。

剂型

商品名	通用名	剂型	价格
Lovaza（Glaxo SmithKline）	Omega-3 脂肪酸	1g（口服的软胶囊）	$1.52 每片
鱼油（多家药品供应商）	Omega-3 脂肪酸	1g（口服的胶囊）	$0.1 每片

正常成人使用的剂量
- Lovaza：4g（4片胶囊）每天一次或 2g（2片胶囊）每天2次。
- 鱼油胶囊，每天 4~12 片胶囊。

特殊人群的使用剂量
肾病患者
- 无须特殊剂量。

肝病患者
- 无数据。

孕妇
- C 类：动物实验无致畸作用。

哺乳期女性
- 无数据。

药物不良反应
一般
- 一般耐受较好。
- 增加体重。

OMEGA-3 脂肪酸（鱼油）

常见
- 增加 LDL 胆固醇（Balk）。

偶见
- 胃肠系统：恶心、腹痛及嗳气。
- 味觉倒错。
- 皮疹。
- 增加 ALT 水平。

药物相互作用
- 数据有限，且尚无人群的研究。
- 阿司匹林：两者同服，可能增加出血时间。
- 华法林：两者同服，可能增加出血时间。虽然在临床研究中 omega-3 脂肪酸未引起明显出血事件，但是二者同服时需对患者严密检测。
- 氯吡格雷：两者同服，可能增加出血时间。
- 普萘洛尔：两者同服，可能增强降压作用。
- 洛匹那韦：两者同服不影响洛匹那韦在血浆中的浓度。

药代动力学
- 吸收：二十碳五烯酸（EPA）和二十二碳六烯酸（DHA）口服后可被吸收。

专家意见
- 鱼油对糖尿病患者而言，是一种安全而有效的降低甘油三酯的方法，但是尚无对鱼油的 I 期研究。
- 和安慰剂相比，有严重高甘油三酯血症（>500mg/dl）的患者口服鱼油可将甘油三酯降低 30%~50%（Balk；Harris）。
- Lovaza：含接近的 90% 长链 omega-3 脂肪酸。价格更贵，但相比口服标准鱼油胶囊，口服少量的 Lovaza 脂肪酸可减少体重或增加上消化道不适的发生。
- 在二级预防方面，有足够证据证明鱼油对预防心血管事件有作用（GISSI；Oikawa）。
- 和贝特类和/或他汀类联用，Lovaza 可进一步降低血清甘油三酯水平，但可能增加 LDL 达 6mg/dl（Balk；Davidson）。
- 鱼油对冠心病的主要益处：预防猝死，可能通过稳定或预防有危险性的心律不齐（GISSI；Rupp；Oikawa）。

参考文献

Rupp H. Omacor(R) (prescription omega-3-acid ethyl esters 90): from severe rhythm disorders to hypertriglyceri- demia. Adv Ther, 2009; Vol. 26: pp. 675–90.

Comments: In addition to lowering triglycerides, Omacor can improve rhythm disorders and reduce cardiovascular events in secondary prevention.

Oikawa S, Yokoyama M, Origasa H, et al. Suppressive effect of EPA on the incidence of coronary events in hyper- cholesterolemia with impaired glucose metabolism: sub-analysis of the Japan EPA Lipid Intervention Study (JELIS). Atherosclerosis, 2009; Vol. 206: pp.

535–9.

Comments: A randomized study involving over 18,000 patients found that treatment with the fish oil eicosa- pentaenoic acid (EPA) plus statin over a 4.5-year period reduced the incidence of coronary artery disease by 22% in hypercholesterolemic individuals with impaired fasting glucose or diabetes.

Davidson MH, Stein EA, Bays HE, et al. Efficacy and tolerability of adding prescription omega-3 fatty acids 4 g/d to simvastatin 40 mg/d in hypertriglyceridemic patients: an 8-week, randomized, double-blind, placebo- controlled study. Clin Ther, 2007; Vol. 29: pp. 1354–67.

Comments: Compared with those taking statin plus placebo, the group taking omega-3 plus statin had signifi- cantly lower non-HDL cholesterol and triglyceride levels along with higher HDL cholesterol.

Balk EM, Lichtenstein AH, Chung M, et al. Effects of omega-3 fatty acids on serum markers of cardiovascular disease risk: a systematic review. Atherosclerosis, 2006; Vol. 189: pp. 19–30.

Comments: In this review of 21 trials fish oil lowered triglycerides by 27 mg/dl and increased HDL cholesterol by 1.6 mg/dl, but increased LDL cholesterol by 6 mg/dl.

Harris WS, Bulchandani D. Why do omega-3 fatty acids lower serum triglycerides? Curr Opin Lipidol, 2006; Vol. 17: pp. 387–93.

Comments: Fish oils reduce triglyceride synthesis in the liver.

Chan DC, Watts GF, Barrett PH, et al. Regulatory effects of HMG CoA reductase inhibitor and fish oils on apoli- poprotein B-100 kinetics in insulin-resistant obese male subjects with dyslipidemia. Diabetes, 2002; Vol. 51: pp. 2377–86.

Comments: Fish oils reduce secretion of VLDL in obese men with insulin resistance.

Gruppo Italiano per lo Studio della Sopravvivenza nell'Infarto miocardico (GISSI). Dietary supplementation with n-3 polyunsaturated fatty acids and vitamin E after myocardial infarction: results of the GISSI-Prevenzione trial. Lancet, 1999; Vol. 354: pp. 447–55.

Comments: During a 3.5-year follow-up, fish oil supplementation, started in patients after an acute myocar- dial infarction, significantly decreased the risk for overall and cardiovascular disease death, particularly for sudden death.

Harris WS. n-3 fatty acids and serum lipoproteins: human studies. Am J Clin Nutr, 1997; Vol. 65: pp. 1645S–1654S.

Comments: This review found that fish oils lowered triglycerides by 25%–30% while increasing both HDL and LDL cholesterol levels by small amounts.

他汀类药物和联合药物

Simeon Margolis, MD, PhD, and Paul A. Pham, PharmD

适应证

FDA

- 高胆固醇血症。
- 动脉粥样硬化（一级和二级预防）。
- 心血管事件（一级和二级预防）。

机制

- 他汀类可抑制胆固醇合成路径中所需的 HMG CoA 还原酶，从而降低肝中的游离胆固醇。
- 继而可激活形成 LDL 受体的基因的表达（尤其在肝中）。
- 细胞膜上 LDL 受体的增加使更多的 LDL 从血中清除，从而降低血中的总胆固醇和 LDL 胆固醇。

成人常用的剂量

- 阿托伐他汀：10~80mg 每天一次（可在一天中的任何时候服用）。
- 氟伐他汀：20~80mg 可不必随餐服用，或氟伐他汀（Lescol）XL 80mg 每天。
- 洛伐他汀：20~80mg 每天一次（睡前）。
- 匹伐他汀：1~4mg 每天一次。
- 普伐他汀：10~80mg 每天一次（可任何时间服用，随餐或不随餐皆可）。
- 瑞舒伐他汀：5~40mg 每天一次（可任何时间服用）。
- 辛伐他汀：10~40mg 每天一次（睡前）。
- 依泽替米贝 + 辛伐他汀：合剂称为 Vytorin，其中两药的含量 10/10mg、10/20mg、10/40mg 或 10/80mg。Vytorin 剂量：每天 1 片（睡前）。
- 烟酸 + 洛伐他汀：合剂称为 Advicor，其中两药的含量 500/20mg、750/20mg、1 000/20mg 或 1 000/40mg。Advicor 剂量：500/20mg~2 000/40mg 每天 1 次。
- 烟酸 + 辛伐他汀：合剂称为 Simcor，其中两药含量 500/40mg、750/20mg、500/20mg。Simcor 剂量：500/20mg~2 000/40mg 每天 1 次。
- 氨氯地平 + 阿托伐他汀：合剂称为 Caduet，其中两药的含量 2.5/10mg、5/10mg、10/10mg、2.5/20mg、5/20mg、10/20mg、2.5/40mg、5/40mg、10/40mg、5/80mg、10/80mg。Caduet 剂量：每天 1 片。

剂型

商品名	通用名	剂型	价格
Lipitor（Pfizer）	阿托伐他汀	10mg（口服片剂） 20、40、80mg（口服片剂）	$3.19 $4.54
Lescol, Lescol XL（Novaris）	氟伐他汀	80mg（口服的缓释片剂） 20、40mg（口服的胶囊）	$3.66 $2.86
Mevacor, Altocor（Merck 及其他一些专利制药商）	洛伐他汀	20、40、60mg（口服的片剂 Altoprev） 10mg（口服的片剂） 20mg（口服的片剂） 40mg（口服的片剂）	$5.00 $0.71 $1.26 $2.21
Livalo(Kowa 制药公司)	匹伐他汀	1、2、4mg（口服的片剂）	$3.62
Pravachol（Bristol-Myers 及其他一些专利制药公司）	普伐他汀	5mg（口服片剂） 10mg（口服片剂） 20mg（口服片剂） 40、80mg（口服片剂）	$2.00 $2.79 $4.73 $4.92
Crestor(AstraZenica)	瑞舒伐他汀	5、10、20、40mg（口服的片剂）	$3.97
Zocor（Merck 和其他一些专利制药公司）	辛伐他汀	5mg（口服的片剂） 10mg（口服的片剂） 20、40、80mg(口服的片剂)	$2.00 $2.79 $4.92
Vytorin（Schering 和 Merck/Schering-Plough 公司）	辛伐他汀 + 依泽替米贝	10/10mg、10/20mg、10/40mg、10/80mg（口服的片剂）	$4.08
Simcor（Abbott 实验室）	辛伐他汀 + 烟酸缓释剂	500/20mg（口服片剂） 750/20mg（口服片剂） 1 000/20mg（口服的片剂）	$2.49 $3.56 $4.41

他汀类药物和联合药物

商品名	通用名	剂型	价格
Caduet（Pfizer）	氨氯地平+阿托伐他汀	10/10mg、2.5/10mg（口服的片剂）	$4.37
		5/20mg、5/40mg、5/80mg、2.5/20mg、2.5/40mg、10/20mg、10/40mg、10/80mg（口服的片剂）	$5.98
		5/10mg（口服的片剂）	$3.21
Advicor 缓释剂（Kos 制药公司）	洛伐他汀+烟酸缓释剂	500/20mg（口服的片剂）	$2.74
		750/20mg（口服的片剂）	$2.94
		1 000/20mg（口服的片剂）	$3.16
		1 000/40mg（口服的片剂）	$3.67

特殊人群的用药剂量

肾病患者
- 无须特殊剂量。

肝病患者
- 活动性肝病或无法解释的血清转氨酶持续升高患者，禁止使用他汀类药。

孕妇
- 孕妇禁服他汀：X 类。
- 孕龄期妇女性只有在使用合适的避孕方式并被告知他汀类药的潜在副作用时，才能给予服用他汀类药。

哺乳期女性
- 哺乳期女性若口服他汀类药，不应进行母乳喂养。

药物不良反应

一般
- 肌痛和肌无力是最常见的症状。
- 严重肌炎不常见但很危险。

常见
- 肌痛。

偶见
- 腹痛。

- 恶心。
- 失眠。
- 头晕。
- 肝转氨酶异常。

罕见
- 严重肌炎、横纹肌溶解及肾衰竭(Joy)。

药物相互作用
- 辛伐他汀、洛伐他汀和阿托伐他汀是CYP3A4的底物。阿托伐他汀也被葡萄糖醛酸化。CYP3A4抑制剂(如大环内酯类抗生素、胺碘酮、氮二烯五环类抗真菌药、HIV蛋白酶抑制剂)可明显升高这些他汀类药的血清浓度。
- 普伐他汀通过多种代谢途径进行首过代谢,尤其是葡萄糖醛酸化(独立于CYP3A4);氟伐他汀主要经CYP2C9代谢;瑞舒伐他汀较少经肝代谢;因此,普伐他汀、瑞舒伐他汀和氟伐他汀和CYP3A4抑制剂的相互作用很小。
- 贝特类,尤其是吉非贝齐和烟酸:可能增加肌病的危险。若它们合用,需严密监测肌病的发生(Joy)。
- 抗生素:红霉素和克拉霉素可能明显增加辛伐他汀和洛伐他汀的血清浓度。考虑可换成其他他汀类药,如普伐他汀和瑞舒伐他汀。
- HIV-蛋白酶抑制剂:禁忌和辛伐他汀及洛伐他汀合用。考虑可用小剂量的阿托伐他汀(10mg)、瑞舒伐他汀(5mg)或普伐他汀。
- 伊曲康唑、酮康唑、伏立康唑、泊沙康唑:可能明显增加辛伐他汀和洛伐他汀的血药浓度。考虑换用其他他汀类药,如普伐他汀和瑞舒伐他汀。
- 香豆素类抗凝药:INR可能升高。若合用,严密监测INR。
- 地尔硫䓬:可能明显增加辛伐他汀和洛伐他汀的血药浓度。考虑换用其他他汀类药,如普伐他汀和瑞舒伐他汀。
- 口服避孕药:瑞舒伐他汀可增加乙炔雌二醇和炔诺孕酮分别达26%和34%。监测潜在的药物不良反应。

药代动力学
- 吸收:普伐他汀:吸收率为34%,生物利用度为17%。洛伐他汀:吸收率为30%,生物利用度为5%(与食物同服)。辛伐他汀:生物利用度为5%。氟伐他汀:吸收率为95%,生物利用度为20%~30%。阿托伐他汀:可快速被吸收,生物利用度为14%。瑞舒伐他汀:吸收率为59%,生物利用度为20%。
- 代谢和排出:普伐他汀:普遍在肝中首过代谢,20%经肾、71%经胆排泄。洛伐他汀:普遍经肝水解称为有活性的代谢产物,10%经肾、83%经胆排出。辛伐他汀:普遍在肝中通过CYP3A4途径代谢,13%经肾、60%经胆排出。氟伐他汀:通过CYP2C9(75%)、CYP3A4(20%)及CYP2D6途径代谢,5%经肾、95%经胆排出。阿托伐他汀:经CYP3A4途径代谢,经胆排出。瑞舒伐他汀:少量经肝代谢,10%经肾、90%经胆排出。

他汀类药物和联合药物

- 蛋白结合率：普伐他汀：43%~55%。洛伐他汀：>95%。辛伐他汀：95%。氟伐他汀：98%。阿托伐他汀：98%。瑞舒伐他汀：88%。
- 最高血药浓度（Cmax）、最低血药浓度（Cmin）、及浓度/时间曲线下面积（AUC）：普伐他汀的 Cmax：15ng/ml；洛伐他汀的 Cmax：5.8ng/ml；氟伐他汀的 Cmax：287ng/nl；阿托伐他汀的 Cmax：25ng/ml；瑞舒伐他汀的 Cmax：37ng/ml。
- 半衰期：普伐他汀和辛伐他汀：约 3 小时。氟伐他汀：<3 小时。阿托伐他汀：7~14 小时。洛伐他汀：4.5 小时。瑞舒伐他汀：13~20 小时。

专家意见

- 他汀类药物是至今最有效且耐受性最好的降总胆固醇和 LDL 胆固醇水平的一类药，也可以降低甘油三脂 10%~25%，增加 HDL 5%~10%。
- 在推荐剂量范围内，他汀类药物的药效强度如下：匹伐他汀＞瑞舒伐他汀＞阿托伐他汀＞洛伐他汀＞辛伐他汀＞普伐他汀＞氟伐他汀，平均降低 LDL 的程度分别为 55%~60%、48%~52%、48%、39~41%、32%、23%（Jones，1998；Jones，2003）。
- 普伐他汀因很少有药物相互作用，常被推荐给服用可抑制 CYP3A4 的药物的患者（这些具有抑制 CYP3A4 作用的药物包括大环内酯类抗生素、HIV-蛋白酶抑制剂、氮二烯五环类抗真菌药），但也可考虑用药效更强的阿托伐他汀（以 10mg 作为慎重使用的起始剂量，慢慢逐渐增加至最大剂量 40mg/d）或瑞舒伐他汀（以 5mg/d 起始）；服用 CYP3A4 抑制剂的患者禁用洛伐他汀和辛伐他汀。
- 服用他汀类药物的患者需被问及有无横纹肌溶解的症状（如肌痛、无力），尤其是当这些患者也同时服用贝特类药物的时候（Joy）。
- 他汀类药物除了降 LDL 胆固醇之外，还有其他功效；这些多方面的功效包括降低血中的炎症标志物（如 C 反应蛋白），并可改善内皮细胞功能，从而帮助预防心血管疾病。
- 他汀药和葡萄汁（＞1 夸脱每天）同服可增加他汀的血药浓度（Li）。
- 有或无糖尿病的人服用他汀类药皆可降低发生心血管事件的风险（Pedersen；Heart Protection Study Collaborative Group）。
- 他汀类药可能使发展为糖尿病的风险增加 9%，但和降低心血管事件相比，这个风险是低的（Sattar）。

参考文献

Sattar N, Preiss D, Murray HM, et al. Statins and risk of incident diabetes: a collaborative meta-analysis of randomised statin trials. Lancet, 2010; Vol. 375 Suppl 9716: pp. 735–42.

Comments: The increased risk of developing diabetes is very small compared with the reduction in cardiovascular events achieved with statins.

Shaw SM, Fildes JE, Yonan N, et al. Pleiotropic effects and cholesterol-lowering therapy. Cardiology, 2009; Vol. 112: pp. 4–12.

Comments: This review provides a critical evaluation of the proposed pleiotropic effects of the statins.

Joy TR, Hegele RA. Narrative review: statin-related myopathy. Ann Intern Med, 2009; Vol. 150: pp. 858–68.

Comments: Myalgia is common; rhabdomyolysis is rare. This review discusses the management of myalgia and the prevention of rhabdomyolysis.

Golomb BA, Evans MA Statin adverse effects: a review of the literature and evidence for a mitochondrial mechanism. Am J Cardiovasc Drugs, 2008; Vol. 8: pp. 373–418.

Comments: This review considers some of the less common adverse effects of statins and the relationship of these effects to statin interactions with mitochondrial mechanisms.

Li P, Callery PS, Gan LS, et al. Esterase inhibition by grapefruit juice flavonoids leading to a new drug interaction. Drug Metab Dispos, 2007; Vol. 35: pp. 1203–8.

Comments: Flavenoids in grapefruit juice interfere with the breakdown of statins in the intestine and can raise blood levels of ingested statin.

Pedersen TR, Kjekshus J, Berg K, et al. Randomised trial of cholesterol lowering in 4444 patients with coro- nary heart disease: the Scandinavian Simvastatin Survival Study (4S). 1994. Atheroscler Suppl, 2004; Vol. 5: pp. 81–7.

Comments: This study (4S) enrolled nearly 4500 subjects with known coronary heart disease. Simvastatin reduced the number of major coronary events and the need for angioplasty or bypass surgery by more than 35% in both men and women.

Jones PH, Davidson MH, Stein EA, et al. Comparison of the efficacy and safety of rosuvastatin versus atorvastatin, simvastatin, and pravastatin across doses (STELLAR* Trial). Am J Cardiol, 2003; Vol. 92: pp. 152–60.

Comments: The STELLAR trial showed that rosuvastatin was more potent than the other available statins.

Heart Protection Study Collaborative Group. MRC/BHF Heart Protection Study of cholesterol lowering with simv- astatin in 20,536 high-risk individuals: a randomised placebo-controlled trial. Lancet, 2002; Vol. 360: pp. 7–22.

Comments: This, the largest randomized, controlled trial of statin therapy, enrolled subjects with known car- diovascular disease, diabetes, or hypertension. The simvastatin group exhibited a 38% fall in nonfatal heart attacks, about a 25% reduction in the rates of stroke and revascularization procedures, and a 13% lower inci- dence of all cause mortality. The benefits extended to women, subjects over the age of 70, and those with a baseline LDL cholesterol less than 100 mg/dl.

Jones P, Kafonek S, Laurora I, et al. Comparative dose efficacy study of atorvastatin versus simvastatin, pravas- tatin, lovastatin, and fluvastatin in patients with hypercholesterolemia (the CURVES study). Am J Cardiol, 1998; Vol. 81: pp. 582–7.

Comments: The CURVES trial determined the relative potencies of five statins.

勃起功能障碍

昔多芬

Ari Eckman, MD, and Paul A. Pham, PharmD

适应证

FDA
- 用于治疗勃起功能障碍。
- 治疗肺动脉高压（WHO Group I）以增强运动能力和减缓病情恶化。

药物机理
- 5型磷酸二酯酶（PDE-5）抑制剂：它是小梁平滑肌中的一种酶，可以通过放松平滑肌来促进勃起。
- PDE-5对于cGMP的降解有催化作用，从而增加细胞内钙浓度和平滑肌的收缩。

成人常用的剂量
- 每天服用一次，每次剂量50mg，在性行为之前1小时（或30分钟至4小时以内）服用；剂量范围：25~100mg，每天一次。最大剂量不得超过100mg/次，1次/天。
- 如果>65岁，并有肝肾疾患，或口服CYP3A4抑制剂的人群，剂量以25mg每次起始。
- 可随餐或不随餐服用，但高脂饮食后该药的起效时间会延长。

剂型

商品名	通用名	剂型	价格
伟哥（辉瑞）	昔多芬	口服药片 25/50/100mg	$18.22
西地那非（辉瑞）	昔多芬	口服药片 20mg	$17.35

特殊人群的剂量

肾脏疾病者
- 内生肌酐清除率（CrCl）≥30ml/min时：不需要做剂量调整。
- CrCl<30ml/min时：起始服药的剂量减为25mg。

肝脏疾病者
- 肝硬化（Child-Pugh A级和B级）：初始剂量减为25mg，48小时以内不要使用超过25mg的单次剂量。

怀孕
- 被FDA归类为危险性分级B类。动物研究尚未显示出会导致胎儿器官畸形。人类研究尚未给出明显的结果。孕妇不可服用。

昔多芬

哺乳期
- 目前还没有明确研究结果报告。哺乳期女性不可服用。

药物不良反应

一般
- 头痛、面红、消化不良、视觉干扰（视觉忽然模糊，光线过敏、视觉偏蓝）
- 心脏疾病者慎用。
- 禁忌与硝酸盐类药物混用。

偶见
- 鼻腔充血、尿路感染、眩晕、腹泻、皮疹。

罕见
- 阴茎异常勃起、心悸、低血压、严重的心血管反应（心肌梗死、休克、心绞痛）、过敏性反应。
- 尚不明确的反应：呼吸道感染、背痛、流感综合征、关节痛、虚弱无力、寒战、血管性水肿、疼痛、休克。
- 突发性听觉障碍。

和其他药物的相互作用
- 强效的肝CYP3A4或2C9同工酶抑制剂会减少昔多芬的清除和代谢，增加其浓度。与以下药品混用时应谨慎或减少剂量（48小时内最大剂量不超过25mg）：考尼伐坦（抗利尿激素受体拮抗药）、红霉素、氟康唑、伊马替尼、伊曲康唑（抗真菌药）、酮康唑、泊沙康唑、咪拉地尔、萘法唑酮、其他大环内酯类抗生素（克拉仙霉素，醋竹桃霉素）、奎尼定（抗心律不齐药）、雷诺嗪（血管扩张药）、施怕沙星（已从美国市场撤出）、伏立康唑（抗真菌药）、扎鲁司特（抗过敏药）、积璐琛（白发抑制药）、地拉夫定、HIV蛋白酶抑制剂（包括利托那韦，沙奎那韦，茚地那韦，达芦那韦，福沙那韦，阿扎那韦，奈非那韦，洛匹那韦，替拉那韦）。
- 中度的肝CYP3A4或2C9同工酶抑制剂，会减少昔多芬的清除和代谢，增加其浓度，需要谨慎使用或减少剂量（48小时内最大剂量不超过25mg）。药品包括：甲氰咪呱（抗消化溃疡）、地尔硫䓬、葡萄柚汁、米非司酮（堕胎）、他克莫司（大环内酯类抗生素）、单胺氧化酶抑制剂（MAOIs）、nilotinib（尼洛替尼，第二代酪氨酸激酶抑制剂）、 环丙沙星、aprepitant(新型止吐药)、fosaprepitant（二甲葡胺，止吐药）、fluoxetine（盐酸氟西汀，抗抑郁）、fluvoxamine(氟伏沙明，抗精神失常)、verapamil（抗心律失常）。
- 肝CYP3A4或2C9同工酶诱导剂：会增进昔多芬的清除和代谢，减少其浓度。药品包括：etravirine(非核苷类逆转录酶抑制剂)、依法韦仑、波生坦、巴比妥类药物、卡马西平（抗癫痫）、 地塞米松、 苯妥英、phosphenytion(抗癫痫)、奈韦拉平、利福布汀、利福平、曲格列酮（已从美国市场撤出）、 奈比洛尔。
- Alpha-阻滞剂：可能会增加低血压的风险。与昔多芬混用时应密切监测血压。服用Alpha-阻滞剂的患者应当在病情稳定时小剂量服用昔多芬。

- 硝酸盐类药物：禁忌。与昔多芬同时服用会导致明显的低血压，因此绝对禁忌。
- 氨氯地平（钙拮抗剂，降血压）：与昔多芬混用时会产生额外的降压效应（临床测得典型值收缩压8mmHg，舒张压7mmHg）。
- 西沙比利（胃肠动力药，已退出美国市场）：是CYP3A4的酶作用物；避免与昔多芬混用或代替昔多芬使用（作为CYP3A4的弱阻滞剂），因为可能会导致心律失常。
- 昔多芬与二氢可待因（镇痛药）混用可能导致长时间勃起。应当谨慎使用。
- 阿司匹林、乙醇、噻嗪类利尿剂、ACE抑制剂、华法林（抗凝血）、抗酸药、甲苯磺丁脲：未见与昔多芬有明显作用。
- 沙丙蝶呤（治疗血苯丙氨酸过高）：辅助合成一氧化氮，与昔多芬混用会舒畅血管而降低血压，须谨慎使用。

药代动力学

- 吸收：口服后就会被身体快速吸收，平均绝对生物药效率41%（25%~63%）。
- 新陈代谢和排泄：通过肝细胞色素CYP3A4（主要）和CYP2C9（次要）代谢。代谢产物中有一种被检测出与原药物成分接近，并具有20%的药效。该活性成分被进一步分解为无活性的化学成分，并通过粪便（80%）和尿液（13%）排出。
- 与蛋白质结合率：96%与血浆蛋白结合，结合率与总的药物浓度无关。
- C_{max}，C_{min}和AUC：空腹口服时，30~120分钟达到最高血药浓度（平均60分钟）；配合高蛋白膳食时，吸收率会降低，平均120分钟达到最高血药浓度（C_{max}），且C_{max}平均降低29%。
- 半衰期：昔多芬及其活性代谢产物的半衰期均为4小时。
- 分布：平均稳态体积分布率为105L，说明在组织中分布广泛。

专家建议

- 昔多芬会增进硝酸盐类药物的降压作用，禁忌混用。
- 左心室流出道梗阻（例如主动脉（瓣）狭窄、特发性肥厚性主动脉瓣下狭窄）和血压控制欠佳的患者慎用。
- 糖尿病患者服用西多芬预期的药效低于非糖尿病人群，但报告显示仍然有50%~80%的糖尿病患者仍然有疗效（Ng；Price；Blonde；Stuckey）。
- 新上市的PDE-5抑制剂，包括vardenafil(盐酸伐地那非，又名Levitra)(Ishii; Goldstein)、Tadalafil（他达拉非，又名Cialis)(Saenz de Tejada)也对治疗糖尿病患者的勃起障碍有疗效，但临床研究比昔多芬少。
- 盐酸伐地那：1小时达到最强药效并持续4~6小时。
- 他达拉非：2小时达到最强药效，并持续36~48小时。

参考文献

Blonde L. Sildenafil citrate for erectile dysfunction in men with diabetes and cardiovascular risk factors: a retro-spective analysis of pooled data from placebo-controlled trials. Curr Med Res Opin, 2006; Vol. 22: pp. 2111–20.

Comments: Retrospective analysis showing 62% of patients with DM had improvement in erections with silde- nafil, compared to 18% with placebo.

Ishii N, Nagao K, Fujikawa K, et al. Vardenafil 20-mg demonstrated superior efficacy to 10-mg in Japanese men with diabetes mellitus suffering from erectile dysfunction. Int J Urol, 2006; Vol. 13: pp. 1066–72.

Comments: Randomized, controlled, 12-week study demonstrating that in Japanese men with DM and ED, vardenafil 10 mg and 20 mg were effective in improving erectile function with comparable safety profiles. Vardenafil 20 mg demonstrated superior efficacy compared with 10 mg, suggesting incremental clinical benefit in using the higher dose in this difficult-to-treat population.

Jackson G. Sexual dysfunction and diabetes. Int J Clin Pract, 2004; Vol. 58: pp. 358–62.

Comments: Reviews common agents used for ED in patients with DM.

Stuckey BG, Jadzinsky MN, Murphy LJ, et al. Sildenafil citrate for treatment of erectile dysfunction in men with type 1 diabetes: results of a randomized controlled trial. Diabetes Care, 2003; Vol. 26: pp. 279–84.

Comments: Randomized, double-blinded clinical study focusing on sildenafil use for ED in patients with T1DM, showing 66% of patients had improvement in erections with sildenafil, compared to 29% in placebo group.

Goldstein I, Young JM, Fischer J, et al. Vardenafil, a new phosphodiesterase type 5 inhibitor, in the treatment of erectile dysfunction in men with diabetes: a multicenter double-blind placebo-controlled fixed-dose study. Diabetes Care, 2003; Vol. 26: pp. 777–83.

Comments: Prospective, randomized, multicenter double-blind placebo-controlled fixed-dose parallel-group phase III trial, 452 patients with type 1 or type 2 DM and ED taking 10 or 20 mg vardenafil or placebo as needed for 12 weeks. Vardenafil statistically improved erectile function and was generally well tolerated in these diabetic patients with ED.

Eardley I, Ellis P, Boolell M, et al. Onset and duration of action of sildenafil for the treatment of erectile dysfunc- tion. Br J Clin Pharmacol, 2002; Vol. 53 Suppl 1: pp. 61S–65S.

Comments: Sildenafil is an effective oral treatment for ED that acts relatively quickly and has a duration of action lasting at least 4 h.

Ng KK, Lim HC, Ng FC, et al. The use of sildenafil in patients with erectile dysfunction in relation to diabetes mellitus—a study of 1,511 patients. Singapore Med J, 2002; Vol. 43: pp. 387–90.

Comments: 78% of patients with DM reported success with sildenafil, compared to 86.5% of patients without DM.

Sáenz de Tejada I, Anglin G, Knight JR, et al. Effects of tadalafil on erectile dysfunction in men with diabetes. Diabetes Care, 2002; Vol. 25: pp. 2159–64.

Comments: Randomized study suggesting that tadalafil therapy significantly enhanced erectile function and was well tolerated by men with diabetes and ED.

Price DE, Gingell JC, Gepi-Attee S, et al. Sildenafil: study of a novel oral treatment for erectile dysfunction in diabetic men. Diabet Med, 1998; Vol. 15: pp. 821–5.

Comments: Improved erections reported by 50% and 52% of patients with DM treated with sildenafil 25 mg and 50 mg, respectively, compared with 10% of those receiving placebo.

胃轻瘫

多潘立酮

Lipika Samal, MD, MPH, and Paul A. Pham, PharmD

适应证

FDA
- 并非 FDA 所批准的胃轻瘫治疗药物。
- 有些医生对那些有胃肠功能紊乱,且对标准疗法具有抗药性的病人开具多潘立酮,FDA 鼓励这些医生通过新药试用审查项目(IND)来申请使用。

非 FDA 批准的用途
- 糖尿病患者的胃轻瘫。
- 胃食管反流病。
- 作为止吐药。

作用机理
- 多潘立酮是一种多巴胺拮抗物(阻断 D_1 和 D_2 受体)。
- 多潘立酮通过抑制 D_1 受体上的多巴胺帮助胃肠平滑肌增加活性,通过阻断 D_2 受体抑制神经元释放乙酰胆碱。
- 成人的常用剂量。
- 治疗胃运动不足:每天可达三次,每次 10~20 毫克。饭前和晚上服用。

剂型

商品名	通用名	剂型	价格
多潘立酮马来酸盐(可通过新药试用审查(IND)来获取,拨打食品与药物管理局电话[301]796-3400)	多潘立酮	口服药片 10 毫克	未知

特殊人群的剂量

肾脏疾病者
- 肾排泄水平较低时可能需要调整剂量。

肝脏疾病者
- 药物广泛参与肝代谢。有严重肝脏疾病时需要慎重使用。

孕妇
- 禁止使用。

哺乳期
- 药物会进入母乳。FDA 建议哺乳期女性不要服用。

药物不良反应
一般
- 大部分研究给病人每日服用多潘立酮 30~60 毫克，持续几个星期的观察之后，显示可能有较小的不良反应。
- 偶尔有不良反应报告，包括口唇干燥，短暂的皮疹和皮肤瘙痒、头痛、腹部痛性痉挛、腹泻、昏睡、精神紧张。

常见
- 中枢神经问题：嗜睡、静坐不能、虚弱无力、焦虑、压抑、反应迟钝。
- 内分泌系统问题：高催乳素血症、男性乳腺增生、乳腺痛、月经紊乱、乳溢。

偶见
- 心脏问题：心室肌纤维颤动[见于大剂量静脉注射时（IV administration）]，QT 间期增长。

罕见
- 中枢神经问题：锥体外系症状（EPS）；抗精神病药的恶性综合征（NMS）；癫痫（更为罕见），因为多潘立酮难以渗透到中枢神经系统。
- 心脏问题：扭转型（室性）心动过速（TdP）。

和其他药物的相互作用
- 锂元素会与多巴胺拮抗剂起反应，特别是氟哌丁苯制剂（Haldol），所以也可能同多潘立酮反应。同时服用会出现身体虚弱、运动障碍、增加锥体外症候群和脑病，所以应当避免，控制锂元素的注入维持在合理的水平。

药物代谢动力学
- 吸收率 13%~17%：（1）服药前先服用甲氰咪呱或碳酸氢钠溶液可以促进吸收；（2）不易通过血脑屏障。
- 代谢和排泄：广泛通过肝脏和肠壁代谢。
- 与蛋白质结合率：91%~93%。
- 半衰期：7~9 小时。

专家建议
- FDA 目前不建议糖尿病胃轻瘫患者使用，但可以作为处方药。
- 对糖尿病型胃轻瘫，当甲氧氯普胺和低剂量乙琥红霉素疗效不佳时，可以考虑使用多潘立酮。
- 多潘立酮和甲氧氯普胺都可以减轻糖尿病型胃轻瘫，但多潘立酮对中枢神经的副作用要小一些（Patterson）。
- 潜在的严重副作用包括心脏骤停和心率紊乱。

参考文献

Sugumar A, Singh A, Pasricha PJ. A systematic review of the efficacy of domperidone for the treatment of diabetic gastroparesis. Clin Gastroenterol Hepatol, 2008; Vol. 6: pp. 726–33.

Comments: A good review on the safety and efficacy of domperidone.

Patterson D, Abell T, Rothstein R, et al. A double-blind multicenter comparison of domperidone and metoclo- pramide in the treatment of diabetic patients with symptoms of gastroparesis. Am J Gastroenterol, 1999; Vol. 94: pp. 1230–4.

Comments: Domperidone and metoclopramide were equally effective in alleviating symptoms of diabetic gas- troparesis, but domperidone resulted in less CNS side effects.

Heykants J, Knaeps A, Meuldermans W, et al. On the pharmacokinetics of domperidone in animals and man. I. Plasma levels of domperidone in rats and dogs. Age related absorption and passage through the blood brain barrier in rats. Eur J Drug Metab Pharmacokinet, 1981a; Vol. 6: pp. 27–36.

Comments: Pharmacokinetics were described in the 1980s.

红霉素

Lipika Samal, MD, MPH, and Paul A. Pham, PharmD

适应证
FDA
- 多种抗感染的适应证。

非 FDA 批准的应用
- 糖尿病型胃轻瘫（低剂量红霉素）。

药物机理
- 增加肠胃的运动能力，特别是在两餐之间。此效应可能是通过激励胃腔和十二指肠的促胃动素受体而实现。
- 促进胃的排空。

成人常用剂量：
- 每次 150~250mg，每日 3~4 次，饭前 30 分钟服用。

剂型

商品名	通用名	剂型	价格
红霉素碱（Abbott Pharmaceuticals 等企业生产）	红霉素	口服药片 250 毫克；500 毫克悬浊液，浓度为 200mg/5ml 或 400mg/5ml	$0.27 $0.41~$0.65

特殊人群的剂量
肾病
- 正常剂量。

孕妇
- B 类。

哺乳期妇女
- 会随乳液排除。美国儿科学会认为哺乳期可以服用。

药物不良反应
一般
- 胃肠道：副作用与剂量有关。所以可以根据临床反应对药物剂量进行调整。

常见
- 胃肠道：腹部疼痛、腹泻、食欲不振、恶心呕吐。

红霉素

常见

胃肠道：肝酶升高、获得性幽门肥厚性狭窄，难辨梭状芽孢杆菌导致的伪膜性肠炎。

皮疹（可逆的）。

心脏：QT间期延长（一般见于大剂量静脉滴注或与强效的肝药酶CYP3A4抑制剂同时使用时）。

耳毒性（一般见于大剂量静脉滴注时）。

罕见

胰腺炎。

皮肤病：多形性红斑型药疹，斯–约二氏综合征（多形糜烂性红斑的一型），中毒性表皮坏死松解症。

加重重症肌无力症状，同时有报告显示可以引发重症肌无力的并发症。

瘀胆型肝炎（特别是在使用红霉素盐制剂时，发生率 1/1 000，具可逆性）。

尖端扭转型室速(TdP)，特别见于女性。

药物相互作用

红霉素是一种酶作用物，也是已知的 P_{450}-3A4 和 1A2 细胞色素抑制剂；它可以和多种药物发生相互作用，任何肝药酶CYP3A4作用物与其同时服用时，作用都会明显增强。强效CYP3A4抑制剂（例如HIV蛋白酶抑制剂和唑类抗真菌剂等）会明显增加红霉素浓度，故应该避免使用。

禁忌与红霉素同时服用的药物包括：西沙比利、特非那定（丁苯哌丁醇）、阿司咪唑（抗组胺药）、匹莫齐特（双氟苯丁哌啶苯并咪唑酮）、麦角生物碱、齐拉西酮（抗精神病药）。

一些他汀类药物（辛伐他汀、洛伐他汀）与红霉素同时服用可能会增加肌病和横纹肌溶解症的风险，所以应当避免；作为替代，可以考虑阿伐他汀、帕伐他丁、罗苏伐他汀，用药时需严密监察。

秋水仙碱、地高辛（强心素）、地尔硫䓬、维拉帕米（异搏停）、胺碘酮、环孢霉素、他克莫司（免疫抑制药）、西罗莫司（免疫抑制药）、皮质醇、丁丙诺啡叔丁啡（镇痛药）、丁螺环酮（抗焦虑药）、茶碱：以上药物与红霉素同时服用时血清浓度会增加，因此需要在谨慎监视下小心服用。

酰胺咪嗪、氯扎平、地西潘（苯甲二氮卓）、舍曲林（抗抑郁药）、雷诺嗪（血管扩张药）：与红霉素同时服用时，血清浓度可能会增加，避免同时服用或谨慎使用。

咪达唑仑和芬太尼：避免同时服用。有报告显示会造成严重的镇静作用和呼吸抑制。

钙离子通道阻断剂（地尔硫䓬、氨氯地平、硝苯地平）：与红霉素同时服用可能会增加血清浓度，因此需要酌情降低剂量。

代动力学

吸收率 20%~50%

新陈代谢和排泄：有一部分会产生去甲基化的代谢产物。而大部分以原型通过粪便排出或以代谢产物的形式经胆排出。只有少部分经尿液排出。

- 与蛋白质结合率：75%~90%
- 半衰期：1~1.5 小时

专家建议

- 一般用于胃轻瘫的长期治疗，但对老年人和同时患有其他疾病的患者使用时应当谨慎。
- 用药时要特别检查与其他药物的相互作用。
- 可能会降低二型糖尿病患者的空腹血糖水平，作用机理还不清楚(Ueno)。

参考文献

Arts J, Caenepeel P, Verbeke K, et al. Influence of erythromycin on gastric emptying and meal related symptoms in functional dyspepsia with delayed gastric emptying. Gut, 2005; Vol. 5 pp. 455–60.

Comments: Describes the effect of erythromycin on gastric emptying.

Maganti K, Onyemere K, Jones MP. Oral erythromycin and symptomatic relief of gastroparesis: a systematic review. Am J Gastroenterol, 2003; Vol. 98: pp. 259–63.

Comments: A good review of low-dose erythromycin for the symptomatic relief gastroparesis.

Boivin MA, Carey MC, Levy H. Erythromycin accelerates gastric emptying in a dose-response manner in healthy subjects. Pharmacotherapy, 2003; Vol. 23: pp. 5–8.

Comments: Mechanism of action of low-dose erythromycin.

Ueno N, Inui A, Asakawa A, et al. Erythromycin administration before sleep is effective in decreasing fasting hyperglycemia in type 2 diabetic patients. Diabetes Care, 2001; Vol. 24: p. 607.

Comments: Erythromycin may reduce fasting glucose levels in patients with type 2 diabetes.

Ueno N, Inui A, Asakawa A, et al. Erythromycin improves glycaemic control in patients with Type II diabetes mellitus. Diabetologia, 2000; Vol. 43: pp. 411–15.

Comments: Low doses of erythromycin significantly improved glycemic control over weeks and lowered fasting blood glucose and fructosamine concentrations.

甲氧氯普胺

Lipika Samal, MD, MPH, and Paul A. Pham, PharmD

适应证

FDA

糖尿病患者的胃轻瘫（口服或静脉滴注）。

增强胃的排空和钡元素的小肠转运，后者用来帮助解决延迟排空干扰放射性检查的问题。

胃食管返流病（GRED）（口服）。

术后和化疗期间的呕吐、恶心（静脉滴注）。

小肠插管使用常规操作方式无法穿过幽门时（静脉滴注）。

非 FDA 批准的用途

诱导泌乳。

打嗝。

偏头痛。

作为放射线的敏化剂，辅助放射疗法治疗非小细胞性肺癌（NSCLC）。

作用机理

甲氧氯普胺增进胆碱能活性，通过以下两种方式：（1）引发节后的神经末梢释放乙酰胆碱；（2）增加平滑肌上的毒蕈碱受体的敏感性。

增进胃收缩的幅度和紧张度，放松幽门括约肌和十二指肠球，增强十二指肠和空肠的蠕动。

阻止中枢和外周神经对多巴胺的摄取。

常用成人剂量

每次 10mg，口服、静脉滴注、肌内注射，每日 4 次，饭前和睡前用药（用药 2~8 周）。在症状减退之前，可能需用药达 10 天。

剂型

商品名	通用名	剂型	价格
Reglan（Invamed 制药公司，及其他一些专利厂商）	盐酸甲氧氯普胺	口服药片 5mg 或 10mg；口服溶液 5mh/ml；静脉／肌肉注射管形瓶 5mg/ml	$0.27~$0.32 $19.27(16 只) $5.58

特殊人群的用药剂量

肾病患者

CrCl（内生肌酐清除率）<40 ml/min：从正常剂量的 50% 开始用药，然后逐渐加量至达效。

- 肝病患者。
- 不需要进行剂量调整。

孕妇
- 妊娠 B 类：动物实验未显示出损害生育能力或对胚胎产生伤害。有限的临床数据表明对于妊娠剧吐使用甲氧氯普胺是安全的。

哺乳期妇女
- 甲氧氯普胺会进入乳汁当中。美国儿科医师学会建议谨慎使用，以免对中枢神经系统产生影响。

药物不良反应

一般
- 中枢神经系统：对迟发性运动障碍的黑箱警告。

常见
- 神经方面问题：嗜睡（口服：2.1%~10%；静脉：大剂量（每次 1~2mg/kg 体重时发生率可达 70%）
- 疲劳。

偶见
- 可逆的锥体外系反应；假性帕金森症（与剂量相关，大于 40mg/d 时发生率普遍化）。
- 高催乳素血症、勃起功能障碍、月经失调。
- 头痛（4.2%~5.2%）。
- 肠胃反应：恶心、呕吐（关联性尚不清楚）。

罕见
- 抗精神病药的恶性综合征。
- 失眠、烦躁不安、抑郁。
- 低血压、高血压、AV 传导阻滞、窦性心动过缓、室上性心动过速（SVT）
- 过敏性反应。

药物相互作用
- 泊沙康唑：与甲氧氯普胺同时服用时，泊沙康唑血清浓度会减小。可在保持高脂肪膳食的情况下使用泊沙康唑，并注意记录治疗效果。
- 文拉法新（抗抑郁药）：可能会偶尔增加血清素综合征的风险。同时用时注意观察记录治疗效果。
- 镇静药物、苯二氮䓬类药物、鸦片麻醉剂：与甲氧氯普胺同时服用可会增加嗜睡。
- 单胺氧化酶抑制剂：同时服用时须要密切观察。
- 地高辛：血清浓度会减轻。与甲氧氯普胺同时服用时应注意观察血清浓度
- 多巴胺受体激动药物 [例如罗平尼哈（治疗帕金森氏症）、金刚烷胺、麦角环肽、左旋多巴、丙基麦角灵、普拉克索]：甲氧氯普胺可能会抵激动剂的活性。同时服用时须要密切观察。

甲氧氯普胺

药代动力学
- 最长吸收时间：口服 1~2 小时；静脉滴注 15 分钟。
- 代谢和排泄：85% 通过肾脏代谢排出，肝代谢的比重最小。
- 与蛋白质结合率：与 alpha-1- 酸糖蛋白结合率大约为 30%。
- 半衰期：5~6 小时。
- 分布：3.5L/kg

专家建议
- 甲氧氯普胺是唯一获得 FDA 认可的治疗胃轻瘫的药物。
- 短期（2~8 周）疗程使用甲氧氯普胺对糖尿病型胃轻瘫有较好的疗效。但有些患者可能会造成嗜睡问题。
- 小规模的前瞻性随机研究表明，对糖尿病型胃轻瘫患者使用甲氧氯普胺会改善胃排空。

参考文献

ata PF, Pigarelli DL. Chronic metoclopramide therapy for diabetic gastroparesis. Ann Pharmacother, 2003; Vol. 37: pp. 122–6.

Comments: Literature review through 2002 concluding that there is limited evidence of long-term efficacy of metoclopramide for diabetic gastroparesis.

atterson D, Abell T, Rothstein R, et al. A double-blind multicenter comparison of domperidone and metoclo- pramide in the treatment of diabetic patients with symptoms of gastroparesis. Am J Gastroenterol, 1999; Vol. 94: pp. 1230–4.

Comments: Prospective randomized trial found metoclopramide to be as effective as domperidone for the treatment diabetic gastroparesis; however, CNS side effects were more severe and more common with meto- clopramide (49% vs 29% after 4 weeks of metoclopramide 40 mg/d).

icci DA, Saltzman MB, Meyer C, et al. Effect of metoclopramide in diabetic gastroparesis. J Clin Gastroenterol, 1985; Vol. 7: pp. 25–32.

Comments: Randomized double-blind crossover design—13 patients received 10 mg metoclopramide 4 times a day. Overall mean symptom reduction of 52.6% for nausea, vomiting, anorexia, fullness, and bloating. 7 patients had improved gastric retention on gastric emptying studies, though these results did not correlate with symptom relief.

cCallum TW, Ricci DA, Rakatansky H, et al. A multicenter placebo-controlled clinical trial of oral metoclo- pramide in diabetic gastroparesis. Diabetes Care, 1983; Vol. 6: p. 463.

Comments: 40 patients with diabetic gastroparesis were randomized in a double-blind study to metoclo- pramide 10 mg tablet 4 times daily or placebo. Treatment significantly reduced postprandial fullness. Mean gastric emptying assessed by radionuclide scintigraphy was significantly improved in the metoclopramide- treated group when compared with their baseline.

nape WJ, Battle WM, Schwartz SS, et al. Metoclopramide to treat gastroparesis due to diabetes mellitus: a double-blind, controlled trial. Ann Intern Med, 1982; Vol. 96: pp. 444–6.

Comments: Randomized, double-blind, controlled trial—10 patients received 10 mg metoclopramide 4 times a day for 3 weeks. Treatment resulted in an increase in the rate of gastric emptying (56.8% ± 7.4%) in contrast to the response to placebo (37.6% ± 7.7%) (p ,0.01).

降糖治疗

α 糖苷酶抑制剂

Nadeen Hosein, MD, MS, and Brian Pinto, PharmD, MBA

适应证

FDA
- 2 型糖尿病患者。

机制
- 竞争性和可逆性抑制酶（α 糖苷水解酶），这种酶可以在小肠刷状缘把多糖分解。
- 延迟了胃肠道单糖的吸收，降低餐后高血糖。
- 几乎不抑制乳糖酶，因此不会造成乳糖不耐受。

成人常用剂量
- 在使用 α 糖苷酶抑制剂（AGI）前，检测基线肝酶，在使用的第一年内每三个月监测一次，以后定期监测。
- AGI 必须随餐第一口嚼服。具体剂量见下文。
- 阿卡波糖起始：25mg 口服，每日一次；可上调至 25mg 每日三次。
- 阿卡波糖维持：50–100mg，每日三次；最大剂量 50mg 每日三次（如果体重 <60kg）或者 100mg 每日三次（如果体重 >60kg）。
- 米格列醇起始：25mg 口服每日三次。
- 米格列醇维持：50mg 每日三次（最大剂量 100mg 每日 3 次）。

剂型

商品名	通用名	剂型	价格
阿卡波糖（Cobalt、Roxane、拜耳和其他）	阿卡波糖	口服片剂 25mg 口服片剂 50mg 口服片剂 100mg	$82/100 片 $88/100 片 $90/100 片
米格列醇（辉瑞）	米格列醇	口服片剂 25mg 口服片剂 50mg 口服片剂 100mg	$88/90 片 $97/90 片 $110/90 片

α 糖苷酶抑制剂

特殊人群用量

肾脏
- GFR<25ml/min 或肌酐 >2mg/dl 时不应使用。

肝脏
- 肝硬化患者禁止使用。

妊娠
- FDA 妊娠分级为 B 级。

哺乳期
- 汤姆森哺乳风险评级：婴儿不应使用。

药物不良反应

整体人群
- 在肾功能衰竭患者（GFR<25ml/min 或肌酐 >2mg/dl）患者不应使用。
- 存在胃肠道疾病，如炎症性肠病、肠梗阻/肠闭塞，存在潜在增加胃肠道胀气的疾病，存在影响消化和吸收的疾病或者慢性消化性溃疡时禁用。
- 如与胰岛素促泌剂联用（磺脲类或格列奈类药物）时可引起低血糖。并只能通过口服葡萄糖（单糖）纠正，而非蔗糖（对蔗糖、双糖的分解被抑制）。
- 阿卡波糖禁用于肝硬化患者。
- 不能应用于糖尿病酮症酸中毒。

常见不良反应
- 许多患者（高达 74%）会出现胃肠道反应（胀气、腹泻、腹胀、腹痛）。

少见不良反应
- 米格列醇可导致一过性皮疹。
- 米格列醇会降低血清中铁水平。

罕见不良反应
- 剂量依赖的肝毒性。因此，在使用的第一年内每 3 个月检查肝酶，随后应规律监测。

药物相互作用
生长激素可能会导致口服降糖药，如阿卡波糖和米格列醇的有效性下降（见表 4-3）。

α 糖苷酶抑制剂

药代动力学

表 4-3 α 糖苷酶抑制剂的药代动力学

	阿卡波糖	米格列醇
吸收	<2% 吸收	25-mg 剂量 100% 被吸收；100-mg 剂量 50%~70% 被吸收
代谢	胃和小肠	不代谢，原型排出
排泄	51% 粪便，34% 肾脏	肾脏
蛋白结合	几乎没有	极少
半衰期	2 小时	2 小时
容量分布	0.32L/kg	0.18L/kg

Courtesy of Paul Pham, PharmD, 约翰·霍普金斯大学医学院。

专家意见

- 预期可使 HbA1c 下降 0.5%~0.7%。
- 不影响体重。
- 单药使用不引起低血糖。
- 如果与磺脲类联用出现低血糖，要以口服葡萄糖纠正，不能使用蔗糖。
- 每日多次给药方案可能导致服药依从性下降。
- 胃肠道反应（胀气、腹泻、腹胀、腹痛）是这类药物在美国没能广泛应用的主要原因。
- 对糖耐量异常人群，阿卡波糖可预防糖尿病和心血管合并症发生。

参考文献

Chiasson JL, Josse RG, Gomis R, et al. Acarbose treatment and the risk of cardiovascular disease and hypertension in patients with impaired glucose tolerance: the STOP-NIDDM trial. JAMA,2003; Vol. 290: pp. 486–94.

Comments:Patients with impaired glucose tolerance who were treated with acarbose had significant reductions in risk for experiencing future myocardial infarctions and for developing hypertension.

Chiasson JL, Josse RG, Gomis R, et al. Acarbose for prevention of type 2 diabetes mellitus: the STOP-NIDDM randomised trial. Lancet,2002; Vol. 359: pp. 2072–7.

Comments: In this prospective study, 1429 patients with impaired glucose tolerance were randomized to either acarbose or placebo therapy. After 3.3 years, the acarbose group had a statistically significant 25% reduction in risk for developing type diabetes mellitus.

Campbell LK, Baker DE, Campbell RK. Miglitol: assessment of its role in the treatment of patients with diabetes

mellitus. Ann Pharmacother,2000; Vol. 34: pp. 1291–301.

Comments:Overview of the pharmacology of miglitol and its use in treating patients with type 2 diabetes mellitus.

DPP-IV 抑制剂

Nadeen Hosein, MD, MS, and Brian Pinto, PharmD, MBA

适应证

FDA

- 2 型糖尿病患者。

机制

- 通过抑制二肽基肽酶 IV（DPP-IV）的活性，抑制肠促胰素如 GLP-1 的降解。使肠促胰素的活性延长，通过多种机制降低血糖。

成人常用剂量

- 西格列汀：推荐剂量为 50~100mg，每日一次；可同餐或非同餐服用。
- 沙格列汀：推荐剂量为 2.5 或 5mg，每日一次；可同餐或非同餐服用。
- 西格列汀 + 二甲双胍：命名为捷诺达 50/500mg，每日两次，同餐服用。可以加量至 50/1 000mg，每日两次，同餐服用（日最大剂量）。
- 沙格列汀 + 二甲双胍缓释：即 Kombiglyze，2.5/1 000mg，5/1 000mg 或者 5/2000mg，每日一次，晚餐服用。
- 当西格列汀或沙格列汀与磺脲类降糖药联用时，可以考虑减少磺脲类降糖药的剂量以减少低血糖风险。
- FDA 批准西格列汀及沙格列汀作为 2 型糖尿病（T2DM）患者的单药治疗。
- 西格列汀或沙格列汀可以与二甲双胍或噻唑烷二酮联用。
- 美国，DPP-IV 抑制剂还没有和胰岛素联用的研究。

剂型

商品名	通用名	剂型	价格
捷诺维（默克）	盐酸西格列汀	25mg 口服 50mg 口服 100mg 口服	30 片 $214 30 片 $214 30 片 $214
安立泽（百时美-施贵宝）	沙格列汀	2.5mg 口服 5mg 口服	30 片 $190 30 片 $190
捷诺达（默沙东）	盐酸西格列汀 + 盐酸二甲双胍	50/500mg 口服 50/1 000mg 口服	60 片 $197 60 片 $196

特殊人群用量

肾脏病

西格列汀

- GFR ≥ 50ml/min，无须调整剂量。

- GFR：30~50ml/min，每日不超过 50mg。
- GFR<30ml/min，每日不超过 25mg。
- 血液透析或腹膜透析的患者，每日不超过 25mg。

沙格列汀
- GFR>50ml/min，无须调整剂量。
- GFR ≤ 50ml/min，每日不超过 2.5mg。
- 进行血液透析的患者，调整至每日 2.5mg。

捷诺达
- GFR ≤ 60ml/min 或的血肌酐 ≥ 1.4mg/dl（女性）或 ≥ 1.5mg/dl（男性）患者禁用。
- 肝脏疾病。
- 除捷诺达外剂量无需调整；避免使用于患肝脏疾病的患者，因会升高发生乳酸酸中毒的风险。

妊娠
- FDA 妊娠分级 B 级。

哺乳期
- 汤姆森哺乳风险评级：婴儿不应使用。

药物不良反应

整体人群
- 禁用于对西格列汀或沙格列汀过敏的患者。
- 不应使用于糖尿病酮症酸中毒患者。
- 不应用于治疗 1 型糖尿病。
- 西格列汀有发生急性胰腺炎的报道——内科医师在开始使用西格列汀或增加剂量时，应严密监测患者有无胰腺炎的症状和体征。
- 捷诺达因含有二甲双胍，禁用于肾脏病患者（见上文）。

少见不良反应
- 低血糖，当与磺脲类联用时更为常见。
- 鼻咽炎或上呼吸道感染。
- 头痛。
- 恶心、腹泻、腹痛。
- 泌尿系感染。
- 水肿。
- 捷诺达：二甲双胍造成的胃肠道反应（恶心、呕吐、腹泻），随餐服用时可以减轻。

罕见不良反应
- 西格列汀可能发生急性胰腺炎。
- Stevens-Johnson 综合征，荨麻疹，剥脱性皮炎和其他超敏皮肤反应。

- 过敏反应。
- 血管性水肿。
- 横纹肌溶解。
- 急性肾衰竭。
- 沙格列汀可能发生骨折。
- 捷诺达因有二甲双胍成分,可能发生乳酸酸中毒。

药物相互作用

- 地高辛:使用地高辛 0.25mg/d 时,口服西格列汀导致地高辛 AUC 轻度(11%)升高和血浆 Cmax 升高(18%)。不推荐对地高辛进行剂量调整,但建议严密监测。

药代动力学

- 吸收:西格列汀:生物利用度 87%;达峰时间 1~4 小时。沙格列汀:达峰时间 2 小时。
- 代谢和排泄:西格列汀:肝脏代谢;87% 经肾脏排出,13% 经粪便排出;透析清除率 13.5%。沙格列汀:肝脏代谢;60% 肾脏排出,22% 经粪便排出;透析清除率 23%。
- 蛋白结合率:西格列汀:38%。沙格列汀:几乎不结合。
- Cmax,Cmin 和 AUC:西格列汀:健康志愿者单次口服 100mg,平均西格列汀血浆 AUC 为 8.52 μM/hr; Cmax 为 950nM。
- $T_{1/2}$:西格列汀:12.4 小时。沙格列汀:2.5 小时。
- 分布:西格列汀:Vd 2.8L/kg。

专家意见

- 西格列汀单药最大剂量(100mg 每日)18 周仅能降低 HbA1c 约 0.6%(0.5%~0.8%)(Raz)。因其价格相对昂贵,故当基线 HbA1c<8% 时,内分泌科医师更愿意把 DPP-IV 抑制剂作为二线或三线降糖药。
- 西格列汀不增加体重。
- 西格列汀在 2006 年 10 月上市,故目前还没有长期的安全性数据。
- 2009 年 7 月,FDA 批准一种新的 DPP-IV 抑制剂,沙格列汀(安立泽)用于治疗 T2DM。
- 其他 DPP-IV 抑制剂(如维格列汀和阿格列汀),目前还未被 FDA 批准(现已被批准,译者注)。
- 在欧洲维格列汀已被广泛被批准应用,西格列汀目前已被批准和胰岛素联用。

参考文献

Rosenstock J, Aguilar-Salinas C, Klein E, et al. Effect of saxagliptin monotherapy in treatment-naïve patients with type 2 diabetes. Curr Med Res Opin,2009; Vol. 25: pp. 2401–11.

Comments:In this double-blind trial, 401 patients were randomized to 2.5 mg, 5 mg, 10 mg of saxagliptin or placebo for 24 weeks. Patients in the saxagliptin groups taking 2.5 mg, 5 mg and 10 mg achieved hemoglobin A1C reductions of 0.43%, 0.46% and 0.54%, respectively, compared to a 0.19% reduction in the placebo group.

Chia CW, Egan JM. Incretin-based therapies in type 2 diabetes mellitus. J Clin Endocrinol Metab,2008; Vol. 93: pp. 3703–16.

Comments: Overview of the role of DPP-IV inhibitors and GLP-1 agonists in treating type 2 diabetes mellitus.

Nauck MA, Meininger G, Sheng D, et al. Efficacy and safety of the dipeptidyl peptidase-4 inhibitor, sitagliptin, compared with the sulfonylurea, glipizide, in patients with type 2 diabetes inadequately controlled on metformin alone: a randomized, double-blind, non-inferiority trial. Diabetes Obes Metab,2007; Vol. 9: pp. 194–205.

Comments: In this noninferiority study, 1172 patients on metformin monotherapy and baseline HbA1c of 7.5% were randomly assigned to receive either sitagliptin 100 mg/day or glipizide 5–20 mg/day. After 1 year, both groups showed a 0.67% HbA1c reduction, demonstrating noninferiority.

Raz I, Hanefeld M, Xu L, et al. Efficacy and safety of the dipeptidyl peptidase-4 inhibitor sitagliptin as monotherapy in patients with type 2 diabetes mellitus. Diabetologia,2006; Vol. 49: pp. 2564–71.

Comments: Sitagliptin monotherapy reduced HbA1c by 0.6% after 18 weeks at its maximum daily dose of 100 mg.

肠促胰素类似物和胰淀粉样多肽类似物

Ana Emiliano, MD, and Brian Pinto, PharmD, MBA

适应证

FDA

- 肠促胰素类似物（艾塞那肽和利拉鲁肽）：2型糖尿病患者（T2DM），目前没有批准和胰岛素联用。
- 胰淀粉样多肽类似物（普兰林肽）：胰岛素治疗的1型糖尿病（T1DM）和T2DM。

机制

- 肠促胰素类似物（艾塞那肽、利拉鲁肽）：刺激血糖依赖的胰岛素分泌，减慢胃排空。抑制胰高血糖素分泌；抑制食欲。

  – 以上两种制剂（艾塞那肽、利拉鲁肽），为胰高糖素样肽激动剂，与GLP-1受体结合，刺激血糖依赖的胰岛素分泌。

- 胰淀粉样多肽类似物（普兰林肽）：减缓胃排空，抑制餐后胰高糖素过度的升高（见T2DM），增加饱感。

  – 普兰林肽：与天然的胃蛋白胰淀粉样多肽作用相似，与胰岛β细胞共同分泌胰岛素。

成人常用剂量

- 启用肠促胰素类似物前需评估肾功能。
- 艾塞那肽：5mcg皮下注射每日两次起始（餐前60分钟内注射），如果患者可以耐受，注射一个月后增加到10mcg每日两次（最大日剂量）。
- 利拉鲁肽：0.6mg皮下注射每日一次起始，一周后增加至1.2mg（最大剂量1.8mg每日一次）。
- 普兰林肽：T1DM患者，15mcg每餐前即刻皮下注射，可减少50%的胰岛素剂量来避免低血糖。如没有明显恶心症状，每3~7天可加量15mcg，推荐剂量为60mcg餐前即刻注射。T2DM患者，60mcg每餐前即刻皮下注射，加量至推荐的120mcg每日两次餐前注射。
- 可以使用注射笔或瓶装制剂皮下注射：将mcg（注射笔）转换为单位（瓶装制剂），即将mcg的剂量除以6即可（如，120mcg=20单位）。

肠促胰素类似物和胰淀粉样多肽类似物

剂型

商品名	通用名	剂型	价格
百泌达（Amylin 制药）	艾塞那肽	10 mcg/0.04 ml；5 mcg/0.02 ml 皮下注射	30 天 $271；30 天 $265
诺和力（诺和诺德）	利拉鲁肽	18 mg/3 ml 皮下注射	2 支 3ml 预填充 $280；3 支 3ml 预填充 $400
Symlin（Amylin 制药）	普兰林肽	600 mcg/ml；1 000 mcg/ml 皮下注射	1 支 5ml $228；一盒共 2 支 2.7ml 预填充 $312

特殊人群用量

肾脏病
- 艾塞那肽：GFR < 30ml/min 的患者不应使用。起始药物治疗或剂量调整时，对 GFR 于 30~50ml/min 的患者需监测血肌酐。
- 利拉鲁肽：慎用与肾功能受损的患者。
- 普兰林肽：不适用于中度到重度的肾脏病（GFR 20~50ml/min）患者。对血液透析的患者其安全性不详。

肝脏疾病
- 艾塞那肽和利拉鲁肽：需慎用。
- 普兰林肽：没有研究证明其在肝脏疾病患者的安全性。

妊娠
- 艾塞那肽、利拉鲁肽和普兰林肽 FDA 妊娠分级为 C 级。

哺乳期
- 肠促胰素类似物和普兰林肽：在人类乳汁中排泄情况未知。在哺乳期因婴儿风险未知应慎用。

药物不良反应

整体人群
- 肠促胰素类似物：胰腺炎不常见。如果严重的腹痛加重，停止用药并除外胰腺炎。FDA 罕见报道重度、坏死和出血性胰腺炎。
- 利拉鲁肽：增加啮齿动物发生甲状腺髓样癌风险。在人类是否暴露于同样的风险目前未知。但不应应用于患有甲状腺髓样癌或有家族史的患者，及患有多发性内分泌腺瘤病 2 型（MEN-2）或有家族史的患者 (http://dailymed.nlm.nih.gov/dailymed/about)。

肠促胰素类似物和胰淀粉样多肽类似物

- 普兰林肽、艾塞那肽和利拉鲁肽:因药物会减慢胃排空,故避免应用于胃轻瘫患者。
- 普兰林肽:黑框警告与胰岛素联用时减少胰岛素剂量以减少严重低血糖。避免应用于无感知低血糖的患者。

常见不良反应
- 肠促胰素类似物和普兰林肽:恶心,通常随使用时间延长有所减轻。
- 普兰林肽:低血糖。

少见不良反应
- 艾塞那肽和利拉鲁肽:腹泻、头痛。
- 普兰林肽:上腹痛、关节痛。

罕见不良反应
- 艾塞那肽:血管性水肿、皮疹。
- 利拉鲁肽:血管性水肿。

药物相互作用
- 与降糖药联用发生低血糖。
- 艾塞那肽和利拉鲁肽:减慢胃排空,可以影响口服药吸收。
- 普兰林肽:可能加强抗胆碱能药物的抗胆碱作用。

药代动力学

表 4-4 肠促胰岛素类似物和胰淀素类似物的药代动力学

药物	吸收	代谢	排泄	半衰期
艾塞那肽	血浆峰值 ~2 小时	全身性作用小	尿液	2.4 小时
利拉鲁肽	血浆峰值 8~12 小时	由内生 DPP-IV	尿液及粪便	~13 小时
普兰林肽	血浆峰值 20 分钟	经肾脏代谢为活性代谢产物	尿液	~48 分钟

Courtesy of Paul Pham, PharmD, 约翰·霍普金斯大学医学院。

专家意见
- 艾塞那肽可以剂量依赖性减轻体重 ~1.4kg;更适用于伴有肥胖的患者 (DeFronzo; Kendall)。
- 普兰林肽体重平均下降 0.5~1.4kg (Ratner; Hollander)。
- 利拉鲁肽体重下降 2~2.5kg (Nauck)。
- 因此,体重下降是此类药物吸引力的主要原因。
- 艾塞那肽和利拉鲁肽可以使 HbA1c 下降 ~1.0% (Nauck),与基线 HbA1c 水平成比例。
- T2DM 患者使用普兰林肽 HbA1c 下降 0.62%(Hollander), T1DM 下降 0.3% (Ratner)。

- 肠促胰素类似物和胰淀粉样多肽类似物通常不作为单药治疗应用。
- 肠促胰素类似物和胰淀粉样多肽类似物只能用于皮下注射，若患者惧怕注射则不建议应用。
- 近期研究发现，艾塞那肽与甘精胰岛素联用可以使血糖正常化并没有严重低血糖发生 (Buse)。

推荐依据

Nauck M, Frid A, Hermansen K, et al. Efficacy and safety comparison of liraglutide, glimepiride, and placebo, all in combination with metformin, in type 2 diabetes: the LEAD (liraglutide effect and action in diabetes)-2 study. Diabetes Care,2009; Vol. 32: pp. 84–90.

Comments: A double-blind, double-dummy, placebo and active-controlled trial for 26 weeks, including 1091 type 2 diabetes patients randomly assigned to 0.6 mg, 1.2 mg, and 1.8 mg daily of liraglutide added to metformin, or placebo added to metformin, or glimepiride added to metformin. While patients in the 1.8-mg and 1.2-mg liraglutide and in the glimepiride groups achieved a hemoglobin A1c reduction of 1%, only patients taking liraglutide achieved a significant weight loss (1.8–2.8 kg), whereas patients in the glimepiride group gained on average 1.0 kg.

DeFronzo RA, Ratner RE, Han J, et al. Effects of exenatide (exendin-4) on glycemic control and weight over 30 weeks in metformin-treated patients with type 2 diabetes. Diabetes Care,2005; Vol. 28: pp. 1092–100.

Comments: Double-blind, randomized, placebo-controlled trial involving 336 subjects with type 2 diabetes, who were given 0 mcg, 5 mcg, or 10 mcg of exenatide for 30 weeks. There was a mean hemoglobin A1c reduction of 0.78 (0.1%) and an average weight loss of 2.8 (0.5 kg) in the group receiving exenatide 10 mcg twice daily.

Kendall DM, Riddle MC, Rosenstock J, et al. Effects of exenatide (exendin-4) on glycemic control over 30 weeks in patients with type 2 diabetes treated with metformin and a sulfonylurea. Diabetes Care,2005; Vol. 28: pp. 1083–91.

Comments: This 30-week double-blind, randomized, placebo-controlled trial including 733 subjects showed that patients on 10 mcg of exenatide twice daily achieved better glycemic control (mean hemoglobin A1c reduction of 0.8 [0.1%]) than patients taking 5 mcg or taking placebo. The weight loss was significant in both 5- and 10-mcg arms of exenatide therapy, averaging 1.6 kg (0.2%).

Ratner RE, Dickey R, Fineman M, et al. Amylin replacement with pramlintide as an adjunct to insulin therapy improves long-term glycaemic and weight control in type 1 diabetes mellitus: a 1-year, randomized controlled trial. Diabet Med,2004; Vol. 21 pp. 1204–12.

Comments: Double-blind, placebo-controlled, randomized, multicenter, 52-week trial of 651 patients with type 1 diabetes, to which placebo injections 3–4 times a day or various doses of pramlintide 3–4 times daily were added to their baseline insulin regimen. Patients taking pramlintide 60 mcg 3–4 times a day achieved a hemoglobin A1c reduction of 0.29% and 0.34%, respectively, compared to the placebo group. The pramlintide group as a whole lost an average of 0.4 kg versus a gain of 0.8 kg in the placebo group.

其他参考文献

Buse JB, Bergenstal RM, Glass LC, et al. Use of twice-daily exenatide in basal insulin-treated patients with type 2 diabetes: a randomized, controlled trial. Ann Intern Med,2010; Vol. 154: pp. 103–12.

Comments: In a multicenter trial of 261 patients with uncontrolled type 2 diabetes receiving insulin glargine, adding twice-daily exenatide injections significantly improves glycemic control without increased hypoglycemia or weight gain compared to placebo (-0.69%).

Joy SV, Rodgers PT, Scates AC. Incretin mimetics as emerging treatments for type 2 diabetes. Ann Pharmacother,2005; Vol. 39: pp. 110–8.

Comments: Review of the physiology, mechanism of action, pharmacology, efficacy, and side effect profile of exenatide and liraglutide.

Hollander PA, Levy P, Fineman MS, et al. Pramlintide as an adjunct to insulin therapy improves long-term glycemic and weight control in patients with type 2 diabetes: a 1-year randomized controlled trial. Diabetes Care,2003; Vol. 26: pp. 784–90.

Comments: In this double-blind, placebo-controlled, 52-week trial, 656 patients with type 2 diabetes on insulin (some patients were also on a sulfonylurea or metformin), were randomized to receive pramlintide 60 mcg, 90 mcg, or 120 mcg twice daily versus placebo. The patients taking 120 mcg of pramlintide had a significant hemoglobin A1c reduction of 0.62% over the placebo group and lost on average 1.4 kg, while patients in the placebo group gained 0.7 kg.

US Food and Drug Administration (FDA). Information for Healthcare Professionals: Exenatide (marketed as Byetta). www.fda.gov/Drugs/DrugSafety/PostmarketDrugSafetyInformationforPatientsandProviders/ucm124713.htm,8/2008 Update. Accessed June 16, 2010.

Comments: Exenatide prescribing information for patients with pancreatitis; recommends that exenatide be discontinued if pancreatitis is suspected.

二甲双胍

Nadeen Hosein, MD, MS, and Brian Pinto, PharmD, MBA

适应证

FDA
- 2 型糖尿病。

非 FDA 批准适应证
- 多囊卵巢综合征。
- 在特定的空腹血糖受损和/或糖耐量受损（糖尿病前期）人群中可预防 2 型糖尿病发生。
- 预防妊娠期糖尿病。

机制
- 减少肝糖生成。
- 减少胃肠道对糖的吸收。
- 增加外周葡萄糖摄取和应用。

成人常用剂量
- 速释片："低开始，慢慢走"，同餐或餐后服用减少胃肠道副作用。
- 如没有开始以低剂量起始，没有缓慢调整剂量或在空腹服用，高达 20% 的患者会出现胃肠道反应。
- 建议以 500mg 晚餐服用起始，2 周后加量到 500mg 早餐和 500mg 晚餐服用 2 周，随后加量至 500mg 早餐，1g 晚餐，2 周后如无副反应，则加量至 1g 早晚餐服用。
- 对速释片常规维持剂量为 1 000~2 550mg 每日，分为 2~3 次口服。最大日剂量 2 550mg。
- 缓释片：500mg 缓释片每日一次，每周增加 500mg。最大日剂量 2 500mg（Fortamet），2 000mg（格华止缓释片和 Glumetza）。

剂型

商品名	通用名	剂型	价格
二甲双胍（非专利保护的）（Sandoz, Ivax, Mylan 和其他公司）	盐酸二甲双胍	500mg 口服 850 mg 口服 1 000 mg 口服	60 片 $13 60 片 $52 60 片 $36
格华止（百时美施贵宝）	盐酸二甲双胍	500mg 口服 850 mg 口服 1 000 mg 口服	60 片 $70 60 片 $113 60 片 $141

二甲双胍

商品名	通用名	剂型	价格
Riomet (Ranbaxy Laboratories)	盐酸二甲双胍	每5ml含500mg的口服液(118ml，473ml)	473ml $100
二甲双胍缓释片（非专利保护的）(Amneal, Ranbaxy, Watson, and others)	盐酸二甲双胍缓释片	500mg 口服 750 mg 口服	90片 $19 90片 $99
格华止 XR（百时美施贵宝）	盐酸二甲双胍缓释片	500mg 口服 750 mg 口服	60片 $70 60片 $108
Fortamet (Sciele Pharmaceutical)	盐酸二甲双胍缓释片	500mg 口服 1 000mg 口服	60片 $134 60片 $302
Glumetza (Depomed)	盐酸二甲双胍缓释片	500mg 口服 1 000 mg 口服	100片 $175 90片 $382

特殊人群用量

肾脏病
- 禁用于肌酐 >1.4mg/dl（女性）或 >1.5mg/dl（男性），因增加发生乳酸酸中毒的风险。

肝脏疾病
- 尽量避免，因会增加发生乳酸酸中毒的风险。

妊娠
- FDA 妊娠分级为 B 级。

哺乳期
- 汤姆森哺乳风险评级：婴儿风险是极低的。
- 在一项 Glueck 的研究中（2006 年），哺乳期女性使用二甲双胍（日剂量 2 550mg）6 个月，对于婴儿的生长、运动和社交能力并无影响。对婴儿 6 个月后的影响目前还没有研究。

药物不良反应

整体人群
- 如同餐或餐后服用耐受性佳（减少了胃肠道不良反应）。
- 禁用于肾功能受损患者（女性肌酐 ≥ 1.4mg/dl），男性 ≥ 1.5mg/dl），因增加发生乳酸酸中毒的风险。
- 如果患者进行影像学检查需使用碘造影剂，则在之前或接受检查当天停用二甲双胍，如果检查后肾功能正常，则在 48 小时后继续使用二甲双胍。
- 避免酒精滥用（增加乳酸酸中毒风险）。
- 不要在糖尿病酮症酸中毒时使用，不用于 1 型糖尿病患者的治疗。

常见不良反应

- 恶心、呕吐、腹泻、腹胀、消化不良;如上文所述,药物以低剂量起始,缓慢加量,可以减少胃肠道反应。
- 维生素 B_{12} 缺乏。
- 无力感(身体虚弱或强度损失)。

罕见不良反应

- 因维生素 B_{12} 缺乏导致的巨幼细胞性贫血;二甲双胍可能导致胃肠道维生素 B_{12} 吸收减少。
- 乳酸酸中毒——罕见,但致命(死亡率达 50%)。在存在以下情况的患者更易发生,包括肾功能不全,脱水,酗酒,肝脏疾病,败血症,充血性心功能衰竭,急性心肌梗死,老年人(尤其是年龄 >80 岁),以及其他导致缺氧和灌注减低的疾病(过度生成乳酸或减少乳酸清除)。二甲双胍增加乳酸生成因此增加血乳酸水平。

药物相互作用

- 碘造影剂加强二甲双胍相关的乳酸中毒的不良反应/毒性。在患者接受碘造影剂之前或当天应暂时停药,在接受检查后 48 小时候再开始应用。再次开始使用二甲双胍前需充分平复肾功能情况。
- 多非利特(一种抗心律失常药)经肾小球滤过及肾小管分泌排出。二甲双胍在此通路上与多非利特竞争,使多非利特清除减少,致其在血液中浓度升高,增加心脏毒性风险。二甲双胍和多非利特同时应用时需谨慎。
- 当二甲双胍与其他可能导致肌酐升高的药物一起应用时需谨慎使用,肌酐一旦超过上述建议应停用二甲双胍。

药代动力学

- 吸收:空腹时生物利用度 50%~60%。食物升高缓释片 AUC 达 38%~73%。
- 代谢和排泄:无代谢产物。90% 经肾排出。可经透析排出。
- 蛋白结合率:几乎不结合。
- Cmax,Cmin 和 AUC:
- 格华止缓释片:虽然 Cmax 和 Tmax 并未改变,但食物增加大约 50% 的吸收(同每 AUC)。
- Fortamet:食物增加大约 60% 的吸收;Cmax 增加 30%,Tmax 延长(6.1 小时 vs 4 小时)。
- Glumetza:与空腹相比,低脂和高脂餐分别增加 AUC 达 38% 和 73%。均延长 Tmax 大约 3 小时,但不影响 Cmax。缓释片达峰时间 7 小时。
- $T_{1/2}$:速释片为 6.2 小时。
- 分布:Vd 为(654±358)L。

专家意见

- 使用最大剂量二甲双胍单药治疗 3 个月,HbA1c 下降 1%~2%。
- 二甲双胍是有效的,在大多数患者均可引起体重下降,价格低廉,单药治疗时不引起低血糖。因此,如果没有禁忌证,是大多数新诊断的超重 2 型糖尿病患者的一线治疗。

- 接受胰岛素治疗的超重 2 型糖尿病患者，通常需要二甲双胍来减少胰岛素剂量，因为二甲双胍有增加胰岛素敏感性的作用。如果停止二甲双胍，会增加胰岛素剂量。
- 如患者接受影像学检查需使用静脉碘造影剂，则在之前或接受检查当天停用二甲双胍，如果检查后肾功能正常，则在 48 小时后继续使用二甲双胍。
- 住院患者，根据病情，可暂停二甲双胍暂时开始胰岛素治疗；出院时如果肌酐符合上文提到的标准，则继续二甲双胍治疗。
- 老年患者需谨慎使用二甲双胍，因其可能肌酐虽在正常范围但肾功能受损。同时老年患者使用多种药物，可能影响肾功能，增加乳酸酸中毒风险。
- 长期使用二甲双胍的患者需监测血液学指标和维生素 B_{12} 水平，尤其是那些长时间使用较高剂量的患者。必要时补充维生素 B_{12}。

参考文献

Mathur R, Alexander CJ, Yano J, et al. Use of metformin in polycystic ovary syndrome. Am J Obstet Gynecol,2008; Vol. 199: pp. 596‑609.

Comments:Metformin has a defined role in treating some women with PCOS.

Nathan DM, Davidson MB, DeFronzo RA, et al. Impaired fasting glucose and impaired glucose tolerance: implications for care. Diabetes Care,2007; Vol. 30: pp. 753–9.

Comments:This consensus statement from the ADA (American Diabetes Association) defines and describes IFG and IGT, and gives specific recommendations on which patients with both IFG and IGT should be selected to receive metformin therapy.

Ting RZ, Szeto CC, Chan MH, et al. Risk factors of vitamin B(12) deficiency in patients receiving metformin. Arch Intern Med,2006; Vol. 166: pp. 1975–9.

Comments:Patients on chronic metformin therapy are at increased risk of developing vitamin B12 deficiency.

Glueck CJ, Salehi M, Sieve L, et al. Growth, motor, and social development in breast- and formula-fed infants of metformin-treated women with polycystic ovary syndrome. J Pediatr,2006; Vol. 148: pp. 628–632.

Comments:In nursing infants of mothers who were taking metformin (mean 2550 mg/day) for PCOS, there was no growth retardation or delayed motor/social development, and there was also no difference in intercurrent illnesses, when compared to formula-fed babies. This study only followed the babies up to 6 months of age, however. Thus, metformin during lactation appears to be safe at least up to 6 months of infancy.

UK Prospective Diabetes Study (UKPDS) Group 34. Effect of intensive blood-glucose control with metformin on complications in overweight patients with type 2 diabetes (UKPDS 34). Lancet, 1998; Vol. 352:pp. 854–65.

Comments:Landmark study: metformin is an excellent first-line drug for treating patients with type 2 diabetes mellitus due to its favorable effects on glycemic control and diabetic complications, and decreased incidence of weight gain and hypoglycemia when compared to sulfonylureas or insulin.

Bailey CJ, Turner RC. Metformin. NEJM,1996; Vol. 334: pp. 574–9.

Comments:Overview of the use of metformin in treating type 2 diabetes mellitus.

Gan SC, Barr J, Arieff AI, et al. Biguanide-associated lactic acidosis. Case report and review of the literature. Arch Intern Med,1992; Vol. 152: pp. 2333–6.

Comments:Lactic acidosis occurs very rarely if metformin is used according to its prescribing guidelines.

磺脲类降糖药和其他促泌剂

Nadeen Hosein, MD, MS, and Brian Pinto, PharmD, MBA

适应证

FDA

- 2 型糖尿病。

非 FDA 批准适应证

- 氯磺丙脲:中枢性尿崩症。

机制

- 磺脲类药物和格列奈类药物(瑞格列奈和那格列奈)刺激胰腺尚有功能的 β 细胞工作,刺激胰岛素第一时相分泌。
- 这两类药物结合于胰腺 β 细胞膜上的钾 –ATP 通道,并使其关闭。进而使细胞膜去极化,钙离子内流,胰岛素外排。
- 磺脲类药物与格列奈类药物结合于不同的膜位点,但细胞内的机制相同。

成人常用剂量

- 氯磺丙脲:100~500mg 每日一次。最大日剂量(TDD)750mg。
- 甲苯磺丁脲:250mg~3g 每日,一次或多次服用。最大 TDD 为 3g。
- 格列吡嗪:5~40mg 每日。如 TDD>15mg,至少分为 2 次服用。最大 TDD 为 40mg。
- 格列吡嗪缓释片:5~10mg 每日一次。最大剂量 20mg 每日。
- 格列苯脲:1.25~20mg 每日一次或分 2 次服用。最大 TDD 为 20mg。
- 格列苯脲微乳化片:0.75~12mg 每日一次或分 2 次服用。最大 TDD 为 12mg。
- 格列美脲:1~4mg 每日一次。最大 TDD 为每日 8mg。
- 瑞格列奈:0.5~4mg 每餐服用。最大 TDD16mg。
- 那格列奈:60~120mg 餐前 1~30 分钟服用。最大剂量为 180mg,每日三次。
- 复方制剂:与二甲双胍共同配制:格列苯脲 + 二甲双胍(Glucovance),格列吡嗪 + 二甲双胍(Metaglip)和瑞格列奈 + 二甲双胍(PrandiMet)。
- 如果起始胰岛素治疗,磺脲类药物则需减量或停用。

剂型

商品名	通用名	剂型	价格
Diabinese (Mylan, Pliva, UDL Labora-tories)	氯磺丙脲	100mg 口服片剂 250 mg 口服片剂	60 片 $17 60 片 $21
Orinase, Tol–Tab (Mylan, UDL Laboratories)	甲苯磺丁脲	500mg 口服片剂	60 片 $26
Riomet (Ranbaxy Laboratories)	格列吡嗪	5mg 口服片剂 10mg 口服片剂	100 片 $20 90 片 $19
Glucotrol XL (Watson, Greenstone, 辉瑞和其他公司)	格列吡嗪缓释片	2.5mg 口服片剂 5 mg 口服片剂 10mg 口服片剂	30 片 $19 30 片 $15 30 片 $20
DiaBeta (赛诺菲, Sandoz, Teva, 和其他公司)	格列苯脲	1.25mg 口服片剂 2.5 mg 口服片剂 5 mg 口服片剂	30 片 $13 30 片 $13 30 片 $12
Glynase PresTabs (辉瑞, Teva, Mylan, 和其他公司)	格列苯脲微乳化片	1.5mg 口服片剂 3 mg 口服片剂 6 mg 口服片剂	90 片 $26 90 片 $15 90 片 $17
亚莫利 (赛诺菲, Mylan, Ranbaxy, 和其他公司)	格列美脲	1 mg 口服片剂 2 mg 口服片剂 4 mg 口服片剂	30 片 $13 90 片 $19 30 片 $15
诺和龙 (诺和诺德)	瑞格列奈	0.5 mg 口服片剂 1 mg 口服片剂 2 mg 口服片剂	30 片 $72 30 片 $73 90 片 $193
唐力 (诺华)	那格列奈	60 mg 口服片剂 120 mg 口服片剂	30 片 $56 30 片 $60

特殊人群用量

肾脏病

- 肾功能不全的患者使用，主要经过肾脏排泄的磺脲类药物会增加低血糖风险，会延长药物的效应时间。
- 建议避免使用这些药物或者使用低剂量的药物以减少低血糖的风险。
- 如肾功能不全患者必须使用磺脲类药物，可选择格列吡嗪（代谢产物无活性）或格列美脲（主要经粪便排泄）。避免使用格列苯脲，因具有部分活性的代谢产物蓄积可能导致严重低血糖。

- 格列奈类药物在肾功能不全的各期几乎都能使用。

肝脏疾病
- 建议使用低剂量（如采用常规起始剂量的 50% 开始治疗）。因大多数这类药物均在肝脏进行代谢，采用低剂量起始可以减少发生低血糖的风险。

妊娠
- 格列苯脲是唯一 FDA 妊娠分级为 B 级的磺脲类药物。
- 其他的磺脲类药物均为 FDA 分级 C 级。
- 格列奈类药物为 FDA 分级 C 级。

哺乳期
- 汤姆森哺乳风险评级：婴儿风险不能除外。

药物不良反应

整体人群
- 禁用于糖尿病酮症酸中毒患者或对药物过敏的患者。
- 不能用于 1 型糖尿病患者的治疗。
- 根据全美糖尿病研究大学协作组 (University group diabetes program, UGDP) 的研究结果，黑框警告可能增加心血管死亡率（见 Key Studies in Diabetes Care：Efficacies of Therapies, p. 29）。
- 患者应避免酗酒（增加低血糖风险）。

常见不良反应
- 低血糖，尤其在肾功能不全、肝功能受损和老年患者更常见。
- 空腹锻炼也会增加低血糖风险。
- 体重增加。
- 氯磺丙脲酒精潮红：高达 15% 使用氯磺丙脲的患者，饮酒后出现明显面部潮红。

少见不良反应
- 恶心、呕吐、腹泻、腹胀和腹痛。
- 氯磺丙脲引起低钠血症。
- 肝酶升高。

罕见不良反应
- 皮肤超敏反应。

药物相互作用
- 加强磺脲类药物活性的药物：NSAIDs、华法令、水杨酸类、磺胺类药物、别嘌呤醇、丙磺舒、胍乙啶、MAOIs、氯霉素、酒精、β 受体阻滞剂。
- 降低磺脲类药物活性的药物：糖皮质激素、利尿剂、烟酸、左旋甲状腺素、雌激素、孕激素、苯妥英、二氮嗪、异烟肼、利福平、吩噻嗪类、拟交感血管活性药。

药代动力学

- 见表 4-5。

表 4-5. 磺脲类和促分泌剂的药代动力学

	氯磺丙脲	甲苯磺丁脲	格列吡嗪	格列苯脲	格列美脲	瑞格列奈	那格列奈
吸收	TTPC 2~4 小时	TTPC 3~4 小时	100%BA XL 为 90%	TTPC 4 小时	100%BA	TTPC 1 小时 56%BA	73%BA
代谢	水解	氧化作用	肝脏	肝脏	肝脏	肝脏	肝脏
排泄	80%~90% 肾脏	75% 肾脏	80% 肾脏	50% 肾脏 50% 粪便	60% 肾脏 40% 粪便	90% 粪便 8% 肾脏	83% 肾脏 10% 粪便
蛋白结合	60%~90%	95%	98%~99%	99%	99.5%	98%	98%
半衰期	36 小时	4.5~6.5 小时	2~4 小时 XL 为 2~5 小时	10 小时	5~9.2 小时	1 小时	1.5 小时
分布 (Vd)	不全具有这样的特性	不全具有这样的特性	10~11L	不全具有这样的特性	8.8L	31L	10L

TTPC=浓度达峰时间;BA=生物利用度;M=新陈代谢;E=排泄;Vd=容量分布,以升为单位(L)。Courtesy of Faul Pham, PharmD, 约翰·霍普金斯大学医学院。

专家意见

- 使用磺脲类降糖药至少 3 个月使 HbA1c 大约下降 1%~2%。
- 格列奈类药物降低 HbA1c 大约 1%~1.5%,瑞格列奈(诺和龙)比那格列奈(唐力)降糖效果强。这类药物对于单纯餐后高血糖的患者十分有效,不适用于空腹血糖受损的患者。
- 不良反应包括因促进胰岛素分泌导致的体重增加和低血糖。
- 第二代磺脲类药物比第一代(氯磺丙脲和甲苯磺丁脲)更受欢迎,因第一代更容易发生药物间相互作用和不良反应。
- 虽然基于 UGDP 研究磺脲类药物存在增加心血管风险的黑框警告,但这类药物目前在许多研究中证实都是安全的,并广泛应用于临床。
- 每年有 5%~10% 使用磺脲类药物治疗的糖尿病患者,因磺脲类药物继发失效需起始胰岛素治疗。

参考文献

Black C, Donnelly P, McIntyre L, et al. Meglitinide analogues for type 2 diabetes mellitus Cochrane Database Syst Rev,2007; CD004654.

Comments:Overview of the role of meglitinides in treating type 2 diabetes mellitus.

Inzucchi SE. Oral antihyperglycemic therapy for type 2 diabetes: scientific review. JAMA 2002; Vol. 287: pp. 360–72.

Comments: Review of different types of oral antidiabetic agents, including sulfonylureas and other secretagogues.

Matthews DR, Cull CA, Stratton IM, et al. UKPDS 26: Sulphonylurea failure in non insulin-dependent diabetic patients over six years. UK Prospective Diabetes Study (UKPDS) Group. Diabet Med,1998; Vol. 15: pp. 297–303.

Comments:In this UKPDS analysis of 1305 newly diagnosed diabetics placed on sulfonylurea monotherapy, 44% experienced sulfonylurea failure by 6 years and had to be switched over to other therapy. Risk factors for secondary sulfonylurea failure included lower pancreatic beta cell reserve to begin with, more hyperglycemia, and younger age.

Skillman TG, Feldman JM. The pharmacology of sulfonylureas. Am J Med,1981; Vol. 70: pp. 361–72.

Comments:Overview of the pharmacology of first- and second-generation sulfonylureas

噻唑烷二酮类药物

Nadeen Hosein, MD, MS, and Brian Pinto, PharmD, MBA

适应证

FDA
- 2型糖尿病。

非FDA批准适应证
- 多囊卵巢综合征(PCOS)。
- NASH(非酒精性脂肪性肝炎/脂肪肝)。

机制
- 噻唑烷二酮类药物(TZDs)是PPAR(过氧化物酶体增殖物激活受体)γ的激动剂。
- 其通过减少肝脏和外周的胰岛素抵抗,增加胰岛素依赖的血糖应用并减少肝糖输出。
- 同时影响脂肪酸代谢。

成人常用剂量
- 使用TZD前需检测肝酶水平。如有活动性肝病或ALT(又名SGPT)升高>2.5倍正常上限,则不要使用。
- 吡格列酮:15~30mg每日口服一次。最大日剂量45mg。
- 罗格列酮:2~4mg口服每日一或两次。最大日剂量8mg。
- 复合制剂:吡格列酮+二甲双胍(Actoplus Met或Actoplus Met缓释片),吡格列酮+格列美脲(Duetact),罗格列酮+二甲双胍(Avandamet)和罗格列酮+格列美脲(Avandaryl)。

剂型

商品名	通用名	剂型	价格
艾可拓(武田,PD-Rx制药)	盐酸吡格列酮	15mg口服片剂 30mg口服片剂 45mg口服片剂	30片 $149 30片 $213 30片 $233
文迪雅(葛兰素史克)	马来酸罗格列酮	2mg口服片剂 4mg口服片剂 8mg口服片剂	30片 $82 30片 $129 30片 $239

特殊人群用量

肾脏
- 不需调整剂量。

噻唑烷二酮类药物

肝脏疾病
- 不建议活动性肝病或 ALT（又名 SGPT）升高大于 2.5 倍正常上限的患者使用。

妊娠
- FDA 分级为 C 级。

哺乳期
- 汤姆森哺乳风险评级：婴儿风险不能除外。

药物不良反应

整体人群
- 吡格列酮：对充血性心功能衰竭提出黑框警告：可能导致或加重充血性心功能衰竭。监测患者的心衰的症状和体征；如果病情进展，考虑停药。禁用于 NYHA 分级 III 级或 IV 级患者。
- 罗格列酮：对充血性心功能衰竭提出黑框警告：可能导致或加重充血性心功能衰竭。监测患者的心衰的症状和体征；如果病情进展，考虑停药。禁用于 NYHA 分级 III 级或 IV 级患者。
- 罗格列酮：对心肌缺血提出黑框警告：包装中显示："一项关于 42 项研究的 meta 分析 ... 显示 [罗格列酮] 与增加心肌缺血事件如心绞痛或心肌梗死风险相关。3 项其他研究 ... 仍未确认或除外此风险。总的来说，关于是否增加发生心肌缺血的风险目前仍未确定。"
- 不用于 1 型糖尿病患者或存在糖尿病酮症酸中毒的患者。
- 所有患者均应监测肝酶，有发生肝炎和肝衰竭的报道（虽是罕见的）。
- 也可发生剂量相关的贫血。

常见不良反应
- 因体液增加和脂肪组织增加而引起体重增加，有证据显示增加外周脂肪（如皮下脂肪）而不是中心脂肪（如内脏脂肪）。

少见不良反应
- 先前无排卵的 PCOS 患者引发排卵。
- 增加骨折，尤其是女性骨折的风险。

罕见不良反应
- 暴发性肝炎导致肝衰竭。
- 肺水肿或胸腔积液。

药物相互作用
- 胆汁酸螯合剂减少 TZDs 的吸收。这两类药应至少间隔 2 小时分开服用。
- 硝酸盐类药物加强罗格列酮的不良反应／毒性。一项对 42 个使用罗格列酮的临床试验的 meta 分析显示，与此类药物联用存在更高的心肌缺血风险。虽然与罗格列酮联用并非禁忌证，但并不被推荐。
- CYP2C8 抑制剂（如吉非罗齐）和诱导剂（如利福平）可能增加或降低 TZDs 的水平。

噻唑烷二酮类药物

药代动力学

表 4-6. 噻唑烷二酮类的药代动力学

	吡格列酮	罗格列酮
吸收	药物达峰时间在 2 小时内	药物达峰时间 1 小时。生物利用度 99%
代谢	大部分经肝脏；小部分不代谢	大部分经肝脏
排泄	肾脏和粪便	64% 肾脏，23% 粪便
蛋白结合	>99%	>99%
半衰期	16~24 小时（老年人更长）	3~4 小时（肝损害病人 +2 小时）
容量分布	(0.63 ± 0.41) L/kg	17.6 L

Courtesy of Paul Pham, PharmD, 约翰·霍普金斯大学医学院。

专家意见

TZDs 降低 HbA1c 约 1%~1.5%。

体重增加非常常见。

体液潴留也很常见。增加心衰风险大约 2 倍。

吡格列酮与罗格列酮相比对血脂有益（降低 TG、升高 HDL）。

罗格列酮是否增加心肌缺血风险目前存在争议，但吡格列酮并不增加其风险。

2010 年 9 月，根据一项 52 个研究的 meta 分析显示罗格列酮增加 ~28% 的心肌缺血风险，FDA 发表声明减少罗格列酮使用 (Nissen)。患者需要签署文件表明其知晓继续用药的风险。

可导致女性骨折风险增加，尤其是四肢远端（前臂、手腕、手、脚、踝关节、胫骨、腓骨）。早期证据显示其减少骨形成活性 (Home；Dormuth)。

报告显示在临床前的动物研究中使用吡格列酮增加膀胱癌风险，但临床研究并未发现，需要进一步研究 (Lewis)。

单药使用不出现低血糖。与胰岛素或胰岛素促泌剂联用时可发生低血糖。

美国无普通片制剂，因此花费不详。

TZDs 可能对 HIV 相关的脂代谢紊乱 / 脂代谢障碍和糖尿病患者有额外获益。

推荐依据

Nissen SE, Wolski K. Rosiglitazone revisited: an updated meta-analysis of risk for myocardial infarction and cardiovascular mortality. Arch Intern Med, 2010; Jun 28 [Epub ahead of print].
Comments: This updated meta-anaylsis of 52 trials found that rosiglitazone was associated with significant 28% increased risk of myocardial infarction but not cardiovascular mortality. This article was the basis of the recent FDA decision to severely restrict access to rosiglitazone in September 2010.

其他参考文献

Lewis JD, Ferrara A, Peng T, et al. Risk of bladder cancer among diabetic patients treated with pioglitazone: interim report of a longitudinal cohort study. Diabetes Care, 2011; Vol. 34: pp. 916–22.

Comments: A preliminary report describing no association of pioglitazone therapy with increased incidence of bladder cancer, although a slightly increased risk with pioglitazone use for more than 2 years was found.

Home PD, Pocock SJ, Beck-Nielsen H, et al. Rosiglitazone evaluated for cardiovascular outcomes in oral agent combination therapy for type 2 diabetes (RECORD): a multicentre, randomised, open-label trial. Lancet, 2009; Vol. 373: pp. 2125–35.

Comments: In this prospective, randomized, open-blind trial which enrolled 4447 patients, after a mean of 5.5 years, those randomly assigned to rosiglitazone had statistically significant increased risk for developing heart failure, with a hazard ratio of 2. Women in the rosiglitazone group also had more distal upper and lower limb bone fractures. This study was not able to demonstrate a statistically significant increase in myocardial infarctions in those using rosiglitazone. Since the publication of this study, re-adjudication case records by the FDA suggest that the initially reported results of this trial may have been biased in favor of rosiglitazone.

Dormuth CR, Carney G, Carleton B, et al. Thiazolidinediones and fractures in men and women. Arch Intern Med, 2009; Vol. 169: pp. 1395–402.

Comments: This prospective cohort study compared peripheral fractures in 10,471 patients exposed to TZDs versus 73,863 patients exposed to sulfonylureas over a period of 1998–2007. The mean age of patients was 59, and 43% were women. There was a statistically significant 28% higher incidence of peripheral fractures in men and women exposed to TZDs compared with sulfonylureas (95%CI, 1.10–1.48). When exposure to each TZD was estimated separately, pioglitazone was associated with a significant increase in peripheral fractures in women compared with sulfonylureas (adjusted HR, 1.77; 95% CI 1.32–2.38), but rosiglitazone was not (adjusted HR, 1.17; 95% CI, 0.91–1.50).

Selvin E, Bolen S, Yeh HC, et al. Cardiovascular outcomes in trials of oral diabetes medications: a systematic review. Arch Intern Med, 2008; Vol. 168: pp. 2070–80.

Comments: In this meta-analysis of 40 articles, rosiglitazone was associated with an increased risk of cardiovascular morbidity and mortality, but it was a statistically nonsignificant finding (OR 1.68, 95% CI, 0.92–3.06).

Grey A, Bolland M, Gamble G, et al. The peroxisome proliferator-activated receptor-gamma agonist rosiglitazone decreases bone formation and bone mineral density in healthy postmenopausal women: a randomized, controlled trial. J Clin Endocrinol Metab, 2007; Vol. 92: pp. 1305–10.

Comments: In this randomized, double-blind placebo controlled trial of 50 postmenopausal women initiated on rosiglitazone 8 mg/day, there was a significant decrease in bone formation, as evidenced by a reduction in osteoblast markers: procollagen type 1 N-terminal propeptide by 13% (p ,0.005), and osteocalcin by 10% (p =0.04), when compared to placebo. Changes were seen as early as 4 weeks into rosiglitazone treatment and persisted for the entire 14-week duration of the study.

Nissen SE, Wolski K. Effect of rosiglitazone on the risk of myocardial infarction and death from cardiovascular causes. NEJM, 2007; Vol. 356: pp. 2457–71.

Comments:This small meta-analysis using pooled data from 42 trials (15,565 patients randomly assigned to receive rosiglitazone versus 12,282 patients randomly assigned to receive comparator drugs), included studies with a duration of at least 24 weeks. The mean age of subjects was 56 years, with a baseline HbA1c of approximately 8.2%. This meta-analysis found an increased risk for myocardial infarction with rosiglitazone, with a statistically significant odds ratio of 1.43 (95% CI, 1.03–1.98, p =0.03). This article was the basis for the revised FDA black box warning for rosiglitazone, which now includes myocardial ischemia.

ki-Järvinen H. Thiazolidinediones. NEJM,2004; Vol. 351: pp. 1106–18.

Comments:Overview of the mechanism of action and use of TZDs in patients with type 2 diabetes mellitus.

onseca V. Effect of thiazolidinediones on body weight in patients with diabetes mellitus. Am J Med, 2003; Vol. 115 Suppl 8A: pp. 42S–48S.

Comments:Mechanism of weight gain in patients with diabetes using TZDs, and strategies to manage/minimize the weight gain.

胰岛素（基础）：中效和长效胰岛素

Nadeen Hosein, MD, MS, and Brian Pinto, PharmD, MBA

适应证

FDA

- 1型糖尿病患者（DM1）。
- 2型糖尿病患者（DM2）。
- NPH胰岛素：妊娠期糖尿病患者（GDM）。

机制

- 长效基础胰岛素是因延缓了其在皮下注射的吸收。
- 促进肌肉和脂肪摄取胰岛素。
- 减少肝糖输出。
- 抑制脂肪分解。
- 抑制蛋白质分解增加蛋白质合成。

成人常用剂量

- TDD=日总剂量，U=胰岛素单位，SQ=皮下。
- 长效基础胰岛素（甘精、地特胰岛素）：SQ每日一次或两次。
- 中效基础胰岛素[中效鱼精蛋白（NPH）胰岛素]：SQ每日两次。
- 一般来说，基础餐时胰岛素方案，TDD的50%为基础胰岛素，50%为餐时胰岛素（分为3餐）。
- 1型糖尿病：起始TDD为0.2~0.5U/(kg·d)，范围为0.4~1U/(kg·d)，用于维持血糖剂量可能更大（见1型糖尿病：胰岛素治疗，第177页）。
- 2型糖尿病：起始TDD为0.1~0.2U/(kg·d)，通常先给予基础胰岛素治疗几周/月后，再给予餐时胰岛素。维持剂量为TDD 0.2~1.5U/(kg·d)或更多，取决于胰岛素抵抗的程度（见2型糖尿病：胰岛素治疗，第197页）。
- 如根据体重计算起始胰岛素治疗，应根据患者的血糖情况调整胰岛素剂量。
- 另一种对没使用过胰岛素的患者起始治疗的方法，给予基础胰岛素1单位每24小时SQ，每2~3天调整2单位至空腹血糖达标。
- 如从每日两次的NPH转换为每日一次的甘精或地特胰岛素，首先计算当天NPH总量，并减少20%后改为甘精或地特胰岛素每24小时SQ一次。
- 一些患者，尤其是那些使用大剂量基础胰岛素的患者（如每日多于5单位），使用甘精或地特胰岛素后血糖控制比每日两次NPH时更佳。
- 用于治疗GDM，见妊娠期糖尿病章节，第138页。

胰岛素(基础):中效和长效胰岛素

剂型

商品名	通用名	剂型	价格
来得时 (赛诺菲)	甘精胰岛素 (重组胰岛素类似物)	SQ 溶液,100U/ml,10ml 装溶液(1 000U) SQ 溶液,100U/ml,3ml 溶液,来得时 SoloStar 预填充笔一盒5支装(15ml,1 500U) SQ 溶液,100U/ml,3ml 溶液,来得时笔芯一盒5支装(15ml,1500U)使用单独购买的 OptiClik 注射笔注射	$104 $188 $191
诺和平 (诺和诺德)	地特胰岛素 (重组胰岛素类似物)	SQ 溶液,100U/ml,10ml 装溶液(1 000U) SQ 溶液,100U/ml,3ml,诺和平 FlexPen 预填充笔一盒5支装(15ml,1 500U)	$103 $191
优泌林 N (礼来)	NPH 胰岛素 (精蛋白重组人胰岛素)	SQ 溶液,100U/ml,10ml 装混悬液(1 000U) SQ 溶液,100U/ml,3ml 混悬液,优泌林 N 预填充笔一盒5支装(15ml,1 500U)	$57 $154
诺和灵 (诺和诺德)	NPH 胰岛素 (精蛋白重组人胰岛素)	SQ 溶液,100U/ml,10ml 装混悬液(1 000U)	$58

特殊人群用量

肾脏病
因胰岛素经肾脏代谢,在肾功能受损的患者半衰期延长,故可能需减少胰岛素剂量。

甘精胰岛素代谢产物有活性,肾功能受损患者可能更易低血糖。

肝脏疾病
因胰岛素在肝脏代谢,同时大部分糖异生在肝脏进行,故需减少剂量。

妊娠
甘精和地特胰岛素:FDA 分级为 C 级。

NPH 胰岛素:FDA 分级为 B 级。这是唯一 FDA 批准用于 GDM 的基础胰岛素。

哺乳期
甘精和地特胰岛素:汤姆森哺乳风险评级:婴儿风险不能除外。

NPH 胰岛素:风险未知。

药物不良反应

整体人群
- 禁用于静脉注射。
- 不能用于胰岛素泵。

常见不良反应
- 低血糖。
- 注射部位疼痛,甘精胰岛素因是酸性溶液,更应关注。
- 体重增加。

少见不良反应
- 注射部位局部反应(发红,瘙痒,肿胀)。
- 注射部位脂肪萎缩(缺少皮下脂肪组织),规律轮换注射部位来避免。
- 注射部位脂肪增生(皮下脂肪组织堆积),规律轮换注射部位来避免。

罕见不良反应
- 超敏反应。
- 低钾血症。
- 药物相互作用。
- 任何降低血糖的药物(如磺脲类)与胰岛素共同使用更容易引起低血糖

药代动力学
- 吸收:受很多因素影响(剂量、运动、体温、按摩注射部位、脂肪增生等
- 代谢和排泄:由肝脏和肾脏代谢和排泄。
- 蛋白结合:极少。

表 4-7. 基础胰岛素的药代动力学

	甘精	地特	NPH
起效	2~3 小时	1~3 小时	1~3 小时
达峰	理论上无峰	6~8 小时	4~10 小时
作用时间	通常 20~24 小时	6~24 小时	10~16 小时

Courtesy of Paul Pham, PharmD, 约翰·霍普金斯大学医学院。

专家意见
- NPH("多云"胰岛素)可以与速效胰岛素安全的混合。做法:建议者:(1)把清亮的速效胰岛素注入干净的注射器中;(2)注入混浊 NPH 胰岛素。告诉患者注入顺序为"先清亮后混浊"。
- 甘精和地特胰岛素不能与其他胰岛素混合,因 pH 的改变会影响其效果
- 基础胰岛素的选择必须考虑到花费,注射次数或患者的接受度。
- NPH 是应用更久且更加便宜的基础胰岛素,如果患者经济条件不佳可考虑。

胰岛素(基础):中效和长效胰岛素

NPH曾是动物源性(猪)的胰岛素,而目前所有可用的基础胰岛素均为人工合成的胰岛素,是与人胰岛素结构相同的(NPH)或是胰岛素类似物(甘精和地特)。

传统的胰岛素是以注射器抽取瓶装的胰岛素进行注射,目前大多数患者已使用胰岛素笔注射(预填充的,或可更换胰岛素可重复使用的)。胰岛素注射针头需单独购买,并不与胰岛素笔包装在一起。

饮酒可能使应用胰岛素治疗的患者发生低血糖,需格外警惕。

无"峰"的长效胰岛素如甘精胰岛素,在临床使用中也并非总是无"峰"。可能存在最大的作用时间,尤其在高剂量时,胰岛素作用可能无法持续24小时。

地特胰岛素平均作用时间<20小时,故通常每日两次注射。

其他基础胰岛素包括中效(lente)和长效(ultralente)胰岛素在美国已停止使用,但其他国家可能仍在使用。

参考文献

Holman RR, Farmer AJ, Davies MJ, et al. Three-year efficacy of complex insulin regimens in type 2 diabetes. NEJM,2009; Vol. 361: pp. 1736–47.

Comments: In this 3-year open-label multicenter trial, 708 patients with suboptimal HbA1c while taking metformin and sulfonylurea therapy were randomly assigned to receive biphasic insulin aspart insulin twice daily, prandial insulin aspart 3 times daily, or basal insulin detemir once (or twice, if needed) daily. After 3 years, median HbA1c levels were similar for all three groups, but fewer patients had a HbA1c of ,6.5% in the biphasic group than in the prandial or basal groups. There were also fewer hypoglycemic episodes and less weight gain in patients adding basal insulin.

Mooradian AD, Bernbaum M, Albert SG. Narrative review: a rational approach to starting insulin therapy. Ann Intern Med,2006; Vol. 145: pp. 125–34.

Comments: Suggestions for how to start insulin in patients with diabetes, depending on their individual blood glucose profiles.

Riddle MC. Timely initiation of basal insulin. Am J Med,2004; Vol. 116 Suppl 3A: pp. 3S–9S.

Comments: This article makes a good case for why basal insulin should be started early in patients with type 2 diabetes mellitus.

DeWitt DE, Hirsch IB. Outpatient insulin therapy in type 1 and type 2 diabetes mellitus: scientific review. JAMA,2003; Vol. 289: pp. 2254–64.

Comments: Overview of the different types of insulins available, their pharmacokinetics, and different types of insulin regimens.

Riddle MC, Rosenstock J, Gerich J, et al. The treat-to-target trial: randomized addition of glargine or human NPH insulin to oral therapy of type 2 diabetic patients. Diabetes Care,2003; Vol. 26: pp. 3080–6.

Comments: In this open-label, parallel, multicenter trial, 756 overweight patients with HbA1c 7.5% on one or two oral agents were randomized to have either bedtime glargine insulin or once-daily NPH insulin added to their oral therapy. After 24 weeks, mean fasting plasma glucose and HbA1c were similar in both groups. However, patients on NPH experienced more episodes of symptomatic hypoglycemia than did those receiving Glargine.

胰岛素（餐时）：速效和短效

Nadeen Hosein, MD, MS, and Brian Pinto, PharmD, MB.

适应证

FDA
- 1型糖尿病患者（T1DM）。
- 2型糖尿病患者（T2DM）。
- 妊娠期糖尿病（GDM）。
- 糖尿病酮症酸中毒（DKA）。
- 在胰岛素泵中使用。
- 皮下或静脉注射。

非FDA批准适应证
- 糖尿病高渗昏迷。
- 高钾血症。

机制
- 促进肌肉和脂肪对葡萄糖的摄取。
- 减少肝糖输出。
- 抑制脂肪分解。
- 抑制蛋白质分解，增加蛋白质合成。

成人常用剂量
- TDD=日总剂量，U=胰岛素单位，SQ=皮下注射。
- 速效胰岛素（门冬、赖脯和赖谷胰岛素）：餐前0~15分钟SQ（推荐）或者开始进餐后20分钟内注射（对一些无法预知进食量的患者）。
- 短效胰岛素（常规胰岛素）：建议餐前30分钟SQ。
- 2型糖尿病患者：胰岛素治疗，见197页。1型糖尿病患者：胰岛素治疗见177页。
- 总体来讲，对于基础-餐时胰岛素方案，TDD 50%为基础胰岛素，50%为餐时胰岛素（分为三餐）。
- 可应用于NPO的糖尿病患者，或接受全肠外营养的患者。医院糖尿病管理的信息见78页。
- 关于胰岛素对GDM的使用（见139页），DKA（见47页）对高深昏迷的使用（见53页）。
- 如以U-500（浓度为500U/ml，译者注）胰岛素代替U-100（浓度100U/ml，译者注）胰岛素，注意需把剂量除以5，因U-500胰岛素U-100胰岛素浓度的5倍。

胰岛素（餐时）：速效和短效

剂型

商品名	通用名	剂型	价格
诺和锐（诺和诺德）	门冬胰岛素（重组胰岛素类似物）	SQ 溶液，100U/ml，10ml 装溶液（1 000U） SQ 溶液，100U/ml，3ml 溶液，诺和锐 FlexPen 预填充笔一盒 5 支装（15ml，1 500U） SQ 溶液，100U/ml，3ml 溶液，诺和锐笔芯一盒 5 支装（15ml，1 500U）使用单独购买的任意一款诺和笔注射	$112 $219 $201
尤泌乐（礼来）	赖脯胰岛素（重组胰岛素类似物）	SQ 溶液，100U/ml，10ml 装溶液（1 000U） SQ 溶液，100U/ml，3ml 溶液，优泌乐 KwikPen 预填充笔一盒 5 支装（15ml，1 500U） SQ 溶液，100U/ml，3ml 溶液，优泌乐新预填充笔一盒 5 支装（15ml，1 500U） SQ 溶液，100U/ml，3ml 溶液，优泌乐笔芯一盒 5 支装（15ml，1 500U）使用单独购买的优伴 Memoir 笔或优伴 Luxura HD 笔注射	$104 $198 $208 $199
艾倍得（赛若菲）	赖谷胰岛素（重组胰岛素类似物）	SQ 溶液，100U/ml，10ml 装溶液（1 000U） SQ 溶液，100U/ml，3ml 溶液，艾倍得 SoloStar 预填充笔一盒 5 支装（15ml，1 500U） SQ 溶液，100U/ml，3ml 溶液，艾倍得笔芯一盒 5 支装（15ml，1500U）使用单独购买的 OptiClik 注射笔注射	$102 $207 $196
诺和灵 R（诺和诺德）	常规胰岛素（重组人胰岛素）	SQ 溶液，100U/ml，10ml 装溶液（1 000U）	$58
尤泌林 R（礼来）	常规胰岛素（重组人胰岛素）	SQ 溶液，100U/ml，10ml 装溶液（1 000U）	$57
尤泌林 R 浓宿 U-500（礼来）	浓缩常规胰岛素（重组人胰岛素）	SQ 溶液，500U/ml，20ml 装溶液（10 000U）	$261

特殊人群用量

肾脏病

因胰岛素经肾代谢，且肾功能受损患者胰岛素的半衰期延长，故需减少剂量。

肝脏疾病
- 因胰岛素经肝脏代谢,同时肝糖合成主要在肝脏进行,故可能需减少剂量

妊娠
- 门冬胰岛素:FDA 分级为 B 级。
- 赖脯胰岛素:FDA 分级为 B 级。
- 赖谷胰岛素:FDA 分级为 C 级。
- 常规胰岛素:FDA 分级为 B 级。

哺乳期
- 门冬、赖脯和赖谷胰岛素:婴儿风险不能除外(汤姆森哺乳风险评级)
- 常规胰岛素:未知。

药物不良反应
常见不良反应
- 低血糖。
- 体重增加。
- 注射部位疼痛,可通过使用更细的针头和使用胰岛素笔注射减轻。

少见不良反应
- 注射部位局部反应(发红、瘙痒、肿胀)。
- 注射部位脂肪萎缩(缺少皮下脂肪组织),规律轮换注射部位来避免。
- 注射部位脂肪增生(皮下脂肪组织堆积),规律轮换注射部位来避免。

罕见不良反应
- 超敏反应。
- 低钾血症。
- 常规胰岛素 U-500(500U/ml)增加胰岛素过和不可逆"胰岛素休克"的风险。需谨慎使用。

药物相互作用
- 任何降低血糖的药物(如磺脲类)与胰岛素联用,可能导致低血糖风险增加。

药代动力学
- 吸收:受诸多因素影响(剂量、运动、温度、按摩注射部位、脂肪营养不良等)。
- 代谢和排泄:经肝脏和肾脏代谢和排泄。
- 见表 4-8。

胰岛素（餐时）：速效和短效

表 4-8. 速效胰岛素的药代动力学

	门冬	赖脯	赖谷	常规
起效	5~15 分钟	5~15 分钟	5~15 分钟	30 分钟~1 小时
达峰	1~2 小时	1~2 小时	1~2 小时	2~4 小时
作用时间	3~5 小时	3~5 小时	3~5 小时	5~8 小时

Courtesy of Paul Pham, PharmD, 约翰·霍普金斯大学医学院。

专家意见

- 餐时胰岛素用来治疗高血糖和/或中和进餐的碳水化合物。
- 因速效胰岛素起效更快，其使用范围更广。短效胰岛素更多的用于经济条件受限的患者。
- 避免两次餐时胰岛素注射时间间隔过近（如 3~4 小时内），以减少活性作用时间相互重叠或"胰岛素蓄积"，可能导致患者出现低血糖。
- 大剂量的常规胰岛素，作用时间可达到 8 小时，可能导致胰岛素蓄积。
- 门冬、赖脯和赖谷胰岛素可在胰岛素泵中使用。
- 与传统的胰岛素注射器相比，绝大多数患者更愿使用胰岛素笔注射（可更换小瓶装胰岛素）。胰岛素针头不与胰岛素笔共同包装，需单独购买。何种胰岛素可装入胰岛素笔中，请参考前面的表格。
- 酒精对使用胰岛素的患者可导致低血糖，需节制并谨慎使用。
- 目前所有的餐时胰岛素均为合成胰岛素，为与人胰岛素结构相同的（常规胰岛素）或类似物（门冬、赖脯、赖谷胰岛素）。

参考文献

Orton ES. Defining the role of basal and prandial insulin for optimal glycemic control. J Am Coll Cardiol, 2009; Vol. 53: pp. S21–7.
Comments: Review of the available preparations of bolus and basal insulins, and recommendations for glycemic goals in patients at risk for cardiovascular disease.

DeWitt DE, Hirsch IB. Outpatient insulin therapy in type 1 and type 2 diabetes mellitus: scientific review. JAMA, 2003; Vol. 289: pp. 2254–64.
Comments: Overview of the different types of insulins available, their pharmacokinetics, and different types of insulin regimens.

Gerich JE. Novel insulins: expanding options in diabetes management. Am J Med, 2002; Vol. 113: pp. 308–16.
Comments: Discussion of the use of recombinant insulins as bolus and basal therapy for patients with diabetes mellitus.

预混胰岛素

Nadeen Hosein, MD, MS, and Brian Pinto, PharmD, MBA

适应证

FDA

- 1型糖尿病患者（T1DM）。
- 2型糖尿病患者（T2DM）。
- NPH/常规预混胰岛素：妊娠期糖尿病（GDM）。

机制

- 预混胰岛素是在小瓶中，将短效（常规）或速效胰岛素类似物与中效胰岛素（NPH）或长效胰岛素类似物混合。
- 胰岛素增加肌肉和脂肪对糖的摄取，增加蛋白质合成；减少肝糖输出；抑制脂肪和蛋白质分解。
- 预混胰岛素覆盖餐后血糖的升高，同时提供两餐之间所需的基础胰岛素。
- NPH和常规胰岛素的预混胰岛素是将NPH和常规胰岛素混合。胰岛素类似物预混（如赖脯、门冬）是将速效胰岛素预先与鱼精蛋白修饰的长效胰岛素进行混合。

成人常用剂量

- TDD=日总剂量，U=胰岛素单位，SQ=皮下。
- 诺和锐30，优泌乐25和优泌乐50：起始治疗为每24小时一次SQ，在主餐前0~15分钟注射。随后增加至每日两次注射，早餐和晚餐前0~15分钟注射。
- NPH/常规胰岛素预混胰岛素：早餐和晚餐前30分钟注射。
- T1DM：起始剂量为0.2U/(kg·d)。维持TDD一般为0.2~0.5U/(kg·d)或更多。大多数患者维持每日至少2次注射。
- T2DM：起始剂量为10U或0.2U/(kg·d)。维持TDD一般超过1U/(kg·d)或更多，取决于胰岛素抵抗的程度。大多数患者维持每日至少2次注射。
- 根据体重计算的剂量随后需根据患者的血糖情况进行调整。
- 如每日2次注射不能良好的控制血糖，可考虑在午餐前0~15分钟增加速效胰岛素类似物（如门冬、赖脯或赖谷胰岛素）。

预混胰岛素

剂型

商品名	通用名	剂型	价格
诺和灵 30R（70/30 诺和诺德）	70%NPH 胰岛素混合 30% 常规胰岛素（重组人胰岛素）	SQ 混悬液 100U/ml，10ml 装	$58
优泌林 70/30（礼来）	70%NPH 胰岛素混合 30% 常规胰岛素（重组人胰岛素）	SQ 混悬液 100U/ml，10ml 装	$56
		SQ 混悬液，100U/ml，3ml 混悬液，优泌林 70/30 预填充笔一盒 10 支装（30ml，3 000U）	$291
诺和锐 30（70/30 诺和诺德）	70% 精蛋白门冬胰岛素混合 30% 门冬胰岛素（重组胰岛素类似物）	SQ 混悬液，100U/ml，10ml 装混悬液	$110
		SQ 混悬液，100U/ml，3ml 混悬液，诺和锐 70/30 FlexPen 预填充笔一盒 5 支装（15ml，1500U）	$206
优泌乐 25（75/25 礼来）	75% 精蛋白赖脯胰岛素混合 25% 赖脯胰岛素（重组胰岛素类似物）	SQ 混悬液，100U/ml，10ml 装（1 000U）	$111
		SQ 混悬液，100U/ml，3ml，优泌乐 25 KwikPen 预填充笔一盒 5 支装（15ml，1 500U）	$200
		SQ 混悬液 100U/ml，3ml，优泌乐 25 新预填充笔一盒 5 支装（15ml，1 500U）	$188
优泌乐 50（50/50 礼来）	50% 精蛋白赖脯胰岛素混合 50% 赖脯胰岛素（重组胰岛素类似物）	SQ 混悬液 100U/ml，10ml 装（1 000U）	$107
		SQ 混悬液 100U/ml，3ml，优泌乐 50 KwikPen 预填充笔一盒 5 支装（15ml，1 500U）	$200
		SQ 混悬液 100U/ml，3ml，优泌乐 50 新预填充笔一盒 5 支装（15ml，1 500U）	$209

特殊人群用量

肾脏病

- 因胰岛素经肾代谢，且肾功能受损患者胰岛素的半衰期延长，故需减少剂量。

肝脏疾病
- 因胰岛素经肝脏代谢，同时肝糖合成主要在肝脏进行，故可能需减少剂量。

妊娠
- NPH/常规胰岛素（诺和灵30R和优泌林70/30）：FDA分级为B级。是唯一FDA批准的可用于治疗GDM的预混胰岛素。
- 诺和锐30：FDA分级为C级。
- 优泌乐25和优泌乐50：FDA分级为B级。

哺乳期
- 母亲在哺乳期需要的胰岛素较前减少，因增加了有效的能量消耗。
- NPH/常规胰岛素（诺和灵30R和优泌林70/30）：风险未知。
- 诺和锐30：婴儿风险不能除外（汤姆森哺乳风险评级）。
- 优泌乐25和优泌乐50：婴儿风险不能除外（汤姆森哺乳风险评级）。

药物不良反应
常见不良反应
- 低血糖，尤其当未进餐或运动增加时。
- 体重增加。

少见不良反应
- 注射部位局部反应（发红、瘙痒、肿胀）。
- 注射部位脂肪营养不良，规律轮换注射部位来避免。

罕见不良反应
- 超敏反应。
- 低钾血症。

药物相互作用
- 任何降低血糖的药物（如磺脲类）与胰岛素联用，可能导致低血糖风险增加。

药代动力学
- 吸收：受诸多因素影响（剂量、运动、温度、按摩注射部位、脂肪营养不良等）。
- 代谢和排泄：经肝脏和肾脏代谢和排泄。
- 见表4-9。

预混胰岛素

表 4-9. 预混胰岛素的药代动力学

	诺和灵 70/30	优泌林 70/30	诺和锐 70/30	优泌乐 75/25	优泌乐 50/50
起效	30~60 分钟	30~60 分钟	5~15 分钟	5~15 分钟	5~15 分钟
达峰	两个峰值	两个峰值	两个峰值	两个峰值	两个峰值
作用时间	10~16 小时	10~16 小时	10~16 小时	10~16 小时	10~16 小时

Courtesy of Paul Pham, PharmD, 约翰·霍普金斯大学医学院。

专家意见

- 预混胰岛素类似物（诺和锐预混和优泌乐预混）除了起效时间更短及更高的胰岛素峰值外，与 NPH/常规胰岛素预混有相似的作用时间。因此，胰岛素预混类似物对于控制餐后血糖更为有效。
- 在速效胰岛素类似物（门冬和赖脯）中加入鱼精蛋白延长了其活性时间，生成的鱼精蛋白胰岛素（门冬鱼精蛋白胰岛素和赖脯鱼精蛋白胰岛素）与 NPH 胰岛素有相似的药代动力学参数。
- 速效胰岛素类似物预混胰岛素应在餐前即刻注射，不应在睡前使用。
- 含有鱼精蛋白的长效胰岛素，在晚餐前注射可能导致夜间低血糖，在这种情况下，晚餐使用快速起效的胰岛素，睡前使用长效胰岛素是十分必要的。
- 预混胰岛素治疗（一般每日 2 次注射）对于那些拒绝使用更加符合生理的基础－餐时胰岛素治疗方案（需每日 4 次注射）的患者，考虑到依从性和花费的时候更为适用。
- 使用预混胰岛素治疗的患者需有更加规律的生活方式（进餐规律，每天在相同的时间运动，并且不能不吃饭）。
- 在午餐额外注射速效胰岛素可以改善使用预混胰岛素治疗患者的午间血糖。
- 生活方式不固定的患者（吃饭不固定，运动时间不固定，每餐进食的量和种类不固定）可能更适合基础－餐时胰岛素治疗方案。
- 患者更愿意使用胰岛素笔注射（不用清洗，可重复使用并可更换胰岛素），但针头必须单独购买。何种胰岛素可装入胰岛素笔中，请参考前面的表格。
- 目前临床随机试验中对于单用基础胰岛素、单用餐时胰岛素还是预混胰岛素治疗糖尿病更加有效的结果并不一致 (Holman；Lasserson)。

参考文献

Holman RR, Farmer AJ, Davies MJ, et al. Three-year efficacy of complex insulin regimens in type 2 diabetes. NEJM,2009; Vol. 361: pp. 1736–47.

Comments: In this open-label, multicenter trial, 708 patients who had suboptimal HbA1c levels while taking metformin and sulfonylurea therapy were randomly assigned to receive biphasic insulin aspart twice daily, prandial insulin aspart 3 times daily, or basal insulin detemir once daily (twice if required). After 3 years, the median HbA1c level was 6.9% (no statistical difference between the groups). However, fewer patients had an HbA1c ,6.5% in the biphasic group (31.9%) than in the prandial group (44.7%, p =0.006) or in the basal group (43.2%, p =0.03). Thus, more patients who added a basal or prandial insulin-based regimen to oral therapy were able to achieve HbA1c ,6.5% than those who added a biphasic insulin-based regimen.

Lasserson DS, Glasziou P, Perera R, et al. Optimal insulin regimens in type 2 diabetes mellitus: systematic review and meta-analyses. Diabetologia,2009; Vol. 52: pp. 1990–2000.

Comments: Found significantly greater reduction in HbA1c in patients with type 2 diabetes when insulin treatment was initiated using a biphasic or prandial insulin rather than basal insulin alone.

Garber AJ. Premixed insulin analogues for the treatment of diabetes mellitus. Drugs,2006; Vol. 66: pp. 31–49.

Comments: Thorough review of the premixed insulin analogs, including their development, pharmacokinetics, efficacy, dosing regimen considerations, and comparison to more traditional insulins.

Rolla AR, Rakel RE Practical approaches to insulin therapy for type 2 diabetes mellitus with premixed insulin analogues. Clin Ther, 2005; Vol. 27: pp. 1113–25.

Comments: Suggestions for initial dosing regimens and subsequent dosage titrations, including titration parameters, when using premixed insulin analogs.

Rubin RR, Peyrot M. Quality of life, treatment satisfaction, and treatment preference associated with use of a pen device delivering a premixed 70/30 insulin aspart suspension (aspart protamine suspension/soluble aspart) versus alternative treatment strategies. Diabetes Care,2004; Vol. 27: pp. 2495–7.

Comments: In this study of the delivery device used with a premixed insulin analog (NovoLog 70/30), insulin pens were overwhelmingly preferred over conventional insulin syringes with vials; patients reported significant improvements in their quality of life with the pens, citing convenience and flexibility.

胰岛素：其他形式和可植入式的胰岛素泵

Christopher D. Saudek, MD, and Brian Pinto, PharmD, MBA

适应证

FDA
- 目前除皮下注射和静脉使用的胰岛素外无批准的其他胰岛素制剂。

非FDA批准适应证
- 只用于科研。

机制
- 吸入式胰岛素在肺泡膜吸收。
- 微球用于加强其吸收(Technosphere)。
- 可植入式胰岛素泵已进行了广泛的研究。
- 口服、经鼻和直肠吸收的胰岛素已进行了动物研究，但其与特定的载体结合如胆汁酸或做成胶囊，限制了其在人体的研究。

药代动力学
- 吸收：随制剂不同而不同，整体来说，肺泡吸收的有效率远低于皮下注射的胰岛素。吸入性胰岛素的吸收率为8%~16%。通过可植入式胰岛素泵腹腔内注射的胰岛素可快速被吸收。
- 代谢和排泄：一经吸收，通过不同路径吸收的胰岛素与皮下注射的胰岛素代谢途径相似。经腹腔注射的胰岛素更易吸收进入肝门系统，与正常胰腺产生的胰岛素代谢路径相似。
- 蛋白结合：可能与皮下注射的胰岛素相同。

专家意见
- FDA批准的并已商业化的吸入式胰岛素，商品名为Exubera，在2006年9月已经过临床试验证明了其有效性。
- 吸入式胰岛素的主要不良反应时肺功能的轻度下降，特别是FEV1的下降。
- 其给药装置繁琐，胰岛素以毫克给药而不是单位，并需要常规的肺功能检查。
- 基于上述原因，辉瑞公司在2007年10月决定终止了吸入式胰岛素的生产。
- 随后，在2008年4月，FDA发布了Exubera可能与肺癌相关的声明；使用Exubera的4 740名患者中，有6名发生了肺癌，而4 292名吸烟患者中仅有一名患者发生了肺癌。
- MannKind公司发明了一种微型胶囊技术(Technoshpere)，并在2009年3月对FDA提交了新药物申请。
- 可植入式的胰岛素泵已经有超过400名患者使用了近20年，绝大多数为法国人。
- 虽然法国已经批准了其应用，但美国FDA仍未批准厂商进行生产。
- 其他的胰岛素给药途径（特别是经过胃肠道吸收的口服和胶囊剂型）仍在开发的早期。

参考文献

Hollander PA, Cefalu WT, Mitnick M, et al. Titration of inhaled human insulin (Exubera) in a treat-to-target regimen for patients with type 2 diabetes. Diabetes Technol Ther,2010; Vol. 12: pp. 185–91.

Comments:24-week treat-to-target comparison of 2-dose escalation schemes. Either lowered A1c from mean 8.6% to 6.8%, with Exubera.

Skyler JS, Hollander PA, Jovanovic L, et al. Safety and efficacy of inhaled human insulin (Exubera) during discontinuation and readministration of therapy in adults with type 1 diabetes: a 3-year randomized controlled trial. Diabetes Res Clin Pract,2008; Vol. 82: pp. 238–46.

Comments: A safety study of pulmonary function changes from Exubera treating type 1 diabetes. Found decreased FEV(1) on the inhaled insulin to be reversible when stopping it.

Rosenstock J, Bergenstal R, Defronzo RA, et al. Efficacy and safety of Technosphere inhaled insulin compared with Technosphere powder placebo in insulin-naive type 2 diabetes suboptimally controlled with oral agents. Diabetes Care,2008; Vol. 31: pp. 2177–82.

Comments:12-week demonstration that the Technosphere delivery of inhaled insulin does lower glucose, A1c dropping by 0.72%.

Rosenstock J, Cefalu WT, Hollander PA, et al. Two-year pulmonary safety and efficacy of inhaled human insulin (Exubera) in adult patients with type 2 diabetes. Diabetes Care,2008; Vol. 31: pp. 1723–8.

Comments:2-year study of 635 patients with type 2 diabetes treated with Exubera versus subcutaneous insulin. FEV1 decreased in nonprogressive manner on Exubera. A1c decrease was maintained on Exubera.

McMahon GT, Arky RA. Inhaled insulin for diabetes mellitus. NEJM,2007; Vol. 356: pp. 497–502.

Comments:An unbiased clinical review of Exubera, describing the pros and cons of using inhaled insulin.

Rave K, Heise T, Pfützner A, et al. Coverage of postprandial blood glucose excursions with inhaled technosphere insulin in comparison to subcutaneously injected regular human insulin in subjects with type 2 diabetes. Diabetes Care,2007; Vol. 30: pp. 2307–8.

Comments:Pharmacokinetic evaluation of Technosphere, demonstrating a far quicker peak insulin concentration (15 minutes) than for regular human insulin (120 minutes). Did not compare to fast-acting insulin analogs, and 19% of patients reported a cough.

Saudek CD, Duckworth WC, Giobbie-Hurder A, et al. Implantable insulin pump vs multiple-dose insulin for noninsulin-dependent diabetes mellitus: a randomized clinical trial. Department of Veterans Affairs Implantable Insulin Pump Study Group. JAMA,1996; Vol. 276: pp. 1322–7.

Comments:The only industry-independent randomized clinical trial of implanted insulin pump (IIP) versus subcutaneously (SC) delivered insulin, in the VA system. Designed to lower A1c to equal levels, IIP had less glycemic variability, less hypoglycemia, and less weight gain than SC insulin.

Duckworth WC, Saudek CD, Henry RR. Why intraperitoneal delivery of insulin with implantable pumps in NIDDM? Diabetes,1992; Vol. 41: pp. 657–61.

Comments:A description of the rationale for intraperitoneally delivered insulin.

升高血糖

糖尿病患者需谨慎使用抗生素

Paul Auwaerter, MD, and Paul A. Pham, PharmD

定义
- 某些抗生素（ABX）会导致糖尿病患者血糖控制的改变（表 4-10）。
- 关于抗生素和胰岛素的相互作用并没有明确的描述。
- 因抑制或诱导了氧化代谢（如细胞色素 P450 系统），降糖制剂，包括格列奈类（瑞格列奈、那格列奈），磺脲类（格列苯脲、格列吡嗪）和噻唑烷二酮类（吡格列酮，罗格列酮）的血清浓度可能改变。
- 特定的细胞色素 P450 底物：瑞格列奈（2C8, 3A4）；那格列奈（2C9>3A4）；格列苯脲和格列吡嗪（2C9）；吡格列酮（3A4>2C8）；罗格列酮（2C8>2C9）。
- 二甲双胍潜在的药物相互作用数量有限。

流行病学
- 门诊和住院患者都存在风险。老年患者和重病患者血糖波动的风险更高。
- 接受肺结核治疗的糖尿病患者可能存在治疗失败的风险，因降糖药物降低了利福平的血药浓度，尤其是 BMI 高的患者。
- 肥胖糖尿病患者可能存在治疗失败的更高风险，如果药物相关的剂量没有根据特定的抗生素进行调整（如万古霉素、达托霉素、氟康唑、卡泊芬净、甲氧苄啶/磺胺甲基异噁唑、头孢菌素类、氨基糖苷类和利福霉素）。

诊断
- 重病患者发生的低血糖或高血糖可能是系统合并症的结果（如败血症、肝功能异常），因此很难区分是否为药物相互作用。

临床治疗

所有抗生素
- 艾塞那肽可能减缓抗生素在胃肠道的蠕动。
- 建议在注射艾塞那肽至少 1 小时前服用抗生素。
- 氟喹诺酮类药物（加替沙星、莫西沙星、左氧氟沙星、环丙沙星）
- 有低血糖和高血糖的报道，但可能为药物剂量依赖和类效应造成。通常很难鉴别是由系统性疾病引起或是药物作用。
- 加替沙星因导致低血糖或高血糖，尤其是对接受口服降糖药的老年糖尿病患者。因此已在美国退市（2006年）。其他的氟喹诺酮类药物也可能出现，一些学者认为这是类效应。
- 低血糖或高血糖效应：加替沙星 > 左氧氟沙星 >> 环丙沙星和阿奇霉素（对比剂）（Aspinall）。虽然莫西沙星比加替沙星和左氧氟沙星相比少有血糖波动的报道，这可能是因为药物使用的问题。
- 可能的机制为氟喹诺酮干扰了胰岛 β 细胞 ATP 敏感的钾通道而增加了

糖尿病患者需谨慎使用抗生素

胰岛素的释放 (Saraya)。
- 血糖控制不稳定或重病的糖尿病患者,可考虑环丙沙星替换左氧氟沙星。环丙沙星对血糖影响较小可以安全使用。莫西沙星可能对血糖的影响也较小,但目前研究较少。

大环内酯类抗生素(红霉素、克拉霉素、阿奇霉素)和酮内酯(泰利霉素)
- 克拉霉素增加瑞格列奈的抑制曲线下面积(AUC)达 40%。考虑减少瑞格列奈的剂量以避免低血糖。
- 这类药物可能增加吡格列酮的浓度,效果不清。
- 这类药物可能增加磺脲类药物的血药浓度。合用时考虑减少磺脲类药物剂量以避免发生低血糖。
- 阿奇霉素无需考虑是否与瑞格列奈和磺脲类共用。

唑类(酮康唑、伊曲康唑、氟康唑)
- 与酮康唑共用时瑞格列奈 AUC 增加 15%。那格列奈与氟康唑共用时 AUC 增加 48%。格列奈类药物与唑类共用时应考虑减少剂量以避免发生低血糖。
- 可能增加磺脲类药物水平。氟康唑增加格列苯脲 AUC44%。与唑类药物共用时考虑减少药物剂量。
- 与酮康唑共用时罗格列酮 AUC 增加 47%。与唑类共用时考虑减少罗格列酮剂量。
- 可能增加吡格列酮水平。

利福霉素类(利福平、利福喷汀、利福布汀)
- 利福霉素类显著诱导色素酶 P450。处方此类药物时需时刻警惕药物相互作用。
- 可以显著降低那格列奈、吡格列酮、罗格列酮、瑞格列奈和磺脲类药物的浓度。
- 利福平减少瑞格列奈和那格列奈 AUC 分别达 31% 和 24%。利福平减少罗格列酮和吡格列酮的 AUC 分别达 66% 和 54%。
- 若作为治疗肺结核药物,尤其对肥胖糖尿病患者应考虑高剂量持续应用,因会降低利福平水平,在这部分人群中增加治疗失败的风险 (Nijland; Ruslami)。对剂量没有推荐,但可考虑在常规剂量基础上增加 300~600mg。

其他抗生素
- 头孢菌素类:增加二甲双胍 AUC24%。临床意义未明。
- 异烟肼:在动物研究和人类研究中有改变胰岛素分泌和低血糖的报道,但仍有争议。
- 喷他脒:全身用药可能因对 β 细胞功能的毒效应和不恰当的胰岛素分泌导致高血糖或低血糖。在长期大量使用药物或者肾功能受损的患者中因药物蓄积而更常见 (Assan)。药物雾化时不会引起这种影响。
- 甲氧苄氨嘧啶:可能通过抑制肾小管分泌增加二甲双胍血药浓度。增加瑞格列奈 AUC61%;增加罗格列酮 AUC31%。考虑调整二甲双胍剂量。

糖尿病患者需谨慎使用抗生素

- 万古霉素：糖尿病患者体内抗生素组织穿透力下降(Skhirtladze)。计算万古霉素剂量时需使用实际体重（ABW）。建议万古霉素剂量，肾功能正常时：15mg/kg ABW 静脉使用 q12h。

专家意见

- 糖尿病患者和高 BMI 的患者当治疗严重感染时需调整抗生素剂量。处方万古霉素、达托霉素、氟康唑、卡泊芬净、青霉素类、头孢菌素类、甲氧苄啶/磺胺甲噁唑、氨基糖苷类和利福霉素药物时，应参考药剂师，或感染性疾病专家的意见。
- 氟喹诺酮类药物常用于治疗糖尿病患者的感染，包括 UTI 和糖尿病足感染。环丙沙星对血糖的影响较小，但左氧氟沙星使用时应警惕对血糖的影响。未确定莫西沙星对血糖的影响。
- 糖尿病患者抗结核治疗效果差。一些证据显示可能是因为改变了药物，尤其是利福平的浓度。目前对糖尿病患者并无药物剂量的推荐；然而，一些学者认为当过渡为日常治疗时应增加利福平剂量。

表 4-10. 抗生素与降糖药物的相互作用

抗生素	相互作用的降糖药物	对血糖的影响	建议
所有的抗生素	艾塞那肽	对血糖没有影响，但可能会延迟 ABX 吸收	使用艾塞那肽前一个小时使用 ABX。
唑类 （酮康唑，伊曲康唑，氟康唑）	瑞格列奈，那格列奈，吡格列酮，罗格列酮，磺脲类药物	低血糖	共用时考虑减少降糖药剂量。
头孢菌素类	二甲双胍	潜在的低血糖	临床意义未明，共用时严密监测血糖。
克拉霉素	瑞格列奈，吡格列酮，磺脲类药物	低血糖	考虑减少降糖药剂量或使用阿奇霉素代替。
加替沙星	—	低血糖和高血糖	避免使用（美国市场召回此药）。
左氧氟沙星 > 环丙沙星	—	低血糖和高血糖	环丙沙星更适合脆性糖尿病患者。
异烟肼	—	低血糖	罕见。

糖尿病患者需谨慎使用抗生素

表 4-10. 抗生素与降糖药物的相互作用（续）

抗生素	相互作用的降糖药物	对血糖的影响	建议
喷他脒		低血糖和高血糖	起始药物后，低血糖更常见。
利福平	瑞格列奈，那格列奈，吡格列酮，罗格列酮，磺脲类药物	低血糖	可能需要更高剂量的降糖药。
甲氧苄氨嘧啶	二甲双胍	潜在的低血糖	临床意义未明，共用时严密监测血糖。

Courtesy of Paul Pham, PharmD, Johns Hopkins University School of Medicine.

参考文献

Ruslami R, Nijland HM, Adhiarta IG, et al. Pharmacokinetics of antituberculosis drugs in pulmonary tuberculosis patients with type 2 diabetes. Antimicrob Agents Chemother,2010; Vol. 54: pp. 1068–74.

  Comments: Authors in follow-up to their 2006 paper (Nijland et al, CID) suggest that treatment failures in diabetic patients may be due to lower rifampin concentrations in continuation rather than acute/daily dosing. Why this occurs is unclear, but may be due to increased body mass or differences in hepatic induction of enzymes in these patients.

Aspinall SL, Good CB, Jiang R, et al. Severe dysglycemia with the fluoroquinolones: a class effect? Clin Infect Dis,2009; Vol. 49: pp. 402–8.

  Comments: Large cohort study of outpatients within the VA system regarding 1.2 million patients receiving a FQ between 2001–2005. For patients with diabetes, the odds ratio for azithromycin were 4.3 (95% CI, 2.7–6.6) for gatifloxacin, 2.1 (95% CI, 1.4–3.3) for levofloxacin, and 1.1 (95% CI, 0.6–2.0) for ciprofloxacin. The odds ratios for hyperglycemia were 4.5 (95% CI, 3.0–6.9) for gatifloxacin, 1.8 (95% CI, 1.2–2.7) for levofloxacin, and 1.0 (95% CI, 0.6–1.8) for ciprofloxacin. The authors conclude that the odds of either hypo- and hyperglycemia were significantly greater with gatifloxacin and levofloxacin, but not ciprofloxacin or azithromycin. It is important to note that this is an outpatient study, and that more severely ill patients may respond differently.

Hall RG, Leff RD, Gumbo T. Treatment of active pulmonary tuberculosis in adults: current standards and recent advances. Insights from the Society of Infectious Diseases Pharmacists. Pharmacotherapy,2009; Vol. 29: pp. 1468–81.

  Comments: TB in diabetes often has worse outcomes. Accumulating data suggest that pharmacokinetic /pharmacodynamic factors should be considered when treating these patients. As of yet, there are no formal recommendations in this regard from the American Thoracic Society.

Lewis RJ, Mohr JF. Dysglycaemias and fluoroquinolones. Drug Saf,2008; Vol. 31: pp. 283–92.

  Comments: Review of available data suggests that likelihood of glycemic dysregulation is dose dependent.

Khamaisi M, Leitersdorf E. Severe hypoglycemia from clarithromycin-repaglinide drug interaction. Pharmacotherapy, 2008; Vol. 28: pp. 682–4.

Comments: Case described with severe hypoglycemia occuring within 2 days of instituting the macrolide clarithromycin for H. pyloritreatment.

Scheen AJ. Drug-drug and food-drug pharmacokinetic interactions with new insulinotropic agents repaglinide and nateglinide. Clin Pharmacokinet, 2007; Vol. 46: pp. 93–108.

Comments: Review article highlights that rifampin reduced the repaglinide area under the plasma concentration-time curve (AUC) by 32%–85% and reduced nateglinide AUC by almost 25%. It should be expected that use of rifampin with these agents will moderate their antihypoglycemic effects. In contrast, azoles, macrolides, and trimethoprim increased the AUC of drugs by 15%–77%. It appears that CYP3A4 impact of the glinides is modest, but that CYP2C8 is most for repaglinide and CYP2C9 is important for nateglinide.

Skhirtladze K, Hutschala D, Fleck T, et al. Impaired target site penetration of vancomycin in diabetic patients following cardiac surgery. AAC, 2006; Vol. 50: p. 1372.

Comments: This observational study compared vancomycin tissue penetration in 6 diabetics and 6 nondiabetics. Vancomycin tissue concentrations in diabetic patients were significantly lower compared to nondiabetics (3.7 mg/L vs 11.9 mg/L; p =0.002). The authors hypothesize that the decreased vancomycin tissue concentrations may be due to impaired microcirculation associated with diabetes.

Nijland HM, Ruslami R, Stalenhoef JE, et al. Exposure to rifampicin is strongly reduced in patients with tuberculosis and type 2 diabetes. Clin Infect Dis, 2006; Vol. 43: pp. 848–54.

Comments: Initial report from Indonesia, suggesting a decreased rifampin plasma concentration in diabetics. Authors suggest that diabetics with increased BMI may need higher doses than the standard 600 mg of rifampin.

Saraya A, Yokokura M, Gonoi T, et al. Effects of fluoroquinolones on insulin secretion and beta-cell ATP-sensitive K+channels. Eur J Pharmacol, 2004; Vol. 497: pp. 111–7.

Comments: Study found that gatifloxacin and temafloxacin had greater effect on stimulating insulin secretion than levofloxacin in this murine model.

Gavin JR, Kubin R, Choudhri S, et al. Moxifloxacin and glucose homeostasis: a pooled-analysis of the evidence from clinical and postmarketing studies. Drug Saf, 2004; Vol. 27: pp. 671–86.

Comments: Analysis of 32 studies using moxifloxacin with over 14,731 patients, found 7 pts (0.1%) receiving moxifloxacin with a hyperglycemic adverse reaction. There were no moxifloxacin hypoglycemic-related events noted.

Kilby JM, Tabereaux PB Severe hyperglycemia in an HIV clinic: preexisting versus drug-associated diabetes mellitus. J Acquir Immune Defic Syndr Hum Retrovirol, 1998; Vol. 17: pp. 46–50.

Comments: Study performed in a Birmingham, AL, HIV clinic found that 2% of their HIV patients suffered from severe hyperglycemia, although this was evenly split between those who had preexisting diabetes and those who had drug-induced explanations. Not surprisingly, corticosteroids and megestrol acetate (with weight-related changes) were among the most common medication-related causes. One patient developed hyperglycemia while receiving pentamidine (plus prednisone) for PCP pneumonia, a not unusual combination and complication of therapy in this era. Pentamidine is now rarely used for treatment, but has been effective for visceral leishmania, although toxicity of the drug now has diminished use, including reports of provoking permanent diabetes in patients receiving the compound (Rev Soc Bras Med Trop, 1995; Vol. 28[4]: pp. 405–7 and J Infect Chemother, 2004; Vol. 10[6]: pp. 307–15).

Assan R, Perronne C, Assan D, et al. Pentamidine-induced derangements of glucose homeostasis. Determinant roles of renal failure and drug accumulation. A study of 128 patients. Diabetes Care,1995; Vol. 18: pp. 47–55.

Comments:Although not a commonly used drug, pentamidine can cause dysglycemia especially due to drugaccumulation (either inordinately high or prolonged dosing) or secondary to renal insufficiency. The drug has toxicity to islet beta-cells and may cause dysfunctional insulin release.

Uzzan B, Bentata M, Campos J, et al. Effects of aerosolized pentamidine on glucose homeostasis and insulin secretion in HIV-positive patients: a controlled study. AIDS,1995; Vol. 9: pp. 901–7.

Comments:No longer a popular approach to PCP prophylaxis, aerosolized pentamidine in this study was not found to significantly affect glucose homeostasis, compared to receiving the drug systemically.

Villaume C, Dollet JM, Beck B, et al. Hyperinsulinemia associated with normal C-peptide levels in a woman treated with isoniazide. Biomed Pharmacother,1982; Vol. 36: pp. 32–5.

Comments:Among several reports attributing INH to altered insulin secretion and hypoglycemia that bolster prior observations including animal studies (BMJ, 1953; Vol. 1: pp. 296–9 and Ind J Physiol Pharmac, 1989; Vol. 33: pp. 277–8). It is not clear from any of these reports that diabetics are more prone to this problem.

Cameron SJ, Crompton GK. Severe hypoglycaemia in the course of treatment with streptomycin, isoniazid and ethionamide. Tubercle,1967; Vol. 48: pp. 307–10.

Comments: Antitubercular agents have been implicated in causing hypoglycemia, mostly in nondiabetic patients. In this report, ethionamide is argued as the cause. Others include less commonly used drugs such as PAS (para-aminosalicylic acid) (Postgrad Med J, 1980; Vol. 56(652): p. 135 and J Pharm Sci, 1968; Vol. 57: pp. 2111–6) and INH (see Villaume ref). One should keep in mind that adrenal insufficiency due to TB would be another explanation (Korean J Intern Med,2004; Vol. 19[1]: pp. 70–3).

抗精神病药

Paul A. Pham, PharmD

适应证

FDA
- 精神分裂症。
- 双相情感障碍。
- 抑郁症。
- 激惹。
- 焦虑症。
- 抗精神病药物的 FDA 推荐适应证见表 4-11。

非 FDA 批准适应证
- 呃逆。
- ICU 谵妄。

机制
- 典型（如吩噻嗪）和非典型抗精神病药在中脑边缘系统阻滞突触后的多巴胺受体，导致去极化阻滞多巴胺束，发挥抗精神病效应。
- 非典型抗精神病药（如阿立哌唑、氯氮平、奥氮平、利培酮、喹硫平、齐拉西酮）同时阻滞 5 羟色胺受体。

表格
- 见表 4-11。

成人常用剂量
- 老年患者和患有肾脏疾病和肝脏疾病的患者需小剂量起始，并缓慢加量。
- 见表 4-12。

表4-11. FDA适应证、代谢、禁忌和抗精神病药物药代动力学

典型抗精神病药物	FDA适应证	代谢/排泄/T½	妊娠/母乳喂养	品牌/仿制药/剂型
氯丙嗪	急性间歇性卟啉病 急性精神病 恶心/呕吐 精神病 抑郁症 精神分裂症 呃逆（打嗝） 破伤风	代谢：肝脏细胞色素P450酶CYP2D6，>100的代谢产物已被确定通过肝肠循环代谢。 排泄：尿，部分经胆汁和粪便。 T½：23-37小时。	妊娠分级为C级。 由于经母乳排泄，不推荐哺乳期女性使用。	通用氯丙嗪 · 注射液：25毫克/毫升 · 口服液：100毫克/毫升 · 口服片剂：10毫克，25毫克，50毫克，100毫克，200毫克 60×10毫克/片×22美元 60×25毫克/片×26美元 60×50毫克/片×18美元 60×100毫克/片×16美元 60×200毫克/片×27美元 氯丙嗪 · 口服片剂：200毫克
氟奋乃静	急性精神病 抑郁性精神病 精神分裂症	代谢：肝脏，50%的代谢物有抗精神病活性，通过肝肠循环。 排泄：尿，部分经胆汁和粪便。 T½：16小时，7~10天（癸酸甲酯）	妊娠分级为C级。 由于经母乳排泄，不推荐哺乳期女性使用。	氟奋乃静 · 注射液：2.5毫克/毫升 5毫升＝65.99美元 10毫升＝125.98美元 盐酸氟奋乃静 · 肌内注射制剂：2.5毫克/毫升 · 口服药剂：2.5毫克/5毫升

抗精神病药

药物	适应证	药代动力学	注意事项	剂型及价格
奋乃静	急性精神病 恶心 / 呕吐 精神病 抑郁症 精神分裂症 呃逆（打嗝）	代谢：胃黏膜和肝脏的首过效应。 排泄：胆道和粪便。 T½：9 小时。	妊娠分级为 C 级。 由于经母乳排泄，不推荐哺乳期女性使用。	口服液：5 毫克 / 毫升 口服片剂：1 毫克，2.5 毫克，5 毫克，10 毫克 90×1 毫克 / 片 = 18 美元 60×2.5 毫克 / 片 = 16 美元 60×5 毫克 / 片 = 19 美元 60×10 毫克 / 片 = 25 美元
奋乃静				口服片剂：2 毫克，4 毫克，8 毫克，16 毫克 60×2 毫克 / 片 = 42 美元 60×4 毫克 / 片 = 56 美元 60×8 毫克 / 片 = 60 美元 60×16 毫克 / 片 = 83 美元
硫利达嗪	激惹 焦虑症 抑郁症 精神病 抑郁症 精神分裂症	代谢：胃黏膜和肝脏的首过效应。 排泄：尿，部分经胆汁和粪便。 T½：24 小时。	妊娠分级为 C 级。 由于经母乳排泄，不推荐哺乳期女性使用。	硫利达嗪 口服片剂：10 毫克，15 毫克，25 毫克，50 毫克，100 毫克，150 毫克，200 毫克 90×10 毫克 / 片 = 22 美元 90×15 毫克 / 片 = 12 美元 90×25 毫克 / 片 = 26 美元 90×50 毫克 / 片 = 30 美元 90×100 毫克 / 片 = 35 美元 90×150 毫克 / 片 = 56 美元 90×200 毫克 / 片 = 82 美元

表 4-11. FDA 适应证、代谢、禁忌和抗精神病药物药代动力学（续）

典型抗精神病药物	FDA 适应证	代谢/排泄/T½	妊娠/母乳喂养	品牌/仿制药/剂型
三氟拉嗪	焦虑症 精神分裂症	代谢：肝脏通过氧化代谢生成多种代谢活性产物。 排泄：尿。 T½: 24 小时。	妊娠分级为 C 级。 由于经母乳排泄，不推荐哺乳期女性使用。	三氟拉嗪 • 口服片剂：1 毫克，2 毫克，5 毫克，10 毫克 60 × 1 毫克/片 = 26 美元 60 × 2 毫克/片 = 30 美元 60 × 5 毫克/片 = 35 美元 60 × 10 毫克/片 = 47 美元
氟哌啶醇	精神分裂症	代谢：部分经肝肠循环代谢。 排泄：尿，部分通过粪便。 T½: 21 小时。	妊娠分级为 C 级。 由于经母乳排泄，不推荐哺乳期女性使用。	• 口服片剂：0.5 毫克，1 毫克，2 毫克，5 毫克，10 毫克，20 毫克 90 × 0.5 毫克/片 = 26 美元 90 × 1 毫克/片 = 20 美元 90 × 2 毫克/片 = 19 美元 90 × 5 毫克/片 = 26 美元 60 × 10 毫克/片 = 72 美元 60 × 20 毫克/片 = 125 美元
洛沙平	精神分裂症	代谢：肝脏。 排泄：尿，部分通过粪便。 T½: 4~12 小时。	妊娠分级为 C 级。 由于经母乳排泄，不推荐哺乳期女性使用。	洛沙平 • 口服胶囊 5 毫克 90 × 5 毫克/片 = 56 美元

哌咪呱酮	精神分裂症	代谢：肝脏。 排泄：尿，部分通过粪便。 T½：< 24 小时。	妊娠分级为 C 级。 由于经母乳排泄，不推荐哺乳期女性使用。	哌咪呱酮片：5 毫克，10 毫克，25 毫克，50 毫克
替沃噻吨	精神病性障碍 精神分裂症	代谢：肝脏。 排泄：尿，部分通过粪便。 T½：34 小时。	妊娠分级为 C 级。 由于经母乳排泄，不推荐哺乳期女性使用。	替沃噻吨 • 口服胶囊：1 毫克，2 毫克，5 毫克，10 毫克 90×1 毫克/粒 = 23 美元 90×2 毫克/粒 = 27 美元 90×5 毫克/粒 = 26 美元 60×10 毫克/粒 = 50 美元 氨砜噻吨 • 口服胶囊：2 毫克，5 毫克，10 毫克，20 毫克
阿立哌唑	自闭症 双相情感障碍 抑郁症 激惹 精神分裂症	代谢：肝脏 CYP2D6，CYP3A4。 排泄：尿（25%）和粪便（55%）。 T½：75 小时（药物原型），94 小时（代谢产物）。	妊娠分级为 C 级。 由于经母乳排泄，不推荐哺乳期女性使用。	阿立哌唑 • 口腔速崩片剂：10 毫克，15 毫克 30×10 毫克/片 = 570 美元 90×10 毫克/片 = 1676 美元 阿立哌唑 • 口服液：1 毫克/毫升 • 口服片剂：2 毫克，5 毫克，10 毫克，15 毫克，20 毫克，30 毫克

表 4-11. FDA 适应证、代谢、禁忌和抗精神病药物药代动力学（续）

典型抗精神病药物	FDA 适应证	代谢 / 排泄 / T½	妊娠 / 母乳喂养	品牌 / 仿制药 / 剂型
氯氮平	复发性分裂情感障碍的自杀行为 精神分裂症	代谢：肝脏 CYP1A2、去甲基化，和 N-氧化。 排泄：尿（50%），部分通过粪便（30%）。 T½：12 小时。	妊娠分级为 B 级。 由于经母乳排泄，不推荐哺乳期女性使用。	氯氮平 • 口服片剂：25 毫克、50 毫克、100 毫克、200 毫克 氯氮平 • 口服片剂：25 毫克、100 毫克 FazaClo • 口腔速崩片剂：12.5 毫克、25 毫克、100 毫克
奥氮平	I 型双相躁郁症 激惹型精神分裂症 I 型双相情感障碍，急性混态或躁狂发作 I 型双相情感障碍，维持治疗 精神分裂症	代谢：肝细胞色素 P450 氧化和葡萄醛酸。 排泄：尿（57%），部分通过粪便（30%）。 T½：30 小时。	妊娠分级为 C 级。 由于经母乳排泄，不推荐哺乳期女性使用。	奥氮平 • 口服片剂：10 毫克 再普乐肌肉注射粉剂 • 肌肉注射粉剂：10 毫克 再普乐 • 口服片剂：2.5 毫克、5 毫克、7.5 毫克、10 毫克、15 毫克、20 毫克 30 × 2.5 毫克 / 片 = 245 美元 30 × 5 毫克 / 片 = 296 美元 30 × 7.5 毫克 / 片 = 358 美元 30 × 10 毫克 / 片 = 440 美元 30 × 15 毫克 / 片 = 639 美元

抗精神病药

喹硫平	双相情感障碍，情绪低落期 双相情感障碍，维持 抑郁症 I型双相情感障碍 精神分裂症	代谢：肝脏CYP3A4。 排泄：尿（73%），部分通过粪便（20%）。 T½：6小时。	妊娠分级为C级，由于经母乳排泄，不推荐哺乳期女性使用。	30×20 毫克/片 = 856美元 再普乐口腔速崩片剂： 5毫克，10毫克，15毫克，20毫克 齐拉西酮 • 口服片剂：25毫克，100毫克，200毫克 思瑞康 • 口服片剂：25毫克，50毫克，100毫克，200毫克，300毫克，400毫克 60×25 毫克/片 = 182美元 100×50 毫克/片 = 501美元 60×100 毫克/片 = 325美元 60×200 毫克/片 = 560美元 60×300 毫克/片 = 788美元 30×400 毫克/片 = 482美元 富马酸喹硫平 • 口服片剂，缓释：50毫克，150毫克，200毫克，300毫克，400毫克 60×50 毫克/片 = 291美元 60×150 毫克/片 = 500美元 30×200 毫克/片 = 560美元

表 4-11. FDA 适应证、代谢、禁忌和抗精神病药物药代动力学（续）

典型抗精神病药物	FDA 适应证	代谢/排泄/T½	妊娠/母乳喂养	品牌/仿制药/剂型
齐拉西酮	I 型双相情感障碍，急性混合或躁狂发作，单药治疗或丙戊酸钠、锂剂双相障碍时对锂剂辅助治疗，精神分裂症	代谢：肝脏。排泄：尿（20%），主要通过粪便（66%）。T½：7 小时（口服）；2-5 小时（肌注）。	妊娠分级为 C 级。由于经母乳排泄，不推荐哺乳期女性使用	齐拉西酮 • 口服胶囊 20 毫克，40 毫克，60 毫克，80 毫克 60×1 毫克上限 = 458 美元 60×2 毫克上限 = 463 美元 60×3 毫克上限 = 550 美元 60×4 毫克上限 = 550 美元
利培酮	精神分裂症	代谢：肝脏。排泄：尿，部分通过粪便。T½：34 小时。	妊娠分级为 C 级。由于经母乳排泄，不推荐哺乳期女性使用。	利培酮 • 口服液：1 毫克/毫升 1 毫克/毫升，30 毫升 = 126 美元 口服片剂：0.25 毫克，0.5 毫克，1 毫克，2 毫克，3 毫克，4 毫克 60×0.25 毫克/片 = 145 美元 60×0.5 毫克/片 = 180 美元

抗精神病药

60×1毫克/片 = 196美元
60×2毫克/片 = 300美元
60×3毫克/片 = 300美元
60×4毫克/片 = 400美元

- 口腔速崩片：
0.25毫克, 0.5毫克, 1毫克, 2毫克, 3毫克, 4毫克

利培酮

- 肌肉注射粉剂, 缓释：12.5毫克, 25毫克, 37.5毫克, 50毫克

维思通

- 口腔速崩片：
0.5毫克, 1毫克, 2毫克

表 4-11. FDA 适应证、代谢、禁忌和抗精神病药物药代动力学（续）

典型抗精神病药物	FDA 适应证	代谢 / 排泄 / T½	妊娠 / 母乳喂养	品牌 / 仿制药 / 剂型
				维思通 • 口腔速崩片： 3 毫克, 4 毫克 利培酮 • 口服液：1 毫克/毫升 1 毫克/毫升, 60 毫升 = 375 美元 • 口服片剂：0.25 毫克, 0.5 毫克, 1 毫克, 2 毫克, 3 毫克, 4 毫克 30×0.25 毫克/片 = 137 美元 30×0.5 毫克/片 = 165 美元 30×1 毫克/片 = 175 美元 30×2 毫克/片 = 271 美元 30×3 毫克/片 = 350 美元 30×4 毫克/片 = 435 美元 利培酮 m-tab • 口腔速崩片： 0.5 毫克, 1 毫克, 2 毫克, 3 毫克, 4 毫克

Courtesy of Paul Pham, PharmD, Johns Hopkins University School of Medicine.

表 4-12. 抗精神病药物剂量

名称	起始剂量	维持剂量	最大剂量
典型抗精神病药			
氟奋乃静	2.5~10 毫克/天；12.5~25 毫克/剂量 肌注或皮下注射	20 毫克/天；50 毫克/剂量 肌注或皮下注射	40 毫克/天，口服；100 毫克/剂量 肌注或皮下注射
奋乃静	20~100 毫克/天 口服	200~400 毫克/天 口服	24 毫克/天 口服
硫利达嗪	30~150 毫克/天 口服	300 毫克/天 口服	300 毫克/天 口服
三氟拉嗪	4~10 毫克/天 口服	15~20 毫克/天 口服	40 毫克/天 口服
氟哌啶醇	1~6 毫克/天 口服	6~15 毫克/天 口服	30 毫克/天 口服
洛沙平	10~25 毫克/天 口服	60~100 毫克/天 口服	250 毫克/天 口服
吗啉吲酮	50~75 毫克/天 口服	15~100 毫克/天 口服	225 毫克/天 口服
替沃噻吨	15 毫克/天 口服	20~30 毫克/天 口服	60 毫克/天 口服
非典型抗精神病药			
阿立哌唑	10~15 毫克/天 口服	30 毫克/天 口服（没有证据表明超过 15 毫克/天有效性更佳）	30 毫克/天 口服
氯氮平	25~50 毫克/天 口服	300~450 毫克/天 口服	600~900 毫克/天 口服

表 4-12 抗精神病药物剂量（续）

名称	起始剂量	维持剂量	最大剂量
奥氮平	5~10 毫克/天 口服 210~300 毫克 肌内注射 每两周一次，或 405 毫克肌注每四周一次	10~20 毫克/天 口服 150~300 毫克 肌注 每两周一次， 300~405 毫克肌注 每四周一次	20 毫克/天 口服
喹硫平		300~400 毫克/天 口服	800 毫克/天 口服
利培酮		1~6 毫克/天 口服；6 毫克/天 肌注	16 毫克/天 口服
齐拉西酮		20~80 毫克/天 口服	200 毫克/天 口服

Courtesy of Paul Pham, PharmD, Johns Hopkins University School of Medicine.

抗精神病药

特殊人群用量

肾脏病
重度肾功能异常患者,起始利培酮 0.5mg 每日两次并缓慢加量。
其他抗精神病药无需调整剂量,但应以最低剂量起始(尤其对同时合并肝功能异常的患者)。

肝脏疾病
以最低剂量起始并缓慢加量。

妊娠
抗精神病药妊娠分级为 C 级(氯氮平为 B 级)。
人类临床数据有限,权衡利弊后使用。

哺乳期
应通过乳汁排泄,不建议哺乳期使用。

药物不良反应

全体人群
与吩噻嗪相比,新的非典型抗精神病药的耐受性更好,但与体重增加和发生糖尿病相关。
所有的抗精神病药对急性精神状态改变的患者应避免或谨慎使用。

常见不良反应
体重增加:治疗 10 周后,与安慰剂相比,估计平均体重增加为 0.5~5.0kg。奥氮平和氯氮平与更多的体重增加和血脂升高相关。
抗胆碱能副作用(如口干、便秘和尿潴留)。与其他药物相比,以下药物更为常见,硫利达嗪 > 氯丙嗪 > 洛沙平。利培酮的抗胆碱能不良反应发生率最低。
初始治疗出现剂量相关的镇静作用,虽使用时间延长有所改善。
出现剂量相关的锥体外系症状(如肌张力障碍和静坐不能、迟发性运动障碍)。高效的吩噻嗪(吩噻嗪、氟哌啶醇和替沃噻吨)比低效(氯丙嗪和硫利达嗪)的和非典型"第二代"抗精神病药(阿立哌唑、奥氮平、利培酮、喹硫平、齐拉西酮)相比更为常见。

少见不良反应
新发糖尿病:奥氮平与奎硫平、氟哌啶醇和利培酮相比更为常见。
增加泌乳素水平。
体位性低血压(继发于 α_1 阻滞)± 反射性心动过速。与氟哌啶醇相比,硫利达嗪和氯丙嗪更为常见。
性功能障碍,包括性欲缺失和性快感缺失。
认知障碍。
LFT 升高和肝炎。

抗精神病药

罕见不良反应
- 抗精神病药物恶性症候群（NMS）表现为意识障碍，发热，心动过速，肌肉强直和血压不稳定。
- QTc 和 PR 间期延长。齐拉西酮、硫利达嗪和氯氮平更为常见。
- 硫利达嗪和氯丙嗪发生视网膜良性色素沉积。
- 在氯氮平最初治疗的 4~6 个月，0.8%（1 年风险）的患者发生粒细胞缺乏。初次使用氯氮平治疗的 6 个月内应每周监测血常规。使用吩噻嗪发生一过性的白细胞减少症也有报道。
- 高热（在天气炎热或运动时更常见）。
- 癫痫：有癫痫病史的患者应慎用。

药物相互作用
- 吩噻嗪和氟哌啶醇经 CYP2D6 首次代谢。非典型抗精神病药经 CYP2D6、CYP3A4 和 CYP1A2 首次代谢。因此这些同工酶的诱导剂和抑制剂可以降低和升高非典型抗精神病药的血药浓度。因此需要根据治疗反应调整药物剂量。
- CYP450 诱导剂（如卡马西平、苯巴比妥、扑痫酮、利福平）：可降低非典型抗精神病药的血药浓度，如吩噻嗪和氟哌啶醇。
- 西咪替丁：可增加氯氮平、利培酮、奥氮平、喹硫平和齐拉西酮的血药浓度。
- CYP1A2 抑制剂（如环丙沙星、西咪替丁、氟伏沙明、氟西汀）：增加氯氮平和奥氮平的血药浓度。可能增加癫痫的发生风险。需谨慎使用。
- CYP3A4 抑制剂 [如红霉素、克拉霉素、唑类抗真菌（酮康唑、伊曲康唑、伏立康唑、泊沙康唑）、HIV 蛋白酶抑制剂]：可能增加氯氮平、喹硫平和齐拉西酮的血药浓度。
- CYP2D6 抑制剂（如安非他酮、氟西汀、帕罗西汀、度洛西汀、奎尼丁、利托那韦）：可能增加硫利达嗪、氟哌啶醇、利培酮的浓度。
- 降压药：与抗精神病药共用可能增加体位性低血压的风险。共用时需密监测。
- 苯二氮䓬类药物：可能增加过度镇静的风险（尤其是氯氮平）。共用需严密监测。
- 有抗胆碱能副作用的药物（如三环类抗抑郁药、抗组胺药）：与抗精神病药共用可能增加抗胆碱能副作用并影响认知。
- 已知延长 QTc 的药物（如高剂量的美沙酮、克拉霉素、红霉素、三环类抗抑郁药）：可能增加 QTc 延长的风险（尤其是齐拉西酮）。避免与长 QTc 的药物共用。
- 甲氧氯普胺：与抗精神病药共用可能增加静坐不能和其他锥体外系的作用。
- 抗精神病药并未发现与口服降糖药存在相互作用。

药代动力学
- 吸收：吸收良好。
- 代谢和排泄：首次经 CYP2D6、CYP3A4 和 CYP1A2 代谢。氯丙嗪

抗精神病药

氟哌啶醇、利培酮、奥氮平、喹硫平为活性代谢产物。

- 蛋白结合：中到高的蛋白结合。
- Cmax，Cmin 和 AUC：不进行常规血浆浓度检测。有限的数据表明氯氮平浓度 >350mcg/ml 与治疗反应存在相关性。
- $T_{1/2}$：半衰期 10~40 小时。除了喹硫平（6 小时）、齐拉西酮（7 小时）和奋乃静（9 小时）。
- 分布：组织中广泛分布。
- 药代动力学见表 4-11。

专家意见

- 非典型抗精神病药目前是治疗精神病的一线用药，因其发生锥体外系和迟发性运动障碍的风险较低，但仍存在体重增加、脂代谢紊乱和新发糖尿病的风险。
- 奥氮平和氯氮平与体重明显增加和增加发生 2 型糖尿病的风险相关（Lambert）。
- 体重增加、糖尿病和脂代谢紊乱：氯氮平，利培酮 > 奥氮平，喹硫平 > 齐拉西酮和阿立哌唑（Lieberman）。
- 对肥胖糖尿病患者，齐拉西酮与其他非典型抗精神病药相比体重增加的风险较小（Komossa）。
- 在起始抗精神病药物之前，应尽早进行基线糖尿病筛查。建议在起始非典型抗精神病药的 4、8 和 12 周或更改治疗时应进行重新评估（Consensus Statement）。
- 典型抗精神病药（如氟哌啶醇），与非典型抗精神病（如奥氮平）药相比导致更少的体重增加和糖尿病。
- 虽然使用抗精神病药物治疗的患者体重增加并存在发生糖尿病的风险，但那些体重没有显著增加的患者也发生了高血糖（Lindenmayer）。
- 已患有糖尿病的患者，上述药物是否会使血糖控制恶化目前仍缺少证据。但糖尿病患者开始使用非典型抗精神病药物（如奥氮平）治疗时需严密监测血糖。

推荐依据

American Diabetes Association. American Psychiatric Association, American Association of Clinical Endocrinologists, and North American Association for the Study of Obesity Consensus Development Conference on Antipsychotic Drugs and Obesity and Diabetes. Diabetes Care,2004; Vol. 27: pp. 596–601.

Comments:Consensus recommendation on monitoring of blood glucose for patients on antipsychotics.

其他参考文献

Komossa K, Rummel-Kluge C, Hunger H, et al. Ziprasidone versus other atypical antipsychotics for schizophrenia.Cochrane Database Syst Rev,2009; CD006627.

Comments:In a review of nine randomized controlled trials involving 3361 patients ziprasidone produced less weight gain and cholesterol increase than olanzapine, quetiapine, and risperidone. However, ziprasidone may be less effective with more patients leaving studies early due to low efficacy compared to olanzapine and risperidone.

Citrome LL, Holt RI, Zachry WM, et al. Risk of treatment-emergent diabetes mellitus in patients receiving antipsychotics. Ann Pharmacother,2007; Vol. 41: pp. 1593–603.

Comments:Attributable risk for atypical antipsychotics relative to first-generation antipsychotics (e.g., phenothiazines, haloperidol) ranged from 40–50 new cases of diabetes per 1000 patients. However, few studies controlled for body weight, race or ethnicity, or the presence of other diabetogenic medications.

Lambert MT, Copeland LA, Sampson N, et al. New-onset type 2 diabetes associated with atypical antipsychotic medications. Prog Neuropsychopharmacol Biol Psychiatry,2006; Vol. 30: pp. 919–23.

Comments: This retrospective analysis evaluated the one-year risk of developing type-2 diabetes between olanzapine, quetiapine, and risperidone when compared to haloperidol. Patients treated with olanzapine, but not quetiapine and risperidone, were significantly at higher risk of developing type-2 diabetes compared to haloperidol (odds ratio 8.4, 95% CI 1.8–38.7).

Lieberman JA, Stroup TS, McEvoy JP, et al. Effectiveness of antipsychotic drugs in patients with chronic schizophrenia. NEJM,2005; Vol. 353: pp. 1209–23.

Comments:1493 patients with schizophrenia were randomized to receive olanzapine, quetiapine, ziprasidone, and perphenazine. Compared to the other antipsychotics, olanzapine was the most effective, but was associated with the highest rates of discontinuation due to greater weight gain and increases in measures of glucose and lipid.

Lindenmayer JP, Czobor P, Volavka J, et al. Changes in glucose and cholesterol levels in patients with schizophrenia treated with typical or atypical antipsychotics. Am J Psychiatry 2003; Vol. 160: pp. 290–6.

Comments:In this prospective randomized trial involving 157 hospitalized patients, clozapine, olanzapine, and haloperidol were all associated with an increase of plasma glucose level (. 125 mg/dl) over 14 weeks.

高血压

血管紧张素转换酶（ACE）抑制剂

Lipika Samal, MD, MPH, and Paul A. Pham, PharmD

指征

FDA

- 糖尿病肾病（卡托普利）。
- 高血压（HTN）。
- 充血性心力衰竭（CHF）。
- ACE 抑制剂其他特殊 FDA 适应证详见表 4-13。

机制

- 与其天然底物血管紧张素 I 相比较，对血管紧张素转换酶有更高的亲和力，以阻断其转换能力、减少血管紧张素 II 的生成。血管紧张素 II 是一种强力的血管收缩物质，对肾素活性有反馈抑制作用。因此减低血浆中血管紧张素 II 水平，可导致血压降低、血浆肾素活性升高。

剂型

- 见表 4-13。

成人常用剂量

- 贝那普利：起始剂量为 10mg qd（不合用利尿剂时）。常用剂量：20~40mg 单剂量或分两次口服。
- 卡托普利：CHF/HTN：6.25~12.5mg tid（合用利尿剂时），目标剂量为 50mg tid。糖尿病肾病：25mg tid。
- 依那普利：CHF/HTN：2.5~5mg qd 逐渐加量至 40mg qd，每 1~2 周加量 2.5mg。静脉：每次 1.25mg，每 6 小时一次，最多 36 小时。
- 福辛普利：CHF/HTN：初始剂量 10mg qd，逐渐滴定加量至有效为止（最大剂量 40mg qd）。常用剂量：20~40mg qd。
- 赖诺普利：HTN：初始剂量 10mg qd（不合用利尿剂时）或 5mg qd（合用利尿剂时）。剂量范围：10~40mg qd。CHF：初始剂量 2.5~5mg qd，以每 2 周加量 10mg 速度滴定加量至目标剂量 20~40mg qd。
- 莫西普利：HTN：7.5mg qd（不合用利尿剂时）或 3.75mg qd（与利尿剂合用时）。餐前 1 小时口服。维持剂量：每日 7.5~30mg，单剂量或分 2 次口服。
- 培哚普利叔丁胺：HTN：起始剂量 4mg qd，每 1~2 周逐渐滴定加量至达到预期药效，最大日剂量 16mg。常用剂量为 4~8mg/d，分 2 次口服。稳定性冠状动脉性心脏病（CAD）：起始剂量 4mg qd 口服 2 周后，如能耐受加量至 8mg qd。
- 喹那普利：HTN：起始剂量 10~20mg qd，如与利尿剂合用则起始剂量需减至 5mg qd。剂量范围：10~40mg qd。CHF：5mg qd 或 bid；

每周滴定加量至预期药效,预期剂量为 20~40mg/d,分 2 次口服。
- 雷米普利:2.5~5mg qd(最大剂量为 20mg/d)。心肌梗死后左室功能不全(LVD):2.5mg bid,如能耐受则滴定加量至 5mg bid。降低卒中、心梗和死亡风险:初始剂量 2.5mg qd 口服 1 周,后第 2~4 周为 5mg qd,后如能耐受则滴定加量至 10mg qd。
- 群多普利:CHF/LVD 起始剂量 1mg/d,如能耐受则逐渐加量至 4mg/d。HTN:起始剂量 1mg/d(黑色人种可予 2mg/d),每周滴定加量至预期药效。

特殊人群中用药剂量

肾脏特殊人群
- 肌酐清除率 10~50ml/min:推荐的起始剂量需减少 25%,后滴定加量至药效。
- 肌酐清除率 < 10ml/min:推荐的起始剂量需减少 50%,后滴定加量至药效。

肝脏特殊人群
- 无须调整剂量。

孕期妇女
- FDA 妊娠 D 类,孕期避免使用。
- ACE 抑制剂有致畸作用,可增加新生儿发病率(心血管疾病和中枢神经系统)和死亡率。

哺乳
- 人乳中浓度约为血清浓度的 1%。哺乳期间避免应用 ACE 抑制剂。

药物不良反应

常见
- 心血管系统:水肿,低血压(对容量较小的患者应低剂量用药、缓慢加量)。

偶见
- 药物相关咳嗽(0.5%~2%)。
- 内分泌/代谢:男性乳腺发育,高钾血症。
- 皮疹。
- 肾衰竭。
- 皮肤:面部、口唇和喉部出现血管性水肿(0.1%)。
- 金属味(卡托普利)。

少见
- 血液系统:粒细胞缺乏症,中性粒细胞减少症。
- 胃肠道:肠道血管性水肿。
- 嗜酸性粒细胞肺炎。
- 光过敏。

血管紧张素转换酶（ACE）抑制剂

药物相互作用

- ACE-I 可能增加胰岛素及其他降糖药物的低血糖作用。
- 保钾利尿剂（如螺内酯）和甲氧苄啶：可能增加高钾血症风险。
- 钾盐：与 ACE-I 合用时应监测血钾、警惕高钾血症。
- ARBs（如洛沙坦、替米沙坦）：可能增加肾衰竭、腹泻、低血压、晕厥和高钾血症的风险。ACE-I 与 ARBs 合用时应密切监测肾功能。
- 锂剂：可能增加锂浓度。与 ACE-I 合用时监测锂浓度。
- 普瑞巴林：与 ACE-I 合用可能增加血管性水肿风险。合用时密切监测。
- 抑酸药：可能使 ACE-I 吸收减少。需分不同时间口服。
- 肾毒性药物（例如对比剂、NSAIDs、氨基糖苷类、两性霉素 B）：可能增加肾毒性风险。合用时需密切监测肾功能。
- 也可能是某种遗传综合征的一部分，包括多发性骨纤维发育不良病，多发性内分泌肿瘤 1 型（MEN-1）综合征和 Carney 综合征。多发性骨纤维发育不良病的特点是由多发骨纤维异常。

药代动力学

表 4-13. ACE-I 的其他特殊 FDA 适应证、剂型和药代动力学

药名	商品名	FDA 适应证	制剂（片、胶囊、静脉）	每剂费用	半衰期	起效/达峰时间	代谢/排出	蛋白结合力
贝那普利	洛汀新	高血压，单用或与其他药物合用	贝那普利/洛汀新 5mg 片剂，10mg 片剂，20mg 片剂，40mg 片剂	贝那普利 5mg 片剂 $1.05，10mg 片剂 $0.95，20mg 片剂 $0.95，40mg 片剂 $1.05；洛汀新 5mg 片剂 $1.73，10mg 片剂 $1.73，20mg 片剂 $1.73，40mg 片剂 $1.73	10~11小时	起效/达峰时间：1~2小时	前药（贝那普利）：肝脏水解；活性代谢产物（贝那普利拉）：肝脏结合葡萄糖醛。排出：前药（贝那普利）：4%以葡萄糖醛结合形式经肾脏排出；活性代谢产物（贝那普利拉）：11%~12%经胆排泄，8%经肾脏排泄。	贝那普利：约97%；贝那普利拉：约95%

血管紧张素转换酶（ACE）抑制剂

卡托普利	开博通	充血性心力衰竭，糖尿病肾病，高血压和伴有心肌功能障碍的左室功能不全	卡托普利 12.5mg 片剂，25mg 片剂，50mg 片剂，100mg 片剂	卡托普利 12.5mg 片剂 $0.69, 25mg 片剂 $0.79, 50mg 片剂 $1.56, 100mg 片剂 $1.50	健康人群中 1.9小时；心衰患者中 2.06小时；无尿患者 20~40 小时	起效/达峰时间：1小时	排出：大于95%经肾脏排出，其中 40%~50%以原型排出	25%~30%
依那普利	Vasotec	治疗高血压，无症状性左室功能不全和症状性心衰	依那普利拉 IV 1.25mg/ml, 依那普利/Vasotec 2.5mg 片剂，5mg 片剂，10mg 片剂，20mg 片剂	依那普利拉 IV 1.25mg/ml（每支 2ml）$3.50；依那普利 2.5mg 片剂 $0.89, 5mg 片剂 $1.02, 10mg 片剂 $1.19, 20mg 片剂 $1.69; Vasotec 2.5mg 片剂 $2.17, 5mg 片剂 $2.51, 10mg 片剂 $2.77, 20mg 片剂 $2.51	前药（依那普利）健康人群 2小时，充血性心力衰竭者 3.4~5.8小时；活性代谢产物（依那普利拉）：35~38 小时	起效时间：1小时，达峰时间：口服 0.5~1.5小时，静脉 3~4.5 小时	代谢：前药经肝脏代谢为依那普利拉 排出：60%~80%经肾脏，部分经粪便排出。	50%~60%

表 4-13. ACE-I 的其他特殊 FDA 适应证、剂型和药代动力学（续）

药名	商品名	FDA 适应证	制剂（片、胶囊、静脉）	每剂费用	半衰期	起效/达峰时间	代谢/排出	蛋白结合力
福辛普利	蒙诺	治疗心衰和高血压，单用或与其他药物联用	福辛普利 10mg 片剂，20mg 片剂，40mg 片剂；蒙诺 10mg 片剂，20mg 片剂，40mg 片剂	福辛普利 10mg 片剂 $1.19, 20mg 片剂 $1.19, 40mg 片剂 $1.19；蒙诺 10mg 片剂 $1.53, 20mg 片剂 $1.53, 40mg 片剂 $1.70	活性代谢产物（福辛普利拉）：12 小时	起效时间：1小时，达峰时间：3小时	代谢：前药（福辛普利）经小肠壁水解为活性代谢产物福辛普利拉，也经肝脏代谢。排出：45%尿中排出，50%经粪便。	95%
赖诺普利	Zestril	单用或联合其他药物治疗高血压，心梗后左心功能不全，急性心梗24小时内且患者情况稳定时，以及心衰的辅助治疗	赖诺普利/Zestril 2.5mg 片剂，5mg 片剂，10mg 片剂，20mg 片剂，30mg 片剂，40mg 片剂	赖诺普利 2.5mg 片剂 $0.65, 5mg 片剂 $0.97, 10mg 片剂 $1.00, 20mg 片剂 $1.07, 30mg 片剂 $1.51, 40mg 片剂 $1.56；Zestril 2.5mg 片剂 $1.02, 5mg	11~12 小时	起效时间：1小时，达峰时间约7小时。	代谢：不经代谢。排出：经肾脏以原型排出。	95%

血管紧张素转换酶（ACE）抑制剂

| 培哚普利叔丁胺 | Ace-on | 治疗高血压，对稳定性冠心病患者的非致命性心梗可减低死亡率 | 培哚普利叔丁胺 Aceon 2mg 片剂, 4mg 片剂, 8mg 片剂 | 片剂 $1.53, 10mg 片剂 $1.58, 20mg 片剂 $1.69, 30mg 片剂 $2.40, 40mg 片剂 $2.48 培哚普利叔丁胺 2mg 片剂 $1.90, 4mg 片剂 $2.21, 8mg 片剂 $2.69; Aceon 2mg 片剂 $2.11, 4mg 片剂 $2.45, 8mg 片剂 $2.98 | 前药 1.5~3 小时, 代谢产物 3~10 小时, 终产物 30~120 小时 | 起效/达峰时间: 1~2 小时 | 代谢: 肝脏水解为活性代谢产物培哚普利拉及其他活性代谢产物。排出: 75% 经尿液排出（4%~12% 为原型）。 | 培哚普利 60%; 培哚普利拉 10%~20% |

血管紧张素转换酶（ACE）抑制剂

表 4-13. ACE-I 的其他特殊 FDA 适应证、剂型和药代动力学（续）

药名	商品名	FDA适应证	制剂（片、胶囊、静脉）	每剂费用	半衰期	起效/达峰时间	代谢/排出	蛋白结合力
喹那普利	Acc-upril	治疗高血压和心衰	喹那普利/Accupril 5mg 片剂, 10mg 片剂, 20mg 片剂, 40mg 片剂	喹那普利 5mg 片剂 $1.22, 10mg 片剂 $1.22, 20mg 片剂 $1.22; Accupril 5mg 片剂 $2.05, 10mg 片剂 $2.05, 20mg 片剂 $2.05, 40mg 片剂 $2.05	前药（喹那普利）：0.8小时；喹那普利拉：3小时；半衰期可能随肌酐清除率增加而升高	起效/达峰时间：1~2小时	代谢：水解为喹那普利拉。排出：50%~60%经尿液。	喹那普利：97%；喹那普利拉
雷米普利	Alta-ce	单用或与其他药物联用治疗高血压，心梗后左室功能不全，减小卒中、心肌梗和死亡风险	雷米普利/Altace 1.25mg 胶囊, 2.5mg 胶囊, 5mg 胶囊, 10mg 胶囊	雷米普利 1.25mg 胶囊 $1.53, 2.5mg 胶囊 $1.71, 5mg 胶囊 $2.04, 10mg 胶囊 $2.10;	雷米普利拉：13~17小时；终产物：>50小时	起效时间：1~2小时 达峰时间：雷米普利约1小时 雷米普利拉 44%	代谢：经肝脏由原药转化为活性代谢产物雷米普利拉。	雷米普利：73%；雷米普利拉：56%

血管紧张素转换酶（ACE）抑制剂

			Altace 1.25mg 胶囊 $1.99, 2.5mg 胶囊 $2.35, 5mg 胶囊 $2.47, 10mg 胶囊 $2.88		排出: 原药和活性代谢产物; 60% 经尿液, 40% 经粪便。
群多普利	Ma-vik	单用或与其他药物联用治疗高血压和心梗后左室功能不全	群多普利 /Mavik 1mg 片剂, 2mg 片剂, 4mg 片剂	群多普利 /Mavik 1mg 片剂 $1.20, 2mg 片剂 $1.20, 4mg 片剂 $1.20; Mavik 1mg 片剂 $1.40, 2mg 片剂 $1.40, 4mg 片剂 $1.40	原药（群多普利）: 6小时 活性代谢产物（群多普拉）: 10小时	起效时间: 1~2 小时 达峰时间: 原药: 1小时; 活性代谢产物: 4~10小时	代谢: 经肝脏由原药转化为活性代谢产物群多普利拉 排出: 33% 经尿液 & 66% 经粪便	80%

Courtesy of Paul Pham, PharmD, Johns Hopkins University School of Medicine.

血管紧张素转换酶（ACE）抑制剂

专家建议

- 无论使用何种降压药物，良好控制血压均有获益。
- 临床中常在糖尿病患者发现存在高血压、蛋白尿或两者皆有时加用 ACE 抑制剂或 ARB。
- 我们不在所有糖尿病患者中加用 ACE 抑制剂以"保护肾脏"。
- 常需合用其他种类降压药物以控制血压。
- 多项临床试验显示 ACE-I 在 1 型和 2 型糖尿病患者中，有降低微量白蛋白尿和减缓糖尿病肾病进展的作用（Viberti；微量白蛋白尿卡托普利研究组；Ravid）。
- 卡托普利是唯一获得 FDA 批准用于糖尿病肾病的 ACE-I，尽管其他 ACE-I 可能同样有效。
- 多项研究显示赖诺普利可有效抑制糖尿病患者尿白蛋白排出（Schhoedt）。赖诺普利降压作用优于氢氯噻嗪，降低收缩压作用与阿替洛尔和美托洛尔基本相同，与降低舒张压方面也与二者相同。
- 在一项血压正常、尿白蛋白正常的 1 型糖尿病患者的对照研究中，20mg 依那普利与安慰剂相比并未减缓糖尿病肾病进展，但减缓了糖尿病视网膜病变的进展（Mauer）。然而，其他临床研究显示依那普利在减缓糖尿病肾病进展方面有获益（Ravid）。
- 在一项随机对照试验中，口服福辛普利的糖尿病肾病患者 24 小时尿蛋白排出、血肌酐和 BUN 均减低（Huang）。
- 在 2 型糖尿病合并高血压患者中，单用群多普利或联用维拉帕米，与单用维拉帕米或安慰剂组相比较，可减低微量白蛋白尿的发生率（Ruggenenti）。

参考文献

Mauer M, Zinman B, Gardiner R, et al. Renal and retinal effects of enalapril and losartan in type 1 diabetes. NEJM, 2009; Vol. 361: pp. 40–51.

Comments: Multicenter, controlled trial of 285 normotensive patients with type 1 diabetes and normoalbuminuria randomly assigned to receive losartan (100 mg daily), enalapril (20 mg daily), or placebo for 5 years. Authors found that enalapril did not slow nephropathy progression but slowed the progression of retinopathy.

Schjoedt KJ, Astrup AS, Persson F, et al. Optimal dose of lisinopril for renoprotection in type 1 diabetic patients with diabetic nephropathy: a randomised crossover trial. Diabetologia, 2009; Vol. 52: pp. 46–9.

Comments: At the Steno Diabetes Center, 49 type 1 diabetic patients with diabetic nephropathy participated in double-masked randomised crossover trial with initial washout period followed by three treatment periods of 2 months each, receiving lisinopril 20, 40, and 60 mg once daily in randomised order in addition to slowrelease furosemide. Compared with lisinopril 20 mg there was a further reduction in urinary albumin excretion rate of 23% with lisinopril 40 mg and 19% with 60 mg, p , 0.05.

Ruggenenti P, Fassi A, Ilieva AP, et al. Preventing microalbuminuria in type 2 diabetes. NEJM, 2004; Vol. 351: pp. 1941–51.

Comments: Multicenter double-blind, randomized Bergamo Nephrologic Diabetes Complications Trial (BENEDICT) in subjects with hypertension, type 2 diabetes mellitus, and normal urinary albumin excretion. 1204 subjects randomly assigned to 3 years of trandolapril plus verapamil, trandolapril alone, verapamil alone or placebo. Trandolapril plus verapamil and trandolapril alone decreased the incidence of microalbuminuria to a similar extent.

Arauz-Pacheco C, Parrott MA, Raskin P, et al. Hypertension management in adults with diabetes. Diabetes Care, 2004; Vol. 27 Suppl 1: pp. S65–7.

Comments: American Diabetes Association recommendations for management of hypertension in diabetes.

Huang YH, Wang HT, Zhu QZ, et al. Combination therapy with losartan and fosinopril for early diabetic nephropathy. Di Yi Jun Yi Da Xue Xue Bao, 2003; Vol. 23: pp. 963–5.

Comments: Fifty-seven patients with diabetic nephropathy were divided equally into group A with treatment with losartan (50 mg) and fosinopril (10 mg) daily, group B with daily losartan treatment (50–100 mg), and group C with fosinopril treatment at the daily dose of 10–20 mg for 6 months. Combined use of losartan and fosinopril decreased blood pressure, 24-h urine protein excretion, serum creatinine, and BUN to a greater extent than the use of either alone.

ACE Inhibitors in Diabetic Nephropathy Trialist Group. Should all patients with type 1 diabetes mellitus and microalbuminuria receive angiotensin-converting enzyme inhibitors? A meta-analysis of individual patient data. Ann Intern Med, 2001; Vol. 134: pp. 370–9.

Comments: Meta-analysis concluding that ACE inhibitors improve microalbuminuria in normotensive patients with type 1 diabetes mellitus.

UK Prospective Diabetes Study Group (UKPDS). Tight blood pressure control and risk of macrovascular and microvascular complications in type 2 diabetes: UKPDS 38. BMJ, 1998; Vol. 317: pp. 703–13.

Comments: Captopril was administered to one of the "tight control" arms of UKPDS and this group had significantly reduced progression of diabetic retinopathy, deterioration in visual acuity, and mortality.

The Microalbuminuria Captopril Study Group. Captopril reduces the risk of nephropathy in IDDM patients with microalbuminuria. Diabetologia, 1996; Vol. 39: pp. 587–93.

Comments: 235 normotensive IDDM patients with microalbuminuria participated in double-blind, randomised, placebo-controlled trials to assess the effects of captopril 50 mg twice daily on the progression to overt clinical albuminuria. The risk of progression over 24 months was significantly reduced by captopril ($p = 0.004$) with a risk reduction of 69.2% (31.7%–86.1%).

Viberti G, Mogensen CE, Groop LC, et al. Effect of captopril on progression to clinical proteinuria in patients with insulin-dependent diabetes mellitus and microalbuminuria. European Microalbuminuria Captopril Study Group. JAMA, 1994; Vol. 271: pp. 275–9.

Comments: Randomized, double-blind, placebo-controlled clinical trial of 2 years' duration including 92 patients with insulin-dependent diabetes mellitus and persistent microalbuminuria but no hypertension. Patients randomly allocated to receive either captopril, 50 mg, or placebo twice per day. Progression to clinical proteinuria was significantly reduced by captopril therapy ($p = .03$ by log-rank test).

Lewis EJ, Hunsicker LG, Bain RP, et al. The effect of angiotensin-converting-enzyme inhibition on diabetic nephropathy. The Collaborative Study Group. NEJM, 1993; Vol. 329: pp. 1456–62.

Comments: Captopril protects against deterioration in renal function in insulin-dependent diabetic nephropathy as compared to other similarly effective treatments.

Ravid M, Savin H, Jutrin I, et al. Long-term stabilizing effect of angiotensin-converting enzyme inhibition on plasma creatinine and on proteinuria in normotensive type II diabetic patients. Ann

Intern Med, 1993;Vol. 118: pp. 577–81.

Comments: 94 normotensive, type 2 diabetic patients with microalbuminuria and normal renal function randomly assigned to receive enalapril, 10 mg per day, or placebo. Difference in rate of change in proteinuria between two groups favored enalapril ($p < 0.05$).

血管紧张素受体阻断剂（ARBs）

Lipika Samal, MD, MPH, and Paul A. Pham, PharmD

指征

FDA
- 糖尿病肾病（厄贝沙坦、洛沙坦）。
- 高血压。
- 减低卒中和心血管风险。
- 充血性心力衰竭。
- ARB 其他特殊 FDA 适应证详见表 4-14。

机制
- 血管紧张素受体阻断剂（ARBs）是 AT1 血管紧张素受体的选择性阻断剂，可阻断血管紧张素 II 与受体结合，减低系统性血管阻力。

成人常用剂量
- 坎地沙坦：高血压：起始剂量 4~32mg qd 后逐渐加量至预期药效。心衰：起始剂量 4mg qd，每 3 周剂量加倍、逐渐加量至预期药效。最大剂量 32mg。
- 依普沙坦：起始剂量 600mg qd（剂量需个体化）。剂量大于 800mg 时较少证据支持。
- 厄贝沙坦：高血压：起始剂量 150mg qd，逐渐加量至 300mg qd。肾病：目标剂量 300mg qd。
- 洛沙坦：高血压：50mg qd 或 bid，剂量范围 25~100mg。糖尿病肾病：起始剂量 50mg qd，根据血压变化可加量至 100mg qd。减低卒中风险：50mg qd，最大剂量 100mg。
- 奥美沙坦：起始剂量 20mg qd，2 周后逐渐加量至预期药效，可加量至 40mg qd。
- 替米沙坦：高血压：起始剂量 40mg qd，常用剂量 20~80mg qd。减低心血管风险：起始剂量 80mg qd。
- 缬沙坦：高血压：起始剂量 80~160mg qd，最大剂量每日 320mg。减低心血管风险：20mg bid，目标剂量 160mg bid。心衰：起始剂量 40mg bid，常用剂量在 80~160mg bid 之间，最大剂量每日 320mg。

剂型
- 具体内容见表 4-14。

特殊人群中用药剂量

肾脏特殊人群
- 肌酐清除率 ≥ 30ml/min：无须调整剂量。
- 除非患者容量不足，成人中无须调整剂量。

肝脏特殊人群
- 起始治疗时予 25mg qd 口服。

孕期妇女
- FDA 妊娠 D 类。孕期避免使用。
- 黑框警告：妊娠中晚期使用可能造成胎儿损伤或死亡。

哺乳
- 洛沙坦或其代谢产物是否经母乳排泄尚不明确，然而在大鼠母乳中药物水平显著升高。故洛沙坦使用期间不推荐哺乳，因为该药对婴儿有潜在的不良反应。

药物不良反应
总体
- 总体上耐受良好。

偶见
- 低血压。
- 消化不良和腹泻。
- 头晕。
- 肌痛和肌阵挛。
- 肾衰竭（CHF 和容量不足是危险因素）。
- 不适感。

少见
- 横纹肌溶解。
- 咳嗽（与 ACE-I 相比发生率较少）。
- 过敏和血管性水肿（与 ACE-I 相比发生率较少）。
- 阳痿。
- 过敏反应。

药物相互作用
- 洛沙坦和厄贝沙坦是 CYP1A2、CYP2C9 和 CYP3A4 的底物。缬沙坦和坎地沙坦仅为 CYP2C9 的底物。这些 CYP 同工酶的抑制剂和诱导剂可能分别增加和减少这些 ARBs 类药物的血清浓度。
- ACE 抑制剂联合应用可能增加腹泻、低血压、晕厥、高钾血症和肾功能不全导致透析和血肌酐倍增的风险。
- 与依普利酮、保钾利尿剂和补钾药物合用可能导致高钾血症。
- 利福平和苯巴比妥可能减低所有 ARBs 的血药浓度。故需监测治疗效果并逐渐加量至预期疗效。
- CYP2C9 抑制剂（例如三唑类抗真菌药物、氟西汀、舍曲林、胺碘酮、西咪替丁）可能增加缬沙坦和坎地沙坦的血药浓度。合用时需从最小剂量起并严密监测。

血管紧张素受体阻断剂（ARBs）

- CYP1A2 抑制剂（例如环丙沙星和氟伏沙明）可能增加洛沙坦和厄贝沙坦的血药浓度。合用时需从最小剂量起并严密监测。
- CYP3A4 抑制剂（例如 HIV 蛋白酶抑制剂、三唑类抗真菌药物、大环内酯类抗生素）可能增加洛沙坦和厄贝沙坦的血药浓度。合用时需从最小剂量起并严密监测。

药代动力学
- 表 4-14. ARBs 的其他特殊 FDA 适应证、剂型和药代动力学。

专家建议
- 仅厄贝沙坦和洛沙坦为 FDA 获准用于糖尿病肾病，然而大多数 ARBs 在治疗糖尿病肾病中都有效（Lewis；Parving；Viberti；Brenner）且为不能耐受 ACE-I（例如咳嗽）的患者提供了很好的选择。
- 尽管 ACE-I 在肾脏保护方面证据更多，一项荟萃分析发现 ARBs 和 ACE-I 药效相近（Sarafadis）。
- 与 ACE-I 相比，ARBs 较少出现咳嗽的不良反应，故当患者应用 ACE-I 后出现咳嗽，ARBs 是一项合理选择或可作为首选。

血管紧张素受体阻断剂（ARBs）

表 4-14. ARBs 的其他特殊 FDA 适应证、剂型和药代动力学

药名	商品名	FDA 适应证	制剂 & 美国每单位剂量费用	半衰期	起效/达峰时间	代谢/排出	蛋白结合力
坎地沙坦	Atacand	单用或与其他药物合用治疗高血压、治疗 NYHA 分级 II-IV 级心衰。	Atacand 4mg 片剂（$2.32），8mg 片剂（$2.32），16mg 片剂（$2.32），32mg 片剂（$3.13）	5~9 小时	起效：2~3 小时 达峰：6~8 小时	经小肠壁细胞代谢为坎地沙坦。排出：经尿液。	99%
依普沙坦	Teveten	单用或与其他药物合用治疗高血压。	Teveten 400mg 片剂（$2.82），600mg 片剂（$3.30）	5~9 小时	达峰：1~2 小时	代谢：少量经肝脏代谢。排出：经粪便（90%），经尿液（7%）。	98%
厄贝沙坦	Avapro	单用或与其他药物合用治疗高血压、治疗 2 型糖尿病肾病。	Avapro 75mg 片剂（$3.08），150mg 片剂	11~15 小时	起效/达峰时间：1~2 小时	代谢：肝 CYP2C9。排出：经粪便（80%），经尿液（20%）。	90%

血管紧张素受体阻断剂（ARBs）

					(\$2.50)，300mg 片剂 (\$3.00)	
洛沙坦	Coz-aar	单用或与其他药物合用治疗高血压，治疗2型糖尿病肾病，高血压和左心室高压中降低卒中风险。	Cozaar 25mg 片剂 (\$1.86)，50mg 片剂 (\$2.39)，100mg 片剂 (\$3.26)	洛沙坦 1.5~2 小时，E3174（活性代谢产物）6~9 小时	起效：6小时 达峰：洛沙坦1小时，E3174（活性代谢产物）6~9小时	代谢：在肝脏（14%）通过 CYP2C9 和 3A4 转化为活性代谢产物 E3174。 排出：经尿液。	与白蛋白高度结合
奥美沙坦	Ben-icar	单用或与其他药物合用治疗高血压。	Benicar 5mg 片剂 (\$2.11)，20mg 片剂 (\$2.29)，40mg 片剂 (\$2.89)	13 小时	达峰：1~2 小时	代谢：在胃肠道水解为有活性的奥美沙坦。排出：经粪便（50%~65%）和经尿液（35%~50%）。	99%

血管紧张素受体阻断剂（ARBs）

表 4-14. ARBs 的其他特殊 FDA 适应证、剂型和药代动力学（续）

药名	商品名	FDA 适应证	制剂 & 美国每单位剂量费用	半衰期	起效 / 达峰	代谢 / 排出	蛋白结合力
替米沙坦	Micardis	单用或与其他药物合用治疗高血压，大于55岁、具有主要心血管事件风险的患者中降低心血管风险。	Micardis 20mg 片剂 ($3.00)，40mg 片剂 ($3.00)，80mg 片剂 ($3.00)	24小时	起效：1~2小时 达峰：0.5~1小时	代谢：在肝脏结合为无活性的代谢产物。 排出：97%经粪便。	99.5%
缬沙坦	Dio-van	单用或与其他药物合用治疗高血压，心梗后左室功能不全的患者中降低心血管风险，治疗 NYHA 分级 II–IV 级心衰。	Diovan 40mg 片剂 ($2.12)，80mg 片剂 ($2.54)，160mg 片剂 ($2.73)	6小时	起效：2小时 达峰：2~4小时	代谢：为无活性代谢产物。 排出：83%经粪便，13%经尿液。	95%

Courtesy of Paul Pham, PharmD, Johns Hopkins University School of Medicine.

血管紧张素受体阻断剂（ARBs）

参考文献

Bilous R, Chaturvedi N, Sjølie AK, et al. Effect of candesartan on microalbuminuria and albumin excretion rate in diabetes: three randomized trials. Ann Intern Med, 2009; Vol. 151: pp. 11–20, W3–4.

Comments: In a placebo controlled study for the treatment of diabetic nephropathy in normotensive type 1 and type 2 diabetics, 32 mg/day of candesartan did not prevent microalbuminuria after 4.7 years of follow-up, but may be due to recruitment of mainly patients with well-controlled hypertension who were at low overall vascular risk, which resulted in a low rate of microalbuminuria.

Tomino Y, Kawamura T, Kimura K, et al. Antiproteinuric effect of olmesartan in patients with IgA nephropathy. J Nephrol, 2009; Vol. 22: pp. 224–31.

Comments: In an observational study, patients were found to have a reduction in urinary protein after a 16-week trial of olmesartan. The reduction in urinary protein was independent of BP-lowering properties.

Sarafidis PA, Stafylas PC, Kanaki AI, et al. Effects of renin-angiotensin system blockers on renal outcomes and all-cause mortality in patients with diabetic nephropathy: an updated meta-analysis. Am J Hypertens, 2008; Vol. 21: pp. 922–929.

Comments: A meta-analysis of 24 studies (20 using ACE inhibitors and 4 using ARBs) found that the use ACE inhibitors was associated with a trend toward reduction of ESRD incidence (RR 0.70; 0.46–1.05) and use of ARBs with significant reduction of ESRD risk (RR 0.78; 0.67–0.91). Both drug classes were associated with reduction in the risk of doubling serum creatinine.

Kaliuzhina EV, Zibnitskaia LI, Surkova LG, et al. The effectiveness of eprosartan in patients with chronic glomerulonephritis. Klin Med (Mosk), 2007; Vol. 85: pp. 58–61.

Comments: Limited data of eprosartan in diabetic nephropathy. A small open label study of 15 patients over 12 weeks showed a potential renal protective (defined as an antiproteinuric and antihematuric) effect at a dose of 600 mg daily.

Arauz-Pacheco C, Parrott MA, Raskin P. The treatment of hypertension in adult patients with diabetes. Diabetes Care, 2002; Vol. 25: pp. 134–47.

Comments: ARBs can be considered in the management of HTN in adult patients with diabetes.

Viberti G, Wheeldon NM, MicroAlbuminuria Reduction With VALsartan (MARVAL) Study Investigators. Microalbuminuria reduction with valsartan in patients with type 2 diabetes mellitus: a blood pressure-independent effect. Circulation, 2002; Vol. 106: pp. 672–8.

Comments: 332 patients with type 2 diabetes and microalbuminuria were randomized to receive valsartan or amlodipine, and the valsartan group reverted to normoalbuminuria at a higher rate (29.9% vs 14.5%; , 0.001).

Lewis EJ, Hunsicker LG, Clarke WR, et al. Renoprotective effect of the angiotensin-receptor antagonist irbesartan in patients with nephropathy due to type 2 diabetes. NEJM, 2001; Vol. 345: pp. 851–60.

Comments: Irbesartan is effective in protecting against the progression of nephropathy in patients with type 2 diabetes.

Parving HH, Lehnert H, Bröchner-Mortensen J, et al. The effect of irbesartan on the development of diabetic nephropathy in patients with type 2 diabetes. NEJM, 2001; Vol. 345: pp. 870–8.

Comments: Irbesartan is renoprotective in patients with type 2 diabetes and microalbuminuria.

Bakris G, Gradman A, Reif M, et al. Antihypertensive efficacy of candesartan in comparison to losartan: the CLAIM study. J Clin Hypertens (Greenwich), 2001; Vol. 3: pp. 16–21.

Comments: When given at the maximum dose, there were statistically significantly (p,0.05) higher proportions of responders in the candesartan treated patients (62.4% and 56.0%, respectively) than in the losartan group.

Brenner BM, Cooper ME, de Zeeuw D, et al. Effects of losartan on renal and cardiovascular outcomes in patients with type 2 diabetes and nephropathy. NEJM, 2001; Vol. 345: pp. 861–9.

Comments: Reduction of Endpoints in NIDDM with the Angiotensin II Antagonist Losartan (RENAAL) study randomized 1513 patients to losartan or placebo, and the losartan group had lower primary endpoint of combined doubling of the creatinine concentration, end-stage renal disease, or death.

β 受体阻滞剂

Paul A. Pham, PharmD

指征

FDA

- 有或无糖尿病,单用或联合其他降压药物治疗高血压(HTN)。
- 控制心绞痛。
- 心肌梗死后二级预防治疗。
- 室上性心动过速。
- 嗜铬细胞瘤。
- 特发性震颤。
- 偏头痛的预防性治疗。
- 肥厚性主动脉瓣下狭窄的对症治疗。
- 缺血性或心肌病导致的轻到重度的心衰(仅对卡维地洛和美托洛尔)。
- 每种 β 受体阻滞剂的其他特殊 FDA 适应证详见表 4-15。

机制

- β 受体阻滞剂与肾上腺素能神经递质(例如儿茶酚胺)竞争性结合交感神经受体,导致心率、心输出量、收缩压以及舒张压减低。

剂型

- 见表 4-15。

成人常用剂量

- JNC 7 种用于治疗高血压时的成人常用剂量(其他适应证的推荐剂量见表 4-15)。
- 阿替洛尔:25~100mg qd。
- 比索洛尔:2.5~10mg qd。
- 美托洛尔:50~100mg/d,分 1~2 次口服;或美托洛尔 XL 50~100mg qd。
- 纳多洛尔:40~120mg qd。
- 普萘洛尔:40~160mg 分 2 次口服,或普萘洛尔 LA 60~180mg qd。
- 噻吗心安:20~40mg 分 2 次口服。
- 卡维地洛:12.5~50mg 分 2 次口服。
- 拉贝洛尔:200~800mg 分 2 次口服。

剂型

- 具体内容见表 4-14。

β 受体阻滞剂

特殊人群中用药剂量

肾脏特殊人群
- 阿替洛尔、比索洛尔、纳多洛尔和噻吗心安（尤其是合并肝损害时）：需在肾衰竭时调整剂量。

肝脏特殊人群
- 美托洛尔、普萘洛尔、噻吗心安、拉贝洛尔和卡维地洛：在肝功能不全时需调整剂量。卡维地洛在严重肝损害时应避免使用。

孕期妇女
- 阿替洛尔为 FDA 妊娠 D 类。其他所有 β 受体阻滞剂均为 FDA 妊娠 C 类，但许多专家建议在孕中期和孕晚期避免使用。

哺乳
- 人类和/或动物数据提示所有 β 受体阻滞剂均经母乳排泄。阿替洛尔需避免用于哺乳期。比索洛尔和卡维地洛仅用于获益大于风险时。美国儿科学会认为美托洛尔、纳多洛尔、普萘洛尔、噻吗心安和拉贝洛尔适用于哺乳期。

药物不良反应

常见
- 哮喘或 COPD 患者出现气道痉挛。
- 乏力。

偶见
- 窦性心动过缓（房室传导阻滞）。
- 低血压。
- 血糖升高。
- 胃肠道（例如腹泻、恶心、呕吐）。
- 中枢神经系统不良反应（例如头晕、眩晕、乏力）。
- 外周血管疾病加重（严重外周血管疾病的患者避免使用 β 受体阻滞剂）。
- 血清甘油三酯轻度升高，HDL 轻度减低（卡维地洛和拉贝洛尔较少见）。
- 抑郁、多梦、幻觉（老年人多见）。

少见
- CHF（尤其是既往存在左室功能不全的患者）。
- 粒细胞缺乏症和血小板减少症。
- 皮疹。

药物相互作用
- 与其他降压药物合用（例如 ACE-I、ARBs、钙通道拮抗剂、可乐定）会出现更强的降压作用。
- 胰岛素、磺脲类药物：β 受体阻滞剂可使低血糖所致心动过速反应不敏感；因对 α 肾上腺素能刺激的不阻断，会加重低血糖时的反应性高血压。

β 受体阻滞剂

- 因阻断 β₂ 受体可减少胰岛素分泌、降低胰岛素敏感性,故非选择性 β 受体阻滞剂(例如普萘洛尔、纳多洛尔、噻吗心安)可减少磺脲类药物如格列苯脲和格列吡嗪的药效。
- CYP2D6 抑制剂(例如利托那韦、胺碘酮、奎尼丁、普罗帕酮、尼卡地平、西酞普兰、氟西汀)可能增加美托洛尔、噻吗心安和普萘洛尔的血药浓度。合用时应予小剂量美托洛尔、噻吗心安和普萘洛尔并缓慢滴定加量。
- CYP2C9 抑制剂(如依曲韦林、氟康唑、酮康唑、吉非贝齐、尼卡地平)可能增加卡维地洛的血药浓度。应用小剂量卡维地洛并缓慢滴定加量。
- CYP3A4 抑制剂(例如蛋白酶抑制剂、三唑类抗真菌药、大环内酯类)可能增加比索洛尔血药浓度。合用时应予小剂量比索洛尔并缓慢滴定加量。
- 利福平可能减小美托洛尔、噻吗心安、普萘洛尔、卡维地洛和比索洛尔的血药浓度。可能需将 β 受体阻滞剂加量。
- 任何抑制房室结传导的药物(例如地高辛、丙吡胺、IC 类抗心律失常药如氟卡尼、普罗帕酮)与 β 受体阻滞剂合用时可能导致房室结传导抑制额外增多。

药代动力学
- 表 4-15 β 受体阻滞剂的其他特殊 FDA 适应证,剂型和药代动力学

β受体阻滞剂

表4-15. β受体阻滞剂的其他特殊FDA适应证、剂型和药代动力学

心脏选择性β受体阻滞剂	FDA适应证	他适应证的成人常用剂量	肾脏或肝脏功能不全时剂量调整	吸收、代谢、排出、半衰期	商品名/制剂/费用
阿替洛尔	单用或与其他药物合用治疗高血压;控制心绞痛;心梗后二级预防	心梗后:静脉给药后,予100mg/d或50mg bid,心梗后6~9天使用。	肌酐清除率15~35ml/min:最大剂量50mg/d肌酐清除率<15ml/min:最大剂量50mg隔日血液透析:透析后给药,或补充剂量25~50mg	吸收:不完全。代谢:部分经肝脏。排出:50%经粪便,40%经尿液。半衰期:肾功能正常者6~9小时,肾损害者延长,ESRD者15~35小时。	Tenormin,可购买无商标产品无商标产品:25mg(90片):$14.99 100mg(90片):$19.99
比索洛尔	单用或与其他药物合用治疗高血压。		肌酐清除率40ml/min:起始剂量2.5mg/d,谨慎加量。不经透析清除。	吸收:快速且几乎完全吸收。代谢:几乎全部经肝脏代谢,20%首过效应。排出:50%。半衰期:肾功能正常者9~12小时,肌酐清除率<40ml/min者27~36小时,肝硬化者8~22小时。	Zebeta,可购买无商标产品无商标产品:5mg(30片)$35.99,10mg(30片)$35.15

β 受体阻滞剂

美托洛尔	治疗心绞痛、高血压或血流动力学稳定的急性心梗。缓释剂：同上，以及降低已经接受 ACE-I、地高辛和/或利尿剂治疗的心衰患者（NYHA 分级 II 和 III 级）的死亡率和住院率	心绞痛：口服；速释剂：起始剂量 50mg bid；常用剂量范围：50~200mg bid；最大剂量 400mg/d；隔周加量至预期药效。缓释剂：起始：100mg/d（最大剂量 400mg/d）。心衰：口服；缓释剂：起始 25mg qd（NYHA 分级大于 II 级）时减至 12.5mg qd（最大剂量耐受每 2 周可加倍 200mg/d）。心梗：急性：静脉：早期治疗心梗于 5mg 每 2 分钟一次，重复 3 次；最后一次，静脉给药后 15 分钟肌内开始每 6 小时给予 50mg 口服，持续 48 小时；后子维持剂量 100mg bid。	肝功能不全者可能需要调整剂量。	吸收：快速而完全。代谢：绝大部分通过 CYP2D6 经肝脏代谢，50% 首过效应。排泄：经尿液（<5%~10%）。半衰期：3~8 小时，与 CYP2D6 代谢速率有关。	Toprol-XL, Lopressor。可购买无商标产品。速释剂：无商标酒石酸美托洛尔：25mg（30 片）$12.99, 50mg(60 片)$12.99, 100mg(60 片)$15.99 无商标琥珀酸美托洛尔：25mg（30 片）$34.99, 50mg（30 片）$33.88, 100mg（30 片）$41.99, 200mg（90 片）$204.58 缓释剂：无商标琥珀酸美托洛尔：25mg

表 4-15. β 受体阻滞剂的其他特殊 FDA 适应证，剂型和药代动力学（续）

心脏选择性 β 受体阻滞剂	FDA 适应证	他适应证的成人常用剂量	肾脏或肝脏功能不全时剂量调整	吸收，代谢，排出，半衰期	商品名/制剂/费用
纳多洛尔	治疗高血压和心绞痛；偏头痛的预防性治疗	心绞痛：口服：起始：40~80mg/d，每 3~7 天逐渐加量 40~80mg 直到获得预期临床反应，心率明显下降。剂量最大 160~240mg/d。	肌酐清除率 31~40ml/min：每 24~36 小时给药一次，或予常规剂量的 50%。肌酐清除率 10~30ml/min：每 24~48 小时给药一次，或予常规剂量的 25%。血液透析：20%~50% 可通过透析，透析后给药或 40mg 补充剂量。肝损害患者不需调整剂量。	吸收：30%~40%。代谢：不经代谢。排出：经尿液。半衰期：正常肾功能者 10~24 小时，ESRD 者 45 小时。	Corgard, 可购买无商标产品。无商标产品 20mg（30 片）$13.99，40mg（30 片）$15.99，80mg（30 片）$19.99，160mg（30 片）$33.59

β 受体阻滞剂

普萘洛尔	治疗高血压,心绞痛,嗜铬细胞瘤,特发性震颤,室上性心动过速和心室性心动过速(如心房颤动和扑动,房室结折返性心动过速),室性心动过速(儿茶酚胺敏感性室速,地高辛中毒)预防二级预防;心梗二级预防;预防偏头痛发展;肥厚性主动脉瓣下狭窄(肥厚心肌病)的对症治疗	肥厚性主动脉瓣下狭窄:口服:20~40mg 3~4次/d,心得安LA:80~160mg qd 预防偏头痛发作:口服:起始 80mg/d,分3~4次/d,每6~8小时口服一次;每3~4周加量20~40mg/剂,至最大剂量 160~240mg/d,分3~4次/d,每6~8小时口服一次。嗜铬细胞瘤:口服30~60mg/d,分多次。减小心梗后死亡率:口服 180~240mg/d,分3~4次/d。稳定型心绞痛:口服 80~320mg/d,分2~4次/d 心得安LA:起始 80mg qd;最大剂量 320mg qd 心动过速:口服 10~30mg/次,每6~8小时一次 静脉:1~3mg/次,慢速静推,每2~5分钟重复一次至总量达 5mg;滴定增加起始剂量至预期药效	药物不通过透析排出,故透析后不需补充剂量。慢性肝病患者使用常用剂量时心率减低明显;予小剂量,规律监测心率	吸收:快速而完全 代谢:通过 CYP2D6 和 CYP1A2 经肝脏代谢为活性和无活性部分。显著首过效应。排出:经尿液 半衰期:速释剂:3~6小时。缓释剂:8~10小时。	心得安,可购买无商标产品。速释剂:无商标产品 10mg(100片)$12.99,20mg(100片)$13.99,40mg(30片)$12.99,60mg(60片)$55.99,80mg(90片)$15.99 缓释剂:无商标产品 60mg(100粒胶囊)$115.97,80mg(100粒胶囊)$134.99,120mg(30粒胶囊)$59.99,160mg(100粒胶囊)$219.99

表 4-15. β 受体阻滞剂的其他特殊 FDA 适应证，剂型和药代动力学（续）

心脏选择性 β 受体阻滞剂	FDA 适应证	他适应证的成人常用剂量	肾脏或肝脏功能不全时剂量调整	吸收，代谢，排出，半衰期	商品名/制剂/费用
噻吗心安	口服：治疗高血压和心绞痛；降低心梗后死亡率；预防治疗偏头痛	心梗后二级预防：口服：起始10mg bid，心梗后1~4周内。预防偏头痛发作：口服：起始10mg bid，加量至最大剂量30mg/d	肌酐清除＜10ml/min：根据临床反应调整剂量，监测血压、血透患者口服20mg/d维持剂量曾出现严重低血压反应。肝损害患者可能需减量（至多50%）。	吸收：快速而完全。代谢：绝大多数经肝脏代谢，首过效应强。排出：经尿液。半衰期：2~2.7小时，肾损害者延长。	可购买无商标产品。无商标产品 5mg(60片) \$22.99, 10mg (60片) \$25.99, 20mg(60片)\$41.99
混合性 α 和 β 受体阻滞剂	FDA 适应证	其他适应证的成人常用剂量	肾脏或肝脏功能不全时剂量调整	吸收，代谢，排出，半衰期	商品名/制剂/费用
拉贝洛尔	治疗轻度或重度高血压	高血压：起始 100mg bid，每 2~3 天可按需加量。常用剂量范围（JNC7）：200~800mg/d，分 2 次	不经透析排出；透析后不需补充剂量。肝脏损害者可能需减低剂量。	吸收：完全。代谢：通过结合葡萄糖醛酸经肝脏代谢，首过效应强。排出：经尿液。半衰期：6~8小时	Trandate 可购买无商标产品。无商标产品 100mg (60片) \$20.99, 200mg (60片) \$28.99, 300mg (60片) \$38.99

β 受体阻滞剂

卡维地洛	缺血性或心肌病导致轻至重度心衰（通常作为辅助用药）；心梗后左室功能不全（临床稳定且 LVEF <40%）；控制高血压	心衰：口服，速释剂：3.125mg bid 共2周，如耐受可加量至 6.25mg bid；每2周剂量加倍至能耐受的最大剂量。最大推荐剂量：轻中度心衰：<85kg：25mg bid；>85kg：50mg bid；重度心衰：25mg bid	肾损害者不需调整剂量。严重肝损害者中为禁忌证。	吸收：快速且完全。代谢：绝大部分经肝脏代谢，通过 CYP2C9、CYP2D6、CYP3A4 和 CYP2C19；3种活性代谢产物；首过效应；在肝硬化患者中血药浓度分别出现 4~7 倍升高。排出：主要经粪便 半衰期：7~10 小时	Coreg 速释剂型有无商标产品，缓释剂仅有商品名。速释剂：无商标产品 3.125mg, 6.25mg (30片) $25.99, 12.5mg (30片) $14.99, 25mg (30片) $16.00 缓释剂：10mg (30粒胶囊) $135.28, 40mg (30粒胶囊) $135.28, 80mg (30粒胶囊) $135.28

Courtesy of Paul Pham, PharmD, Johns Hopkins University School of Medicine.

β 受体阻滞剂

专家建议

- β 受体阻滞剂可掩盖低血糖症状（如震颤、心动过速、心悸）。低血糖导致的排汗症状大多不被掩盖。
- 卡托普利和阿替洛尔低血糖发生率相近（UKPDS 39），提示 β 受体阻滞剂对无症状低血糖并无不良反应。
- 心脏选择性 β 受体阻滞剂（例如阿替洛尔、美托洛尔）有选择性地与 B_1 受体结合、多于 B_2 受体。较小剂量应用时，对糖尿病和外周血管疾病患者更倾向于使用心脏选择性 β 受体阻滞剂。
- 选择性 β 受体阻滞剂（例如阿替洛尔、美托洛尔）可能也在血糖控制方面有较小的不良反应。
- 尽管 β 受体阻滞剂可能对血糖控制有轻度负面效应，但这点可经降糖治疗被轻易解决，而在糖尿病患者中使用 β 受体阻滞剂已被证实有降低心血管疾病和心梗后死亡率的获益。
- β 受体阻滞剂在药代动力学和药效学作用方面各有不同，但其降压效果基本相同。
- 具有内在拟交感活性的 β 受体阻滞剂（例如醋丁洛尔、吲哚洛尔和喷布洛尔）总体上不推荐使用，因其减少心血管事件作用不如其他 β 受体阻滞剂。
- β 受体阻滞剂可用于近期心肌梗死病史的患者。
- β 受体阻滞剂可能增加发展为糖尿病的风险，在使用 6 年后该风险升高可能高达 28%（Gress, Dahlof）。

参考文献

Dahlöf B, Devereux RB, Kjeldsen SE, et al. Cardiovascular morbidity and mortality in the Losartan Intervention For Endpoint reduction in hypertension study (LIFE): a randomised trial against atenolol. Lancet, 2002; Vol. 359: pp. 995–1003.

Comments: 9193 patients with hypertension and LVH were randomized to receive losartan-based or atenololbased antihypertensive regimen for at least 4 years. Blood pressure reduction was comparable between the two groups with SBP and DBP decrease of ~30 and 17 mmHg, respectively. However, higher proportion of losartan versus atenolol-.treated pts had fatal or nonfatal stroke (0·75, p = 0·001). Losartan was associated with less cardiovascular morbidity and death compared to atenolol. New-onset diabetes was less frequent with losartan.

Gress TW, Nieto FJ, Shahar E, et al. Hypertension and antihypertensive therapy as risk factors for type 2 diabetes mellitus. Atherosclerosis Risk in Communities Study. NEJM, 2000; Vol. 342: pp. 905–12.

Comments: In an observational study, development of diabetes in patients treated with a beta-blocker was increased by 28% at six years.

Freemantle N, Cleland J, Young P, et al. Beta blockade after myocardial infarction: systematic review and meta regression analysis. BMJ, 1999; Vol. 318: pp. 1730–7.

Comments: In this meta-analysis, beta-blockers with intrinsic sympathomimetic activity (ISA) had a reduction in cardioprotective benefit. The authors recommend against the use of beta-blocker with ISA properties (e.g., acebutolol, penbutolol, pindolol).

UK Prospective Diabetes Study Group (UKPDS) 39. Efficacy of atenolol and captopril in reducing risk of macrovascular and microvascular complications in type 2 diabetes: UKPDS 39. BMJ, 1998; Vol. 317: pp. 713–20.

Comments: 1148 hypertensive patients with type 2 DM were randomized to receive captopril or atenolol to tightly control BP to a goal of ,150/,85 mmHg. Captopril and atenolol were equally effective in reducing blood pressure to a mean of 144/83 mmHg and 143/81 mmHg, respectively. In addition, captopril and atenolol were equally effective in reducing the risk of macrovascular outcomes, retinopathy, and clinical grade albuminuria $300 mg/L. More significant weight gain was observed in the atenolol-treated patients (3.4 kg vs 1.6 kg). Although undetected hypoglycemia is a concern in beta-blocker–treated patients, the incidence was not different between captopril and atenolol.

钙通道阻滞剂

Brian Pinto, PharmD, MBA

指征

FDA
- 高血压。
- 钙通道阻滞剂的其他特殊适应证详见表4-14。

非FDA获准使用
- 糖尿病肾病（地尔硫䓬）。

机制
- 尽管化学结构不同，所有的钙通道阻滞剂都可抑制心肌和血管平滑肌细胞膜外钙离子内流。
- 分类包括二氢吡啶类（氨氯地平、非洛地平、硝苯地平）和非二氢吡啶类（维拉帕米、地尔硫䓬）。

剂型
- 见表4-16。

成人常用剂量
- 氨氯地平：起始剂量5mg/d，最大剂量10mg/d。
- 硝苯地平（缓释剂）：起始剂量30或60mg qd；最大剂量90~120mg/d。
- 地尔硫䓬缓释剂（每日1次）：起始剂量180~240mg qd，14天后可能需调整剂量，最大剂量480mg/d。
- 维拉帕米（速释剂）：80~320mg/d，分两次口服。
- 维拉帕米（缓释剂）：120~480mg/d，分1~2次口服。

特殊人群中用药剂量

肾脏特殊人群
- 进展期肾衰竭的患者维拉帕米肾脏清除率可能减低。
- 地尔硫䓬不经透析排出，故无须补充剂量。

肝脏特殊人群
- 维拉帕米剂量需减低至正常剂量的30%。
- 氨氯地平在高血压患者中起始剂量需减至2.5mg/d口服。
- 肝硬化患者的硝苯地平清除率减低，可能导致过度药物暴露。
- 肝硬化患者地尔硫䓬的半衰期延长。

孕期妇女
- 氨氯地平、硝苯地平、非洛地平、维拉帕米和地尔硫䓬为妊娠C类。

钙通道阻滞剂

哺乳
- 地尔硫䓬和硝苯地平已被证实经母乳排出。

药物不良反应

常见
- 水肿（氨氯地平、硝苯地平、非洛地平）。
- 心动过缓（维拉帕米、地尔硫䓬）。
- 便秘（维拉帕米）。

药物相互作用
- CYP3A4 的强效抑制剂可能显著抑制二氢吡啶类钙通道阻滞剂的代谢，导致该类药物药效增强或延长。
- 西柚汁应避免与硝苯地平合用。研究证明合用时可显著增加硝苯地平血药浓度。

药代动力学

表4-16. 钙通道拮抗剂的其他特殊FDA适应证、剂型和药代动力学

二氢吡啶类	FDA适应证	药代动力学	妊娠期风险分类/哺乳	费用与制剂
氨氯地平	治疗高血压；治疗慢性稳定型心绞痛	吸收：口服约65%。 代谢：绝大部分氧化代谢。 排出：60%经尿液，25%经粪便。 半衰期：30~50小时。	妊娠分类C类。 是否经母乳排出不明确。	无商标产品 2.5mg（30片）：$5.69, 5mg（30片）：$7.67, 10mg（30片）：$8
硝苯地平	治疗高血压	吸收：65~90%。 代谢：经肝脏通过CYP3A4。 排出：60%~80%经尿液。 半衰期：7小时。	妊娠C类。 代谢入母乳（美国儿科学会认为适合使用）。	无商标缓释剂 30mg(30片)$38,60mg(30片)$60,90mg(30片)$68
非洛地平	治疗高血压	吸收：100%。 代谢：CYP3A4底物，首过效应强。 排出：70%经尿液以代谢产物形式。 半衰期：10~16小时。	妊娠C类。 代谢入母乳，哺乳期不推荐使用。	无商标产品 2.5mg(30片)$43,5mg(30片)$50,10mg(30片)$57.72

钙通道阻滞剂

非二氢吡啶类	FDA 适应证	药代动力学	妊娠期风险分类/哺乳	费用与制剂
维拉帕米	治疗高血压,心绞痛,室上性心动过速	吸收:90%。 代谢:经多种 CYP 同工酶代谢,首过效应强。 排出:70%经尿液以代谢产物形式。 半衰期:5~12小时,14~16小时(严重肝损害者)。	妊娠 C 类。 代谢入母乳。 WHO 评级:适合使用。 美国儿科学会评级:多数情况适合使用。	无商标产品维拉帕米, 24小时胶囊 100mg(100):$149.98, 120mg(30片):$27.31, 180mg(30):$26.99, 200mg(30):$72.91, 240mg(30):$27.43, 300mg(30):$,104.09, 360mg(30):$62.99
地尔硫䓬	治疗高血压,慢性稳定型心绞痛,或冠脉痉挛导致的心绞痛	吸收:约 95%。 代谢:首过效应强。 排出:35%经尿液。 半衰期:5~7小时。	妊娠 C 类。 代谢入母乳。 美国儿科学会评级:适合使用。	无商标产品胶囊 120mg(30):$23.99, 180mg(30):$27.99, 240mg(30):$43.99, 300mg(30):$75.99

Courtesy of Paul Pham, PharmD, Johns Hopkins University School of Medicine.

钙通道阻滞剂

专家建议

- 二氢吡啶类钙通道阻滞剂（如硝苯地平和氨氯地平）可能加重蛋白尿，与之相反的是非二氢吡啶类钙通道阻滞剂（如地尔硫䓬和维拉帕米）可能减少糖尿病肾病的显性蛋白尿（Bakris；Smith；Remuzzi）。
- 非二氢吡啶类钙通道阻滞剂被认为是糖尿病肾病的二线治疗，可与ACE-I 联合使用最佳（Ruggenenti）。
- 硝苯地平和尼索地平的速释剂型不能用于急性血压降低者，因其不良事件（例如死亡、卒中、急性心肌梗死）发生率增高（Estacio）。
- 钙通道阻滞剂（如维拉帕米、地尔硫䓬）可能出现血糖升高，也是一项不常见的不良反应；然而其强大降压作用的获益使其在糖尿病患者中的应用并未受到阻碍（Louters, Levine）。

参考文献

Louters LL, Stehouwer N, Rekman J, et al. Verapamil inhibits the glucose transport activity of GLUT1. J Med Toxicol, 2010; 6: 100–5.
Comments: Discusses the association of verapamil with hyperglycemia, and contribution in a dose-dependent manner of GLUT1 transport activity inhibition.

Levine M, Boyer EW, Pozner CN, et al. Assessment of hyperglycemia after calcium channel blocker overdoses involving diltiazem or verapamil. Crit Care Med, 2007; 35: 2071–5.
Comments: Severity of calcium channel blocker (dilitazem, verapamil) overdose correlated directly with resulting serum glucose concentrations, with a median increase in blood glucose of 71%.

Ruggenenti P, Fassi A, Ilieve AP, et al. Preventing microalbuminuria in type 2 diabetes. N Engl Med. 2004; 351: 1941–51.
Comments: In persons with type 2 diabetes and hypertension but with normoalbuminuria, the use of trandolapril plus verapamil and trandolapril alone were similarly associated with a lower incidence of microalbuminuria. The effect of verapamil alone was no different from placebo.

Remuzzi G, Schieppati A, Ruggenenti P. Clinical practice. Nephropathy in patients with type 2 diabetes. N Engl J Med, 2002; 346: 1145–51.
Comments: Discusses treatment of diabetic nephropathy with various agents including calcium channel blockers.

Estacio RO, Jeffers BW, Hiatt WR, et al. The effect of nisoldipine as compared with enalapril on cardiovascular outcomes in patients with non-insulin-dependent diabetes and hypertension. N Engl J Med, 1998; 338: 645–52.
Comments: In a population of patients who had diabetes and hypertension, calcium channel blockers (nisoldipine) were associated with a higher incidence of fatal and nonfatal myocardial infarction compared to enalapril.

Smith AC, Toto R, Bakris GL. Differential effects of calcium channel blockers on size selectivity of proteinuria in diabetic glomerulopathy. Kidney Int, 1998; 54: 889–96.
Comments: This study found that use of diltiazem, but not nifedipine, led to sustained reductions in proteinuria in diabetic nephropathy, by improving glomerular size.

Bakris GL. Renal effects of calcium antagonists in diabetes mellitus. An overview of studies in animal models and in humans. Am J Hypertens, 1991; 4: 487S–93S.
Comments: Reviews use of calcium channel blockers in diabetes.

利尿剂

Lipika Samal, MD, MPH, and Paul A. Pham, PharmD

指征

FDA
- 高血压。
- 充血性心力衰竭。
- 利尿剂其他特殊FDA适应证详见表4-17。

机制
- 利尿剂根据其机制分类为：噻嗪类利尿剂，袢利尿剂，远曲小管或保钾利尿剂，渗透性利尿剂和碳酸酐酶抑制剂。
- 噻嗪类利尿剂通过抑制肾小管上皮的钠离子跨膜转运、同时抑制氯离子重吸收，从而增加钠、氯和水的排出。
- 袢利尿剂通过抑制氯离子与$Na^+/K^+/2Cl^-$共转运体的结合，从而抑制钠和氯离子的重吸收。
- 保钾利尿剂：与醛固酮作用无关（阿米洛利和氨苯蝶啶）或通过拮抗醛固酮（螺内酯），抑制远端肾小管的钠-钾交换作用。
- 渗透性利尿剂增加肾小球滤出液中的渗透压，抑制水和溶质的重吸收。
- 碳酸酐酶抑制剂可减少肾小管腔内的氢离子浓度，增加碳酸氢根、钠离子、钾离子和水的排出。

成人常用剂量
- 氢氯噻嗪：12.5~50mg/d。
- 氯噻嗪：起始剂量125~250mg/d，可逐渐加量至500mg/d。
- 美托拉宗：2.5~10mg qd（水肿患者最大剂量20mg qd）；高血压：2.5~5mg qd。
- 螺内酯：25~200mg/d，分1~2次（水肿患者）；高血压：25~50mg/d，分1~2次；心衰（NYHA分级Ⅲ，Ⅳ）：12.5~25mg/d（最大剂量50mg）。
- 氨苯蝶啶：50~100mg/d（最大300mg/d）。
- 呋塞米：治疗水肿/心衰，起始剂量20~80mg/次（水肿/心衰）；如治疗反应不理想，可加量至每次20~40mg、每6~8小时重复（最大剂量600mg/d）。
- 布美他尼：治疗水肿/心衰，起始剂量0.5~2mg/次、每日1~2次（最大剂量10mg/d）。

剂型
- 具体内容见表4-17。

利尿剂

药物不良反应

偶见
- 低钾血症,低钠血症和低氯性碱中毒(噻嗪类和袢利尿剂)。
- 高钾血症(保钾利尿剂)。
- 光过敏。
- 过强的利尿作用可导致脱水和肾前性急性肾小管坏死(多见于袢利尿剂)。
- 男性乳腺发育(螺内酯)。
- 血糖控制不佳(噻嗪类利尿剂)。

少见
- 磺胺类交叉过敏。
- 耳毒性(袢利尿剂,尤其是与氨基糖苷类药物合用)。
- 高尿酸血症(袢利尿剂)。

药代动力学
- 表4-17. 利尿剂的其他特殊FDA适应证,剂型和药代动力学

药物相互作用
- 锂剂:所有利尿剂都可能升高锂剂血药浓度。合用时需严密监测锂剂毒性和血药浓度。
- 噻嗪类与袢利尿剂联合胺碘酮:低钾血症可能减低胺碘酮药效,或可能增加其致心律失常作用。
- 噻嗪类与袢利尿剂联合多非利特:电解质紊乱可导致药物性心律失常事件。合用时多非利特清除率减低16%。
- 保钾利尿剂(如螺内酯、氨苯蝶啶)相互作用:与依普利酮、血管紧张素II受体拮抗剂、ACE-I、他克莫司、甲氧苄啶和环孢素可导致高钾血症。合用时严密监测血钾。锂剂清除率可能因合用保钾利尿剂而减低。
- 呋塞米与胆汁酸螯合剂:考来替泊和消胆胺可使呋塞米的生物利用度分别减少80%和95%。避免合用。
- 呋塞米和硫糖铝:硫糖铝可显著减低呋塞米血药浓度。
- 呋塞米和利培酮:多项临床研究显示呋塞米联合利培酮可增加痴呆相关精神病的老年患者的死亡率。
- 引起电解质消耗的药物(如两性霉素、磷甲酸)合用利尿剂时可加重低钾血症。

表 4-17. 利尿剂的其他特殊 FDA 适应证，剂型和药代动力学

噻嗪类利尿剂	FDA 适应证	药代动力学	妊娠期风险分类/哺乳	费用与制剂
氢氯噻嗪	治疗轻至中度高血压；治疗心衰或肾病综合征引起的水肿。	吸收：约 50%~80%。 代谢：极少被代谢。 排出：经尿液。 半衰期：5.6~14.8 小时。	妊娠 B 类。 代谢入母乳/慎用。	无商标产品 12.5mg(30 粒胶囊)：$36.71, 25mg (100 片)：$12.99, 50mg (100 片)：$15.99
氯噻嗪	治疗轻至中度高血压；水肿的辅助治疗。	吸收：较少。 代谢：可达饱和，单剂量 250mg 或 500mg 系统吸收程度相等。 排出：经尿液。 半衰期：1~2 小时。	妊娠 C 类，但大多数专家不推荐使用。 代谢入母乳，慎用。	片剂可选择无商标产品，口服混悬剂仍为商品名 250mg (30 片)：$12.99, 500mg (30 片)：$13.99
美托拉宗	治疗轻至中度高血压；治疗心衰或肾病综合征引起的水肿，肾功能不全	吸收：40%~65%。 代谢：极少被代谢。 排出：经尿液。 半衰期：20 小时。	妊娠 B 类。 代谢入母乳/哺乳期不推荐使用。	无商标产品 2.5mg (30 片) $42.99, 5mg (30 片) $37.37

表 4-17. 利尿剂的其他特殊 FDA 适应证,剂型和药代动力学(续)

保钾利尿剂	FDA 适应证	药代动力学	妊娠期风险分类/哺乳	费用与制剂
螺内酯	治疗与醛固酮分泌过多有关的水肿;高血压;原发性醛固酮增多症;低钾血症;肝硬化合并水肿或腹水;肾炎综合症;严重心衰(NYHA 分级 III-IV),在标准治疗基础上加用以增加生存率,降低再住院率。	吸收:73%。 代谢:经肝脏,多种代谢产物。 排出:经尿液和粪便。 半衰期:1.3~2 小时,活性代谢产物半衰期 > 10 小时。	妊娠 C 类(动物试验中有致畸作用)。 代谢入母乳。	无商标产品 25mg(30 片):$15.99, 50mg(30 片):$21.99
氨苯蝶啶	单用或与其他利尿剂合用治疗水肿和高血压;减少排钾利尿剂引起的钾排出。	吸收:快速。 代谢:快速代谢。 排出:小于 50% 经尿液,其余经胆道/粪便。 半衰期:1-2 小时。	妊娠 C 类。 是否进入母乳尚无证据支持。	暂无可购买的无商标产品 商品名:Dyrenium 50mg(30 粒胶囊):$44.09, 100mg(30 粒胶囊):$67.24

利尿剂

样利尿剂	FDA 适应证	药代动力学	妊娠期风险分类 / 哺乳	费用与制剂
呋塞米	治疗心衰和肝脏或肾脏疾病引起的水肿；急性肺水肿；控制高血压（单用或与其他降压药物合用）	吸收：不稳定。 代谢：少量经肝脏代谢。 排出：经尿液，粪便。 半衰期：0.5~2 小时。	妊娠 C 类。 代谢入母乳/慎用。	无商标产品为片剂和溶液制剂 10mg/ml（60ml）：$17.99, 10mg/ml（120ml）：$15.98, 20mg（100 片）：$13.99, 40mg（100 片）：$13.99, 80mg（30 片）：$12.99
布美他尼	治疗心衰或肝肾疾病继发的水肿，包括肾炎；可单用或与其他降压药物合用治疗高血压；可用于呋塞米过敏者	吸收：85%~95%。 代谢：部分经肝脏。 排出：经尿液。 半衰期：1~1.5 小时。	妊娠 C 类（根据制药商），D 类（根据专家评价）。 不明确是否代谢入母乳，慎用。	无商标产品 0.5mg（90 片）：$17.00, 1mg（90 片）：$28.97, 2mg（30 片）：$20.99, 2mg（100 片）：$82.39

Courtesy of Paul Pham, PharmD, Johns Hopkins University School of Medicine.

专家建议

- 无论使用何种降压药物，严格控制血压都有获益，目标血压总体上建议 <130/80mmHg。
- 利尿剂可轻度降低 HDL。
- 噻嗪类利尿剂，尤其是合并低钾血症时可能加重胰岛素抵抗，故可能需加强降糖治疗。
- 一系列研究显示常规剂量噻嗪类利尿剂可降低胰岛素敏感性（Pollare）。
- 然而噻嗪类利尿剂对高血压的获益被认为大于血糖相关的轻微不良反应。
- 然而有研究比较小剂量噻嗪类利尿剂（苄氟噻嗪）与常规剂量相比，其药效相近而代谢方面不良反应较少（Harper）。

参考文献

ACCORD Study Group, Cushman WC, Evans GW, et al. Effects of intensive blood-pressure control in type 2 diabetes mellitus. NEJM, 2010; Vol. 362: pp. 1575–85.

Comments: The ACCORD study randomly assigned people at high risk for CVD with diabetes to target more or less tight BP control. With average systolic BP 119, there was no added benefit over average systolic BP 133 mmHg.

Barzilay JI, Davis BR, Cutler JA, et al. Fasting glucose levels and incident diabetes mellitus in older nondiabetic adults randomized to receive 3 different classes of antihypertensive treatment: a report from the Antihypertensive and Lipid-Lowering Treatment to Prevent Heart Attack Trial (ALLHAT). Arch Intern Med, 2006; Vol. 166: pp. 2191–201.

Comments: A post hoc analysis that suggested that chlorthalidone causes impaired glucose metabolism in people who do not have preexisting diabetes.

Kasiske BL, Ma JZ, Kalil RS, et al. Effects of antihypertensive therapy on serum lipids. Ann Intern Med, 1995; Vol. 122: pp. 133–41.

Comments: A meta-analysis that suggested that diuretics produce a small (0.08 mmol/L) deleterious effect on HDL cholesterol level in patients with diabetes.

Harper R, Ennis CN, Heaney AP, et al. A comparison of the effects of low and conventional-dose thiazide diuretic on insulin action in hypertensive patients with NIDDM. Diabetologia, 1995; Vol. 38: pp. 853–9.

Comments: A small trial reporting similar efficacy and decreased metabolic side effects using low-dose thiazide diuretic (bendrofluazide) as compared to a conventional dose.

Pollare T, Lithell H, Berne C A comparison of the effects of hydrochlorothiazide and captopril on glucose and lipid metabolism in patients with hypertension. NEJM, 1989; Vol. 321: pp. 868–73.

Comments: A small trial showing that hydrochlorothiazide decreases insulin sensitivity at conventional dose.

肾病

乙酰半胱氨酸

Lipika Samal, MD, MPH, and Paul A. Pham, PharmD

指征

FDA
- 对于肺气肿、结核、支气管炎等呼吸系统疾病引起的异常、浓稠的黏性分泌物起到辅助化痰作用,同时也可用于治疗囊性纤维化或气管切开术后的并发症。

机制
- 与其天然底物血管紧张素 I 相比较,对血管紧张素转换酶有更高的亲和力,以阻断其转换能力、减少血管紧张素 II 的生成。血管紧张素 II 是一种强力的血管收缩物质,对肾素活性有反馈抑制作用。因此减低血浆中血管紧张素 II 水平,可导致血压降低、血浆肾素活性升高。

非 FDA 的获准使用
- 预防肾毒性(本章重点)。
- 对乙酰氨基酚过量。

成人常用剂量
- 慢性肾功能不全的患者(包括糖尿病患者)在使用非离子、低渗对比剂的 CT 检查前起到预防肾毒性作用:600mg bid 口服,在应用对比剂前一天及当日(共 4 次)。
- 拟行血管成形术的患者(包括糖尿病患者)预防对比剂相关肾病:血管成形前 1 200mg 静推,术后 48 小时 1 200mg bid 口服。

剂型

商品名	通用名	剂型	价格
Mucomyst (Bristol-Myers Squibb 和其他多种制造商)	乙酰半胱氨酸	口服/吸入 每剂 30ml 20% 或 200mg/ml 10% 或 100mg/ml	$12.00 $6.49
Acetadote (Cumberland pharmaceutical)	乙酰半胱氨酸	静脉 200mg/ml (30ml)	$181.25

特殊人群中用药剂量

肾脏特殊人群
- 常规剂量。

肝脏特殊人群
- 尽管在肝硬化患者中乙酰半胱氨酸血浆浓度多出现 3 倍升高,但剂量方面并不推荐减量。

孕期妇女
- FDA 孕期用药分类 B 类。不经胎盘转运;有报道称,孕妇应用乙酰半管氨酸治疗对乙酰过量被证明安全且有效。

哺乳
- 避免哺乳。乙酰半胱氨酸是否分布于人乳还属未知。

药物不良反应
常见
- 臭鸡蛋样异味在许多患者中可导致味觉倒错。在口服前按推荐方法稀释可减轻异味。
- 胃肠道:腹泻,恶心(2%~7%),呕吐(9%~12%)。

偶见
- 输注过程中出现突发面红和皮肤红斑。无须干预。
- 呼吸系统:气道痉挛和呼吸窘迫(吸入乙酰半胱氨酸时)。患者有气道痉挛或哮喘病史时应用吸入剂型需谨慎。
- 过敏反应(0.1%~19%):多发生于单剂量静推乙酰半胱氨酸的第一小时中。可应用苯海拉明和减慢输注速度至 1 小时以上。

少见
- 神经系统:癫痫持续状态(关系不明确)。
- 心血管系统:心电图异常,心功能减退(关系不明确)。
- 皮肤:瘙痒和风团。

药物相互作用
- 硝酸甘油:增强硝酸酯类药效。合用应密切监测。
- 活性碳:可能减低乙酰半胱氨酸血药浓度。

药代动力学
- 吸收:6% 到 10%(经口)。
- 代谢和排出:经肝脏代谢,30% 经肾排出。
- 蛋白结合率:83%。
- 半衰期:5.6 小时。
- 分布:表观分布体积 Vd=0.47L/kg。

专家建议
- 又名 N-乙酰半胱氨酸或 N 乙酰 L 半胱氨酸(缩写为 NAC)。
- 糖尿病肾病患者常需行多种诊断性对比剂检查(如 CT、心导管检查),在这些患者中,乙酰半胱氨酸可被用于预防对比剂相关肾病,可能时还需适量水化并在使用造影剂后密切监测肾功能。

乙酰半胱氨酸

- 对于容量负荷过重的患者（如合并充血性心力衰竭）不能完善检查前后水化，本药对此类患者可能能更好地预防对比剂相关肾病。
- 慢性肾功能不全患者在口服乙酰半胱氨酸后对比剂相关肾病发病率较安慰剂组患者显著减低（2%vs21%；Tepel）。
- 同样，血管成形术前静脉应用乙酰半胱氨酸可有效预防对比剂相关肾病（8%vs15%；Marenzi）。

参考文献

Marenzi G, Assanelli E, Marana I, et al. N-acetylcysteine and contrast-induced nephropathy in primary angioplasty. NEJM, 2006; Vol. 354: pp. 2773–82.

Comments: In patients undergoing angioplasty (large contrast load) after acute myocardial infarction, lower incidence of nephrotoxicity (Scr increased . 25% from baseline) was observed with high-dose (1200 mg twice daily) acetylcysteine group compared to standard-dose (600 mg twice daily) group (15% vs 8%, p , 0.001).

Tepel M, van der Giet M, Schwarzfeld C, et al. Prevention of radiographic-contrast-agent-induced reductions in renal function by acetylcysteine. NEJM, 2000; Vol. 343: pp. 180–4.

Comments: In patients with chronic renal insufficiency, acetylcysteine (600 mg twice daily ′ 48 hrs) plus hydration were effective in preventing contrast-induced nephropathy compared to control (2% vs 21%, p = 0.01).

神经病变

神经性疼痛的治疗

Michael Polydefkis, MD, MHS, and Brian Pinto, PharmD, MBA

指征

FDA
- 普瑞巴林可用于缓解糖尿病多神经病变(DPN)的疼痛症状。
- 度洛西汀可用于缓解糖尿病多神经病变的疼痛症状。

非 FDA 的获准使用
- 加巴喷丁是最常用的非 FDA 获准使用的药物(Backonja)。
- 非 FDA 获准使用的缓解糖尿病多神经病变疼痛的药物包括抗抑郁药、阿片类药物或阿片样制剂,以及抗癫痫药物。
- 抗抑郁药包括三环类抗抑郁药(阿米替林、去甲替林)和选择性五羟色胺去甲肾上腺素再摄取抑制剂(SNRIs:文拉法辛、度洛西汀)。
- 抗癫痫药物包括加巴喷丁、丙戊酸、拉莫三嗪、卡马西平、苯妥英和拉科酰胺。
- 阿片类药物或其衍生物包括羟考酮、硫酸吗啡、氢吗啡酮、芬太尼和曲马多。
- 其他制剂包括外用药物(利多卡因乳膏、利多卡因贴片),营养调节药物(Metanx、α 硫辛酸)以及器械(脊柱刺激器、经皮电子神经刺激器)。

机制
- 普瑞巴林:GABA 类似物,对电压门控钙通道的 α2-δ 亚单位具有亲和力。
- 度洛西汀:选择性五羟色胺去甲肾上腺素再摄取抑制剂。
- 加巴喷丁:未知。

成人常用剂量
- 普瑞巴林:起始量 50mg tid,如能耐受 1 周后逐渐滴定加量至 100mg tid。普瑞巴林等效剂量约为加巴喷丁的 6 倍(例如,1 800mg 加巴喷丁 =300mg 普瑞巴林),且起效更迅速。可每天两次使用。
- 度洛西汀:起始量 30mg,如有需要一周后可加量至 60mg。每日剂量大于 60mg 会相对增强疼痛缓解作用,但可能增加不良反应。启动治疗后 1~2 周即可出现获益,但 4~6 周后会达到平台期。建议每日早晨服用,因为睡前服用可导致失眠。
- 加巴喷丁:起始量为 300mg(1 片)睡前,每 2~3 天逐渐加量,首先可于早晨加用一次,然后下午加用一次。患者感到疼痛缓解或出现镇静等不良反应时需停止加量。常规有效剂量为日总量 1 800mg,分三次口服,即每次 600mg。更大剂量(日总量大于 5g)难以提高更多药效。
- 三环类抗抑郁药:阿米替林为代表,6~8 周较长时间缓慢加量后起效(Wernicke)。
- 抗癫痫药物:疼痛缓解作用与加巴喷丁和普瑞巴林相似,但不良反应更多 [如

神经性疼痛的治疗

苯妥英（Sindrup）]。许多较陈旧制剂因为存在潜在骨髓抑制和多种药物相互作用，还需监测血药浓度。

- 阿片类或阿片样制剂：可单用或与对乙酰氨基酚联用以起到协同作用，从而在减少阿片类药物剂量的同时获得同样的缓解疼痛效果。
- 外用制剂：不吸收入机体，以减少药物不良反应及药物相互作用。辣椒素可每天 2~4 次外用于疼痛部位。利多卡因贴片按每 12 小时用药 / 无药周期外用于疼痛部位。
- 营养调节药物：此类物没有系统地在控制 – 对照临床试验中研究过。但 α 硫辛酸除外，该药在神经病变症状严重程度中体现获益，当药理剂量的 α 硫辛酸每日剂量大于 600mg 时症状有改善趋势（美国未被获准）（Ziegler）。
- 器械：脊髓刺激器械是一项有创且昂贵的操作，但无系统性不良反应，仍需更多研究支持（Tesfaye）。其他研究进展包括近红外线疗法。因其有潜在的不恰当营销而未受 FDA 程序获准。

剂型

商品名	通用名	剂型	价格
Lyrica（辉瑞）	普瑞巴林	口服胶囊 25mg, 50mg, 75mg, 100mg, 150mg, 200mg, 225mg, 300mg	$225（90 片）
Cymbalta（礼来）	度洛西汀	口服胶囊 20 mg 口服胶囊 30 mg 口服胶囊 60 mg	$300（60 片） $168（30 片） $168（30 片）
Neurontin（辉瑞及其他制药公司）	加巴喷丁	口服胶囊 100 mg 口服胶囊 300 mg 口服胶囊 400 mg 口服胶囊 600 mg 口服胶囊 800 mg 口服胶囊 250/5ml	$53（100 片） $133（100 片） $160（100 片） $73（90 片） $93（90 片） $160（470ml）

特殊人群中用药剂量

肾脏特殊人群

- 度洛西汀不推荐用于 GFR < 30ml/min 人群中。
- 加巴喷丁和普瑞巴林肾功能不全剂量调整分别见表 4-19 和表 4-20。

肝脏特殊人群

- 度洛西汀经肝脏代谢，故慎用于肝病患者。

神经性疼痛的治疗

孕期妇女
- 所有药物（加巴喷丁、普瑞巴林、度洛西汀）均为妊娠 C 类。

哺乳
- 所有药物：婴儿受累风险仍不能除外（Thomson）。

药物不良反应
总体
- 度洛西汀禁忌与单胺氧化酶抑制剂联用，且因其存在增加自杀观念的风险而在儿科患者中有黑框警告。度洛西汀还禁用于未控制的闭角型青光眼患者。其他不良反应包括肝毒性、体位性低血压和出血倾向。
- 普瑞巴林不良反应包括血管性水肿、过敏反应、撤药时抽搐发作、自杀行为和外周性水肿。
- 加巴喷丁不良反应包括自杀行为、撤药时抽搐发作，以及在临床前试验中有潜在的致癌作用和其他未明临床作用。

常见
- 普瑞巴林：水肿、体重增加、便秘、食欲增加、镇静和头晕。
- 加巴喷丁：水肿、镇静、头晕、乏力和发热。
- 度洛西汀：便秘、头晕、头痛、镇静、乏力、恶心和口干。

偶见
- 普瑞巴林：血管性水肿（尤其与 ACEI 合用时）可能较严重。
- 加巴喷丁：Stevens-Johnson 综合征、自杀观念和药物介导的昏迷

药物相互作用
- 加巴喷丁和普瑞巴林没有明确的药物相互作用，无需调整剂量。
- 度洛西汀禁忌与单胺氧化酶抑制剂合用（例如异卡波肼、利奈唑胺、吗氯贝胺、奋乃静、甲基苄肼、雷沙吉兰、司来吉兰、百乐明）
- 肝药酶 CYP1A2 抑制剂（如西咪替丁、喹诺酮类抗生素）和 CYP2D6 抑制剂（如氟西汀）应避免合用。
- 普瑞巴林与 ACEI 同时应用可增加血管性水肿风险。

药代动力学
表 4-18. 药代动力学

药物	吸收	代谢	排出	半衰期
普瑞巴林	>90%	极少量经肝脏代谢。	90% 经肾脏原型排出。	6.3 小时
度洛西汀	吸收良好	经肝药酶 CYP1A2、2D6 代谢以灭活代谢产物。	约 70% 经肾脏原型排出，20% 由粪便排出。	12 小时
加巴喷丁	50%~60%	不经肝脏代谢。	经肾脏原型排出。	5~7 小时

Courtesy of Paul Pham, PharmD, Johns Hopkins University School of Medicine.

神经性疼痛的治疗

表 4-19. 普瑞巴林肾功能不全剂量调整

GFR（ml/min）	每日总剂量（mg）	药物用法
> 60	150~600	每日 2 次或每日 3 次
30~60	75~300	每日 2 次或每日 3 次
15~30	50~150	每日 1~2 次
< 15	25~75	每日 1 次

Courtesy of Paul Pham, PharmD, Johns Hopkins University School of Medicine.

表 4-20. 加巴喷丁肾功能不全剂量调整

GFR（ml/min）	每日总剂量（mg）	药物用法
> 60	300~1200	每日 3 次
0~60	200~700	每日 2 次
15~30	200~700	每日 1 次
< 15	100~300	每日 1 次

Courtesy of Paul Pham, PharmD, Johns Hopkins University School of Medicine.

专家建议

- 总体原则：起始量为最低有效剂量，逐渐加量；较大剂量可能增加不良反应。
- 治疗应着重于减低患者疼痛级别 [例如在由 0 级到 10 级的视觉近似评价标尺（VAS）中疼痛级别约为 3 级]，以改善生活质量、减轻功能受限，而非不切实际地企图完全解除疼痛。
- 总体来说，需治疗人数流行病学分析提示神经病变药物的药效近似，因此不良反应、调整剂量方案、潜在的药物相互作用和花费常常在药物选择中起到重要作用。
- 2011 年美国神经内科学会推出的新指南中提出普瑞巴林在糖尿病多神经病变中有效并应加用；文拉法辛、度洛西汀、阿米替林、加巴喷丁、丙戊酸、阿片类药物（硫酸吗啡、曲马多和羟考酮控释剂）以及辣椒素在糖尿病多神经病变中可能有效，可考虑加用。
- 加巴喷丁和普瑞巴林不经肝脏代谢，故可能较吸合并肝病的患者。
- 普瑞巴林与噻唑烷二酮类药物合用时可能增加水肿和体重升高的发生率。
- 度洛西汀可能与空腹血糖及 HbA1c 轻度升高有关。不同类型药物合剂可引起协同作用（Gilron, 2005; Gilron, 2009），从而使阿片类药物、抗抑郁药和抗癫痫药物的用量减少。
- 治疗炎性疼痛较有效的抗炎药物一般对神经性疼痛无效。
- 选择性五羟色胺再摄取抑制剂（SSRIs）对糖尿病多神经病的疼痛无效。

神经性疼痛的治疗

推荐依据

Bril V, England H, Franklin GM, et al. Evidence-based guideline: Treatment of painful diabetic neuropathy: Report of the American Academy of Neurology, the American Association of Neuromuscular and Electrodiagnostic Medicine, and the American Academy of Physical Medicine and Rehabilitation. Neurology, 2011. Prepublished online before print April 11, 2011.

Comments: New consensus guidelines on effective treatments for DPN based on a systematic review of the literature between 1960–2008.

Wernicke JF, Pritchett YL, D'souza DN, et al. A randomized controlled trial of duloxetine in diabetic peripheral neuropathic pain. Neurology, 2006; Vol. 67: pp. 1411–20.

Comments: One of the registration trials for duloxetine.

Rosenstock J, Tuchman M, LaMoreaux L, et al. Pregabalin for the treatment of painful diabetic peripheral neuropathy: a double-blind, placebo-controlled trial. Pain, 2004; Vol. 110: pp. 628–38.

Comments: One of the FDA registration trials for pregabalin.

Backonja M, Beydoun A, Edwards KR, et al. Gabapentin for the symptomatic treatment of painful neuropathy in patients with diabetes mellitus: a randomized controlled trial. JAMA, 1998; Vol. 280: pp. 1831–6.

Comments: The first trial to demonstrate pain relief with gabapentin. Many subsequent trials adopted the same design.

其他参考文献

Gilron I, Bailey JM, Tu D, et al. Nortriptyline and gabapentin, alone and in combination for neuropathic pain: a double-blind, randomised controlled crossover trial. Lancet, 2009; Vol. 374: pp. 1252–61.

Comments: Similar to the Backonja et al. study but with gabapentin and a tricyclic agent.

Ziegler D, Ametov A, Barinov A, et al. Oral treatment with alpha-lipoic acid improves symptomatic diabetic polyneuropathy: the SYDNEY 2 trial. Diabetes Care, 2006; Vol. 29: pp. 2365–70.

Comments: A well-designed study of alpha lipoic acid.

Gilron I, Bailey JM, Tu D, et al. Morphine, gabapentin, or their combination for neuropathic pain. N Engl J Med, 2005; Vol. 352: pp. 1324–34.

Comments: Landmark publication showing that combination of morphine and gabapentin was better than either agent alone.

Sindrup SH, Jensen TS. Pharmacologic treatment of pain in polyneuropathy. Neurology, 2000; Vol. 55: pp. 915–20.

Comments: A nice comparison of different classes of agents.

Tesfaye S, Watt J, Benbow SJ, et al. Electrical spinal-cord stimulation for painful diabetic peripheral neuropathy. Lancet, 1997; Vol. 348: pp. 1698–701.

Comments: A nice early report of spinal cord stimulators in painful diabetic neuropathy.

Max MB, Lynch SA, Muir J, et al. Effects of desipramine, amitriptyline, and fluoxetine on pain in diabetic neuropathy. N Engl J Med, 1992; Vol. 326: pp. 1250–6.

Comments: A classic reference on tricyclic agents and neuropathic pain in diabetes.

肥胖

奥利司他

Reza Alavi, MD, MHS, MBA, and Paul A. Pham, PharmD

指征
FDA
- 对肥胖治疗起到减轻和保持体重的作用,适用于体重指数(BMI)≥ 30kg/m² 或 ≥ 27kg/m² 且同时具有其他危险因素(比如高血压、糖尿病、脂代谢紊乱)的患者。

机制
- 奥利司他通过抑制胃肠道脂肪酶,阻断食物中脂肪类的吸收。

成人常用剂量
- 120mg(1粒胶囊)口服 tid,每次进食含有脂肪的主餐时口服一次,每次于餐中或餐后1小时口服。
- 用量大于 120mg tid 时未显示有更多获益。

剂型

商品名	通用名	剂型	价格
Xenical(罗氏制药)	奥利司他	口服胶囊 120mg	90粒胶囊:$284.33

特殊人群中用药剂量
肾脏特殊人群
- 常用剂量。

肝脏特殊人群
- 可同常用剂量。

孕期妇女
- 妊娠B类。

哺乳
- 无相关数据,总体上不推荐使用。

药物不良反应
总体
- 胃肠道不良反应最为常见,尤其是高脂饮食者(每日总能量 > 30% 由脂肪类提供)。

常见
- 腹胀、排气。
- 排便急迫感、失禁。
- 脂肪泻。
- 油性斑点和油样排泄物。
- 排便增多。

偶见
- 腹痛。
- 恶心、呕吐。
- 头晕。
- 感染性腹泻。
- 下腹痛。

少见
- 过敏反应:瘙痒、红斑(无特异性)、风团、血管性水肿、气道痉挛和其他过敏反应。
- 大疱样皮疹或泛发皮疹。
- 肝酶升高。
- 碱性磷酸酶升高。

药物相互作用
- 因奥利司他的作用机制,故可能存在对脂溶性药物和营养补充制剂潜在的吸收不良。
- 维生素 A、维生素 D、维生素 E、维生素 K 和 β 胡萝卜素:脂溶性维生素补充制剂(和类似物)应在口服奥利司他前后至少 2 小时后应用。
- 华法林:因维生素 K 吸收不良,INR 可能继发性升高。故华法林剂量可能需相应减量。
- 环孢素:因减少环孢素吸收,故应在口服奥利司他前后 2 小时后应用环孢素。
- 胺碘酮和普罗帕酮:可能会减少吸收,故应在口服奥利司他前后 2 小时应用。
- 左甲状腺素:可能会显著减少吸收,故需在口服奥利司他前后 4 小时应用。
- 普伐他汀、地高辛、苯妥英、口服避孕药、硝苯地平和格列苯脲:与奥利司他合用不会影响药代动力学。

药代动力学
- 吸收:小于 1%。
- 代谢和排出:在胃肠壁内代谢,形成无活性的代谢产物。约 97% 经粪便排出,其中 83% 以原型排出;小于 2% 经尿液排出。
- 半衰期:48 小时。

奥利司他

专家建议

- 与安慰剂相比,奥利司他有适度减轻体重的作用,4年中体重约减轻3kg。
- 应强烈建议患者同时口服脂溶性维生素(A、D、E和K)的复合补充制剂。
- 可能对调整脂代谢有获益。
- 奥利司他未见有增加心血管疾病风险的报道,此点与另一类减肥药物西布曲明不同,而后者已退出北美市场。
- 奥利司他禁用于慢性吸收不良综合征或胆汁淤积的患者。

参考文献

Siebenhofer A, Horvath K, Jeitler K, et al. Long-term effects of weight-reducing drugs in hypertensive patients.Cochrane Database Syst Rev, 2009; (3): CD007654.

Comments: A meta-analysis of orlistat trials showed safe cardiovascular profile and an average reduction in systolic blood pressure of 2.5 mmHg.

Chou KM, Huang BY, Fanchiang JK, et al. Comparison of the effects of sibutramine and orlistat on obese, poorly controlled type 2 diabetic patients. Chang Gung Med J, 2008; Vol. 30: pp. 538–46.

Comments: This study found that sibutramine treatment produced greater reduction in weight than orlistat in obese, poorly controlled type 2 diabetic patients.

Rucker D, Padwal R, Li SK, et al. Long term pharmacotherapy for obesity and overweight: updated meta-analysis. BMJ, 2007; Vol. 335: pp. 1194–9.

Comments: A meta-analysis of 3 pharmacologic agents for weight loss.

苯丁胺

Reza Alavi, MD, MHS, MBA, and Paul A. Pham, PharmD

指征

FDA
- 短期应用（数周），作为运动减重方案、生活方式调整和能量摄入限制的辅助治疗，适用于初始 BMI ≥ 30kg/m^2 或 BMI ≥ 27kg/m^2 且同时具有其他危险因素（比如高血压、糖尿病、高脂血症）的患者。

机制
- 为拟交感胺类药物，药理属性与安非他明类药物相似。
- 抑制食欲的作用可能继发于对中枢神经系统的作用，包括刺激下丘脑释放去甲肾上腺素。

成人常用剂量
- 口服：18.75~37.5mg/d（盐酸苯丁胺）或 15~30mg/d（苯丁胺树脂）。
- 早餐前或早餐后 1~2 小时口服。
- 在睡前 10~14 小时口服，以减轻失眠的不良反应。

剂型

商品名	通用名	剂型	价格
Adipex-P (Gate Pharmaceuticals 和其他制造商)	苯丁胺	口服胶囊 37.5mg；口服片剂 37.5mg	$1.52~$2.19；$1.52~$2.15
Lonamin（UCB Pharmaceuticals 和其他制造商）	苯丁胺	口服胶囊 15mg，30mg	$1.25

特殊人群中用药剂量

肾脏特殊人群
- 肾功能不全者中应减量。

肝脏特殊人群
- 慎用，肝功能不全者需考虑减量。

孕期妇女
- 妊娠 C 类。

哺乳
- 避免使用，该药在母乳婴儿中有潜在的严重不良反应。

苯丁胺

药物不良反应

总体
- 与安非他明类药物相比,苯丁胺有较少的致欣快作用,也有较少的中枢神经系统或心血管毒性。

常见
- 心悸、心动过速、血压升高。
- 中枢神经系统:过度刺激、烦躁不安、头晕、失眠、欣快、焦虑、震颤、头痛。

偶见
- 泌尿生殖/内分泌系统:阳痿,性欲改变。
- 胃肠道:口干,异常口味,腹泻,便秘。
- 皮肤:过敏性风团。

少见
- 黑框警告:原发性肺动脉高压(PPH)在合用芬氟拉明或右旋芬氟拉明的患者中有较多报道,但单用苯丁胺的患者中鲜有PPH的报道。
- 黑框警告:严重的心脏瓣膜病如二尖瓣、主动脉瓣和/或三尖瓣反流可见报道于合用芬氟拉明或右旋芬氟拉明的患者,但单用苯丁胺的患者中鲜有心脏瓣膜病的报道。
- 精神异常(与超过推荐剂量范围应用相关)。

药物相互作用
- 胍乙啶、胍环定、甲基多巴和利血平:可能减低以上药物的降压效果。
- 单胺氧化酶抑制剂(MAOIs,例如奋乃静)、呋喃唑酮:合用可能导致高血压危象和颅内出血。MAOIs或有单胺氧化酶抑制活性的药物应用后14天内不应加用苯丁胺。
- 选择性五羟色胺再摄取抑制剂(SSRI,例如氟西汀):可能增加苯丁胺的拟交感活性,也会增加出现五羟色胺综合征的风险,故须避免合用。
- 三环类抗抑郁药:可能增加苯丁胺的升压作用,应避免合用。
- 吩噻嗪类:可能减低苯丁胺药效,可能的话避免合用。
- 任何具有拟交感活性药物(例如安非他明、右苯丙胺、麻黄碱类药物和麻黄)可能导致其他交感兴奋的不良反应(例如高血压危象、心律失常、严重焦虑不安)。避免合用。

药代动力学
- 吸收:吸收良好,树脂制剂吸收较慢。
- 代谢和排出:经肝脏代谢;无显著生物转化作用。主要经肾脏排出(70%~80%以原型排出);酸化尿液后排出增多。
- 半衰期:19~24小时。

苯丁胺

专家建议

- 严重动脉硬化、心血管疾病、中高度高血压、甲亢和青光眼患者为使用禁忌。
- 药物依赖:长期用药可能出现精神性和躯体性药物依赖,此类药物已被广泛滥用。
- 有药物滥用史的患者应避免使用本药。
- 与安非他明类产品相比,苯丁胺有同等程度的减体重效果,而有较少的致欣快作用,也有较少的中枢神经系统或心血管毒性。
- 应用苯丁胺数周后可能出现对其抑制食欲作用的耐受。此时可将药物加量,最大剂量37.5mg/d,但如已加量至最大推荐剂量时仍有耐受则需停用药物。
- 在糖尿病患者中慎用,降糖药物使用条件可能因本药抑制食欲和相应的饮食控制而改变。
- 与安慰剂相比,6个月平均体重减轻约为3.6kg。
- 目前研究中本药可与托吡酯组成合剂,小剂量应用时可出现协同作用。

参考文献

Snow V, Barry P, Fitterman N, et al. Pharmacologic and surgical management of obesity in primary care: a clinical practice guideline from the American College of Physicians. Ann Intern Med, 2005; Vol. 142: pp. 525–31.

Comments: Guidelines on the management of obesity.

Li Z, Maglione M, Tu W, et al. Meta-analysis: pharmacologic treatment of obesity. Ann Intern Med, 2005; Vol. 142: pp. 532–46.

Comments: Excellent meta-analysis of obesity medications including phentermine.

McTigue KM, Harris R, Hemphill B, et al. Screening and interventions for obesity in adults: summary of the evidence for the U.S. Preventive Services Task Force. Ann Intern Med, 2003; Vol. 139: pp. 933–49.

Comments: Pharmacogic therapy appears safe in the short term; long-term safety has not been as strongly established.

Abenhaim L, Moride Y, Brenot F, et al. Appetite-suppressant drugs and the risk of primary pulmonary hypertension. International Primary Pulmonary Hypertension Study Group. NEJM, 1996; Vol. 335: pp. 609–16.

Comments: When phentermine is coadministered with fenfluramine for .3 months, there is a 23-fold increased risk of primary pulmonary hypertension.

泌尿系统

氨甲酰甲胆碱

Lipika Samal, MD, MPH, and Paul A. Pham, PharmD

指征
FDA
- 治疗急性术后或产后非梗阻性(功能性)尿潴留,以及尿潴留膀胱的神经性弛缓。

非 FDA 获准用药
- 肠梗阻。
- 胃液反流。

机制
- 具有拟副交感活性,直接激动泌尿道毒蕈碱(胆碱能)受体,从而提高膀胱收缩力。
- 也可刺激胃肠道活动性。

成人常用剂量
- 对神经源性膀胱弛缓:初始剂量 5~10mg 口服,间隔每小时逐渐加量至最大剂量 50mg。常用维持剂量:10~50mg 口服,每日 3~4 次。

剂型

商品名	通用名	剂型	价格
氯贝丁酯(Abrika Pharmaceuticals 和其他制造商)	氯贝丁酯	口服片剂 5mg	$0.71
		口服片剂 10mg	$1.33
		口服片剂 25mg	$1.78
		口服片剂 50mg	$2.85

特殊人群中用药剂量
肾脏特殊人群
- 无须调整剂量。

肝脏特殊人群
- 暂无针对性指南推荐。

孕期妇女
- FDA 妊娠 C 类。

哺乳
- 本药是否经哺乳排出尚不清楚。

氨甲酰甲胆碱

药物不良反应

总体
- 胆碱能激动剂可导致皮肤潮红、温暖、瞳孔缩小、多汗、流泪、唾液分泌增多和气道痉挛。

常见
- 泌尿生殖系统：尿急迫、尿频。
- 消化系统：腹痛/腹部绞痛、腹泻、腹胀、恶心/呕吐以及腹部鸣响（胃部咕噜声）。

偶见
- 视物模糊（继发于瞳孔缩小）。
- 头痛。
- 尿液逆流。
- 体位性低血压或高血压患者突发血压降低。

少见
- 抽搐发作。
- 低体温。

药物相互作用
- M受体阻断剂：麦普替林、美卡拉明、三环类抗抑郁药、吩噻嗪类、氯氮平、安非他酮、氯氮平、丙吡胺、奥氮平、普鲁卡因胺和奎尼丁可显著降低本药药效。可能时避免合用。
- 止泻药：卡比沙明、氯丙嗪、氯马斯汀、苯海拉明、美索达嗪、奥氮平、阿片类药物、拟副交感活性药物、普马嗪、异丙嗪、奎尼丁和拟交感活性药物也可影响本药作用。可能时避免合用。

药代动力学
- 吸收：几乎不被吸收，起效时间为30~90分钟。
- 半衰期：活性时间约维持1小时。

专家建议
- 可用于治疗糖尿病神经源性膀胱（Frimodt-Moller）。
- 可有效治疗尿潴留，与α受体阻断剂联用可能更加有效；但本药因存在胆碱样作用不良反应如腹泻、腹部绞痛而应用受限（Yamanishi）。
- 应用本药之前，临床医师须除外膀胱或泌尿系梗阻可能。
- 心动过速、低血压和冠心病患者中存在用药禁忌。甲状腺功能减退、发作性癫痫和帕金森患者亦应避免使用本药，因其会使上述疾病加重。
- 避免哮喘或COPD患者使用本药，因为有潜在的气道阻塞可能。

参考文献
Taylor JA, Kuchel GA. Detrusor underactivity: clinical features and pathogenesis of an underdiagnosed geriatric condition. J Am Geriatr Soc, 2006; Vol. 54: pp. 1920-32.
  Comments: A good review of the clinical features of detrusor underactivity.

Yamanishi T, Yasuda K, Kamai T, et al. Combination of a cholinergic drug and an alpha-blocker is more effective than monotherapy for the treatment of voiding difficulty in patients with underactive detrusor. Int J Urol, 2004; Vol. 11: pp. 88–96.

Comments: Total urinary symptom scores (International Prostate Symptom Score, IPSS) remained unchanged after the cholinergic therapy, but were significantly lower after the alpha-blocker treatment and the combination therapy ($p = 0.0001$). Combination therapy with a cholinergic drug and an alpha-blocker appears to be more useful than monotherapy for the treatment of underactive detrusor.

Frimodt-Møller C, Mortensen S. Treatment of diabetic cystopathy. Ann Intern Med, 1980; Vol. 92: pp. 327–8.

Comments: Describes treatments for diabetic cystopathy including bethanechol.

奥昔布宁

Lipika Samal, MD, MPH, and Paul A. Pham, PharmD

指征
FDA
- 未抑制或反射性神经源性膀胱（比如尿急、尿频、尿漏、急迫性尿失禁、排尿困难）。

机制
- 奥昔布宁是一种叔胺酯,具有抗胆碱(阿托品样)和解痉(罂粟碱样)作用,从而抑制平滑肌表面乙酰胆碱作用。反射性神经源性膀胱中，奥昔布宁可抑制逼尿肌反射亢进。

成人常用剂量
- 非高龄成年人：奥昔布宁速释剂 5mg 口服，每日 4 次；可根据药效和耐受情况调整剂量，每周可加量 5mg。
- 老年人：根据 Beers 标准，奥昔布宁缓释剂 5mg qd 口服更适用于高龄患者。
- 最大剂量 30mg/d。
- 透皮贴：3.9mg/d, 每周 2 次外用于腹部、髋部或臀部的干燥、无破损皮肤。
- 10% 外用凝胶：将小袋中剂量外用于腹部、上臂/肩部或大腿的干燥、无破损皮肤。
- 贴剂和凝胶需要患者轮换外用部位。

剂型

商品名	通用名	剂型	价格
Ditropan (Major Pharmaceuticals Inc. 和其他制造商)	盐酸奥昔布宁	口服片剂 5mg	$0.61
Ditropan XL (Ortho Womens Health & Urology: a Division of OMP 和其他制造商)	盐酸奥昔布宁缓释剂	口服缓释剂 5mg 口服缓释剂 10mg 口服缓释剂 15mg	$3.30 $3.30 $3.40
Ditropan (Pharmaceutical Association Inc. 及其他制造商)	盐酸奥昔布宁	口服糖浆 5mg/5ml	$66.32（每16盎司）
Oxytrol Transdermal System (Watson Pharmaceuticals)	盐酸奥昔布宁	透皮贴 3.9mg/24 小时	$19.53
Gelnique 10% 凝胶 (Watson Pharmaceuticals)	盐酸奥昔布宁	10% 外用凝胶	$4.78

奥昔布宁

特殊人群中用药剂量

肾脏特殊人群
- 奥昔布宁缓释剂型未在严重肾功能不全患者中评估,故不推荐使用。

肝脏特殊人群
- 本药几乎全部经肝脏代谢,故在肝病患者中应减量。
- 奥昔布宁缓释制剂未在该类患者中评估,故不推荐使用。

孕期妇女
- 尽管奥昔布宁在 FDA 中被归为妊娠 B 类,在孕期使用的安全性证据并不充分。

哺乳
- 奥昔布宁是否在母乳中排出仍不明确。奥昔布宁速释剂在市场后研究中有抑制泌乳的报道。

药物不良反应

总体
- 不良反应与本药在胃肠道平滑肌的抗胆碱能及抗毒蕈碱作用有关。

常见
- 胃肠道:便秘、胃肠炎、恶心、口干。
- 中枢神经系统:头晕、头痛、嗜睡。

偶见
- 心脏:心悸、窦性心动过速、液体潴留、外周水肿。
- 内分泌:血糖升高。

少见
- 严重过敏反应、风团。

药物相互作用
- 奥昔布宁主要通过肝脏及胃肠壁的细胞色素 P450 3A4 同工酶代谢。
- CYP450 3A4 的强抑制剂(例如 HIV 蛋白酶抑制剂、唑类抗真菌药、大环内脂类抗生素)需避免合用。
- CYP450 3A4 的诱导剂(例如卡马西平、苯妥英、苯巴比妥、利福平、奈韦拉平、依法韦仑)可减弱奥昔布宁药效。

药代动力学
- 吸收:1.6%~10.9% 速释。
- 代谢和排出:绝大部分经肝脏代谢,少量经肠壁代谢;很少经肾脏排出。
- 半衰期:速释剂 2~3 小时;10mg 缓释剂 12~19 小时。

专家建议
- 常用于门诊糖尿病患者膀胱过度激惹的治疗,有证据表示可在高龄患者中减少日间排尿频率。

- 因其对胃肠道平滑肌的作用，故糖尿病胃轻瘫患者慎用。禁用于尿潴留和 / 或膀胱流出道梗阻患者。
- 闭角型青光眼和尿潴留为绝对禁忌证。
- 对糖尿病自主神经病变患者的味觉相关出汗及严重腹泻症状可能有效。

参考文献

Abrams P, Cardozo L, Chapple C, et al. Comparison of the efficacy, safety, and tolerability of propiverine and oxybutynin for the treatment of overactive bladder syndrome. Int J Urol, 2006; Vol. 13: pp. 692–8.

Comments: Oxybutynin 15 mg was more effective than propiverine 20 mg in reducing symptomatic and asymptomatic involuntary detrusor contractions.

Blair DI, Sagel J, and Taylor I. Diabetic gustatory sweating. South Med J, 2002; Vol. 95: pp. 360–2.

Comments: Oxybutinin can be considered for diabetic gustatory sweating.

Szonyi G, Collas DM, Ding YY, et al. Oxybutynin with bladder retraining for detrusor instability in elderly people: a randomized controlled trial. Age Ageing, 1995; Vol. 24: pp. 287–91.

Comments: Oxybutynin is effective in controlling overactive bladder.

Chideckel EW. Oxybutynin for diabetic complications. JAMA, 1990; Vol. 264: p. 2994.

Comments: The author reports successful treatment of diabetic gustatory sweating and severe diarrhea with oxybutynin.

第五部分

临床试验

骨骼系统	609
内分泌系统	617
消化系统	623
血糖监测	626
血液系统	640
免疫学	643
血脂	652
肾脏	656

骨骼系统

骨骼矿物质密度

Kendall F. Moseley, MD, and Todd T. Brown, MD, PhD

概念
- 骨骼矿物质密度（BMD）可测定某指定部位骨骼的矿物质含量。
- 骨质疏松是一种系统性骨骼疾病，以骨密度减低和骨组织细微结构退行性病变为特点，并继发骨骼脆性及骨折易患性增加。
- 骨骼结构由矿物质（钙、磷）、I型胶原和蛋白组成，而矿物质在其中形成羟磷灰石结晶。
- 1型糖尿病（T1DM）：其BMD较同龄健康人群低，较同龄人骨折风险更高（Schwartz）。
- 2型糖尿病（T2DM）：其BMD较同龄健康人群高，但尽管BMD较高仍可能有较高骨折风险（Schwartz；Brandi）。

实验室检查
- 双能X线吸收法（DXA）测定腰椎、全髋关节、股骨颈和前臂的BMD被认为是临床的金标准。
- DXA可定量测定以克为单位的骨矿物质含量（BMC）和以平方厘米为单位的骨面积（BA），而BMD等于BMC/BA，单位为克每平方厘米。
- 对于高危患者亦应评价椎体骨折情况。
- 定量计算机体层成像（CT）测定每体积骨密度而非面积密度（由DXA测定），但价格昂贵，不作为临床常规检查（Khoo）。
- 足跟超声、放射吸收法和单能X线吸收法也可用于BMD计算（Nayak）。
- 新的影像学技术[MICRO CT和磁共振成像（MRI）]正在发展中，以更好地为临床评价骨骼微结构和质量。

适应证
- 对1型或2型糖尿病患者的BMD测量还没有针对性的指南，需使用为同年龄、性别健康人群建立的指南。
- 国家骨质疏松基金会（NOF）推荐大于65岁女性和大于70岁男性，无论有无骨折危险因素均需筛查BMD（Heinemann）。
- 建议更年轻的绝经后女性和有其他骨折危险因素的50~69岁男性考虑评价DXA。根据NOF，糖尿病也被认为是一项骨折的危险因素。
- 其他推荐评估BMD的临床危险因素包括BMI减低，髋部骨折家族史，烟酒嗜好，慢性炎性疾病（类风湿关节炎、溃疡性结肠炎等），长期使用激素或抗癫痫药物，激素代谢异常（长期维生素D缺乏症、甲状旁腺功能亢进、性腺功能不全、甲状腺功能亢进、Cushing综合征等）（Kanis）。
- 无论年龄大小、出现脆性骨折（从直立身高或更低高度摔倒导致的骨折）

的患者和使用抗骨质疏松药物（双磷酸盐、特立帕肽、SERMs 等）或被认为应进行抗骨质疏松药物治疗的患者，均需评价 DXA。
- 使用噻唑烷二酮类药物可能引起低 BMD 和骨折。

鉴别诊断
- 骨密度测量可定义正常、骨量减少和骨质疏松等一系列临床情况（见下面分析一节）。

分析
- DXA 测定腰椎、全髋关节、股骨颈和前臂的 BMD 以 T 值和 Z 值表示（在某些机构可能要求分别测定）。
- T 值计算方法为：小于 30 岁的参考人群的平均 BMD 减去患者测定 BMD，后除以年轻人群的标准差（SD）。
- Z 值计算方法为：同年龄、性别参考人群的平均 BMD 减去患者测定 BMD，除以该人群 SD。
- 正常骨密度定义为 T 值 > –1.0。
- 骨量减少定义为 T 值为 –1~–2.5。
- 骨质疏松定义为 T 值 ≤ –2.5。
- 重度骨质疏松定义为 T 值 ≤ –2.5 同时出现一次或多次脆性骨折。
- 经连续多次 DXA 测定可提示骨密度改变，需在标准机构和器械上测定某特定部分且出现显著性百分比改变（Baim）。
- 在绝经前女性和小于 50 岁男性应以 Z 值而非 T 值评价。Z 值 ≤ –2.0 时认为骨密度减低，但不能单独作为启动治疗的根据。

局限性和难点
- DXA、定量 CT 及其他提到的显像模式近描述骨量，而非骨质量（在评价骨折风险中同样重要）。
- DXA 的准确性与精密度与器械校准、技工能力，以及对影像和 BMD 数据的准确解读（Kanis）。
- 准确的 BMD 要求患者在扫描床上取合适体位，也是密度测定中最常见误差。
- 脊柱侧弯患者无法在扫描床上取正确体位，故其脊柱 BMD 测量结果无效。
- 局部结构性和退行性变（骨赘、压缩性骨折、主动脉钙化、脊椎强直等）可能导致局部 BMD 测定有误。
- 人工制品如外科小钳夹、金属首饰和 X 线不透过的药片等可能使 BMD 数值假性升高。
- 肥胖患者，如 T2DM 患者可能无法良好适应扫描床，故可使用半身 DXA 扫描仪。
- 在测量骨骼局部的过多肌肉或脂肪含量（肥胖个体）可增加 DXA 法测定 BMD 的不准确性（Bolotin）。

专家建议
- BMD 可预测骨折风险，但不能替代临床决策，在可能存在骨质量减低（例如骨骼细微结构和力学结构受损）的糖尿病患者中也不能替代危险因素评估（Burghardt）。
- 对于进行骨质疏松药物治疗的患者和有较高骨折风险、可能需药物治疗的患者，在首次 DXA 筛查后需测定骨密度 1~2 年。
- 骨折风险评估工具（http://www.shef.ac.uk/FRAX/）将股骨颈 BMD 和患者骨质疏松危险因素综合为一个多因素模型，可用于计算 10 年内发生任何重要的骨质疏松性骨折和髋部骨折的概率；1 型糖尿病在 FRAX 模型中被认为是骨丢失的一项危险因素（Kanis）。

推荐依据

National Osteoporosis Foundation. Clinician's Guide to Prevention and Treatment of Osteoporosis. Washington, DC: National Osteoporosis Foundation; 2010. Available at: http://www.nof.org/sites/default/files/pdfs/NOF_ ClinicianGuide2009_v7.pdf. Accessed 4/25/11.

Comments: Consensus guidelines on the management of osteoporosis in postmenopausal women and men.50 years.

其他参考文献

Brandi ML Microarchitecture, the key to bone quality. Rheumatology (Oxford), 2009; Vol. 48 Suppl 4: pp. iv, 3–8.

Comments: Bone as comprised of a macrostructure and microstructure, and the imaging techniques used for measuring each one.

Burghardt AJ, Issever AS, Schwartz AV, et al. High-resolution peripheral quantitative computed tomographic imaging of cortical and trabecular bone microarchitecture in patients with type 2 diabetes mellitus. J Clin Endocrinol Metab, 2010; Vol. 95: pp. 5045–55.

Comments: Describes increased BMD but impaired bone strength in patients with type 2 diabetes.

Khoo BC, Brown K, Cann C, et al. Comparison of QCT-derived and DXA-derived areal bone mineral density and T scores. Osteoporos Int, 2009; Vol. 20: pp. 1539–45.

Comments: Quantitative CT compared to gold standard DXA was found to accurately diagnose osteoporosis.

Baim S, Binkley N, Bilezikian JP, et al. Official positions of the International Society for Clinical Densitometry and executive summary of the 2007 ISCD Position Development Conference. J Clin Densitom, 2008; Vol. 11: pp. 75–91.

Comments: Position paper highlighting current recommendations, standards, and guidelines in the clinical use of densitometry testing.

Schwartz AV, Sellmeyer DE. Diabetes, fracture, and bone fragility. Curr Osteoporos Rep, 2007; Vol. 5: pp. 105–11.

Comments: Description of low BMD in T1DM and high BMD in T2DM with speculation as to why both groups are at higher risk for fracture.

Kanis JA, Oden A, Johnell O, et al. The use of clinical risk factors enhances the performance of BMD in the prediction of hip and osteoporotic fractures in men and women. Osteoporos Int, 2007; Vol. 18: pp. 1033–46.

Comments: Meta-analysis serving as foundation of WHO risk factor assessment tool (FRAX).

Nayak S, Olkin I, Liu H, et al. Meta-analysis: accuracy of quantitative ultrasound for identifying patients with osteoporosis. Ann Intern Med, 2006; Vol. 144: pp. 832–41.

Comments: Meta-analysis to evaluate the sensitivity and specificity of calcaneal ultrasound (US) in detecting osteoporosis compared to gold standard DXA.

Kanis JA, Borgstrom F, De Laet C, et al. Assessment of fracture risk. Osteoporos Int, 2005; Vol. 16: pp. 581–9.

Comments: Discussion of additional risk factors for bone loss which, combined with BMD, aid in determining a patient's risk for fracture.

Bolotin HH, Sievänen H, Grashuis JL. Patient-specific DXA bone mineral density inaccuracies: quantitative effects of nonuniform extraosseous fat distributions. J Bone Miner Res, 2003; Vol. 18: pp. 1020–7.

Comments: Discussion of inaccuracies in BMD interpretation caused by fat mass and lean mass attenuation artifacts.

维生素 D

Kendall F. Moseley, MD, and Todd T. Brown, MD, PhD

概念
- 据分析,世界范围内约10亿人存在维生素 D 缺乏或不足(Holick 2007)。
- 1 型糖尿病(T1DM)和 2 型糖尿病(T2DM)患者维生素 D 缺乏症的患病率仍在研究中,初步数据提示其患病率在 T2DM 患者中可能高达 30%(Targher)。
- 维生素 D 促进小肠对钙和磷的吸收,以维持骨骼矿物质含量。
- 维生素 D 的来源包括日光照射、食物摄入和食物补充成分。
- 经日光照射或食物来源的维生素 D 在肝脏代谢形成 25-羟维生素 D(25(OH)D)。
- 25-羟维生素 D 在肾脏由 1-α-羟化酶转化为活性形式,即 1,25-羟维生素 D(1,25(OH)D)。
- 成人维生素 D 缺乏症可导致骨量减少、骨质疏松和/或骨软化症;肌无力;以及较高的骨折和跌倒风险(Holick 2007)。
- 维生素 D 在人体健康中可能有其他作用,包括调节免疫和减少炎症反应。

实验室检查
- 金标准:高效液相色谱法,但昂贵而不方便(Holick 2009)。
- 常用的两种测定方法:免疫分析和液相色谱-质谱(LC-MS)。免疫分析可测定总 25(OH)D,而 LC-MS 可测定血清 D2 和 D3,其总和即为总 25(OH)D 浓度。这两种方法的相对准确性存在争议。
- 放射免疫分析(RIA)目前在临床实践中用于测定 1,25(OH)D2 和 1,25(OH)D3。
- 在疑诊低钙血症时,同时测定钙和甲状旁腺素(PTH)浓度也有意义。

适应证
- 在健康人群或糖尿病患者中对维生素 D 缺乏或不足的筛查尚无明确指南。
- 25(OH)D 水平决定个体的维生素 D 储备和状态(Holick 2009)。
- 在高龄或日光暴露较少、过度使用防晒霜、乳制品摄入较少、深色皮肤、肥胖或营养不良的人群中,可考虑筛查 25(OH)D 水平。
- 骨质疏松患者继发因素、疑诊或确诊乳糜泻的患者或有其他吸收不良情况(溃疡性结肠炎、胃旁路术后等)的患者可考虑检查 25(OH)D 水平(Taxel)。
- 常规抽血发现低钙血症或出现手足搐搦、感觉异常或肌阵挛症状时可进一步查维生素 D 水平。
- 如乏力、肌无力和骨痛等症状可能无特异性。

鉴别诊断
- 合成减少导致 25(OH)D 减低:深色皮肤色素沉着,使用隔离霜,高龄,冬季,高纬度,肝脏疾病(Holick 2007)。
- 吸收减少导致 25(OH)D 减低:乳糜泻,囊性纤维化,Whipple 病,胃旁路术后,肥胖(维生素 D 分布于脂肪组织中)。

- 摄入减少导致 25(OH)D 减低。
- 分解增多导致 25(OH)D 减低：HIV 治疗，抗排异药物，抗癫痫药物，激素。
- 1,25(OH)D 增多而 25(OH)D 减低：原发性甲状旁腺功能亢进，肉芽肿性疾病，淋巴瘤。

分析
- 对于 25(OH)D 正常范围或定义维生素 D 缺乏和不足的界值尚无明确共识（Holick 2009）。
- 25(OH)D 水平在 30~40ng/ml 之间时 PTH 到达稳态，故定义正常血清维生素 D 水平应大于 30ng/ml。
- 维生素 D 不足：20~30ng/ml。
- 维生素 D 缺乏：< 20ng/ml。
- 维生素 D 中毒：25(OH)D 水平 > 150ng/ml，与高钙血症、高尿钙和高磷血症有关。

局限性和难点
- 免疫分析和 LC-MS 分析最为常用，但应用不同方法测定可能出现差异；正在为规范检测手段做出努力。
- 1,25(OH)D 尽管是具有生物活性的维生素 D 形式，但因其半衰期短（4~6 小时）而不能较好地评价维生素 D 水平。
- 维生素 D 缺乏的患者因继发甲状旁腺功能亢进、PTH 升高，可能出现一过性 1,25(OH)D 升高。
- 尽管 25(OH)D 水平 > 30ng/ml 被认为正常，但每个个体都有自己的维生素 D 正常的界值，在当前 PTH 正常（无继发甲状旁腺功能亢进证据）时更为可靠。
- 25(OH)D 在维生素 D 缺乏或不足范围内时，可能 PTH 水平仍正常（无继发甲状旁腺功能亢进证据）。

专家建议
- 血清 25(OH)D 是评价维生素 D 水平的最高指标。
- 患有 T1DM 的儿童和青少年出现乳糜泻的患病率可能高达 10%（成人中为 8%）；在 T1DM 患者中，医师可考虑筛查乳糜泻相关抗体（抗组织谷氨酰氨基转移酶抗体、抗肌内膜抗体、抗麦胶蛋白抗体）和维生素 D 吸收不良情况（25(OH)D 水平）（Larsson）。
- 孕期和儿童早期补充维生素 D 可能通过减少胰岛自身抗体而减少患 T1DM 的风险，但这一点仍有争议（Hyppönen）。
- 在观察性研究中看到，血清 25(OH)D 水平减低与心血管疾病、肥胖、β 细胞功能障碍、胰岛素抵抗、糖耐量减退、代谢综合征和 T2DM 有关，但机制仍不清楚（Cheng；Chiu；Pittas；Chonchol）。
- T1DM 与 T2DM 都与骨折风险增高有关；故维生素 D 缺乏和不足的患者应进行维生素 D 筛查和适当的补充治疗，以减小骨折风险。
- 诊断维生素 D 不足或缺乏后需给予较大剂量维生素 D 治疗（例如骨钙化醇 50 000IU 口服，每周 1 次，共 8 周；如维生素 D 水平仍 < 30ng/ml 需重复治疗）。

- 适量补充钙剂是保证维生素 D 功能的基础，也可用于优化治疗。
- 近期医学研究所 2011 年报道指出，目前证据提示维生素 D 促进骨骼健康，但对骨骼外预后报道并不一致。当维生素 D 水平 > 20ng/ml 时，对于年龄 1~70 岁的患者推荐日剂量为 600IU，大于 70 岁患者为 800IU。

参考文献

Ross AC, Manson JE, Abrams SA, et al. The 2011 Report on Dietary Reference Intakes for Calcium and Vitamin D from the Institute of Medicine: What Clinicians Need to Know. J Clin Endocrinol Metab; epub ahead of print November 29, 2010.

Comments: Summarizes the new IOM report on dietary requirements for calcium and vitamin D. Suggests that vitamin D level of .20 ng/ml is adequate and that levels .50 ng/ml may be associated with adverse effects.

Holick MF. Vitamin D status: measurement, interpretation, and clinical application. Ann Epidemiol, 2009; Vol. 19: pp. 73–8.

Comments: Overview of vitamin D synthesis, sources, assays, degrees of sufficiency, and treatment recommendations.

Cheng S, Massaro JM, Fox CS, et al. Adiposity, cardiometabolic risk, and vitamin D status: the Framingham Heart Study. Diabetes, 2010; Vol. 59: pp. 242–8.

Comments: 25(OH)D levels positively correlated with insulin sensitivity, negatively correlated with beta-cell function in T2DM.

Holick MF. The vitamin D deficiency pandemic and consequences for nonskeletal health: mechanisms of action. Mol Aspects Med, 2008; Vol. 29: pp. 361–8.

Comments: Role of vitamin D in multiple organ systems and nonskeletal consequences that deficiency might precipitate.

Chonchol M, Cigolini M, Targher G. Association between 25-hydroxyvitamin D deficiency and cardiovascular disease in type 2 diabetic patients with mild kidney dysfunction. Nephrol Dial Transplant, 2008; Vol. 23: pp. 269–74.

Comments: Inverse association between vitamin D levels and CVD prevalence in T2DM with mild renal dysfunction.

Larsson K, Carlsson A, Cederwall E, et al. Annual screening detects celiac disease in children with type 1 diabetes. Pediatr Diabetes, 2008; Vol. 9: pp. 354–9.

Comments: Because celiac disease with 10% prevalence in T1DM, recommended screening at time of diagnosis and yearly for minimum of 2 years.

Smyth DJ, Plagnol V, Walker NM, et al. Shared and distinct genetic variants in type 1 diabetes and celiac disease. NEJM, 2008; Vol. 359: pp. 2767–77.

Comments: T1DM and CD share common alleles (HLA-DR3, HLA-DQ2) and genetic variations, suggestive that the diseases have common pathogenesis.

Holick MF. Vitamin D deficiency. NEJM, 2007; Vol. 357: pp. 266–81.

Comments: Review article highlighting vitamin D metabolism, conditions associated with deficiency, and hypovitaminosis D as potentially causal in other disease states.

Pittas AG, Lau J, Hu FB, et al. The role of vitamin D and calcium in type 2 diabetes. A systematic review and meta-analysis. J Clin Endocrinol Metab, 2007; Vol. 92: pp. 2017–29.

Comments: Calcium and vitamin D as positive mediators of glycemic control, while deficient states associated with progression to metabolic syndrome and T2DM.

Levin A, Bakris GL, Molitch M, et al. Prevalence of abnormal serum vitamin D, PTH, calcium, and phosphorus in patients with chronic kidney disease: results of the study to evaluate early kidney disease. Kidney Int, 2007; Vol. 71: pp. 31–8.

Comments: Vitamin D and other mineral metabolism disrupted at varied levels of GFR.

Pittas AG, Dawson-Hughes B, Li T, et al. Vitamin D and calcium intake in relation to type 2 diabetes in women. Diabetes Care, 2006; Vol. 29: pp. 650–6.

Comments: Prospective Nurse's Health Study showing . 1200 mg calcium and . 800 IU vitamin D intake associated with 33% lower risk of developing T2DM.

Targher G, Bertolini L, Padovani R, et al. Serum 25-hydroxyvitamin D3 concentrations and carotid artery intimamedia thickness among type 2 diabetic patients. Clin Endocrinol (Oxf), 2006; Vol. 65: pp. 593–7.

Comments: Hypovitaminosis D independently associated with increased carotid intima-media thickness in T2DM.

Chiu KC, Chu A, Go VL, et al. Hypovitaminosis D is associated with insulin resistance and beta cell dysfunction. Am J Clin Nutr, 2004; Vol. 79: pp. 820–5.

Comments: 25(OH)D levels inversely associated with visceral and subcutaneous adiposity, the fat mass that contributes to cardiovascular disease.

Hyppönen E, Läärä E, Reunanen A, et al. Intake of vitamin D and risk of type 1 diabetes: a birth-cohort study. Lancet, 2001; Vol. 358: pp. 1500–3.

Comments: Cohort study indicating that vitamin D supplementation following birth could reduce risk of T1DM development.

Taxel P, Kenny A. Differential diagnosis and secondary causes of osteoporosis. Clin Cornerstone, 2000; Vol. 2: pp. 11–21.

Comments: Vitamin D as a component of secondary osteoporosis workup.

Lampasona V, Bonfanti R, Bazzigaluppi E, et al. Antibodies to tissue transglutaminase C in type I diabetes. Diabetologia, 1999; Vol. 42: pp. 1195–8.

Comments: 10% prevalence of CD and 30% anti-tissue transglutaminase antibodies in T1DM; possible that the antibody may arise from pancreatic beta-cell destruction.

内分泌系统

醛固酮减少症

Amin Sabet, MD

概念
- 醛固酮缺乏或抵抗状态,常与高钾血症和轻度非AG增高型代谢性酸中毒有关。
- 在糖尿病肾病患者中与4型肾小管酸中毒(RTA)有关。
- 也可见于糖尿病合并高血压患者应用ACE抑制剂、ARBs或保钾利尿剂治疗时。
- 在某些自身免疫病如1型糖尿病的患者中,可能与原发性肾上腺皮质功能不全有关。

实验室检查
- 血管紧张素I在37℃血浆温育后用放射免疫分析(RIA)可测定血浆肾素活性(PRA)。
- 经RIA或化学发光免疫分析(CLIA)测定血清醛固酮和皮质醇水平。
- 测定血钾、尿钾及血尿渗透压以计算跨肾小管钾浓度梯度(TTKG)。
- TTKG=(尿钾 × 血渗透压)/(血钾 × 尿渗透压)

适应证
- 除外其他明显诱因如急性肾衰竭或严重疾病继发血管内容量大量丢失(如严重充血性心力衰竭、脱水),持续或反复出现高钾血症;而上述情况常加重糖尿病患者的高钾血症。

鉴别诊断
- 醛固酮减少症总体上说有3种病因(低肾素性醛固酮减少症、原发性醛固酮分泌不足、醛固酮抵抗)。
- 低肾素性醛固酮减少症:原因包括糖尿病肾病、慢性间质性肾炎、药物(NSAID、ACE-I、ARB、环孢素)和HIV。
- 原发性醛固酮分泌不足:原因包括原发性肾上腺皮质功能不全(Addison病),先天性肾上腺皮质增生症中的某些类型(CAH,以21羟化酶缺陷症最多见),醛固酮合成酶缺陷症(少见)或使用肝素。
- 醛固酮抵抗:原因包括保钾利尿剂(螺内酯、依普利酮、阿米洛利、氨苯蝶啶),甲氧苄啶,喷他脒,假性醛固酮减少症(少见)。

分析
- 高钾血症时,醛固酮应促进钾离子排出,导致TTKG > 10。
- 高钾血症同时TTKG < 6提示醛固酮减少症(Choi)。应查上游PRA、血清醛固酮及皮质醇水平以进一步分析。
- 低PRA、低醛固酮和正常皮质醇水平提示低肾素性醛固酮减少症。

- 低皮质醇、低醛固酮和高 PRA 水平提示原发性肾上腺皮质功能不全或 CAH。
- 低醛固酮、正常水平皮质醇和高 PRA 符合醛固酮合成酶缺陷症表现（见于反复低血容量、生长发育停滞的婴儿）。
- 高 PRA 和高醛固酮水平提示假性醛固酮减少症。

局限性和难点

- TTKG 在尿钠浓度 < 25mEq/L 时不可信，因为钠离子向肾单位远端转运时可能限制钾离子排出速率。
- TTKG 在尿渗透压 < 血渗透压时亦不可信，因为理想的钾离子排出还需 ADH 参与。

专家建议

- 低肾素性醛固酮减少症是年龄 > 50 岁的糖尿病患者高钾血症的常见原因，可能同时存在轻到中度肾病、应用使高钾加重的药物（如 ACE-I）或急性疾病（如脱水）。
- 因醛固酮减少症导致高钾血症的患者常合并肾功能不全，伴随的容量负荷过多可能在使用盐皮质激素（氟氢可的松）后加重。
- 多数低肾素性醛固酮减少症患者对低钾饮食反应良好，必要时可加用袢利尿剂以促进钾离子排出。

参考文献

Nyirenda MJ, Tang JI, Padfield PL, et al. Hyperkalaemia. BMJ, 2009; Vol. 339: p. b4114.
  Comments: Clinical review of hyperkalemic disorders.

Choi MJ, Ziyadeh FN. The utility of the transtubular potassium gradient in the evaluation of hyperkalemia. J Am Soc Nephrol, 2008; Vol. 19: pp. 424–6.
  Comments: TTKG , 6 indicates impaired aldosterone action as a cause of hyperkalemia.

White PC. Disorders of aldosterone biosynthesis and action. NEJM, 1994; Vol. 331: pp. 250–8.
  Comments: Review of disorders of mineralocorticoid deficiency and resistance including CAH, aldosterone synthase deficiency, and pseudohypoaldosteronism.

Ethier JH, Kamel KS, Magner PO, et al. The transtubular potassium concentration in patients with hypokalemia and hyperkalemia. Am J Kidney Dis, 1990; Vol. 15: pp. 309–15.
  Comments: Defined expected values for TTKG in hypokalemia and hyperkalemia.

West ML, Marsden PA, Richardson RM, et al. New clinical approach to evaluate disorders of potassium excretion. Miner Electrolyte Metab, 1986; Vol. 12: pp. 234–8.
  Comments: Described the use of TTKG in assessing renal mineralocorticoid action.

性激素

Ana Emiliano, MD, and Rita Rastogi Kalyani, MD, MHS

概念

- 睾酮（T）和雌二醇（E2）对不同性别具有不同的重要代谢活性（性别异质性）。
- 性激素结合球蛋白（SHBG）是一种糖蛋白，可以调控有生物活性的性激素水平，多数T和E2在其结合状态下进行循环。
- 在所有T中，54%不稳定结合于白蛋白和其他类型蛋白，44%与SHBG结合，2%未结合（即游离T）（Dunn）。
- 在育龄女性，所有T的三分之一直接由卵巢分泌，而三分之二在外周由雄烯二酮转化而来。
- 雄烯二酮可由卵巢直接分泌，也可在外周由肾上腺分泌的硫酸脱氢表雄酮（DHEA-S）转化而来。
- 男性性腺功能不全（例如前列腺癌的激素去势治疗）与代谢综合征、2型糖尿病有关，且有较多可能患心血管病（Basari）。
- 女性中高雄激素血症[例如多囊卵巢综合征（PCOS）患者]与代谢综合征、2型糖尿病和心血管病有关（Moran）。绝经后女性雄激素水平升高也是2型糖尿病的易患因素（Ding 2006；Kalyani）。
- 男性和绝经后女性自体产生E2增多提示较多可能患2型糖尿病（Ding 2006；Kalyani）。
- 低SHBG在男性和女性中都是2型糖尿病的危险因素之一。

实验室检查

- 总睾酮：多用化学发光免疫分析或放射免疫分析法测定；液相色谱-质谱（LC-MS）为测定的金标准。LC-MS在睾酮浓度低的标本中尤其重要，例如女性和青春期前个体；而免疫分析法在睾酮浓度低的标本中测定不佳（Wang）。
- 有生物活性的睾酮：即可被生物利用、有活性的睾酮；包括游离T和白蛋白结合T，可测定SHBG和白蛋白结合T后计算得出。同时也可直接通过硫酸铵沉淀法测出，该法可使SHBG和SHBG结合T沉淀。
- 游离睾酮：金标准为直接由平衡透析法测定。也可通过总T和SHBG水平计算得出（Vermeulen）。
- 雌二醇：多用化学发光免疫分析或放射免疫分析法测定，但金标准也为LC-MS（Kushnir）。
- SHBG：化学发光免疫分析、放射免疫分析和硫酸铵沉淀法。
- DHEA-S：由肾上腺分泌的生物惰性的类固醇，在外周被转化为雄烯二酮后具有活性，后被转化为睾酮。用化学发光免疫分析、放射免疫分析或LC-MS测定。
- LH和FSH：化学发光免疫分析或放射免疫分析法测定。

性激素

适应证
- 男性性腺功能不全：性功能不全（包括勃起功能障碍）、肌无力、抑郁、认知功能障碍和骨质疏松。测定清晨总T（和游离T），需在两天早晨重复测定。应测 LH 和 FSH 水平以鉴别原发性和继发性性腺功能不全。
- 女性月经周期紊乱：月经不规律或闭经，低生育力和高雄激素血症表现（在疑诊 PCOS 的患者中）。测总 T、DHEA-S、LH、FSH、泌乳素、E2 和甲状腺功能检查。
- 中或重度多毛症：测总 T、游离 T 和 DHEA-S。
- 绝经后状态：测 FSH。

鉴别诊断
- SHBG 升高见于：增龄，甲状腺功能亢进，使用雌激素，慢性炎症状态
- SHBG 减低见于：肥胖，高胰岛素血症（如2型糖尿病），肝脏疾患，雄激素过量，甲状腺功能减退，使用糖皮质激素，肾病综合征。
- T 升高见于：卵巢肿瘤，卵巢滤泡膜细胞增生症，肾上腺皮质腺癌，非经典型先天性肾上腺皮质增生症。
- T 减低见于：增龄，激素去势治疗，2型糖尿病男性（Dhindsa）。
- E2 升高见于：妊娠，卵巢性索间质肿瘤。
- E2 减低见于：绝经，闭经。
- LH 和 FSH 升高见于：原发性性腺功能不全，绝经。
- LH 和 FSH 减低见于：继发性性腺功能不全。
- DHEA-S 升高见于：PCOS，肾上腺皮质腺癌。

分析
- T 或 DHEA-S 升高，FSH/LH 减低：雄激素分泌性肿瘤。
- T 和 DHEA-S 升高，LH/FSH 比值升高：符合 PCOS，但不是诊断该病的必要条件。
- T 减低，FSH/LH 升高：原发性男性性腺功能不全，该病可见于2型糖尿病患者。
- T 减低，FSH/LH 减低：继发性男性性腺功能不全，更多见于2型糖尿病患者。
- E2 减低，FSH/LH 升高：原发性女性性腺功能不全，绝经。
- E2 减低，FSH/LH 减低：继发性女性性腺功能不全。
- E2 升高，FSH/LH 减低：妊娠，卵巢性索间质肿瘤。

局限性和难点
- 检测 T 水平应在早8点左右取标本，因为 T 水平会在日间波动，而最高点出现在清晨。
- 育龄女性 E2 在滤泡早期最低，在月经中期最高。

专家建议
- 在非超重的2型糖尿病个体中，测定总 T（免疫分析或 LC-MS）可较好地用于评价男性性腺功能不全。

- 对超重或肥胖者,考虑男性性腺功能不全时需测定游离T、总T和SHBG。游离T可经平衡透析法及Vermeulen法测定。
- 尽管男性性腺功能不全在2型糖尿病患者中较多见,除非存在症状,总体上不推荐应用雄激素替代治疗,应用时则需个体化。
- 通过测定激素水平评价糖尿病易感性仍是一项正在研究中的课题。

参考文献

Moran LJ, Misso ML, Wild RA, et al. Impaired glucose tolerance, type 2 diabetes and metabolic syndrome in polycystic ovary syndrome: a systematic review and meta-analysis. Hum Reprod Update, 2010; Vol. 16 Supp. 4: pp. 347–63.

Comments: A systematic review and meta-analysis of the literature on prevalence and incidence of impaired glucose tolerance, type 2 diabetes, or metabolic syndrome in women with and without PCOS, concluding that women with PCOS have a higher prevalence of impaired glucose tolerance, type 2 diabetes and metabolic syndrome。

Kalyani RR, Franco M, Dobs AS, et al. The association of endogenous sex hormones, adiposity, and insulin resistance with incident diabetes in postmenopausal women. J Clin Endocrinol Metab, 2009; Vol. 94: pp. 4127–35.

Comments: Prospective study of 1612 postmenopausal women aged 45–84, not taking hormone replacement therapy, which showed that women with higher quartiles of bioavailable T and E2 and lower quartiles of SHBG had a greater risk for developing type 2 diabetes.

Ding EL, Song Y, Manson JE, et al. Sex hormone-binding globulin and risk of type 2 diabetes in women and men. NEJM, 2009; Vol. 361: pp. 1152–63.

Comments: A nested case-control study of postmenopausal women in the Women's Health Study not on hormone therapy showed that a low circulating SHBG is associated with a higher risk of type 2 diabetes in men and women.

Kushnir MM, Rockwood AL, Bergquist J, et al. High-sensitivity tandem mass spectrometry assay for serum estrone and estradiol. Am J Clin Pathol, 2008; Vol. 129: pp. 530–9.

Comments: This study describes the use of a high-sensitivity liquid chromatography-tandem mass spectrometry assay for measurement of E2, showing its superiority over radioimmunoassay and chemiluminescent immunoassay.

Basaria S, Muller DC, Carducci MA, et al. Hyperglycemia and insulin resistance in men with prostate carcinoma who receive androgen-deprivation therapy. Cancer, 2006; Vol. 106: pp. 581–8.

Comments: Cross-sectional study of 18 men with prostate cancer who had received androgen deprivation therapy (ADT), 17 age-matched controls with prostate cancer who had not received ADT, and 18 age-matched healthy controls, showed that men in the ADT group had higher fasting blood glucose, insulin level, and leptin level, and a higher HOMA-IR.

Ding EL, Song Y, Malik VS, et al. Sex differences of endogenous sex hormones and risk of type 2 diabetes: a systematic review and meta-analysis. JAMA, 2006; Vol. 295: pp. 1288–99.

Comments: Systematic review and meta-analysis of 43 prospective and cross-sectional studies, including 6974 women and 6427 men, found that high T levels are associated with an increased risk for type 2 diabetes in females but a lower risk in males; and an inverse correlation between SHBG level and type 2 diabetes risk in males but stronger in females.

Wang C, Catlin DH, Demers LM, et al. Measurement of total serum testosterone in adult men: comparison of current laboratory methods versus liquid chromatography-tandem mass spectrometry. J Clin Endocrinol Metab, 2004; Vol. 89: pp. 534–43.

Comments: The comparison of automated immunoassay instruments, manual immunoassay methods, and liquid chromatography-tandem mass spectrometry (LC-MS) showed that LC-MS had a much greater accuracy and precision, especially in the detection of low levels of T.

Dhindsa S, Prabhakar S, Sethi M, et al. Frequent occurrence of hypogonadotropic hypogonadism in type 2 diabetes. J Clin Endocrinol Metab, 2004; Vol. 89: pp. 5462–8.

Comments: Cross-sectional study that evaluated total T, free T, SHBG, LH, and FSH of 103 male patients with type 2 diabetes, showing that 33% of patients were hypogonadal.

Vermeulen A, Verdonck L, Kaufman JM. A critical evaluation of simple methods for the estimation of free testosterone in serum. J Clin Endocrinol Metab, 1999; Vol. 84: pp. 3666–72.

Comments: Study showing that calculation of free T based on total testosterone and SHBG as determined by immnunoassay is a reliable index of bioavailable T and comparable to free T measured by equilibrium dialysis.

Dunn JF, Nisula BC, Rodbard D. Transport of steroid hormones: binding of 21 endogenous steroids to both testosterone-binding globulin and corticosteroid-binding globulin in human plasma. J Clin Endocrinol Metab, 1981; Vol. 53: pp. 58–68.

Comments: Study describing the plasma distribution of steroid hormones into fractions bound to sex-hormone binding globulin, albumin-bound and unbound under equilibrium conditions using a solid phase method.

消化系统

肝功能

Mariana Lazo, MD, ScM, PhD, and Jeanne M. Clark, MD, MPH

定义
- 多种血清生化检验可以评估肝功能指标以及是否受损。
- 化验指标（1）肝炎：ALT（丙氨酸转氨酶）和 AST（天冬氨酸转氨酶）；（2）胆汁淤积或胆管阻塞：胆红素（包括总胆红素、直接及间接胆红素），ALP（碱性磷酸酶），和 GGT（r-谷氨酰胺转移酶）；（3）合成功能：白蛋白和 PT（凝血酶原时间）。
- 糖尿病患者异常的肝功能大部分源自非酒精性脂肪肝（NAFLD）（见281页）。

测定
- 可以直接使用分光光度计测量血清 ALT、AST、ALP 和胆红素（总胆红素和直接胆红素）。
- PT，即国际标准比值（INR），使用含枸橼酸的取血管抽取全血测定：蓝帽采血管，轻轻混匀。管里须有合适量的血与抗凝剂达到合适的比例。

适应证
- 提示肝脏疾病的症状：黄疸、尿色加深、大便颜色变浅、食欲不振、乏力、呕血、鲜血便或黑便、腹痛或腹胀、无原因的体重下降。
- 提示肝脏疾病的体征：肝大、腹水。
- 用药史：使用过可能造成肝损伤的药物（如 HMG Co-A 还原酶抑制剂、噻唑烷二酮类药物）。
- 曾与病毒性肝炎的患者接触。
- 过量的酒精摄入。
- 合并症：在患有糖尿病、肥胖、高甘油三酯血症、酒精摄入的人更易造成肝损害。
- 患有肝脏疾病的患者监测治疗反应和监测疾病过程。

鉴别诊断
- AST 升高：原发性肝病、急性心肌梗死、肌肉损伤和肌肉病、胰腺炎、胃肠道手术、烧伤、肾梗死和肺栓塞。
- ALT 升高：原发性肝病、胆道梗阻和胰腺炎。
- ALT>AST 病毒性肝炎；AST>ALT 酒精性肝病。
- ALP 升高：胆道梗阻、原发性肝病（与 GGT 变化相平行）、浸润性肝病、骨病、甲状旁腺功能亢进症、甲状腺功能亢进症。
- GGT 升高：胆道梗阻、原发性肝病（与 ALP 变化相平行）、酗酒、胰腺炎。

- 胆红素升高：胆道阻塞、原发性肝病、溶血性贫血、甲状腺功能减退症。
- 药物因肝毒性和胆汁淤积可能造成一项或多项肝脏指标升高 [全部药物见 American Gastroenterological Association（AGA） Technical 的综述]。

解释
- ALT 和 AST 在肝脏中大量存在，AST 同时存在心肌中。
- ALP 几乎在所有组织都存在，尤其是骨骼和肝脏。
- GGT 在肝脏、肾脏、胰腺和肠道中大量存在。
- ALT 和 AST 的正常值在不同的实验室不同，大多数为 <40U/L。
- 轻度 ALT 和 AST 升高 [ALT 和 AST 升高小于 5 倍正常值上限（ULN）]，在进一步检查前应先复查。可能的病因：慢性的乙型或丙型肝炎，急性肝炎，NAFLD，血色病，自身免疫性肝炎，药物性肝损害，酒精性肝损伤，Wilson 病。
- 中度 ALT 和 AST 升高（ALT 和 AST 升高 5~15 倍 ULN）应立即明确病因而不必再确定 ALT 异常是否存在。可能的病因：所有的肝脏疾病均可造成 ALT 和 AST 轻度或重度的升高。
- 重度 ALT 和 AST 升高（ALT 和 AST 升高 >15 倍 ULN）提示严重的急性肝细胞损伤：急性病毒性肝炎，缺血性肝病或其他血管性疾病，毒素介导肝炎，急性自身免疫性肝炎。
- 胆红素是血红素的降解产物，在胆汁中排泄。在分泌前于肝脏结合。
- GGT 升高：酒精性肝损伤。
- ALP 和 GGT 升高：胆道梗阻，原发性胆汁性肝硬化，原发性硬化性胆管炎，良性复发性胆汁淤积，肝浸润性疾病（结节病、淋巴瘤、转移性肿瘤）。
- 仅 ALP 升高（肝外疾病）：骨病、妊娠、慢性肾功能衰竭、淋巴瘤、充血性心衰。
- 高胆红素血症：确定是直接（结合）胆红素还是间接（非结合）胆红素。肝前原因（生成增多，肝摄取降低）导致间接胆红素升高。肝内或肝后原因（肝脏分泌减少）导致直接胆红素升高。生成增加：溶血。肝摄取减少：Gilbert 综合征，5% 的人群发生，为良性。肝脏分泌减少：胆道梗阻，原发性胆汁性肝硬化，原发性硬化性胆管炎，良性复发性胆汁淤积，肝炎，肝硬化，药物使用，败血症，全肠外营养，Dubin-Johnson 综合征，药物使用相关。（全部药物见 AGA Technical 的综述。）
- PT 异常（可继发 INR 异常）和白蛋白水平异常：提示严重的肝脏合成功能障碍和肝硬化进展及肝衰竭的发生。
- 其他常用的评估肝脏疾病病因的检查包括：病毒指标（IgA 甲型肝炎、HBsAg、抗-HBc、IgM 抗-HBc、抗丙型肝炎抗体），自身免疫性指标（ANA、SMA、抗-LKM-1、AMA），遗传性疾病（遗传性血色病：转铁蛋白饱和度，铁蛋白，肝铁指数；Wilson 病：血清铜蓝蛋白，尿铜；α-1-抗胰蛋白酶缺乏症：血清电泳），肝细胞癌指标（AFP：甲胎蛋白）和影像学检查（超声、CT、MRI）。

局限性
- ALT 和 AST 水平与肝纤维化之间无明显的相关性。患有肝硬化的患者 ALT 可能为正常或仅仅轻度升高。
- 溶血可以导致 ALT、AST、ALP 和胆红素明显升高。标本需保存在

0~4℃，1~3 天。
- ALT 和 AST：进行剧烈运动和肌肉损伤时也会升高，进餐对 ALT 和 AST 无影响。
- ALT 在 BMI 升高时也会升高。
- ALP 水平在进食、妊娠和吸烟时也会升高。
- 胆红素水平在空腹时升高。暴露在光线下使胆红素下降。

专家意见

- 患有 2 型糖尿病的患者 (T2DM)，肝脏疾病是导致死亡的一个原因。
- 另外，T2DM 的患者与正常人相比，不仅仅 NAFLD 有更高的发病率和患病率，同时丙型肝炎和肝细胞癌的发病率和患病率也较高。
- 肝脏的指标特异性并不是很高，因为在肝外也存在。
- 肝脏化验检查的正常并不能排除存在肝脏疾病。

推荐依据

Green RM, Flamm S. AGA technical review on the evaluation of liver chemistry tests. Gastroenterology ,2002; Vol.123:pp.1367–84. Available online from the American Gastroenterological Association at http://www. Gastro.org.

Comments: Formal recommendations on how to interpret liver function tests and comprehensive list of medications that may cause liver toxicity or injury.

其他参考文献

Dufour DR, Lott JA, Nolte FS, et al. Diagnosis and monitoring of hepatic injury. I. Performance characteristics of laboratory tests. Clin Chem,2000; Vol. 46: pp. 2027–49.

Comments:Very detailed review of the characteristics of all liver tests, reference values, individual factors influencing their levels. An approved guideline not only by the National Academy of Clinical Biochemistry but also by the American Association for the Study of Liver Diseases.

Dufour DR, Lott JA, Nolte FS, et al. Diagnosis and monitoring of hepatic injury. II. Recommendations for use of laboratory tests in screening, diagnosis, and monitoring. Clin Chem,2000; Vol. 46: pp. 2050–68.

Comments: Detailed review of the different patterns of liver injuries and their laboratory findings. An approved guideline by the National Academy of Clinical Biochemistry.

血糖监测

动态血糖监测

Ari Eckman, MD, and Christopher D. Saudek, MD

定义
- 动态血糖监测（CGM）系统包括感应器、传送器和接收器，可提供实时数据、图、血糖趋势、血糖水平和对患者直接进行血糖的报警。
- 通过自测血糖进行校准，来提示即刻的组织间液血糖，以及全天血糖的高低情况。
- 对组织间液的血糖进行实时的监测，在更换探头前可最多显示5~7天血糖情况。
- 在外部的显示设备或胰岛素泵上显示结果。
- 每5~10分钟报告血糖一次，有些CGM可以每分钟报告血糖。

测定
- 将小巧、灵活的葡萄糖氧化酶探头植入腹部或上臂的皮下，用来测定组织液中的葡萄糖水平。位于皮肤上防水的传送器将葡萄糖通过无线方式传送到接收器，再下载到电脑上，最终生成血糖信息。
- 探头移出后会残留部分膜的聚合物。无其会影响健康的报道，目前还未确定长期会有怎样的影响。
- 目前可用的设备：雅培Free Style Navigator动态血糖仪，DexCom公司的SEVEN Plus动态血糖监测仪，美敦力Guardian Real-Time动态血糖监测仪和MiniMed Paradigm和Revel实时系统。

适应证
- 目前适应证并不明确，应建议血糖不稳定的糖尿病患者进行，以改善血糖控制。
- 对进行强化血糖控制（未）使用胰岛素泵的1型糖尿病患者，用来发现血糖波动和波动原因。
- 可以用于评估存在一些特殊临床情况患者的血糖情况，如妊娠期糖尿病或重症监护室的患者。
- 对于无症状低血糖、反复发作重度低血糖或未发现低血糖的患者非常有用。
- JDRF(Juvenile Diabetes Research Foundation，青少年糖尿病研究基金会)研究发现，儿童和青少年患者使用相对较少，并未发现获益。

解释
- JDRF研究表明6个月内更加频繁的使用CGM与HbA1c的下降相关(Tamborlane)。
- 成人（>25岁）糖尿病患者与儿童和青少年相比，更多的使用CGM。

- 规律的使用 CGM，血糖在目标值 71~180 mg/dl 内的时间更多。
- 使用 CGM 的患者血糖在低血糖和高血糖范围的时间较少，并存在较少发生夜间低血糖（Garg）。
- 指导治疗方案调整的价值：更改餐时推注剂量，调节基础率，调整胰岛素碳水化合物比值等。
- 用于诊断和预防餐后低血糖。

局限性

- 结果没有自我血糖监测准确。平均误差约 15%。
- 毛细血管血糖和组织间液探头测定数据存在达 4~10 分钟的生理性滞后，取决于血糖改变的速率（Boyne）。
- 动态血糖监测不能替代 SMBG，读数异常的高或低应该在 CGM 结果改变之前通过 SMBG 快速检测。
- 在探头植入的部位会出现感染，轻度出血，罕见感染。
- 基于 CGM 的品牌，应该每 3~7 天对探头进行更换，在旧探头移除的同时必须植入新的探头。
- 接收器必须要在探头的 1.5~3 米之内，以保证接受到无线信号。
- 新探头植入后需要进行首次校正，在预热阶段（不同 CGM 仪器设备的预热期在 2~10 小时之间不等）没有数据生成。
- 只有当血糖水平没有快速波动时进行校正，所以在空腹状态或者在餐后 2~3 小时进行校正。
- 对于那些无法掌握操作的人并不是一个好的选择，对存在视觉障碍的人不适用。
- 价格昂贵，在使用 CGM 之前应确认患者可以报销。

专家意见

- 对于那些可以掌握操作的高度自主的糖尿病患者中 CGM 可以帮助加强自我管理。
- 可以更广泛应用于使用胰岛素治疗但血糖控制不佳的患者中。
- 通过增加血糖测量次数，可以提供血糖控制情况的全图。帮助患者调整更适合的胰岛素治疗，饮食和运动方案。
- CGM 在 1 型和 2 型糖尿病患者中对于检测无症状低血糖非常有效。
- 帮助高自主性的患者进行自我管理，直观告诉患者是什么原因（胰岛素剂量、饮食、运动）导致了高血糖和低血糖。
- 对控制每日血糖波动很有价值，但可能并不能改善 HbA1c。

参考文献

Juvenile Diabetes Research Foundation Continuous Glucose Monitoring Study Group. Factors predictive of use and of benefit from continuous glucose monitoring in type 1 diabetes. Diabetes Care, 2009; Vol. 32 Suppl 11: pp. 1947–53.

Comments: Factors associated with greater CGM use was age 25 years and more frequent self-reported prestudy blood glucose meter measurements per day. More frequent CGM use associated with greater reduction in HbA1c after 6 months, in all age groups.

Juvenile Diabetes Research Foundation Continuous Glucose Monitoring Study Group. Sustained benefit of continuous glucose monitoring on HbA1c, glucose profiles, and hypoglycemia in adults with type 1 diabetes. Diabetes Care,2009; Vol. 32 Suppl 11: pp. 2047–9.

Comments: Evaluated long-term effects of CGM in intensively treated adults with type 1 diabetes. CGM use and benefit sustained for 12 months in this population.

Juvenile Diabetes Research Foundation Continuous Glucose Monitoring Study Group. The effect of continuous glucose monitoring in well-controlled type 1 diabetes. Diabetes Care,2009; Vol. 32: pp. 1378–83.

Comments: Study examined CGM benefits for patients with type 1 diabetes who have already achieved HbA1c levels 7.0 %. Most outcomes, including those combining A1c and hypoglycemia, better with CGM group.

Juvenile Diabetes Research Foundation Continuous Glucose Monitoring Study Group, Tamborlane WV, Beck RW, et al. Continuous glucose monitoring and intensive treatment of type 1 diabetes. NEJM,2008; Vol. 359: pp. 1464–76.

Comments: Landmark study evaluating the value of CGM in management of type 1 diabetes mellitus. Results suggested CGM can be associated with lower HbA1c levels in adults with T1DM.

Garg S, Zisser H, Schwartz S, et al. Improvement in glycemic excursions with a transcutaneous, real-time continuous glucose sensor: a randomized controlled trial. Diabetes Care,2006; Vol. 29: pp. 44–50.

Comments: Study revealed patients using CGM spent less time in hypoglycemic and hyperglycemic range, more time at target glucose range, and had less nocturnal hypoglycemia; no difference in A1C levels.

Klonoff DC. Continuous glucose monitoring: roadmap for 21st century diabetes therapy. Diabetes Care, 2005; Vol. 28: pp. 1231–9.

Comments: Real-time recognition of both the absolute magnitude of glycemia and trend patterns provides enormous, useful information to patient.

Tanenberg R, Bode B, Lane W, et al. Use of the Continuous Glucose Monitoring System to guide therapy in patients with insulin-treated diabetes: a randomized controlled trial. Mayo Clin Proc,2004; Vol. 79: pp. 1521–6.

Comments: Study revealed fewer hypoglycemic events per day (1.4 +1.1 vs 1.7 +1.2; p =.30) as well as a shorter duration of the event (49.4 +40.8 minutes per event vs 81.0 +61.1 minutes per event; p =.009) in a group of patients using the CGM as compared to a control group using SMBG.

Chico A, Vidal-Ríos P, Subirà M, et al. The continuous glucose monitoring system is useful for detecting unrecognized hypoglycemias in patients with type 1 and type 2 diabetes but is not better than frequent capillary glucose measurements for improving metabolic control. Diabetes Care,2003; Vol. 26: pp. 1153–7.

Comments: CGM useful for detecting unrecognized hypoglycemias in type 1 and type 2 diabetic subjects, but not better than standard capillary glucose measurements for improving metabolic control of type 1 diabetic subjects.

Boyne MS, Silver DM, Kaplan J, et al. Timing of changes in interstitial and venous blood glucose measured with a continuous subcutaneous glucose sensor. Diabetes,2003; Vol. 52: pp. 2790–4.

Comments: Physiological lag between capillary blood glucose data and interstitial fluid sensor data can be as much as 4–10 minutes, depending on rate of glucose change.

果糖胺，血清 1,5-AG

Vanessa Walker Harris, MD, and Rita Rastogi Kalyani, MD, MHS

定义

- 果糖胺是 1-氨基酸-脱氧果糖的常用名称。
- 果糖胺是血浆中的蛋白质分子（主要是白蛋白）和果糖通过糖基化过程形成的一种酮胺（Armbruster）。
- 由于白蛋白的半衰期是 14~21 天，果糖胺可以反应 2~3 周前的平均血糖水平（Armbruster；Goldstein；Austin；Baker, 1985；Baker, 1984）。
- 1,5-脱水葡萄糖醇（1,5-AG）——葡萄糖的 1-脱氧形式，一种代谢的惰性多醇，主要由小肠从食物和水中吸收的六碳单糖合成。
- 1,5-AG 与葡萄糖在肾脏竞争性重吸收。当葡萄糖浓度升高（>180mg/dl），哪怕时间很短，1,5-AG 都可从尿中排出，使循环的 1,5-AG 水平降低。
- 1,5-AG 水平与血糖快速波动相关，在 24 小时内即可反应（Buse）。
- 日本近十年来已经将测量 1,5-AG 应用于临床评估短期血糖控制情况。

测定

- 果糖胺：第一代测定方法特异性较差，缺乏实验室的标准化，容易受到高血脂的干扰，并不容易校准。
- 但是，第二代检测果糖胺的方法快捷，价格低廉，特异性高，而且解决了尿酸和甘油三酯的干扰（Austin）。
- 果糖胺检测现在常用硝基蓝四氮唑比色法，这种方法可以分离糖化与非糖化的细胞。
- 大量研究表明血浆果糖胺的水平和 HbA1c 高度相关（相关系数，$r=0.76$）。果糖胺和 HbA1c 一样也可以反应血糖水平（Gebhart；Negoro）。
- 果糖胺是否应校正总蛋白或白蛋白目前仍存在争论，目前尚没有被正式推荐的校正方法（Goldstein）。
- 果糖胺测试结果可以当天在门诊由自动检测设备检查（Austin；Goldstein）。
- 1,5-AG：在美国，1,5-AG 可以由 GlycoMark 提供自动商业化检验（Dungan）。
- GlycoMark 检验包含两步酶促法：第一步葡萄糖激酶使葡萄糖转变为葡萄糖-6-磷酸盐从而避免干扰第二步反应；第二步，1,5-AG 被吡喃糖氧化酶氧化，使用过氧化氢比色法检出（Dungan）。
- 血清或血浆样本均可检测果糖胺和 1,5-AG。

适应证

- 与 HbA1c，空腹血糖，或自我血糖监测不同，关于使用果糖胺或 1,5-AG 来作为衡量血糖的辅助方法，目前并没有明确的指南。(Goldstein)。
- 考虑到患者体内的果糖胺和患者在一个月内来看病。因为白蛋白和其他血清蛋白的半衰期短于血红蛋白，故果糖胺水平比 HbA1c 改变更快。果糖胺可以被看做是中期血糖控制的指标（Armbruster）。
- 患有血红蛋白病的患者可以考虑检测果糖胺（如地中海贫血或血红蛋白变异），因这些疾病可能导致 HbA1c 出现假性的升高或降低(Saudek)。

- 患有可能造成红细胞寿命改变或会导致 HbA1c 出现假性升高或降低疾病（如肾病，肝病，溶血性贫血，HIV，缺铁性贫血，再生障碍性贫血）的患者，可考虑检测果糖胺 (Saudek)。
- 果糖胺可能对评估孕妇短期血糖状况的改变有益。
- 与空腹血糖相比，果糖胺和 1,5-AG 与餐后血糖更具相关性 (Herdzik; Dungan)，对疑有餐后高血糖的患者可能更为有益。
- 当监测每日血糖改变 (Yamanouchi)，或作为自我血糖监测的辅助手段来确定稳定的血糖控制时 (Buse) 1,5-AG 可能是最有帮助的手段。
- 1,5-AG 可能比 HbA1c 和果糖胺在检测接近正常的血糖和血糖波动方面更有优势。

鉴别诊断
- 高果糖胺：提示之前的 2~3 周存在高血糖，同时自我血糖监测和 / 或空腹或随机血糖检测也提示高血糖。
- 低果糖胺：肝功能不全导致的低白蛋白血症和 / 或低蛋白血症，蛋白丢失性肠病或肾病综合征 (Armbruster; Austin)。
- 低 1,5-AG：之前的 24 小时内出现高血糖。
- 低血糖对 1,5-AG 影响不大，并且 1,5-AG 可以更好的区分那些 HbA1c 水平相似，但血糖波动不同的患者。

解释
- 果糖胺水平取决于患者的年龄和性别。
- 通常情况下果糖胺水平正常值为 <265μmol/L，>350μmol/L(大约相当于 HbA1c7.5%~8.0%) 时则认为血糖控制不佳。
- 果糖胺水平随时间的变化趋势可能比绝对值更为重要。
- 正常 1,5-AG 浓度：女性 6.8~29.3 mcg/ml，男性 10.7~32.0 mcg/ml (Dungan)。
- 糖尿病患者的果糖胺也与微血管病变的发生相关 (Selvin)。

局限性
- 血清果糖胺水平是否需要校正蛋白和 / 或白蛋白目前仍不明确。
- 血清果糖胺的变化比 HbA1c 明显，这就意味着果糖胺水平在可以检测到显著变化前就已大幅改变 (Howey)。
- 家庭果糖胺检测的临床有效性研究产生了不同的结果。一项研究发现 HbA1c 能更好的预测前 2 周的平均血糖。此外，当作为家庭血糖监测的辅助方法，每周测定果糖胺并未改善 HbA1c 水平 (Saudek; Goldstein)。
- 高果糖胺可以导致高水平的糖化免疫球蛋白，尤其是 IgA。
- 与 HbA1c 相似，果糖胺和 1,5-AG 在肾病时使用受限 (Chen)。
- 1,5-AG 在妊娠期糖尿病患者中临床效果有限 (Buse)。
- 中药远志含有一种天然的 1,5-AG，会人为增加 1,5-AG 水平。

专家意见
- 很多研究建议，在大量应用血清果糖胺前，应谨慎解释其意义。

- 在就诊前一周或两周内，患者增加其依从性，就可以改善其果糖胺水平 (Goldstein)。
- 血清果糖胺作为血糖控制的临床中期有效指标，目前仍存在争议。也许应用于特定亚群的糖尿病患者是较好的选择，如患有血红蛋白病或红细胞寿命异常的患者，因其HbA1c并不能完全反映血糖情况。
- 对监测门诊的糖尿病患者，果糖胺也许特别适用，至少可作为其他血糖测定方法的有益补充。
- 果糖胺测定价格低廉并且测定方便，在发展中国家可以作为一种可供选择的替代HbA1c的方法。
- 1,5-AG可作为自我血糖监测的辅助，反应血水平的每日变化。

参考文献

Selvin E, Francis LM, Ballantyne CM, et al. Nontraditional markers of glycemia: associations with microvascular conditions. Diabetes Care, 2011; Vol. 34: pp. 960–7.
Comments: This study examined the association of fructosamine, glycated albumin, and 1,5-AG versus standard glycemic markers with risk of microvascular conditions associated with diabetes. Fructosamine and glycated albumin were as or more strongly associated with microvascular conditions as HbA1c.

Chen HS, Wu TE, Lin HD, et al. Hemoglobin A(1c) and fructosamine for assessing glycemic control in diabetic patients with CKD stages 3 and 4. Am J Kidney Dis, 2010; Vol. 55: pp. 867–74.
Comments: This study suggests that estimated average glucose calculated from HbA1c and fructosamine underestimates mean blood glucose in patients with CKD stages 3–4.

Dungan KM. 1,5-anhydroglucitol (GlycoMark) as a marker of short-term glycemic control and glycemic excursions. Expert Rev Mol Diagn, 2008; Vol. 8: pp. 9–19.
Comments: Comprehensive review of 1,5-AG as a marker of short-term glycemia.

Saudek CD, Derr RL, Kalyani RR. Assessing glycemia in diabetes using self-monitoring blood glucose and hemoglobin A1c. JAMA, 2006; Vol. 295: pp. 1688–97.
Comments: Literature review assessing the evidence underlying the use of self-monitored blood glucose and hemoglobin A1c.

Dungan KM, Buse JB, Largay J, et al. 1,5-anhydroglucitol and postprandial hyperglycemia as measured by continuous glucose monitoring system in moderately controlled patients with diabetes. Diabetes Care, 2006; Vol. 29: pp. 1214–9.
Comments: Describes utility of 1,5-AG in assessing postprandial hyperglycemia in patients with diabetes.

Goldstein DE, Little RR, Lorenz RA, et al. Tests of glycemia in diabetes. Diabetes Care, 2004; Vol. 27: pp. 1761–73.
Comments: Technical review of the tests most widely used in monitoring blood glucose control by the National Academy of Clinical Biochemistry and published as a position statement by the American Diabetes Association.

Buse JB, Freeman JL, Edelman SV, et al. Serum 1,5-anhydroglucitol (GlycoMark): a short-term glycemic marker. Diabetes Technol Ther, 2003; Vol. 5: pp. 355–63.
Comments: Describes clinical utility of 1,5-AG.

Herdzik E, Safranow K, Ciechanowski K. Diagnostic value of fasting capillary glucose, fructosamine and glycosylated haemoglobin in detecting diabetes and other glucose tolerance abnormalities compared to oral glucose tolerance test. Acta Diabetol,2002; Vol. 39: pp. 15–22.

Comments: This study found that fructosamine correlated better with 2h-post-load glucose than fasting glucose values.

Austin GE, Wheaton R, Nanes MS, et al. Usefulness of fructosamine for monitoring outpatients with diabetes.Am J Med Sci, 1999; Vol. 318: pp. 316–23.

Comments: Prospective case-control study evaluating impact of same-day serum fructosamine levels on clinical decision making.

Yamanouchi T, Akanuma Y. Serum 1,5-anhydroglucitol (1,5 AG): new clinical marker for glycemic control. Diabetes Res Clin Pract,1994; Vol. 24 Suppl: pp. S261–8.

Comments Good review of 1,5-AG.

Gebhart SS, Wheaton RN, Mullins RE, et al. A comparison of home glucose monitoring with determinations of hemoglobin A1c, total glycated hemoglobin, fructosamine, and random serum glucose in diabetic patients. Arch Intern Med, 1991; Vol. 151: pp. 1133–7.

Comments Study comparing four objective measures of glycemic control with home glucose monitoring in diabetic patients.

Howey JE, Bennet WM, Browning MC, et al. Clinical utility of assays of glycosylated haemoglobin and serum fructosamine compared: use of data on biological variation. Diabet Med,1989; Vol. 6: pp. 793–6.

Comments Describes the relative variation of HbA1c and fructosamine with changes in glycemia.

Negoro H, Morley JE, Rosenthal MJ. Utility of serum fructosamine as a measure of glycemia in young and old diabetic and non-diabetic subjects. Am J Med,1988; Vol. 85: pp. 360–4.

Comments Comparison of fructosamine levels with other measures of glycemia in young and old diabetic and nondiabetic subjects.

Armbruster DA. Fructosamine: structure, analysis, and clinical usefulness. Clin Chem, 1987; Vol. 33: pp. 2153–63.

Comments Details the mechanisms, usefulness, and limitations of available fructosamine assays.

Baker JR, Metcalf PA, Holdaway IM, et al. Serum fructosamine concentration as measure of blood glucose control in type I (insulin-dependent) diabetes mellitus. BMJ (Clin Res Ed), 1985; Vol. 290: pp. 352–5.

Comments Evaluation of fructosamine as a measure of glycemia in type 1 diabetics.

Baker JR, Johnson RN, Scott DJ. Serum fructosamine concentrations in patients with type II (non-insulin-dependent) diabetes mellitus during changes in management. BMJ (Clin Res Ed),1984; Vol. 288: pp. 1484–6.

Comments: Prospective study evaluating usefulness of fructosamine in monitoring metabolic control in noninsulin-dependent diabetics during changes in management.

糖化血红蛋白

Christopher D. Saudek, MD

定义

- 糖化血红蛋白（HbA1c）是糖稳定结合在血红蛋白的 β 链上形成的加合物 [N-（1-脱氧果糖）血红蛋白]。
- 当血红蛋白暴露在葡萄糖环境中，进行不可逆、翻译后、非酶催化的反应所形成。
- 替代词：A1c（一般用于和患者交流时），糖化的血红蛋白（最准确的术语），糖基化血红蛋白。
- 通常表示为糖基化血红蛋白的比例（或者表示为每摩尔总血红蛋白中毫摩尔糖基化的血红蛋白）。
- 是糖尿病患者最佳的监测血糖控制情况的指标(Saudek，2006)。
- 虽与近期血糖水平所占的权重不同，但可以反应之前 3 个月的平均血糖水平(Tahara)。
- 对发生糖尿病慢性合并症是非常有效的指标，尤其对视网膜病变、神经病变和肾病(DCCT)。
- 虽然血糖水平对发生 CVD 的风险没有血脂、血压和吸烟的高，但 HbA1c 也是发生心血管（CVD）疾病风险的指标(Selvin)。
- 目前 HbA1c>6.5% 已经作为诊断糖尿病的指标（国际专家委员会； 美国糖尿病协会；Saudek，2008）。

测定

- 有很多特异性的方法，根据电荷分类 [阳离子交换高效液相色谱法（HPLC）、电泳法等电聚焦法]，根据结构分类 [硼酸亲和层析法、免疫测定] 或化学分析（质谱法）。美国最常用的方法是 HPLC 和免疫测定法。
- 医院或商用的实验室需要通过美国国家糖化血红蛋白标准化计划(NGSP)进行标准化，这是一项严格的质控系统。
- 即时检测（POC）器材适用于临床和行政部门，需要标准化和质量控制，通常用于糖尿病筛查系统(LentersWestra)。
- 一般说来，POC 和 HbA1c 有很好的相关性。但 18% 实验室检测 HbA1c ≥ 7% 的糖尿病患者没有被 POC 检测到 (Schwartz)。
- 因缺乏质控，并不推荐家用的检测试剂盒。

适应证

- 建议用于所有糖尿病患者血糖情况的监测。
- 建议每 3~6 个月检测一次，如果治疗方案更改频繁可以增加检测次数。
- 可以用于糖尿病高危人群进行糖尿病筛查和诊断（国际专家委员会）。

解释

- 与最近 3 个月的平均血糖直接相关。

- 正常（非糖尿病）范围是 4%~6%；目前的标准建议 A1c 5.7%~6.4% 的个体是发生糖尿病的高危人群（国际专家委员会）。
- 建议对于绝大多数糖尿病患者，A1c 目标为 <6.5%~7%，根据不同的临床情况确定不同的治疗目标。
- A1c 超过 8% 则认为血糖控制差，超过 10% 则血糖控制非常差。
- 表 5-1 描述了 A1c 和平均血糖的关系。
- A1c 与估测平均血糖的公式（eAG）：eAG（mg/dl）=28.7×A1c - 46.7；eAG（mmol/L）=1.59×A1c - 2.59。
- 需要警惕混杂因素（见局限性章节，延伸阅读见 NGSP 网页）。
- 作为平均血糖水平的指标，A1c 不受血糖的变异度影响（Derr）。

更多

表 5-1. A1c 与估测平均血糖的关系 *

HbA1c（%）	eAG（平均血糖）	
	(mmol/L)	(mg/dl)
5	5.4 (4.2~6.7)	97 (76~120)
6	7.0 (5.5~8.5)	126 (100~152)
7	8.6 (6.8~10.3)	154 (123~185)
8	10.2 (8.1~12.1)	183 (147~217)
9	11.8 (9.4~13.9)	212 (170~249)
10	13.4 (10.7~15.7)	240 (193~282)
11	14.9 (12.0~17.5)	269 (217~314)
12	16.5 (13.3~19.3)	298 (240~347)

* 括号里的数据是 95%CI

来源：Nathan DM, Kuenen J, Borg R, et al. Translating the A1C assay into estimated average glucose values. Diabetes Care, 2008; Vol. 31(8:) pp. 1473-8. Epub 2008 Jun 7. Reproduced with permission of The American Diabetes Association.

局限性

- 任何降低红细胞生存时间（如溶血性贫血）在不影响血糖的情况下降低 A1c。
- 相反的，任何升高红细胞生存时间的情况（如再生障碍性贫血）在不影响血糖的情况下升高 A1c。
- 异常血红蛋白病在一些化验中干扰 A1c。
- 完整的影响因素见分析方法，NGSP 网址 (http://www.ngsp.org/interf.asp)。

专家意见

- 甚至在异常血红蛋白病时，如果红细胞生存时间正常，测定 A1c 是最常用有效反映血糖情况的指标。
- 实验室质量控制非常重要。

- A1c 是临床上最常用的提示何时需要强化控制血糖的指标。
- 并不建议 A1c 用于评估妊娠期血糖情况，因为 A1c 变化较慢。妊娠期，血糖控制应尽快达标。
- 目前使用 A1c 确诊糖尿病仍处于初期并存在争议。是否把其作为诊断标准应根据种族/民族情况决定。
- ADA 在 2007 年发表声明建议全球使用国际临床化学联合会（IFCC）提出的新的质谱法用于 A1c 的标准化；同时建议实验室以传统的 % 形式报告结果，也可以使用 mmol/mol。
- 尽管 ADA 在 2007 年发表了声明，大多数临床医生仍以 % 形式报告结果。

推荐依据

American Diabetes Association. Standards of medical care in diabetes—2011. Diabetes Care, 2011; Vol. 34 Suppl 1: pp. S11–61.

Comments.Most recent summary of the standards of medical care in diabetes from the American Diabetes

Association including recommendations for annual measurement of renal function. International Expert Committee. International Expert Committee report on the role of the A1C assay in the diagnosis of diabetes. Diabetes Care, 2009; Vol. 32: pp. 1327–34.

Comments: An expert committee report recommending the use of hemoglobin A1c be the preferred method of diagnosing diabetes.

其他参考文献

National Glycohemoglobin Standardization Program. HbA1c methods and Hemoglobin Variants (HbS, HbC, HbE and HbD traits). http://www.ngsp.org/prog/index3.html,Updated 2/2010, accessed 3/16/2011.

Comments: National Glycohemoglobin Standardization Program website, providing comprehensive list of factors that interfere with HbA1c by measurement method.

Lenters-Westra E, Slingerland RJ. Six of eight hemoglobin A1c point-of-care instruments do not meet the general accepted analytical performance criteria. Clin Chem,2010; Vol. 56: pp. 44–52.

Comments:A careful comparison of 8 different point-of-care devices used to measure HbA1c. Valuable information in choosing POC equipment.

Schwartz KL, Monsur J, Hammad A, et al. Comparison of point of care and laboratory HbA1c analysis: a MetroNet study. J Am Board Fam Med,2009; Vol. 22: pp. 461–3.

Comments: In five clinical practices which performed paired point-of-care and laboratory A1c tests on 99 samples, correlation was good (coefficient =0.88) but 18% of individuals with A1c 7% using laboratory assays missed by point-of-care testing.

Nathan DM, Kuenen J, Borg R, et al. Translating the A1C assay into estimated average glucose values. Diabetes Care,2008; Vol. 31: pp. 1473–8.

Comments:A discussion of the various options for reporting results of HbA1c.

Saudek CD, Herman WH, Sacks DB, et al. A new look at screening and diagnosing diabetes mellitus. J Clin Endocrinol Metab,2008; Vol 93: pp. 2447–53.

Comments:Results of a consensus panel, reviewing the rationale for use of hemoglobin A1c in screening and diagnosing diabetes.

American Diabetes Association, European Association for the Study of Diabetes, International Federation of Clinical Chemistry and Laboratory Medicine, and the

International Diabetes Federation. Consensus Committee statement on the worldwide standardization of the hemoglobin A1C measurement. Diabetes Care,2007; Vol. 30: pp. 2399–400.
Comments:Consensus statement on use of IFCC reference method to standardize A1c assay.

Saudek CD, Derr RL, Kalyani RR. Assessing glycemia in diabetes using self-monitoring blood glucose and hemoglobin A1c. JAMA,2006; Vol. 295: pp. 1688–97.
Comments:A review of the use of hemoglobin A1c and self-monitoring in clinical diabetes care.

Sacks DB, ADA/EASD/IDF Working Group of the HbA1c Assay Global harmonization of hemoglobin A1c. Clin Chem,2005; Vol. 51: pp. 681–3.
Comments:Discusses the issue of hemoglobin A1c being reported in various ways: using conventional DCCTvalidated units (% of total hemoglobin), as Average Blood Glucose, or as mmol/mol hemoglobin.

Selvin E, Marinopoulos S, Berkenblit G, et al. Meta-analysis: glycosylated hemoglobin and cardiovascular disease in diabetes mellitus. Ann Intern Med,2004; Vol. 141: pp. 421–31.
Comments:A meta-analysis describing the statistically significant association between hemoglobin A1c and macrovascular (cardiovascular) disease.

Derr R, Garrett E, Stacy GA, et al. Is HbA(1c) affected by glycemic instability? Diabetes Care,2003; Vol. 26: pp. 2728–33.
Comments:A demonstration that hemoglobin A1c reflects average, not variability, of blood glucose.

UK Prospective Diabetes Study (UKPDS) Group. Intensive blood-glucose control with sulphonylureas or insulin compared with conventional treatment and risk of complications in patients with type 2 diabetes (UKPDS 33). Lancet,1998; Vol. 352: pp. 837–53.
Comments:The UKPDS description of the relationship between intensive glycemic control and complication
risk in type 2 diabetes. One of many UKPDS publications.

The Diabetes Control and Complications Trial Research Group. Hypoglycemia in the Diabetes Control and Complications Trial. Diabetes,1997; Vol. 46: pp. 271–86.
Comments:The DCCT description of adverse effect of intensive blood glucose control: the increase in hypoglycemic events as hemoglobin A1c is lowered.

Tahara Y, Shima K. Kinetics of HbA1c, glycated albumin, and fructosamine and analysis of their weight functions against preceding plasma glucose level. Diabetes Care,1995; Vol. 18: pp. 440–7.
Comments:A study of the kinetics of hemoglobin glycation, indicating that about 50% of the value of HbA1c is determined by the previous 30 days'glycemia.

The Diabetes Control and Complications Trial Research Group (DCCT). The effect of intensive treatment of diabetes on the development and progression of long-term complications in insulin-dependent diabetes mellitus. NEJM,1993; Vol. 329: pp. 977–86.
Comments:The main DCCT article describing the relationship of intensive glycemic control, as assessed by hemoglobin A1c, to microvascular complications (retinopathy, nephropathy, and neuropathy) in type 1 diabetes. One of many DCCT publications.

Koenig RJ, Peterson CM, Jones RL, et al. Correlation of glucose regulation and hemoglobin Alc in diabetes mellitus. NEJM,1976; Vol. 295: pp. 417–20.
Comments:An early description of the relationship between hemoglobin A1c and blood glucose.

自我血糖监测

Christopher D. Saudek, MD

定义
- 自我血糖监测(SMBG)是指患者将自己的一滴指血滴于试纸条测定血糖。
- 血糖水平的数值即刻显示在仪器上。
- 血糖仪和试纸条千差万别,有各自的缺点和长处。
- 尽管有些仪器可以通过测定其他部位如前臂的血,但通常取手指血进行测定。
- 测定的结果与日期、时间一同储存在血糖仪里,并可通过软件下载;一些血糖仪可以在胰岛素泵上显示血糖值("smart pumps")。

化验
- 葡萄糖氧化酶或葡萄糖脱氢酶提前置于试纸条上,通过测定过氧化氢或电子生成来测定血糖。
- 精确度依赖于技术,理想状况是 ±10%,与实验室测定值相比,精确度一般在 ±10%~15%。
- 虽测定的是全血样本,但大多数血糖仪校正显示为血浆血糖值。
- SMBG 不如实验室测定的血浆血糖精确,但其可以在家重复测定,因此更加实用。
- 试纸条必须很好地包装和储存,一些血糖仪需要输入试纸条瓶上的编码。

适应证
- 医师一致认为 1 型糖尿病患者应规律和频繁地进行自我血糖监测(如一天几次)。
- 对胰岛素依赖的糖尿病患者,不论是 1 型(T1DM)或是 2 型(T2DM)糖尿病,证据显示规律 SMBG 可以使其获益(Soumerai)。
- 对非胰岛素依赖的 2 型糖尿病患者,SMBG 的成本效益分析存在一些争议,如果持续较长时间进行 SMBG 可能更加有效(Tunis)。
- 非胰岛素依赖的 2 型糖尿病患者,一项 meta 分析显示可以适当(-0.16%)改善 A1c(St. John)。

解释
- 医疗保健专业人员必须评估 SMBG 的结果并对患者进行反馈。
- 患者必须理解结果的意义,并知道如何处理高血糖或低血糖。
- 下载结果并以图形显示,可以非常容易的对结果进行解释。
- SMBG 可以明确一些症状是否因高血糖或低血糖造成,而且可以了解更改的治疗方案是否有效。
- 是否或何时进行餐前或餐后的 SMBG 更加有效,目前仍存在争议。

局限性
- 使用者操作失误是最常见导致精确度严重下降的原因(Bergenstal)。
- 试纸条在购买时应检验是否有效,不正确地在一些极端的温度或湿度条件下储存时可能会失效。

- 在血糖过低（<50mg/dl）或过高（>300mg/dl）时准确度虽会下降，但在这些情况下准确度也是可以满足需要的。
- 保证准确度同时需要测定的手是清洁、干燥的且没有接触糖类，并要保证测定的血标本体积充足。
- 许多血糖仪需要将试纸条瓶上的编码输入仪器进行校准。
- 很少有干扰血糖值测定的情况出现。葡萄糖氧化酶试纸条可能受到大剂量的对乙酰氨基酚、水杨酸、抗坏血酸或低氧干扰测定。葡萄糖脱氢酶试纸条可能受患者腹透时用到的麦芽糖或半乳糖所干扰。

专家意见

- 只有测定的血糖值用来进行治疗方案更改时，规律进行 SMBG 才能帮助糖尿病患者进行自我管理。
- SMBG 使患者参与到自我管理中，并知道何时血糖水平是高或低。
- 鼓励 1 型糖尿病患者每天至少测定 2~4 次血糖。
- 对 2 型糖尿病患者，我们建议 SMBG 在血糖不稳定和治疗方案更改时进行。
- 尤其建议 2 型糖尿病患者当 A1c 明显升高，或治疗方案更改时进行 SMBG。
- 我们通常建议餐前和睡前进行检测，除非怀疑存在孤立性餐后高血糖。
- 一天中不同时间的血糖数据只对比有相同时间的血糖值更有意义。
- 强烈建议对已下载的血糖仪中的数据进行回顾，可以显示全面数据（如平均血糖和血糖标准差；每天检测血糖的次数；每天、每周、每月血糖变化的情况；严重高或低血糖发生的频率和时间）。
- 当 SMBG 与 A1c 水平不匹配，则需考虑存在的干扰因素和进行更加频繁的监测（包括餐后血糖和夜间血糖测定）或者进行动态血糖监测。

参考文献

St John A, Davis WA, Price CP, et al. The value of self-monitoring of blood glucose: a review of recent evidence. J Diabetes Complications,2010; Vol. 24: pp. 129–141.

Comments:Meta-analysis and review of SMBG in type 2 diabetes, finding SMBG-related decrease in hemoglobin A1c.

Neeser K, Weber C. Cost impact of self-measurement of blood glucose on complications of type 2 diabetes: the Spanish perspective. Diabetes Technol Ther,2009; Vol. 11: pp. 509–16.

Comments:A Spanish study showing cost savings in the use of SMBG.

Murata GH, Duckworth WC, Shah JH, et al. Blood glucose monitoring is associated with better glycemic control in type 2 diabetes: a database study. J Gen Intern Med,2009; Vol. 24: pp. 48–52.

Comments:Increasing use of SMBG along with intensification of treatment was associated with better glycemic control.

Towfigh A, Romanova M, Weinreb JE, et al. Self-monitoring of blood glucose levels in patients with type 2 diabetes mellitus not taking insulin: a meta-analysis. Am J Manag Care,2008; Vol. 14: pp. 468–75.

Comments: A recent meta-analysis of SMBG in non-insulin-requiring type 2 diabetes; found small benefit but such studies are hard to interpret because people with more unstable or worse glycemic control tend to monitor more often.

Simon J, Gray A, Clarke P, et al. Cost effectiveness of self monitoring of blood glucose in patients with non-insulin treated type 2 diabetes: economic evaluation of data from the DiGEM trial. BMJ,2008; Vol. 336: pp. 1177–80.

Comments: A health economics group evaluated cost benefit of SMBG in non-insulin-treated type 2 diabetes, found no benefit.

Kristensen GB, Monsen G, Skeie S, et al. Standardized evaluation of nine instruments for self-monitoring of blood glucose. Diabetes Technol Ther,2008; Vol. 10: pp. 467–77.

Comments: Evaluation of 9 meters, showing improvement in recent years but still the need for using an evaluation protocol.

SMBG International Working Group. Self-monitoring of blood glucose in type 2 diabetes: an inter-country comparison. Diabetes Res Clin Pract,2008; Vol. 82: pp. e15–8.

Comments: A multinational study, finding unexpectedly high use of SMBG in non-insulin-treated diabetes.

Tunis SL, Minshall ME. Self-monitoring of blood glucose in type 2 diabetes: cost-effectiveness in the United States. Am J Manag Care,2008; Vol. 14: pp. 131–40.

Comments: Positive cost effectiveness of SMBG, especially over a longer (10-year) time frame.

Farmer A, Wade A, Goyder E, et al. Impact of self monitoring of blood glucose in the management of patients with non-insulin treated diabetes: open parallel group randomised trial. BMJ,2007; Vol. 335: p. 132.

Comments: Randomized trial, no improvement with SMBG in non-insulin-treated type 2 diabetes.

Saudek CD, Derr RL, Kalyani RR. Assessing glycemia in diabetes using self-monitoring blood glucose and hemoglobin A1c. JAMA,2006; Vol. 295: pp. 1688–97.

Comments: Review of the use of SMBG and hemoglobin A1c.

Diabetes Research in Children Network (Direcnet) Study Group, Buckingham BA, Kollman C, et al. Evaluation of factors affecting CGMS calibration. Diabetes Technol Ther,2006; Vol. 8: pp. 318–25.

Comments: A detailed study of calibration approaches.

Moreland EC, Volkening LK, Lawlor MT, et al. Use of a blood glucose monitoring manual to enhance monitoring adherence in adults with diabetes: a randomized controlled trial. Arch Intern Med,2006; Vol. 166: pp. 689–95.

Comments: Joslin Diabetes Center randomized clinical trial of SMBG in type 1 diabetes, discusses use of their manual.

Davidson MB, Castellanos M, Kain D, et al. The effect of self monitoring of blood glucose concentrations on glycated hemoglobin levels in diabetic patients not taking insulin: a blinded, randomized trial. Am J Med,2005; Vol. 118: pp. 422–5.

Comments: Randomized trial of SMBG in a large inner-city diabetes center, found no benefit to its use.

Soumerai SB, Mah C, Zhang F, et al. Effects of health maintenance organization coverage of self-monitoring devices on diabetes self-care and glycemic control. Arch Intern Med,2004; Vol. 164: pp. 645–52.

Comments: Evaluation of policy that provided SMBG equipment and instruction for insulin-treated diabetes. Use of SMBG reduced HbA1c by 0.63%.

Bellazzi R, Arcelloni M, Bensa G, et al. Design, methods, and evaluation directions of a multi-access service for the management of diabetes mellitus patients. Diabetes Technol Ther,2003; Vol. 5: pp. 621–9.

Comments: A multicenter trial of alternate site testing.

Bergenstal R, Pearson J, Cembrowski GS, et al. Identifying variables associated with inaccurate self-monitoring of blood glucose: proposed guidelines to improve accuracy. Diabetes Educ,2002; Vol. 26: pp. 981–9.

Comments: Demonstrated that various errors in user technique are common and correctable by good education.

血液系统

贫血

Nisa M. Maruthur, MD, MHS

定义
- 男性血红蛋白 <13g/dl，女性 <12g/dl(WHO 标准)。
- 糖尿病患者出现贫血最常见的原因是慢性肾脏病造成的贫血。

测定
- 全血细胞计数及分类（包括平均红细胞）：电阻抗。
- 网织红细胞计数：流式细胞仪。
- 外周血涂片：光镜。
- 其他实验室检测：基础代谢法来评估肾小球滤过率。

适应证
- 贫血的症状：疲劳，乏力，头晕，气短，胸痛，四肢末梢寒冷。
- 存在糖尿病肾病。
- 存在出血的情况，常见月经出血及胃肠道出血（呕血、便血或黑便）。
- 限制饮食（如素食）。
- 糖化血红蛋白(反应血糖水平)比预期的偏低时提示可能存在溶血性贫血。
- 缺铁性贫血与糖化血红蛋白升高存在相关性，但并没有显著影响糖尿病患者的 HbA1c 水平 (Ford)。

鉴别诊断
- 慢性肾脏病。
- 营养缺乏（如维生素 B_{12} 和叶酸）。
- 炎症（"慢性病贫血"）包括急性感染、肿瘤、自身免疫性疾病。
- 出血（如胃肠道）或吸收不良（如腹腔疾病）引起的铁缺乏。
- 骨髓疾病。
- 获得性溶血性贫血（如药物诱发）。
- 血红蛋白病（如地中海贫血、镰状细胞性贫血）。
- 其他：甲状腺疾病、肝脏疾病、HIV 感染。

解释
- 小细胞性贫血：平均红细胞体积减低，红细胞宽度增加提示缺铁性贫血。平均红细胞体积减低，红细胞宽度正常提示地中海贫血。
- 大细胞性贫血：平均红细胞体积增加提示维生素 B_{12} 缺乏、叶酸缺乏、甲状腺功能减退、酗酒或肝脏疾病。
- 正常细胞性贫血：平均红细胞体积正常提示慢性肾脏病、炎症性贫血、

贫血

镰状细胞性贫血或者骨髓病变。
- 铁相关检查、网织红细胞计数、外周血涂片可以用来评估铁缺乏、炎症性贫血和骨髓疾病。
- 贫血严重程度分级见表5-2。

更多

表5-2. 贫血严重程度

严重度	Hb范围（g/dl）	症状	医疗
轻度	9.5~13.0	通常无症状及体征	通常未经治疗
中度	8.0~9.5	可能存在症状	需要通过治疗来减少并发症出现
重度	<8.0	通常有症状	可能是危及生命的，需要立刻处理

来源：Elsevier Oncology. The Elsevier Guide to Oncology Drugs & Regimens. New York: Elsevier Health; 2006. Reprinted with permission of Elsevier.

局限性
- 脱水可以掩盖贫血。
- 近期输血会影响红细胞指标和外周血涂片的结果。
- 缺铁性贫血与HbA1c升高有关。
- 高血红蛋白浓度与HbA1c升高相关(Ford)。

专家意见
- 溶血性贫血（如红细胞寿命缩短）可以与HbA1c假性降低有关。
- 长期使用二甲双胍治疗的巨幼红细胞性贫血患者，应考虑存在维生素B_{12}缺乏。
- 当肾小球滤过率<60 ml/(min·1.73m^2)时需定期（肾功能下降时至少每年检查）检测全血细胞分析。
- 目前对于贫血时何时输血并没有太多的临床数据。
- 一般来讲，促红素治疗只应用于慢性肾脏病的肾性贫血中（维持血红蛋白11~12g/dl）。

参考文献

American Diabetes Association. Standards of medical care in diabetes—2011. Diabetes Care, 2011; Vol.34 Suppl 1:pp. S11–61.
   Comments:American Diabetes Association report on general standards of diabetes care, which suggests the potential for HbA1c to be misleading in the presence of anemia or chronic kidney disease.
Ford ES, Cowie CC, Li C, et al. Iron-deficiency anemia, non-iron-deficiency anemia and HbA1c among adults in the US.J Diabetes,2011; Vol. 3: pp. 67–73.
   Comments:This cross-sectional national study found higher mean adjusted HbA1c

in persons with iron deficiency versus those without (5.56% vs. 5.46%; p=0.095). Higher hemoglobin concentration was also associated with higher HbA1c.

Thomas DR. Anemia in diabetic patients. Clin Geriatr Med,2008; Vol. 24: pp. 529–40, vii.
Comments:Review of approach to anemia in diabetes patients emphasizing importance of diabetic nephropathy in development of anemia.

Saudek CD, Derr RL, Kalyani RR. Assessing glycemia in diabetes using self-monitoring blood glucose and hemoglobin A1c. JAMA,2006; Vol. 295: pp. 1688–97.
Comments:A review of methods, use, and interpretation of HbA1c and self-monitoring of blood glucose.

Weiss G, Goodnough LT. Anemia of chronic disease. NEJM,2005; Vol. 352: pp. 1011–23.
Comments:Review of pathophysiology, laboratory testing, and management of anemia of inflammation.

Panzer S, Kronik G, Lechner K, et al. Glycosylated hemoglobins (GHb): an index of red cell survival. Blood,1982; Vol. 59: pp. 1348–50.
Comments:Study showing that glycosylated hemoglobins are lower in patients with hemolytic anemia compared with those with nonhemolytic anemia or in normal controls.

World Health Organization. http://whqlibdoc.who.int/publications/2008/9789241596657_eng.pdf. Accessed March 5, 2010.
Comments:Report of worldwide anemia based on WHO Global Database on anemia.

National Kidney Foundation. http://www.kidney.org/professionals/KDOQI/guidelines_anemia/cpr21.htm. Accessed March 5, 2010.
Comments:National Kidney Foundation Disease Outcomes Quality Initiative (NKF KDOQI) practice guideline on anemia related to chronic kidney disease

免疫学

1型糖尿病的自身免疫性抗体

Shivam Champaneri, MD, and Christopher D. Saudek, MD

定义

- 1型糖尿病患者有4个针对β细胞的自身免疫性抗体：胰岛细胞抗体（ICA）是针对β细胞中胞质蛋白的抗体，谷氨酸脱羧酶抗体（GAD65），胰岛素自身免疫性抗体（IAA）和针对蛋白酪氨酸磷酸酶（Taplin）的胰岛抗原-2抗体（IA-2A）。
- 在80%的1型糖尿病患者都可检测到针对GAD65的自身免疫性抗体(Isermann)。
- ICA和IA-2A在1型糖尿病患者中的存在的比例分别为69%~90%和54%~75%(Winter)。
- IAA的患病率与患糖尿病的发病年龄呈负相关；通常是青少年发生糖尿病风险性的第一个标志（Franke），并且在青少年诊断1型糖尿病时大约有70%的患者存在IAA(Bingley)。

测定

- 放射性免疫法(RIA)比酶联免疫吸附法(ELISA)有更好的敏感性和特异性(Greenbaum)。
- 糖尿病自身免疫性抗体标准化程序2000工作组，用ELISA法测定胰岛素自身抗体（IAA）的敏感为4%~42%；与GAD或IA-2A抗体相比，胰岛素自身抗体测定的标准化具有更大的挑战(Greenbaum)。

适应证

- 当糖尿病分型不清时，如因胰岛细胞功能快速衰竭时（如成人<2年）考虑成人迟发性自身免疫性糖尿病（LADA），或一些患者不符合2型糖尿病的表型(Falorni)。
- 评估妊娠期糖尿病患者发展为1型糖尿病的风险；在分娩时存在自身免疫性抗体的患者，既不是1型糖尿病也没有发展为1型糖尿病的风险(Füchtenbusch)。
- 对高危人群筛查可能存在的早期1型糖尿病，如1级亲属患有1型糖尿病的人群。
- 对胰腺移植或β细胞移植的患者监测自身免疫性抗体，与预测移植物的存活率同时进行(Shapiro)。

鉴别诊断

- 糖尿病患者存在一个或多个自身免疫性抗体阳性提示为1型糖尿病。
- 对于筛查发现存在一个或多个抗体的非糖尿病患者，并不能说明其会发展为糖尿病。发生的风险取决于抗体的数量及滴度(Achenbach)。

解释

- 抗体可以在患者发生高血糖前数年即已经存在,提示自身免疫反应在逐年进展。
- 在存在多个抗体阳性及高滴度胰岛素抗体的患者,胰岛素分泌第一时相缺乏提示其存在早期的 β 细胞衰竭 (Achenbach, Keskinen)。
- 糖尿病预防试验(DPT1)中,882 名 1 型糖尿病患者的 1 级亲属测定了 GAD,IAA 和胰岛素抗体。在 11 年的随访中,有两个或两个以上抗体的个体发生糖尿病的 5 年风险度为 68%,有 3 个抗体的个体则 100% 发生了糖尿病 (Verge)。
- DPT1 研究中,存在 GAD 抗体的个体中,91% 存在其他抗体 (Verge)。
- GAD 抗体的敏感性为 84%,对成人发生 1 型糖尿病有更高的敏感性;与胰岛素抗体不同,当患者甚至不再分泌 C 肽时 GAD 抗体仍可保持高滴度 (Yu)。
- IAA 对于诊断 1 型糖尿病的敏感性为 49%~92%(Yu)。

局限性

- 在 DIPP(Finnish Type I Diabetes Prediction and Prevention; Kimpimäki) 和 DAISY (Diabetes Autoimmunity Study in the Young; Barker) 队列研究中发现,人们可以有短暂的自身抗体消失,数月或数年后并未发生糖尿病。
- 当使用胰岛素治疗的患者产生胰岛素自身抗体,IAA 测定对这些患者并无益处 (Falorni)。
- 抗体可能通过胎盘从 1 型糖尿病的母亲传给胎儿,因此要向其认真说明(Ziegler)。
- 一小部分 2 型糖尿病患者可能存在 GAD 抗体和 IA-2A(Umpaichitra)。

专家意见

- 当自身抗体阳性时可确诊 1 型糖尿病,当患者无法明确是 1 型还是 2 型糖尿病时测定自身免疫性抗体。
- 大多数抗体在诊断 1 型糖尿病数年后逐渐转阴,因此在起病数年后测定抗体对于诊断帮助不大。

参考文献

Bingley PJ. Clinical applications of diabetes antibody testing. J Clin Endocrinol Metab,2010; Vol. 95: pp. 25–33.

Comments:This 2009 review provides a summary of literature review and consensus statements on diabetes antibody testing.

Taplin CE, Barker JM. Autoantibodies in type 1 diabetes. Autoimmunity,2008; Vol. 41: pp. 11–8.

Comments:This 2008 review provides a basic overview of the described antibodies associated with type 1 diabetes and their role as a predictive marker for overt diabetes.

Yu L, Eisenbarth GS. Humoral autoimmunity. In Eisenbarth GS (Ed.) Type 1 diabetes: molecular, cellular, and clinical immunology.Denver: Barbara Davis Center for Childhood Diabetes; 2007.

Comments:This review examines the immunologic basis underlying type 1 diabetes.

Isermann B, Ritzel R, Zorn M, et al. Autoantibodies in diabetes mellitus: current utility and perspectives. Exp Clin Endocrinol Diabetes,2007; Vol. 115: pp. 483–90.

Comments:This review focuses on knowledge about antibody assays for diabetes associated autoimmunity, their clinical value, and their role in diagnosing and predicting autoimmune-associated diabetes mellitus.

Shapiro AM, Ricordi C, Hering BJ, et al. International trial of the Edmonton protocol for islet transplantation. NEJM,2006; Vol. 355: pp. 1318–30.

Comments:This international, multicenter trial looked at 36 type 1 diabetes patients who underwent islet cell transplantation and reported cases of long-term restoration of endogenous insulin production.

Falorni A, Brozzetti A. Diabetes-related antibodies in adult diabetic patients. Best Pract Res Clin Endocrinol Metab,2005; Vol. 19: pp. 119–33.

Comments:This 2005 review provides an overview of different markers of autoimmunity in type 1 diabetes and their role in the clinical setting.

Pihoker C, Gilliam LK, Hampe CS, et al. Autoantibodies in diabetes. Diabetes,2005; Vol. 54 Suppl 2. pp. S52–61.

Comments:This 2005 article is a review of the different autoantibodies seen in diabetes and pathogenesis and clinical significance of autoimmunity in type 1 diabetes.

Franke B, Galloway TS, Wilkin TJ. Developments in the prediction of type 1 diabetes mellitus, with special reference to insulin autoantibodies. Diabetes Metab Res Rev,2005; Vol. 21: pp. 395–415.

Comments:This 2005 review provides an overview of antibodies in type 1 diabetes and assays for its detection.

Achenbach P, Warncke K, Reiter J, et al. Stratification of type 1 diabetes risk on the basis of islet autoantibody characteristics. Diabetes,2004; Vol. 53: pp. 384–92.

Comments:The study found a strong association between risk of developing type 1 diabetes and high titer, with the highest risks associated with high-titer IA-2A and IAA, IgG2, IgG3, and/or IgG4 subclass of IA-2A and IAA, and antibodies to the IA-2-related molecule IA-2beta.

Barker JM, Goehrig SH, Barriga K, et al. Clinical characteristics of children diagnosed with type 1 diabetes through intensive screening and follow-up. Diabetes Care,2004; Vol. 27: pp. 1399–404.

Comments:This study assessed whether earlier diagnosis of diabetes in prospectively followed autoantibodypositive children lowered onset morbidity and improved the clinical course after diagnosis, and the authors found that such patients did have a milder clinical course in the first year after diagnosis.

Barker JM, Barriga KJ, Yu L, et al. Prediction of autoantibody positivity and progression to type 1 diabetes: Diabetes Autoimmunity Study in the Young (DAISY). J Clin Endocrinol Metab,2004; Vol. 89: pp. 3896–902.

Comments:This prospective study reveals that determination of islet autoantibodies in 1972 children found a large number of individuals being either false or transiently positive.

Umpaichitra V, Banerji MA, Castells S. Autoantibodies in children with type 2 diabetes mellitus. J Pediatr Endocrinol Metab,2002; Vol. 15: Suppl 1: pp. 525–30.

Comments:In 37 children and adolescents with type 2 diabetes who had positive meal-stimulated C-peptide levels, 10.8% also had positive GAD and/or IA2 antibodies.

Keskinen P, Korhonen S, Kupila A, et al. First-phase insulin response in young healthy children at genetic and immunological risk for Type I diabetes. Diabetologia,2002; Vol. 45: pp. 1639–48.

Comments:This study noted a decreased first-phase insulin response as potentially an early phenomenon in the course of prediabetes in young children, implying a rapid autoimmune destruction or loss of function of beta cells as well as possible metabolic compensation mechanisms.

Winter WE, Harris N, Schatz D. Type 1 diabetes islet autoantibody markers. Diabetes Technol Ther,2002; Vol. 4: pp. 817–39.

Comments:This 2002 article provides a basic overview of antibodies seen in type 1 diabetes and their diagnostic role in the clinical setting.

Kimpimäki T, Kupila A, Hämäläinen AM, et al. The first signs of beta-cell autoimmunity appear in infancy in genetically susceptible children from the general population: the Finnish Type 1 Diabetes Prediction and Prevention Study. J Clin Endocrinol Metab,2001; Vol. 86: pp. 4782–8.

Comments: In this population-based prospective cohort study, monitoring for the appearance of diabetes associated autoantibodies and development of type 1 diabetes from birth was performed. The authors noted children with a strong human-leukocyte-antigen-DQ-defined genetic risk of type 1 diabetes show signs of beta-cell autoimmunity proportionally more often than those with a moderate genetic risk with generally IAA emerging as the first detectable antibody more commonly than any other antibody.

Ziegler AG, Hummel M, Schenker M, et al. Autoantibody appearance and risk for development of childhood diabetes in offspring of parents with type 1 diabetes: the 2-year analysis of the German BABYDIAB Study. Diabetes,1999; Vol. 48: pp. 460–8.

Comments:This prospective trial of 1353 offspring of parents with type 1 diabetes looked at the development of autoantibodies. They noted a cumulative risk for disease of 1.8% by 5 years of age and a 50% risk for offspring with more than one autoantibody in their 2-year sample.

Füchtenbusch M, Ferber K, Standl E, et al. Prediction of type 1 diabetes postpartum in patients with gestational diabetes mellitus by combined islet cell autoantibody screening: a prospective multicenter study. Diabetes,1997; Vol. 46: pp. 1459–67.

Comments:This prospective multicenter study of 437 gestational diabetes patients assessed the predictive value of autoantibody markers for the development of type 1 diabetes. The authors noted the risk for type 1 diabetes 2 years postpartum increased with the number of antibodies present at delivery from 17% (6%–28%) for one antibody, to 61% (30%–91%) for two antibodies, and to 84% (55%–100%) for 3 antibodies.

Verge CF, Gianani R, Kawasaki E, et al. Prediction of type I diabetes in first-degree relatives using a combination of insulin, GAD, and ICA512bdc/IA-2 autoantibodies. Diabetes,1996; Vol. 45: pp. 926–33.

Comments:This study looked at 882 first-degree relatives of patients with type 1 diabetes, 50 of whom later developed diabetes with a median follow-up of 2.0 years. The authors concluded that the presence of 2 or more autoantibodies (out of IAAs, GAAs, and ICA512bdcAAs) is highly predictive of the development of type 1 diabetes among relatives.

Greenbaum CJ, Palmer JP, Kuglin B, et al. Insulin autoantibodies measured by radioimmunoassay methodology are more related to insulin-dependent diabetes mellitus than those measured by enzyme-linked immunosorbent assay: results of the Fourth International Workshop on the Standardization of Insulin Autoantibody Measurement. J Clin Endocrinol Metab,1992; Vol. 74: pp. 1040–4.

Comments: This report compares the measurement of insulin autoantibodies(IAA) using RIA and ELISA assays, with the finding of labs that used RIA had a much higher percentage of sera to be IAA positive among both newly diagnosed patients and healthy individuals who later developed diabetes than laboratories using ELISA.

胰岛素抗体

Shivam Champaneri, MD, and Christopher D. Saudek, MD

定义
- 对外源性胰岛素产生抗体在胰岛素治疗的患者中非常常见,但一般并无临床意义。
- IgG 抗体最为常见,IgE 抗体是导致胰岛素过敏的抗体 (Fineberg)。
- 高滴度的 IgG 抗体会影响胰岛素的活性,可能延迟或减少胰岛素的作用。
- 极少数情况下,抗体会激动胰岛素受体,而引起低血糖(通常为餐后低血糖)(Koyama)。
- 抗体的增殖取决药物的纯度、分子结构和胰岛素的储存条件,同时也受患者自身因素如年龄、HLA 分型和给药途径影响 (Fineberg)。
- 对使用牛或猪胰岛素的患者产生抗体极为常见,比使用人胰岛素和胰岛素类似物的患者明显增多。
- 对胰岛素类似物或未经修饰的人胰岛素反应相同。
- 在之前没有使用过胰岛素的患者体内出现胰岛素自身抗体,是一项预测未来发展为 1 型糖尿病的提示。

测定
- 放射配体结合 (RLB) 分析是最常用的测定胰岛素自身抗体的方法 (Fineberg)。
- 标准免疫沉淀法和凝集分析法不能用于测定胰岛素抗体,因为胰岛素抗体免疫复合物并不能沉淀 (Fineberg)。
- 测定胰岛素自身抗体需要高敏感性,因为其浓度比外源性胰岛素产生抗体的浓度低很多 (Greenbaum)。

适应证
- 严重的胰岛素抵抗,对高剂量的胰岛素治疗无反应。
- 评估胰岛素过敏的可能性:IgE 抗体出现在快速的 1 型超敏反应,而 IgG 出现在迟发的 III 型超敏反应中 (Heinzerling)。
- 评估可能存在的假性低血糖:没有糖尿病的患者使用胰岛素,可通过测定发现胰岛素抗体而诊断。
- 确诊自身免疫性低血糖:很罕见但需与胰岛细胞瘤进行鉴别 (Koyama)。

鉴别诊断
- 存在胰岛素抗体并不能说明其导致了胰岛素抵抗或低血糖。
- 可溶性胰岛素,如常规胰岛素,比中效或长效胰岛素相比更不容易过敏 (Chance)。
- 血循环中针对胰岛素的 IgE 抗体对动物源性胰岛素,可导致皮肤或系统性过敏反应 (Fineberg)。
- 需要区分对鱼精蛋白锌(用于使长效胰岛素延长吸收时间)还是对胰岛素本身过敏 (Feinglos)。
- 自身免疫性低血糖是由于对胰岛素的内源性抗体或对胰岛素受体的抗体出现 (Koyama)。

胰岛素抗体

解释

- 大多数研究并未发现胰岛素自身抗体与糖尿病并发症相关，如肾病、视网膜病变和神经病变 (Fineberg)。
- 极其罕见的，抗体对不同种类的胰岛素结合程度不同，临床上可以通过更换胰岛素剂型减少抗体 (Grammer)。
- 临床研究未发现胰岛素剂量与胰岛素自身抗体产生相关。
- 高滴度的抗体仅是发生胰岛素抵抗的一个原因 (Fineberg)。
- 对严重胰岛素抵抗的患者，出现胰岛素抗体可以考虑更换胰岛素配方、糖皮质激素治疗，极少数情况下可考虑血浆置换 (Kahn；Koyama)。
- 胰岛素过敏可以使用抗组胺药来控制症状，更换胰岛素或免疫脱敏治疗 (Heinzerling)。
- 自身免疫性低血糖可以通过逐渐减少糖皮质激素来抑制内源性胰岛素抗体 (Redmon)。

局限性

- 没有标准化的胰岛素抗体量化测定试剂盒 (Fineberg)。
- 仅有 IgE 抗体并不能诊断胰岛素过敏，因为其可以在没有明显过敏的患者体内存在 (Fineberg)。
- 少量证据显示，对使用胰岛素治疗的患者，存在胰岛素抗体和低血糖之间存在因果关系。
- 抗体在病毒性疾病、其他自身免疫性疾病、副肿瘤综合征或可能发生 1 型糖尿病的患者中也会出现。

专家意见

- IgG 胰岛素抗体一般并不致病，因此仅当抗体滴度很高且除外其他常见致胰岛素抵抗的原因时，才考虑自身抗体导致了胰岛素抵抗。

参考文献

Radermecker RP, Renard E, Scheen AJ. Circulating insulin antibodies: influence of continuous subcutaneous or intraperitoneal insulin infusion, and impact on glucose control. Diabetes Metab Res Rev, 2009; Vol. 25 Suppl 6: pp. 491–501.
Comments:This 2009 reference discusses the significance of different modalities of insulin administration toward development of insulin antibodies and its potential implications toward management.

Heinzerling L, Raile K, Rochlitz H, et al. Insulin allergy: clinical manifestations and management strategies. Allergy,2008; Vol. 63: pp. 148–55.
Comments:This review provides an overview of insulin allergy, including presentation, diagnosis, and immunotherapy.

Fineberg SE, Kawabata TT, Finco-Kent D, et al. Immunological responses to exogenous insulin. Endocr Rev,2007; Vol. 28: pp. 625–52.
Comments:This reference provides an overview of the immunologic factors in the development of insulin antibodies and reviews its relationship toward diabetes complications.

Koyama R, Nakanishi K, Kato M, et al. Hypoglycemia and hyperglycemia due to insulin antibodies against therapeutic human insulin: treatment with double filtration plasmapheresis and prednisolone. Am J Med Sci,2005; Vol. 329: pp. 259–64.

Comments:This article discusses the role of plasmapheresis and subsequent use of steroid therapy to lower insulin antibodies to achieve better glycemic control by insulin.

Redmon JB, Nuttall FQ. Autoimmune hypoglycemia. Endocrinol Metab Clin North Am,1999; Vol. 28: pp. 603–18, vii.

Comments:This excellent review describes the clinical significance, pathogenesis, evaluation, and management of autoimmune hypoglycemia.

Salardi S, Cacciari E, Steri L, et al. An 8-year follow-up of anti-insulin antibodies in diabetic children: relation to insulin autoantibodies, HLA type, beta-cell function, clinical course and type of insulin therapy. Acta Paediatr,1995; Vol. 84: pp. 639–45.

Comments:This trial studied 105 children and adolescents with insulin-dependent diabetes and noted an inverse relationship between insulin autoantibodies and age at diagnosis; they compared levels of antibodies to A1c values, insulin requirement, HLA, and presence of early complications and concluded that antibodies did not have significant effects on the clinical course of the disease.

Greenbaum CJ, Palmer JP, Kuglin B, et al. Insulin autoantibodies measured by radioimmunoassay methodology are more related to insulin-dependent diabetes mellitus than those measured by enzyme-linked immunosorbent assay: results of the fourth International Workshop on the Standardization of Insulin Autoantibody Measurement. J Clin Endocrinol Metab,1992; Vol. 74: pp. 1040–4.

Comments:This summarizes the findings of the fourth International Workshop on the Standardization of Insulin Autoantibody Measurement with the finding that the data suggest that insulin autoantibodies measured by radioimmunoassay are more disease related than those measured by enzyme-linked immunosorbent assay.

Sutton M, Klaff LJ, Asplin CM, et al. Insulin autoantibodies at diagnosis of insulin-dependent diabetes: effect on the antibody response to insulin treatment. Metabolism,1988; Vol. 37: pp. 1005–7.

Comments:This study assessed whether insulin antibody response over the first year of treatment with insulin was different in individuals with or without insulin autoantibodies. They noted that patients with insulin autoantibodies at diagnosis develop higher insulin antibody measurements when subsequently treated with exogenous insulin.

Grammer LC, Roberts M, Patterson R. IgE and IgG antibody against human (recombinant DNA) insulin in patients with systemic insulin allergy. J Lab Clin Med,1985; Vol. 105: pp. 108–13.

Comments:This paper notes the presence of IgE and IgG antibodies to human insulin as well as bovine and porcine insulin in patients found to have systemic insulin allergy.

Kahn CR, Rosenthal AS. Immunologic reactions to insulin: insulin allergy, insulin resistance, and the autoimmune insulin syndrome. Diabetes Care,1980; Vol. 2: pp. 283–95.

Comments:This is a review from 1980 (one of the original papers) that provides a summary of insulin allergy and insulin resistance and what was known about the mechanisms at that time.

Feinglos MN, Jegasothy BV. "Insulin" allergy due to zinc. Lancet,1979; Vol. 1: pp. 122–4.

Comments:This 1979 paper describes the phenomenon of allergy to zinc in commercially prepared insulins.

Chance RE, Root MA, Galloway JA. The immunogenicity of insulin preparations. Acta Endocrinol Suppl(Copenhagen), 1976; Vol. 205: pp. 185–98.

Comments:This review assessed antibody formation from differently prepared insulins (porcine and bovine) with the finding that more purely prepared insulins had less immunogenecity.

Schlichtkrull J, Brange J, Christiansen AH, et al. Clinical aspects of insulin—antigenicity. Diabetes,1972; Vol. 21: pp. 649–56.

Comments:This is one of the original papers that describes the antigenicity of insulin

血脂

血脂

Simeon Margolis, MD, PhD

定义
- 通常来说血脂包括总胆固醇（TG）、甘油三酯、高密度脂蛋白（HDL-C）和低密度脂蛋白（LDL-C）。
- 载脂蛋白和脂蛋白脂酶的活性可以检测。
- 乳糜微粒携带脂肪由小肠吸收。
- 高LDL-C（"坏胆固醇"）是风险最高的心血管疾病因素。
- 低HDL-C（"好胆固醇"）也是心血管疾病的高危因素。
- 高TG也与心血管疾病相关，但不如高LDL-C和低HDL-C的影响大。
- 严重的高甘油三酯血症易引起胰腺炎。

测定
- 最重要的化验是使用标准的生化分析仪对空腹血进行化验，通常包括一台全自动分析仪，可以检验总胆固醇、甘油三酯和高密度脂蛋白（并计算得出低密度脂蛋白）。
- 免疫检测法可以检测出载脂蛋白（APO）A、B，C-II、C-III和E，还包括载脂蛋白E的三种亚型。
- 冷藏过夜的血清上层可见白色的脂肪层，可以测定乳糜微粒。

适应证
- 2型糖尿病一经确诊应进行空腹抽血化验血脂，并在2型糖尿病治疗过程中应每年至少化验一次。
- 如果LDL-C高于70mg/d或者患者患有心血管疾病（CVD）应检测载脂蛋白B，判断是否需要更积极的降脂治疗或增加烟酸，因为这些是小而密的致动脉粥样硬化的LDL颗粒(Pischon；Contois)。

鉴别诊断
- Fredrickson分类法可用来区分不同亚型的高脂血症，尽管这个分类系统本身并不常用。主要的亚型描绘如下。
- 高乳糜微粒血症：非常高的空腹甘油三酯（通常>1 000mg/dl），在冷藏过夜的血清中可以看到大量的乳糜微粒。家族性高乳糜微粒血症是由于缺乏脂蛋白脂酶或其活化剂载脂蛋白（ApoCII）。两者可通过测定apoCII进行鉴别。严重的胰岛素缺乏可导致高乳糜微粒血症。
- 高胆固醇血症（HCH）：LDL-C升高。TG可能正常也可能升高。LDL受体缺乏是家族性高胆固醇血症的主要原因。原发的HCH也可能由其他遗传缺陷造成。其他代谢紊乱及过量饮食也会造成HCH。
- 家族性复合高脂蛋白血症：LDL-C、甘油三酯和ApoB升高(Veerkamp)。

血脂

- 血 β 脂蛋白异常：几乎同等升高的胆固醇和 TG 可以提示，通过载脂蛋白 E2：E2 异构体确诊（Kane）。
- 家族性高甘油三酯血症：极低密度脂蛋白（VLDL）升高且 LDL-C 水平正常或轻度升高。
- 混合型高甘油三酯血症：VLDL 和乳糜微粒升高。血清冷藏过夜，可以看到乳糜微粒层出现在浑浊血清的上方。
- 家族性混合性高脂血症：家族成员中可见高水平的胆固醇、甘油三酯和 / 或 ApoB。家族成员中的血脂异常情况不同 (Veerkamp)。获得性混合性高脂血症在糖尿病患者中多见。
- 确定患者是否患有家族性高胆固醇血症、血 β 脂蛋白异常和家族性混合性高脂血症非常重要，因为患者存在发生 CVD 极高的风险。建议对家族成员进行筛查。
- 2 型糖尿病患者最常见的血脂紊乱是胆固醇和甘油三酯升高，同时 HDL 下降（混合性高脂血症）。

解释

- LDL-C 通常不能直接测定，但可通过 Friedewald 等式估算（如 TG 低于 400mg/dl）：低密度脂蛋白 = 总胆固醇 - 甘油三酯 /5 - 高密度脂蛋白。
- 当治疗高甘油三酯血症时使用非 HDL 胆固醇。通过以下进行计算：非 HDL 胆固醇 = 总胆固醇 - 高密度脂蛋白。
- 对 2 型糖尿病患者 LDL-C 的目标值为 < 100mg/dl，对于高危的患者则小于 70mg/dl。2 型糖尿病患者非 HDL-C 的目标值为 < 100 mg/dl 或 < 130mg/dl。
- 高甘油三酯血症通常合并低 HDL-C，及更多的致动脉粥样化的小而密 LDL。
- 存在乳糜微粒可能提示为非空腹血标本。
- 当 TG 超过 1 000 mg/dl 增加急性胰腺炎风险。

局限性

- 当 TG 超过 400mg/dl 及存在血 β 脂蛋白异常时不能用 Friedewald 等式来正确估算 LDL-C，这些情况下可直接测定 LDL-C。
- 如 TG 明显升高，血淀粉酶及脂肪酶通常不能用来确诊急性胰腺炎。
- 不佳的血糖控制情况会导致高乳糜微粒血症，并增加急性胰腺炎的风险。
- 甘油三酯和 HDL-C 在血糖控制更好的时候会有很大改善。
- 运动或血糖控制对 LDL-C 影响不大。
- 血脂应在空腹状态下测定，原因是甘油三酯会随最近一次进食情况不同而产生很大变化。
- 总胆固醇和 LDL-C 随禁食或进食状态变化不大，除非甘油三酯明显升高。
- HDL-C 水平与空腹状态关系不大。

专家意见

- 虽然更建议空腹状态下检测血脂（尤其对甘油三酯），但是否空腹对总胆固醇、HDL-C 和 LDL-C 水平影响不大。
- LDL-C 升高目前被认为是发生心血管疾病风险最高的危险因素。

- 然而，非HDL胆固醇，总胆固醇：HDL，尤其是ApoB可能是心血管疾病风险更好的预测因素；ApoB的改变是额外评估降脂治疗有效性的指标(Pischon；Contois)。
- ApoB可以确定LDL颗粒的数量和致动脉粥样化性的小而密的LDL颗粒。
- 除了ApoB，对脂蛋白脂酶的活性和载脂蛋白的测定目前已经成为科研热点，但很少用于临床(Mora)。
- 开始降脂治疗前，对患者的基线测定应包括血脂谱及TSH和肝酶，但不需要测定CK；但当患者出现肌痛或乏力时必须检测。
- 最近的研究表明，非空腹的甘油三酯水平比空腹状态下测定的对心血管风险的预测价值更高，但非空腹状态下甘油三酯检测的上限还未确定(Bansal；Nordestgaard)。

参考文献

Mora S. Advanced lipoprotein testing and subfractionation are not (yet) ready for routine clinical use. Circulation,2009; Vol. 119: pp. 2396–404.
Comments:It is not necessary to measure apoproteins or particle size and number to determine risk of cardiovascular disease or to follow treatment outcomes in most patients with type 2 diabetes.

Mora S, Otvos JD, Rifai N, et al. Lipoprotein particle profiles by nuclear magnetic resonance compared with standard lipids and apolipoproteins in predicting incident cardiovascular disease in women. Circulation,2009; Vol. 119: pp. 931–9.
Comments:At least in healthy women, lipoprotein profiles evaluated by nuclear magnetic resonance (NMR) were comparable but not superior to measurements of standard lipids or apolipoproteins.

Contois JH, McConnell JP, Sethi AA, et al. Apolipoprotein B and cardiovascular disease risk: position statement from the AACC Lipoproteins and Vascular Diseases Division Working Group on Best Practices. Clin Chem,2009; Vol. 55: pp. 407–19.
Comments: This paper from clinical chemists recommends the use of apo B rather than LDL-C to assess cardiovascular disease risk.

Martin SS, Qasim AN, Mehta NN, et al. Apolipoprotein B but not LDL cholesterol is associated with coronary artery calcification in type 2 diabetic whites. Diabetes,2009; Vol. 58: pp. 1887–92.
Comments:Plasma apo B, but not LDL cholesterol, levels were associated with coronary artery calcification scores in type 2 diabetic whites.

El Harchaoui K, van der Steeg WA, Stroes ES, et al. Value of low-density lipoprotein particle number and size as predictors of coronary artery disease in apparently healthy men and women: the EPIC-Norfolk Prospective Population Study. J Am Coll Cardiol,2007; Vol. 49: pp. 547–53.
Comments:The additional value of LDL particle number was comparable to non-HDL-C, and it was abolished after adjusting for triglycerides and HDL-C.

Ingelsson E, Schaefer EJ, Contois JH, et al. Clinical utility of different lipid measures for prediction of coronary heart disease in men and women.JAMA,2007; Vol. 298: pp. 776–85.
Comments: During a 15-year follow-up of subjects from the Framingham study, results did not support measurement of apo B or apo A-I to predict risk of coronary heart disease in clinical practice when total cholesterol and HDL-C measurements are available.

Nordestgaard BG, Benn M, Schnohr P, et al. Nonfasting triglycerides and risk of myocardial infarction, ischemic heart disease, and death in men and women. JAMA,2007; Vol. 298: pp. 299–308.

Comments:Nonfasting triglycerides were as good or better than fasting triglycerides for predicting risk of coronary heart disease events and death.

Bansal S, Buring JE, Rifai N, et al. Fasting compared with nonfasting triglycerides and risk of cardiovascular events in women. JAMA,2007; Vol. 298: pp. 309–16.

Comments:Nonfasting triglycerides were more effective than fasting triglycerides in predicting cardiovascular events in women.

Pischon T, Girman CJ, Sacks FM, et al. Non-high-density lipoprotein cholesterol and apolipoprotein B in the prediction of coronary heart disease in men. Circulation,2005; Vol. 112: pp. 3375–83.

Comments:In this study of men, the plasma concentration of atherogenic lipoprotein particles (measured by apo B) was more predictive for the development of CHD than LDL-C or the cholesterol carried by atherogenic particles, measured by non-HDL-C.

Veerkamp MJ, de Graaf J, Hendriks JC, et al. Nomogram to diagnose familial combined hyperlipidemia on the basis of results of a 5-year follow-up study. Circulation,2004; Vol. 109: pp. 2980–5.

Comments:Familial combined hyperlipidemia is associated with a very high risk of cardiovascular complications. Identification of the disorder can be made from detailed family information, but it is also possible to identify the disorder in an individual patient by measuring total cholesterol, triglcerides, and apo B.

Huang ES, Meigs JB, Singer DE. The effect of interventions to prevent cardiovascular disease in patients with type 2 diabetes mellitus. Am J Med,2001; Vol. 111: pp. 633–42.

Comments:Improvement in cholesterol levels reduce the risk of cardiovascular disease in patients with type 2 diabetes.

Kane JP, Havel RJ. Disorders of the biogenesis and secretion of lipoproteins containing the B apoproteins. In Scriver CR, Beaudet AL, Sly WS, Valle DS, (Eds.), The Metabolic and Molecular Bases of Inherited Disease,8th edition. New York: McGraw-Hill; 2001: pp. 2717–62.

Comments:Description of normal and abnormal production and metabolism of B-containing lipoproteins—VLDL and LDL—along with criteria for diagnosis of dysbetalipoproteinemia.

肾脏

肾功能

Donna I. Myers, MD

定义

- 血肌酐：实用并易于测定的监测肾功能的指标。但血肌酐处于正常范围并不能反映肾小球滤过率（GFR）正常，因同时还应考虑年龄、性别和肌肉量情况。
- 血清肌酐倒数曲线是非常有用的指标，但计算起来却十分繁琐，并随肌酐变化。斜率突然变大表示可能存在潜在的可逆因素，如容量耗竭导致慢性肾脏病急性加重。同样的，良好的血压和血糖控制使曲线变平。
- GFR：最简单测定肾功能的指标，不需留取 24 小时尿。GFR 升高提示高滤过，可提示早期的糖尿病肾病。随肾脏病进展 GFR 逐渐下降。4 变量的 MDRD 公式计算 GFR 基于血肌酐、年龄、种族和性别。6 变量的 MDRD 公式除了以上 4 项外还包括了血尿素氮（BUN）和血清白蛋白。Cockcroft-Gault 公式计算 GFR 基于血肌酐、体重、性别和年龄。但对于肥胖患者，因体重并不能反映肌肉容量，因此 Cockcroft-Gault 公式更适用于体型偏瘦的患者。
- BUN：与 GFR 呈反向变化，但比 GFR 的影响因素更多（见第 657 页，局限性章节）。
- 微量白蛋白尿：是糖尿病肾病最早期的指征，尤其对于 1 型糖尿病患者，糖尿病患者应规律监测。
- 随机尿白蛋白：肌酐比值评价微量白蛋白尿，通常用于监测治疗干预后的治疗效果，如使用肾素－血管紧张素阻滞剂后尿蛋白变化的情况。几乎不需要 24 小时尿蛋白定量收集。
- 显微镜下尿液分析：在肾前性或肾后性肾功能不全时可见到沉淀物。肾小球肾炎：血尿、蛋白尿，并可见形态不整的红细胞（RBC）、红细胞管型、颗粒管型和脂肪尿。肾病：蛋白尿、脂肪尿。感染：试纸法测定阳性的白细胞（WBC）及亚硝酸盐，脓尿、血尿、细菌尿、伴或不伴白细胞管型，尿培养阳性。急性间质性肾炎：非感染性的白细胞尿和白细胞管型。如发现嗜酸性粒细胞则更支持过敏性因素所致急性间质性肾炎。急性肾小管坏死：可见棕色颗粒管型。
- 影像学检查：包括肾脏和膀胱的超声检测，功能性核素扫描测定分肾功能、GFR 及有无梗阻。以及 CT 血管造影、肾脏 MRA、多普勒超声检测有无肾动脉狭窄（见第 657 页，局限性章节）。

测定

- 血肌酐和 BUN：血肌酐采用碱性苦味酸法测定，是一种比色测定方法。
- GFR[ml/（min·1.73m^2）]：绝大多数的实验室采用基于血肌酐、性别、种族和年龄估测的 GFR（MDRD）。
- 尿白蛋白和肌酐（用于测定微量白蛋白尿）：见蛋白尿，661 页。

肾功能

适应证
- 确诊 2 型糖尿病后每年预防性测定微量蛋白尿，在诊断 1 型糖尿病 5 年后每年测定（ADA 标准）。
- 不论尿蛋白排泄率情况，所有成人糖尿病患者每年至少测定一次血肌酐，以便使用 GFR 进行慢性肾脏病（CKD）的分期（ADA 标准）。
- 肾功能衰竭的症状和体征包括泡沫尿、水肿、不可控制的高血压、充血性心功能衰竭和尿毒症。
- 电解质紊乱常常与慢性肾功能不全一同出现（如高钾血症、低钠血症、低钙血症、高磷血症和代谢性酸中毒）或贫血。
- 潜在肾毒性药物（如二甲双胍）或受肾脏清除率影响显著的药物（如胰岛素、磺脲类降糖药）。

鉴别诊断
- 血肌酐升高：肾前性、肾性或肾后性肾功能不全，药物反应（见下文）。
- BUN 升高：肾前性、肾性或肾后性肾功能不全，非肾性因素（见下义）。
- GFR 下降：肾前性、肾性或肾后性肾功能不全，24 小时尿收集有误。
- 尿蛋白增加：肾小球疾病导致的微量或大量蛋白尿，肾静脉血栓，充血性心功能衰竭，发热，良性体位性蛋白尿。

解释
- 慢性肾脏病以 GFR 及尿蛋白进行分期：1 期：蛋白尿，GFR ≥ 90ml/min；2 期：蛋白尿，GFR=60~89ml/min；3 期：GFR=30~59ml/min；4 期：GFR=15~29ml/min；5 期：GFR < 15ml/min。
- 血肌酐的倍增导致 GFR 减半，基础血肌酐 0.6mg/dl，随访发现升至 1.2mg/dl，虽然血肌酐水平仍在实验室检查的"正常"范围，但已提示肾脏病进展。
- 肌酐曲线和 GFR 呈非线性关系。在曲线下端血肌酐的轻度升高导致 GFR 的巨大改变，在曲线上端血肌酐轻度变化对 GFR 没有显著影响。对肌酐取倒数可以回避这种影响。但了解肌酐的倍增会导致 GFR50% 的下降是非常有用的。血肌酐从 0.6mg/dl 升至 1.2mg/dl 与从 4.0mg/dl 升至 8.0mg/dl 的变化是同样重要的。
- 以肌酐的倒数对时间作图，这可用于预测患者何时到达 CKD5 期，但何时启动维持性透析治疗取决于患者的并发症和症状。
- 随机尿蛋白：肌酐比位于 30~300mg/g 肌酐提示微量蛋白尿，>300mg/g 肌酐提示大量蛋白尿。

局限性
- MDRD 公式并不适用于 GFR>60ml/min 的患者（均报道为">60ml/min"，而非其他特定数值）。
- 碱性苦味酸法测定肌酐会受一些肌酐色原的影响，如糖尿病酮症酸中毒，可使肌酐假性升高达 2mg/dl。
- 血肌酐可因肾前性因素波动，如容量状态、心功能情况和胶体渗透压。运动引起的肌肉量增加或消耗及截肢引起的肌肉量的减少会引起血肌酐的变化，但不影响 GFR。

肾功能

- 当进食大量肉类或出现肌肉损伤（横纹肌溶解）导致大量肌酐释放会引起血肌酐升高。
- 消耗性疾病引起的重度营养不良（肝硬化、肿瘤、暴食症、低蛋白摄入）会使肌酐（肌肉量减少）及 BUN 位于较低水平，甚至在如肝肾综合征引起的急性肾功能衰竭时。
- 影响近曲小管分泌肌酐的药物，会造成肌酐升高的假象，但并不会使 GFR 下降，如复方新诺明和西咪替丁。
- 脱水时血尿素氮会升高（肾前性氮质血症），当大量蛋白质在饮食中增多（一种风行一时的食谱），胃肠道（消化道出血），败血症或大量使用激素的状态引起分解作用时也会增高。肾前性氮质血症定义为：BUN：血肌酐 ≥ 20:1。
- 确诊尿微量蛋白应收集两次尿液进行化验，因其易受运动及高代谢状态影响，如发热和心功能不全。
- 对于肌酐大于 1.8mg/dl 的患者应避免进行增强 CT 检查，尤其对于那些患有糖尿病、蛋白尿及心脏病的患者。如果需要增强 CT 检查，建议在之前使用 N-乙酰半胱胺酸和静脉输液。
- 禁忌在 GFR<60ml/min 时，对肾动脉进行增强 MRI 检查时使用钆造影剂，因与发生肾源性系统性纤维化的风险相关。
- 多普勒超声评估肾动脉是否存在狭窄对于肥胖患者和技术不熟练的操作人员使用受限。

专家意见

- 确诊糖尿病肾病的最早证据是微量蛋白尿（30~300mg/d），一般在确诊糖尿病 10 年后出现。如果没有良好的血糖控制和血管紧张素系统阻滞剂的治疗（ACEI 或 ARB），则会在数年后进展为大量蛋白尿（>300mg/d），进而在 3~5 年内出现 GFR 下降、高血压和肾功能衰竭。
- 仅有 25% 的糖尿病患者出现典型的糖尿病肾病（糖尿病性肾小球硬化或毛细管间性肾小球硬化症）。在 20 年后也未必发生。糖尿病患者长期生存，会逐渐出现动脉硬化性肾脏疾病（肾硬化），表现虽为无蛋白尿，但是缓慢进展。
- 肾血管疾病（RAS）常与糖尿病肾病同时存在。对那些有外周血管疾病的患者，伴或不伴血管杂音，起始 ACEI 或 ARB 治疗后肌酐突然升高，双肾大小不对称，出现一过性肺水肿（双侧 RAS）的患者均要怀疑 RAS。
- 与肾功能直接相关的电解质紊乱包括低钠血症、高钾血症和代谢性酸中毒。早期 CKD 的糖尿病患者出现高钾血症应考虑低肾素-低醛固酮（IV 型肾小管酸中毒）（见醛固酮减少症，第 617 页）。
- 日常血肌酐的轻度波动反应了容量改变及脱水状态。
- 医生应避免过度使用利尿剂，尤其与 RAAS 阻断剂合用。
- 钠排泄分数（FENa）或尿素排泄分数（FEurea）可以帮助医生鉴别急性肾损伤和容量不足，但对评估稳定的肾功能状态并没有太大帮助。
- 尿干化学分析无法进行肾功能判断，但对泌尿系统感染（白细胞酯酶和亚硝酸盐阳性）、肾炎、肾病有直接证据。
- 在每一次随访时都应评估是否存在体位性低血压。

- 对CKD3期的患者应考虑肾科咨询。

推荐依据

Levey AS, Schoolwerth AC, Burrows NR, et al. Comprehensive public health strategies for preventing the development, progression, and complications of CKD: report of an expert panel convened by the Centers for Disease Control and Prevention. Am J Kidney Dis, 2009; Vol. 53: pp. 522–35.

Comments:Physician awareness of the patient's GFR is recommended for timely referral and appropriate management of CKD.

High WA, Ayers RA, Chandler J, et al. Gadolinium is detectable within the tissue of patients with nephrogenic systemic fibrosis. J Am Acad Dermatol,2007; Vol. 56: pp. 21–6.

Comments:The toxicity of gadolinium in patients with kidney disease was suspected when gadolinium was detected in tissue of a number of patients with nephrogenic systemic fibrosis (NSF). This association has been confirmed and new guidelines established for the use of this agent.

Schwab SJ, Christensen RL, Dougherty K, et al. Quantitation of proteinuria by the use of protein-to-creatinine ratios in single urine samples. Arch Intern Med,1987; Vol. 147: pp. 943–4.

Comments:This article describes the utility of single voided urine samples to measure protein-to-creatinine ratios, an observation that obviated the need, in most instances, of a 24-hr urine collection.

其他参考文献

American Diabetes Association. Standards of medical care in diabetes—2011. Diabetes Care, 2011; Vol. 34 Suppl 1: pp. S11–61.

Comments:Most recent summary of the standards of medical care in diabetes from the American Diabetes Association including recommendations for annual measurement of renal function.

Kanbay M, Kasapoglu B, Perazella MA. Acute tubular necrosis and pre-renal acute kidney injury: utility of urine microscopy in their evaluation—a systematic review. Int Urol Nephrol,2010; Vol. 42 Suppl 2: pp. 425–33.

Comments:Urine microscopy is useful for the diagnosis of acute kidney injury.

Tanemoto M. Treatment for hyperkalemia in hyporeninemic hypoaldosteronism. Kidney Int,2009; Vol. 75: p. 1113; author reply 1113–4.

Comments:Type IV RTA, which is prevalent in diabetic patients, may limit the ability to treat proteinuria with renin-angiotensin blocking agents such as ACE-I and ARB therapy.

Diskin CJ, Stokes TJ, Dansby LM, et al. The comparative benefits of the fractional excretion of urea and sodium in various azotemic oliguric states. Nephron Clin Pract,2009; Vol. 114: pp. c145–c150.

Comments:This compares the utility of FENa versus FEurea in oliguric azotemia.

Miller WG. Reporting estimated GFR: a laboratory perspective. Am J Kidney Dis,2008; Vol. 52: pp. 645–8.

Comments:Setting up estimated GFR from a laboratory's perspective.

Levey AS, Bosch JP, Lewis JB, et al. A more accurate method to estimate glomerular filtration rate from serum creatinine: a new prediction equation. Modification of Diet in Renal Disease Study Group. Ann Intern Med,1999; Vol. 130: pp. 461–70.

Comments:Historical derivation of the MDRD equation following analysis of the Modification of Diet in Renal Disease Study.

Geyer SJ. Urinalysis and urinary sediment in patients with renal disease. Clin Lab Med,1993; Vol. 13: pp. 13–20.

Comments:Patterns on microscopic examination also help distinguish chronic injury based on findings of red cells, white cells, tubular cells, and various casts.

Webb JA. Ultrasonography in the diagnosis of renal obstruction. BMJ, 1990; Vol. 301 pp. 944–6.

Comments:Ultrasonography is a valuable tool in diagnosing renal disease as it has no risk. (Author's comment: CT scan without intravenous contrast is more costly, exposes the patient to radiation, and in general is not necessary in the workup of medical renal disease.)

蛋白尿

Donna I. Myers, MD

定义
- 微量蛋白尿定义为，蛋白：尿肌酐比值（ACR）在 30~300mg/g。
- 大量蛋白尿定义为 ACR > 300mg/g。
- 首次发现蛋白尿除外泌尿系感染后，应在 3~6 个月至少 3 次标本中的 2 次尿蛋白阳性以确诊。

测定
- 免疫化学法不论对于 24 小时尿或是随机尿化验，均作为测定尿蛋白的高度敏感、特异的方法。
- 免疫法测定尿蛋白是利用与白蛋白结合的抗体进行。如果尿中存在白蛋白，可测定抗体 白蛋白复合物。
- 4 个方法可测定抗体 – 白蛋白复合物：（1）比浊法（易于操作但费用较高）；（2）放射性免疫测定（RIA）；（3）ELISA 法（操作相对费力）；（4）放射免疫扩散法。
- 免疫比浊法（ITA）目前已用做商业用途。罗氏公司的"The Albumin Tina-Quant"就是个例子，因为是线性检验，尿蛋白从 3~400mg/L 甚至到 4 400mg/L 均可检验。当 >4 400mg/L 时，可以最多稀释 20 倍后进行测定。
- "Point-of-care"检验利用免疫反应，如 DCA2000（拜耳分析仪）和 HemoCue Albumin 201 系统，可快速出报告（7 分钟）。
- 分光光度法通过测定有颜色的终产物来测定 24 小时尿总蛋白（vs 白蛋白）。
- 尿常规中，尿蛋白用四溴酚试剂棒测定，白蛋白与蓝色的二价阴离子结合，使指示剂从黄色变到绿色、蓝色。利用比色仪（反射光谱法），其敏感性达到 10mg/dl，特异性 97%。校正板用于对尿的本色进行补充。
- 试纸条测定随机尿蛋白是临床中非常有用的一种监测方法。
- 磺基水杨酸 3% 浊度检验是对总尿蛋白的一种半定量检测方法，测定白蛋白、球蛋白及本周氏蛋白。这种方法对于初步诊断肾病范围内的蛋白尿非常有效，表现为在检测试管底部的白色厚团块。
- 高效液相色谱法（HPLC）可以准确测定尿蛋白，但因为耗时，目前只用于科研。

适应证
- 指南建议在确诊 2 型糖尿病（T2DM）时或确诊 1 型糖尿病（T1DM）的 5 年后，每年进行慢性肾脏病的筛查。
- 筛查慢性肾脏病应包括血肌酐的测定及 GFR 和随机尿测定尿蛋白：肌酐比值（ACR）。
- 24 小时尿蛋白测定则很少应用。
- 对患有糖尿病和高血压的患者，微量及大量蛋白尿（肾病水平的蛋白尿）除了是肾病的预测指标外，也均是心功能衰竭的预测指标。

- 对患有糖尿病或有过心血管疾病的患者，微量蛋白尿增加发生心功能不全的风险高达2倍。
- 存在大量蛋白尿（≥3g/g肌酐）的2型糖尿病患者与低水平的大量蛋白尿（<1.5g/g）患者相比，发生心功能衰竭的风险增加了3倍。
- 在一般人群中，微量蛋白尿增加发生高血压、糖尿病和心血管疾病的风险。微量尿蛋白应为健康人发生心血管疾病风险的一项指标。
- 现场及时检验（Point-of-care testing）可以在咨询的当时提供检验结果，可以提供额外的心血管疾病风险评估，使临床医生在随访当时即可帮助患者制定合适的生活方式改变方案。

局限性

- 高水平的结合胆红素（>66mg/dl）、溶血（>300mg/dl）和高脂血症会干扰"The Albumin Tina-Quant"测定，会使测定尿蛋白的水平偏低或者呈阴性。
- 如果尿中有高水平的酮体、抗坏血酸、钙、肌酐、糖、血红蛋白、尿素及尿酸也会干扰Tina-Quant测定。
- 患有尿酸性肾结石的患者通常存在高尿酸尿（男性>800mg/d），会干扰Tina-Quant检测中高达10%的准确性。
- 只有尿中没有白细胞、亚硝酸盐或潜血时才可以使用现场即时检验。
- 用只对白蛋白敏感的方法来检测尿蛋白会遗漏尿中的肾小管来源的蛋白成分，如本周氏蛋白，可能漏诊多发性骨髓瘤。
- 比色法分析尿蛋白是半定量的方法，对白蛋白比本周氏蛋白和球蛋白有更高的敏感性；但需要新鲜的标本（冷藏<4小时）；在碱性尿（pH>8）、血红蛋白尿和造影剂存在时可能导致假阳性结果。
- 试纸法的另一项局限性是观察者间的差异性。
- 留取24小时尿是繁琐的，因此很少使用，要求严格按照要求留取，充足的水化并且排尿即时和完整留取。对检测尿肌酐非常有用，并对于特定的患者非常稳定，除非体重改变。

专家意见

- 对于早期糖尿病肾病，检测尿蛋白是至关重要的。尿微量白蛋白对1型糖尿病相对特异，但对2型糖尿病患者出现糖尿病肾病没有那么强的特异性。
- 推荐随机尿蛋白：肌酐比值用于检查是否存在蛋白尿。
- 对健康人群及风险人群，微量和大量蛋白尿均与心血管疾病风险增加相关。
- 蛋白尿与心血管疾病相关的原因未明，可能与内皮细胞功能受损有关。
- 蛋白尿对肾脏和心血管保护是重要的治疗指标。

推荐依据

National Kidney Foundation-Kidney Disease Outcomes Quality Initiative (NFK-KDOQI). NFK- KDOQI Clinical Practice Guidelines and Clinical Practice Recommendations for Diabetes and Chronic Kidney Disease. Am J Kidney Dis,2007; Vol. 49: pp. S12–154.
Comments:Comprehensive practice guidelines for diabetes and chronic kidney disease by the National Kidney Foundation-Kidney Disease Outcomes Quality

Initiative (NFK-KDOQI).

Arnlöv J, Evans JC, Meigs JB, et al. Low-grade albuminuria and incidence of cardiovascular disease events in nonhypertensive and nondiabetic individuals: the Framingham Heart Study. Circulation,2005; Vol. 112: pp. 969–75.

Comments:Urinary albumin:creatinine ratios below normal (< 30 mg/g) predicted the development of de novo cardiovascular disease in a population healthy at baseline.

其他参考文献

Guy M, Borzomato JK, Newall RG, et al. Protein and albumin-to-creatinine ratios in random urines accurately predict 24 h protein and albumin loss in patients with kidney disease. Ann Clin Biochem,2009; Vol. 46: pp. 468–76.

Comments:Evidence that a random spot urinary albumin to creatinine ratio is adequate to detect proteinuria.

Dobre D, Nimade S, de Zeeuw D. Albuminuria in heart failure: what do we really know? Curr Opin Cardiol,2009; Vol. 24: pp. 148–54.

Comments: A comprehensive review article of the association of albuminuria with cardiovascular disease citing many important references.

Sarafidis PA, Riehle J, Bogojevic Z, et al. A comparative evaluation of various methods for microalbuminuria screening. Am J Nephrol,2008; Vol. 28: pp. 324–9.

Comments:HemoCue system was compared to a central laboratory system for measuring urine albumin and found to be comparable.

Lambers Heerspink HJ, Witte EC, Bakker SJ, et al. Screening and monitoring for albuminuria: the performance of the HemoCue point-of-care system. Kidney Int,2008; Vol. 74: pp. 377–83.

Comments:The HemoCue system using a first voided urine of the day accurately measures urinary albumin. It does not provide a urinary albumin:creatinine determination.

Contois JH, Hartigan C, Rao LV, et al. Analytical validation of an HPLC assay for urinary albumin. Clin Chim Acta,2006; Vol. 367: pp. 150–5.

Comments:The immunoturbidimetric assay (ITA) was compared to the high-performance liquid chromatography (HPLC) assay. HPLC has the advantage of measuring immunounreactive urinary albumin species and may provide earlier detection of microalbuminuria in diabetic subjectsde Zeeuw D, Remuzzi G, Parving HH, et al. Albuminuria, a therapeutic target for cardiovascular protection in type 2 diabetic patients with nephropathy. Circulation,2004; Vol. 110: pp. 921–7.

Comments:In the RENAAL Study (Reduction in End Points in NIDDM with Losartan) albuminuria was the strongest predictor of cardiovascular outcome.

Arnold JM, Yusuf S, Young J, et al. Prevention of Heart Failure in Patients in the Heart Outcomes Prevention Evaluation (HOPE) Study. Circulation,2003; Vol. 107: pp. 1284–90.

Comments:In this trial to prevent heart failure in 9297 patients, microalbuminuria has a risk ratio of 1.82.

Collins AC, Vincent J, Newall RG, et al. An aid to the early detection and management of diabetic nephropathy: assessment of a new point of care microalbuminuria system in the diabetic clinic. Diabet Med,2001; Vol. 18: pp. 928–32.

Comments:This study describes a point of care microalbuminuria detection system (DCA2000) in a clinic setting with rapid and reliable results.

附录

附录 1：2 型糖尿病高血糖治疗路径	667
附录 2：GFR 和白蛋白尿网格	668
附录 3：2015 ADA EASD 立场声明对 2 型糖尿病降糖治疗的推荐	670
附录 4：2015 AACE/ACE 血糖控制流程图	672

附录1：2型糖尿病高血糖治疗路径

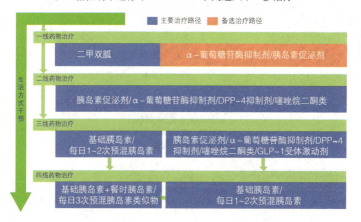

注：HBA1c：糖化血红蛋白

2型糖尿病高血糖治疗路径。蓝色路径是根据药物卫生经济学、疗效和安全性等方面的临床证据以及我国国情等因素权衡考虑后推荐的主要药物治疗路径，与国际上大部分糖尿病指南中建议的药物治疗路径相似，橙色路径为与蓝色路径相应的备选路径。

摘自：中华医学会糖尿病学分会.中国2型糖尿病防治指南（2013年版）.中华糖尿病杂志，2014,6（7）：447-498

附录2：GFR和白蛋白尿网格

以GFR和白蛋白尿分类的监测频率（每年监测次数）建议			持续白蛋白尿分类描述及范围		
			A1 正常至轻度升高	A2 中度升高	A3 重度升高
GFR分类 ml(min·1.73m²)	G1	正常或增高 ≥90	1（如存在CKD）	1	2
	G2	轻度降低 60~89	1（如存在CKD）	1	2
	G3a	轻度至中度降低 45~59	1	2	3
	G3b	中度至重度降低 30~44	2	3	3
	G4	重度降低 15~29	3	3	4+
	G5	肾衰竭 <15	4+	4+	4+

来源：Handelsman Y, et al. American Association of Clinical Endocrinologists and Amecircan College of Endocrinology – Clinical Practice Guidelines for Developing a Diabetes Mellitus Comprehensive Care Plan –2015. Endocrine Practice, 2015, 21(S1):1–87

GFR和白蛋白尿网格，以颜色强度显示风险进展。每格内的数字表示监测频率（每年监测次数）。绿色提示稳定，如存在CKD，每年随访监测1次；黄色提示谨慎，每年需监测≥1次；橙色提示每年须监测2次；红色提示每年须监测3次，而深红色提示密切监测，每年须监测≥4次（每1~3个月至少1次）。这些参数是基于专家意见，在应用时必须考虑到潜在的合并症和疾病状态，并考虑到在进行患者个体管理时加以调整的可能性。CKD：慢性肾脏病；GFR：肾小球滤过率。推荐频率来自KDIGO CKD工作组。

附录3：2015 ADA EASD 立场声明对

健康饮食 控制体重

单药治疗	二甲双胍		
有效性	高		
风险性	低		
对体重的影响	中性/降低		
副作用	胃肠反应/乳酸中毒		
价格	低		

如果单一药物治疗3个月后糖化血红蛋白不达标，改为两种药物联

两药联合治疗*	二甲双胍+ 磺硫脲类	二甲双胍+ 噻唑烷二酮类	二甲双胍+ DPP-4抑制剂
有效性	高	高	中
风险性	中	低	低
对体重的影响	增加	增加	中性
副作用	低血糖	水肿/心衰/骨折	极少
价格	低	低	高

如果两药联合治疗3个月后糖化血红蛋白不达标，改为三种药物联

三种药物联合治疗*	二甲双胍+ 磺硫脲类 噻唑烷二酮类 DPP-4抑制剂 SGLT2抑制剂 GLP-1受体激动剂 基础胰岛素[5]	二甲双胍+ 噻唑烷二酮类 磺硫脲类 DPP-4抑制剂 SGLT2抑制剂 GLP-1受体激动剂 基础胰岛素[5]	二甲双胍+ DPP-4抑制剂 磺硫脲类 噻唑烷二酮类 SGLT2抑制剂 基础胰岛素[5]

如果三药联合治疗3个月后糖化血红蛋白不达标，
（1）单纯口服三药联合，则开始胰岛素治疗；
（2）包括GLP-1受体激动剂的三药联合治疗，则增加基础胰岛素治疗；
（3）包括基础胰岛素的三药联合治疗，则增加GLP-1受体激动剂或餐

药物联合胰岛素治疗	基础胰岛素+餐时胰岛素或GLP-1受体激动剂

摘自：Inzucchi, SE, et al. Management of Hyperglycemia in Type 2 Diabetes, 2015: A Patient-Centered Approach Update to a Position Statement of the American Diabetes Association and the European Association for the Study of Diabetes. Diabetes Care 2015, 38:140-149.

2 型糖尿病降糖治疗的推荐

体育锻炼 患者教育

合应用（注：应考虑患者的实际情况灵活操作）

二甲双胍 + SGLT2 抑制剂	二甲双胍 + GLP-1 受体激动剂	二甲双胍 + 基础胰岛素
中	高	最高
低	低	高
降低	降低	增加
泌尿系统反应/脱水	胃肠反应	低血糖
高	高	不等

合应用（注：应考虑患者的实际情况灵活操作）

二甲双胍 + SGLT2 抑制剂	二甲双胍 + GLP-1 受体激动剂	二甲双胍 + 基础胰岛素
磺脲类	磺脲类	噻唑烷二酮类
噻唑烷二酮类	噻唑烷二酮类	DPP-4 抑制剂
DPP-4 抑制剂	基础胰岛素[5]	SGLT2 抑制剂
基础胰岛素[5]		GLP-1 受体激动剂

时胰岛素，如果仍难以达标，则考虑使用噻唑烷二酮类药物或 SGLT2 抑制剂。

附录4：2015 AACE/ACE 血糖控制流程图

生活方式干预

就诊时HbA1c＜7.5%

单药治疗*

- ✓ 二甲双胍
- ✓ GLP-1受体激动剂
- ✓ SGLT2抑制剂
- ✓ DPP-4抑制剂
- ✓ α-糖苷酶抑制剂
- ⚠ TZD
- ⚠ SU/GLN

若3个月后HbA1c未能达标(仍＞6.5%)，则两药联合治疗 ➡

就诊时HbA1c≥7.5%

两药联合治疗*

二甲双胍或其他一线药物 **加**：

- GLP-1受体激动剂 ✓
- SGLT2抑制剂 ✓
- DPP-4抑制剂 ✓
- TZD ⚠
- 基础胰岛素 ⚠
- 考来维仑 ✓
- 快速释放型
- α-糖苷酶抑制剂
- SU/GLN ⚠

若3个月后未能达标，则三药联合治疗 ➡

*所列药物顺序是按用药等级进行建议

摘自：Garber AJ, et al. AACE Comprehensive Diabetes Management Algorithm 2013. Endocrine Practice, 2013, 19(2):327-336

（包括医疗干预减轻体重）

就诊时HbA1c＞9.0%

无症状 → 两药联合治疗 或 三药联合治疗

有症状 → 胰岛素 ± 其他药物 → 加药或胰岛素强化治疗

三药联合治疗*

二甲双胍或其他一线药物

 加

- GLP-1受体激动剂 ✓
- SGLT2抑制剂 ✓
- DPP-4抑制剂 ✓
- TZD ⚠
- 基础胰岛素 ⚠
- 考来维仑 ✓
- 快速释放型 ✓
- α-糖苷酶抑制剂 ✓
- SU/GLN ⚠

若3个月后未能达标，则胰岛素强化治疗 ➡

图例

✓ = 较少的不良事件或可能获益   ⚠ = 谨慎使用

病情进展 →

临床医师口袋工具书系列（感染专业）

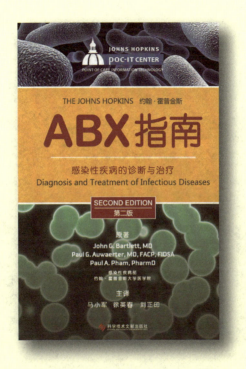

《约翰·霍普金斯 ABX指南——感染性疾病的诊断与治疗》

原　　著：巴特利特（Bartlett J.G.）　奥威特（Auwaerte P.G.）　范（Pharn P.A.）
主　　译：马小军　徐英春　刘正印
出 版 社：科学技术文献出版社
定　　价：168.00元

　　本书由约翰·霍普金斯大学医学院的专家编著，中文版由北京协和医院感染科专业医师团队编译。本书重点阐述了专家推荐意见、临床和诊断决策技术以及药物相互作用。为临床医师提供关于抗菌药物、感染性疾病和常见病原体的最新、最权威、最全面的信息，是一本临床各科室医师必备的用药速查手册和学习工具。

临床医师口袋工具书系列（感染专业）

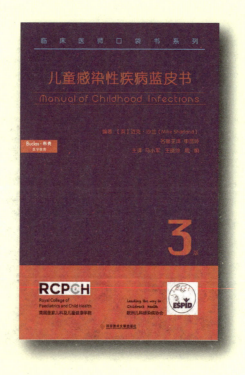

《儿童感染性疾病蓝皮书》

原　　著：迈克·莎兰（Mike Sharland）
名誉主译：申昆玲
主　　译：马小军　王晓玲　周炯等
出 版 社：科学技术文献出版社
定　　价：168.00元

  本书原著由牛津大学出版社出版，是英国儿科与儿童健康皇家学院、欧洲儿童感染性疾病学会合作完成的重要文献。经150余位国际专家共同撰写120余章节，涵盖了针对新生儿和儿童近百种主要抗感染药物的用药信息。提供全部主要感染的流行病学、临床特点和管理措施的关键点，具有易查、循证、实用性强的特点。

临床医师口袋工具书系列（感染专业）

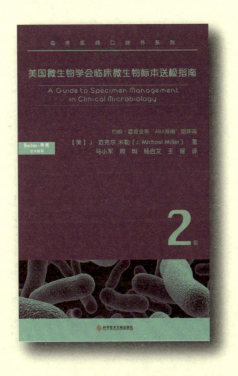

《美国微生物学会临床微生物标本送检指南》

原　著：J·迈克尔·米勒（J. Michael Miller）
主　译：马小军　周炯　杨启文　王瑶
出版社：科学技术文献出版社
定　价：85.00元

　　本书为《约翰·霍普金斯 ABX指南：感染性疾病的诊断与治疗》的姊妹篇。涵盖临床微生物标本从对象选择、采集到报告全流程规范操作的经典指南。是有效连接对感染性疾病诊疗负有责任的各个部门、团队、人员的核心纽带。

临床医师口袋工具书系列(内分泌专业)

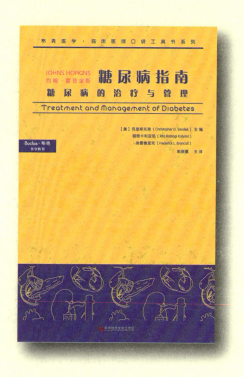

《约翰·霍普金斯 糖尿病指南 —— 糖尿病的治疗与管理》

原　著：克里斯托弗(Christopher D. Saudek)　　卡利亚尼(Rita Rastogi Kalyani)
　　　　弗雷德里克(Frederick L. Brancati)
主　译：郭晓蕙
出版社：科学技术文献出版社
定　价：168.00元

　　本书由150余个主题组成,由超过40名不同专业的临床专家撰写,其中包括临床医师、药剂师、糖尿病足病专家、营养学专家和教育护士。
　　本书根据循证证据结果编写,提供丰富的糖尿病相关信息,是可以快速参考的临床指南,方便临床操作。而这是其他参考书籍很难做到的。相关主题以章节目录列出:包括总论、管理、并发症、药物和临床检验。专家意见部分则对如何在临床实践中有效治疗和管理糖尿病提出了独特的视角。

临床医师口袋工具书系列(心血管专业)

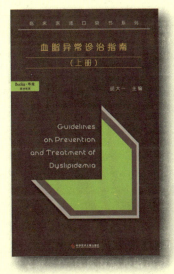
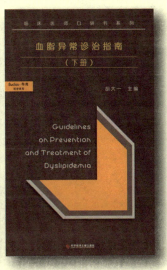

《血脂异常诊治指南:全2册》
主　　编:胡大一
出版社:科学技术文献出版社
定　　价:116.00元

本书汇聚最新、最权威的国内外血脂异常诊治指南,指南解读与专家共识,重要研究的解读。如通过解读39个国家参与的IMPROVE-IT研究,分析阐述降脂药物他汀联用胆固醇抑制吸收剂的临床获益。还收录《2014美国国家脂质协会关于他汀安全性的评估建议》,为临床医师掌握他汀剂量、科学使用降血脂药物提供最新、最准确的循证医学依据。

临床医师口袋工具书系列（心血管专业）

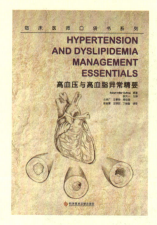

《高血压与高血脂异常精要》

原　　著：Robert Miller Guthrie
主　　译：胡大一
出版社：科学技术文献出版社
定　　价：48.00元

本书探讨和介绍两类疾病的危险分层和药物干预。重点和详细阐述了各类降压药物和调脂药物的特点和临床实用。这本小册子体现出的循证医学特别是循证用药的理念和去伪存真的思想值得提倡和推崇。现在翻译和出版这本书有利于提高广大医务人员对高血压和高血脂的认识，将高血压和血脂异常防治的指南更好地贯彻到临床实践中去，转化为疾病干预实际效果，从而更好地服务于患者。

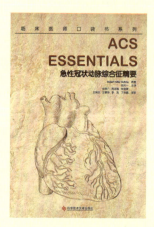

《急性冠脉综合征精要》

原　　著：Robert M.Califf 和 Matthew.Roe
主　　译：胡大一
出版社：科学技术文献出版社
定　　价：58.00元

该书系统讲述了不稳定性心绞痛和急性心肌梗死的诊断、评估和治疗，既全面、系统，又简洁和清晰，实用性强。全书涵盖基本药物治疗、溶栓治疗和介入治疗，疾病的急诊处理、院内诊疗和出院时处理，专章讲述并发症识别和处理，并对诊疗过程中的误区分别进行剖析等。所涉及的诊疗策略尤其是治疗策略的选择是建立在循证医学基础之上，具有普遍指导意义。

临床医师口袋工具书系列（心血管专业）

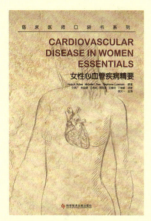

《女性心血管疾病精要》

原　著：Kevin A. Bybee　Stephanie L. Lawhorn
原版著：Michelle L. Dew　Tracy L. Stevens
主　译：胡大一
出版社：科学技术文献出版社
定　价：39.00元

本书围绕心血管病防治问题，体现了女性心血管病的鲜明特征。该书从流行病特点，非侵入性检查特点，冠心病治疗特点，及女性激素、危险因素、特有心血管病处理特点等方面全面介绍女性心血管健康问题。

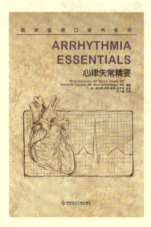

《心律失常精要》

原　著：Brian Olshansky　Mina K. Chung
原　著：Steven M. Pogwizd　Nora Goldschlager
主　译：胡大一
出版社：科学技术文献出版社
定　价：58.00元

本书是一本实时、准确、细化的心律失常指南。内容涵盖了心脏电生理基础知识，心律失常发生机制，各型心律失常的病因、诊断、治疗，常见抗心律失常药物的使用原则，以及起搏治疗、植入型心律转复除颤器（ICD）和心脏再同步治疗（CRT）等新兴治疗技术，同时穿插大量的心电图图片和实例，多角度论述临床常见心律失常诊治的相关问题。

临床医师口袋工具书系列（心血管专业）

ISCP（国际心血管药物治疗学会）现代心血管治疗系列丛书
Juan Carlos Kaski 教授主编　胡大一 教授主译

- 广泛适用临床
- 全面指导各科室医生心血管用药
- ISCP旨在全球范围内倡导心血管药物临床应用研究及规范化使用。
- 指导临床医生心血管用药的重要教育工具书之一。
- 丛书主题包含主要临床心血管情况，由相关领域的专家编辑和撰写。

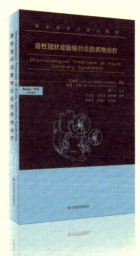
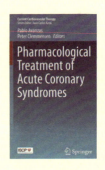

《急性冠脉综合征的药物治疗》
《Pharmacological Treatment of Acute Coronary Syndromes》
Pablo Avanzas, Peter Clemmensen 著　　胡大一 主译

临床医师口袋工具书系列(心血管专业)

ISCP现代心血管治疗系列丛书

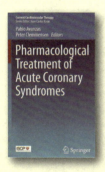

《急性冠脉综合征的药物治疗》

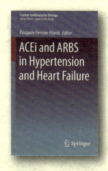

《肾素血管紧张素系统抑制剂与高血压及心力衰竭》

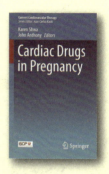

《妊娠期心脏用药》

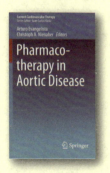

《主动脉疾病的药物治疗》

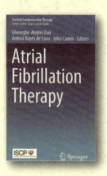

《心房颤动的治疗》

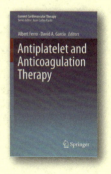

《抗血小板和抗凝治疗》

Buclas·布克 医学教育事业部

临床医师口袋工具书系列（解剖·影像）

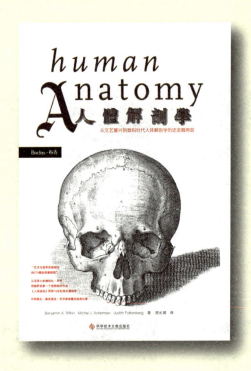

《人体解剖学》

原　著：Benjamin A. Rifkin
主　译：周长满 等
出版社：科学技术文献出版社
定　价：128.00元

　　艺术与医学完美结合的274幅珍贵解剖图。从亚里士多德到达·芬奇，到维萨里第一个里程碑的作品《人体结构》，再到19世纪格氏解剖学……是一部值得外科及其他临床医生、艺术家珍藏的经典著作。

临床医师口袋工具书系列(解剖·影像)

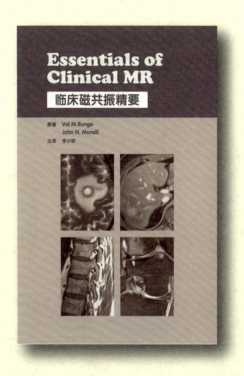

《临床磁共振精要》
原 著:Val M.Runge,John N. Morelli
主 译:李小明
出版社:科学技术文献出版社
定 价:85.00元

　　本书按系统进行分类,图文对照、病例齐全、描述细腻,对全身各系统疾病的MRI表现特征及要素进行了细致的解读,包括了临床诊断中常见疾病的磁共振诊断要领。650多幅图片清楚阐明了各种疾病的MRI表现特征,还包括了有关对比剂和对比增强MRA的最新信息。

国际指南临床医师口袋手册系列

心脑血管、内分泌国际指南
临床口袋手册中文版隆重上市（APP、Android 版即将上线）

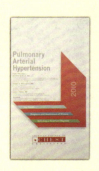
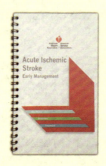
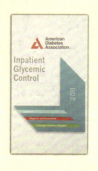
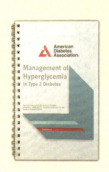
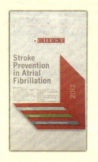
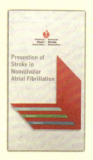

全球 30 多个协会 100 多个国际指南临床口袋卡

请联系布克公司销售团队或各赞助商、制药企业、器械公司的市场和销售人员

Buclas·布克 医学教育事业部

国际指南临床医师口袋手册系列

协会分类	国际指南临床医师口袋手册
美国胸科医师协会（ACCP）	静脉血栓栓塞的抗血栓治疗指南口袋手册 心血管疾病预防指南口袋手册 冠状动脉疾病指南口袋手册 深静脉血栓形成指南口袋手册 肝素诱发的血小板减少症指南口袋手册 外周动脉疾病指南口袋手册 预防血栓形成指南口袋手册 骨科手术的静脉血栓栓塞的预防指南口袋手册 肺动脉高压指南口袋手册 瓣膜病指南口袋手册 ST段抬高型心肌梗死指南口袋手册
美国心脏协会（AHA）	基于设备的疗法指南口袋手册 机械循环支持指南口袋手册 ST段抬高型心肌梗死指南口袋手册 稳定缺血性心脏病指南口袋手册 非ST段抬高型心肌梗死指南口袋手册
美国糖尿病协会（ADA）	临床实践建议口袋手册 成人糖尿病指南口袋手册 高血糖管理口袋手册 住院患者血糖控制指南口袋手册
美国临床内分泌医师学会（AACE）	糖尿病指南口袋手册
欧洲心脏病学会（ESC）	关于心肌梗死定义的第三次国际共识指南口袋手册 心脏瓣膜病指南口袋手册 伴随ST段抬高的急性心肌梗死指南口袋手册 急慢性心力衰竭指南口袋手册 血脂异常的管理指南口袋手册 无持续性ST段抬高的急性冠脉综合征指南口袋手册 成人先天性心脏病的管理指南口袋手册 外周动脉疾病指南口袋手册 糖尿病，糖尿病前期和心血管疾病指南口袋手册 稳定性冠状动脉疾病指南口袋手册 心脏起搏和心脏再同步治疗指南口袋手册 高血压管理指南口袋手册 心房颤动的管理指南口袋手册 妊娠期心血管病管理指南口袋手册 心血管病防治临床实践指南口袋手册
美国内分泌学会（ENDO）	雄激素缺乏症指南口袋手册 减重手术指南口袋手册 先天性肾上腺增生症指南口袋手册 高血糖指南口袋手册 高甘油三酯血症指南口袋手册 低血糖症指南口袋手册 有代谢性危险因素的患者中预防心血管疾病和2型糖尿病指南口袋手册
美国国家脂质协会（NLA）	家族性高胆固醇血症指南口袋手册

临床医生口袋诊断工具卡

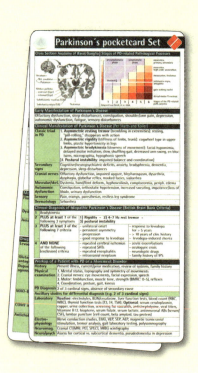

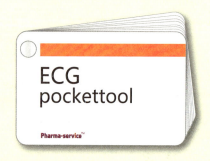

胡大一健康工作室

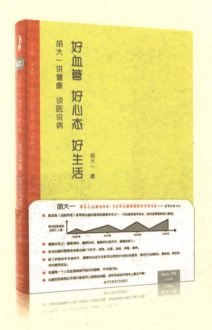

胡大一讲健康

《胡大一讲健康 谈医说病：好血管 好心态 好生活》

著　者：胡大一
出版社：科学技术文献出版社
定　价：128.00元

本书送予心脑血管疾病患者最棒的五个处方帮助您：

- 用好药物
- 避免不必要的支架
- 调节心情，提高生活质量
- 落实健康的生活方式

送礼送健康，送礼送爱心，家庭必备图书

- 孝敬父母，关爱家人
- 关爱自己，关爱客户
- 关爱亲朋好友，关爱同事

Buclas·布克　健康科普出版及健康教育

胡 大 一 健 康 工 作 室

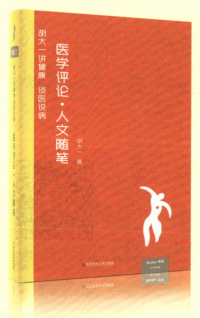

胡大一讲健康

《胡大一讲健康 谈医说病：医学评论·人文随笔》

著　　者：胡大一
出 版 社：科学技术文献出版社
定　　价：88.00元

- "谨以此书追思、纪念亲爱的母亲和父亲。学习母亲和父亲，做一名热爱职业、热爱临床工作、有良知良心的医生"。
- "看的是病，救的是心，开的是药，给的是情"。
- "并以此书推动医学回归人文、回归临床和回归基本功"。

Miss Grey · 格蕾 医学沟通工具

Miss Grey · 格蕾 医患沟通手册（门诊 · 手术 · 随诊 · 患教）

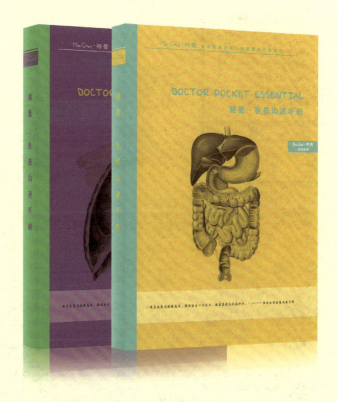

Buclas · 布克 医学教育事业部

Miss Grey · 格蕾 医学沟通工具

Miss Grey · 格蕾 医学解剖图谱（挂图 · 桌垫 · 台历）

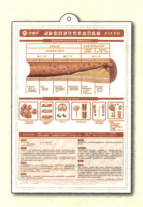

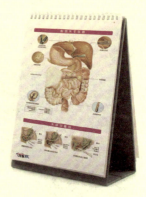

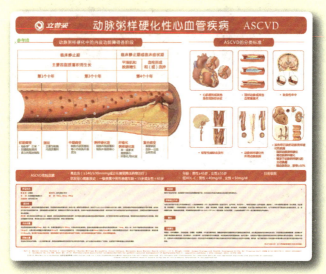

Buclas · 布克 医学教育事业部

Miss Grey · 格蕾 医学沟通工具

Miss Grey · 格蕾 医学教育模型

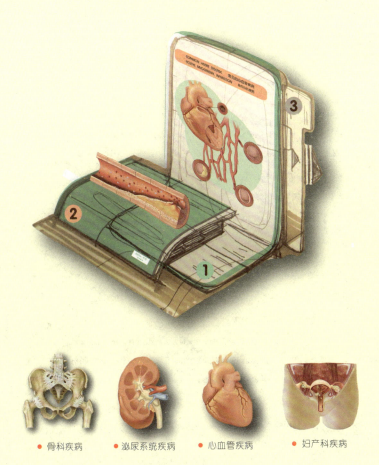

- 骨科疾病
- 泌尿系统疾病
- 心血管疾病
- 妇产科疾病

Buclas · 布克 医学教育事业部

Pharma-service

- **Buclas·布克** 医学出版
  - 指南与共识临床口袋手册（国内、国际30多个医学协会）
  - 指南与共识制定及全国巡讲项目
  - 临床医师口袋工具书
  - 临床医生口袋诊断工具卡
  - 医学策略服务

- **Buclas·布克** 健康科普出版及健康教育
  - 胡大一讲健康 谈医说病
  - 健康科普出版

- **Buclas·布克** 医学学术项目（医学会、基金会、杂志社）
  - "心脑血管·内分泌·感染·风湿……"

- **Miss Grey·格蕾** 医学沟通工具
  - 医患沟通手册（门诊·手术·随诊·患教）
  - 医学解剖图谱（挂图·台历·桌垫）
  - 医学教育模型

- **Happy Doctor 快乐医师** 专业医学礼品
  - 临床医师诊断工具
  - 医学礼品
  - 品牌提示物
  - 临床科室医学装饰画

- **We Talk** 医学视频与新媒体
  "分享最干货的临床经验，提高临床技能"
  - We Talk pro 医学视频 我们说医学 我们说健康 www.ropemd.com
  - We Talk Issue 医学临床杂志
  - We Talk Health 健康纪录片
  - 胡大一讲健康 谈医说病

- **胡大一健康工作室及长缨** 健康管理
  - 健康管理与培训（个人·家庭·企业）

Buclas·布克 医学教育

www.buclas.com　　www.pharma-service.com.cn

图书及健康礼品淘宝订购：布克的礼物

http://buclas.taobao.com　+86-10-51284280